Pharmacology in
MIDWIFERY

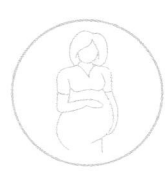

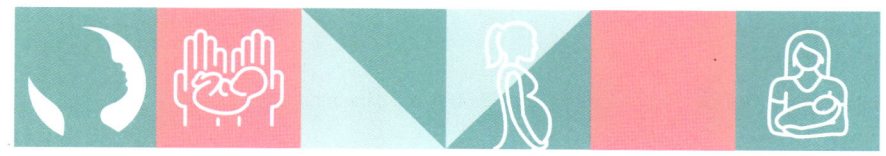

Pharmacology in
MIDWIFERY

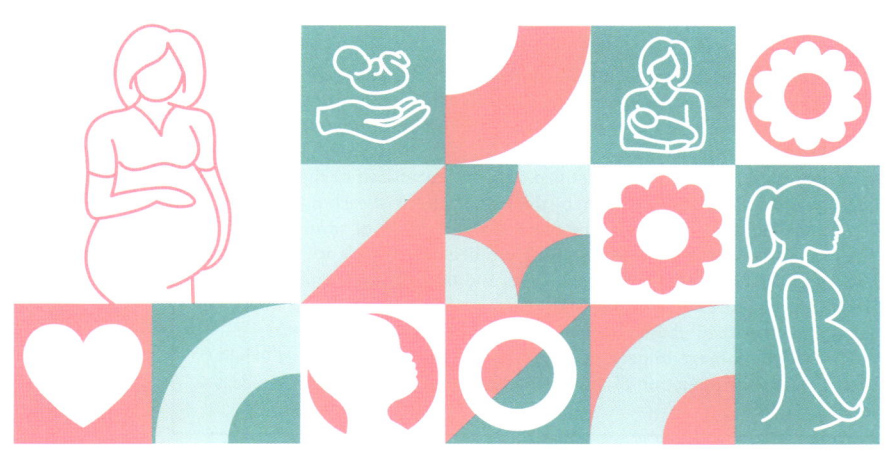

ROSLYN **DONNELLAN-FERNANDEZ** | MARYAM **BAZARGAN**

CLARE **DAVISON** | MICHELLE **GRAY** | KIRSTEN **SMALL**

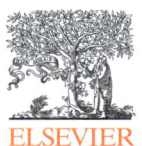

ELSEVIER

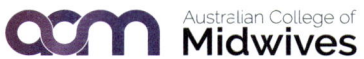

Australian College of
Midwives

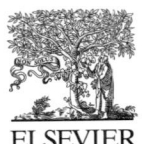

ELSEVIER

Elsevier Australia. ACN 001 002 357
(a division of Reed International Books Australia Pty Ltd)
475 Victoria Avenue, Chatswood, NSW 2067

ISBN: 978-0-7295-4460-3

National Library of Australia Cataloguing-in-Publication Data

A catalogue record for this book is available from the National Library of Australia

Content Strategist: Melinda McEvoy
Content Project Manager: Shubham Dixit
Edited by Claire Linsdell
Proofread by Annabel Adair
Copyrights Coordinator: Gobinaath Palanisamy
Cover Designer: Gopalakrishnan Venkatraman
Index by Innodata
Typeset by GW Tech
Printed in Chennai by Multivista Global Pvt. Ltd.

Last digit is the print number: 9 8 7 6 5 4 3 2 1

Contents

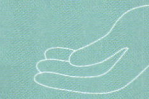

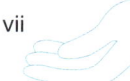

About the authors

Dr Roslyn Donnellan-Fernandez BN, RN, RM, Grad Cert MID (Pharm), IBCLC MNg (Women's Health), PhD Community Midwife

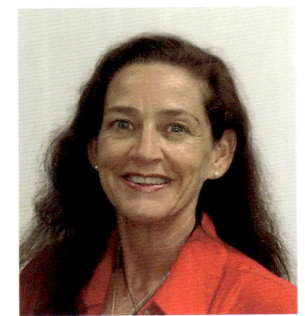

Dr Roslyn Donnellan-Fernandez is a passionate senior midwifery leader and academic with 30 years of experience spanning such diverse contexts as clinical practice, education, policy development, regulation, maternity services implementation/change management, professional advocacy, and research. Roz is Director of the postgraduate Primary Maternity Care suite of programs at Griffith University, and has experience in teaching and curriculum development at three Australian universities. She is actively engaged in strategic, policy and funding initiatives aimed at scaling up 'continuity of midwifery' models so they can become the primary public health strategy, thereby providing access and equity for under-served groups. Roz's teaching and research are informed by critical emancipatory social theory, principles of lifelong learning, advocacy, and political and professional engagement that facilitate transformation of people, structures, and communities towards social justice, health equity, and gender equality. Two decades ago, Roz co-led implementation of the sustained public health midwifery group practice model in South Australia, later completing a PhD supported by a Midwifery Fellowship through the Women's & Children's Hospital Foundation: 'Midwifery Group Practice and Standard Hospital Care – a cost and resource study of women with complex pregnancy' (2016). Roz maintains clinical currency as well as Commonwealth Medicare (MBS) and Midwifery Prescribing (PBS) endorsement. Since 2018 she has reviewed, taught and co-developed curriculum to inform midwifery pharmacology and prescribing practice across the childbearing continuum, supporting comprehensive, high-quality care for women and their babies. She has published several book chapters, peer-reviewed journal articles, and contributed to the inaugural undergraduate textbook, *Midwifery Preparation for Practice*, including several revised editions. Roz presents regularly at national and international conferences and provides peer review for several high-impact journals. She is committed to developing and improving high-quality resources that support midwifery knowledge in pharmacology, and safe midwifery prescribing practice. Roz gratefully acknowledges the superb team who have worked diligently to make *Pharmacology for Midwifery* a reality.

Dr Maryam Bazargan RM, MSc Medical (Human) Physiology, PhD

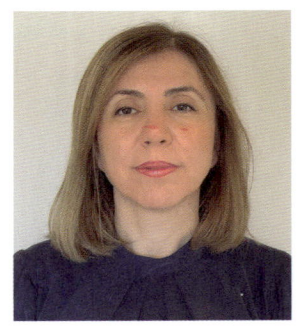

Dr Maryam Bazargan is a Senior Lecturer in Midwifery at the University of Canberra's Faculty of Health, and holds a Bachelor of Midwifery, an MSc in Human Physiology, and a PhD in Pharmacology. Maryam is both a scientist and a midwife. Having completed her first midwifery degree (BSc/Midwifery) in 1996 in Iran, and with a strong interest in science, she commenced her master's degree in human physiology in 2003 and since then has contributed to numerous research projects in medical sciences in both Iran and Australia. Maryam has resided in Australia since 2008, and in 2015 completed her PhD, focusing on drug disposition between mother and fetus. Maryam has worked as a researcher at several universities and also at CSIRO in Adelaide. She completed a second midwifery degree in Australia to attain registration with AHPRA, and is a clinically active midwife while also being an academic. By combining her extensive knowledge of human physiology, pharmacology, and clinical midwifery, Maryam is able to provide a comprehensive and informed approach to her teaching and research.

Dr Clare Davison RM, RN, PG Diploma (Midwifery), MPhil, PhD

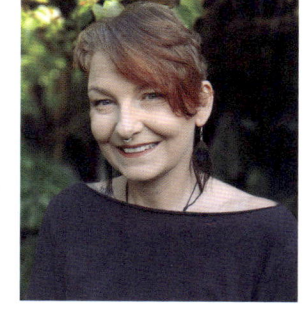

Dr Clare Davison is a clinician, academic and feminist researcher in midwifery, specialising in enabling midwives to work to their full scope of practice, and in supporting and promoting normal physiological birth. Clare is an experienced midwifery academic with a background in clinical midwifery. She has worked in higher education since 2013 and holds two higher degrees by research, having completed her Master of Philosophy in Midwifery in 2014, and PhD in 2019. She has extensive experience in teaching and developing curriculums in both undergraduate and postgraduate midwifery, women's reproductive health, public health and research. Clare's research interests are feminist qualitative research, women and midwives' qualitative research, the history of midwifery, midwives working to their full scope of practice, and supporting and promoting normal physiological birth.

Clare wrote the first prescribing course for midwives in Western Australia, and believes it is essential that midwives can work to their full scope of practice, and that all women should have access to midwifery-led care. She combines her academic work with working as an endorsed midwife in private practice, providing continuity of midwifery care to all risk women in the home and hospital setting.

Dr Michelle Gray SFHEA, RN, RM, BSC(Hons) Midwifery, PGDE, Master Professional Learning, PhD

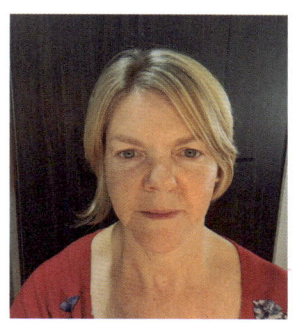

Dr Michelle Gray is Associate Professor of Nursing and Midwifery Education at the University of Newcastle and has adjuncts at the University of the Sunshine Coast, University of Queensland, and Edith Cowan University, where she supervises ongoing higher degree by research students. Michelle is originally from the UK and has resided in Australia since 2006. She has been a nurse since 1990, a midwife since 1995, and an academic since 2007. Michelle is a Senior Fellow of the Higher Education Academy in England, has a master's degree in Education, and completed her PhD in Midwifery in 2016 for which she examined midwives' perspectives on the move to national registration standards in Australia in 2010. Michelle's research interests focus on midwifery practice and education and making learning engaging for students, such as through a case-based learning curriculum. Her research has included evaluating the use of electronic resources in midwifery education, such as Eportfolios and the use of 3D technology. Michelle has published several book chapters, and was lead editor of *Starting Life as a Midwife: An international review of transition from student to practitioner* (Springer Books, 2019) which examines the transition of new graduates to practice globally, covering 12 countries.

Dr Kirsten Small BMedSc, MBBS, MReproMed, GradDipHlthRes, PhD

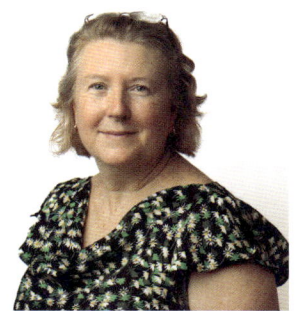

Dr Kirsten Small is an obstetrically trained educator and researcher. Both her parents were retail pharmacists, and she grew up helping in their pharmacy and pinching jellybeans when she thought no one was watching. While she didn't recognise it at the time, learning all those drug names would prove useful in later life. After a successful clinical career as an obstetrician, gynaecologist, and fertility specialist, Kirsten moved into academia. She wrote the first course for midwives seeking endorsement for scheduled medicines in Australia, then went on to write and then teach a second course at Griffith University. Kirsten has recently launched an online education business where she continues to provide pharmacology updates for midwives. In addition to her role as an educator, Kirsten published the first research about midwifery prescribers in Australia and has provided expert advice to policy makers about midwifery prescribing. She remains committed to the strengthening of relationship based and woman-centred maternity care provision.

Foreword from Australian College of Midwives (ACM)

This first edition *Pharmacology in Midwifery* textbook is a thorough and comprehensive resource, with clearly laid-out chapters covering medication administration principles, clinical, ethical, and legal foundations, complementary and alternative therapies, and pharmacology across the childbearing continuum.

Governance, safety and quality, a midwife's role and scope of practice, and mental health are also addressed, making this a well-rounded contemporary resource within the Australian context of practice. Critical thinking scenarios enhance engagement and learning, and review exercises consolidate readers' understanding of the content. This textbook will be an invaluable resource for students as well as experienced midwives and is proudly endorsed by the Australian College of Midwives.

Alison Weatherstone
Chief Midwife
Australian College of Midwives (ACM)

Reviewers

Rowena Shakes Bachelor of Midwifery, Master of Primary Maternity Care
School of Nursing and Midwifery
Griffith University
Gold Coast QLD Australia

Joclyn Neal Registered Nurse, Registered Midwife, Master of Midwifery, Grad Cert Neonatal Care
Lecturer in Midwifery & Midwifery Clinical Coordinator
School of Nursing, Midwifery and Paramedicine
Australian Catholic University
Virginia QLD Australia

Hazel Clarke BNursing/BArts, International Studies, Grad Cert Critical Care Nursing, Grad Dip Public Health, Grad Dip Midwifery
Australian College of Midwives
University of Technology Sydney
Canberra ACT Australia

Gill Harris Dip Adult Nursing, BNSc (Hons) Community Nurse Specialist, BNSc (Hons) Registered Midwife, Master of Midwifery, Grad Cert Education (Academic Practice)
Lecturer – Midwifery & Nursing
College of Healthcare Sciences I Academy
James Cook University
Townsville QLD Australia

Carolyn Ross Bachelor of Midwifery, Registered Midwife, Master of Primary Maternity Care, Bachelor of Business (Accounting)
Faculty of Health Science
School of Nursing, Midwifery & Paramedicine
Australian Catholic University
Fitzroy VIC Australia

Anne Barnes Registered Nurse – Hospital Certificate, Midwife – Hospital Certificate; Grad Dip Midwifery; Prescribing for Midwives; Endorsed Midwife, Master of Primary Maternity Care; IBCLC
Griffith University
Brisbane QLD Australia

Farnoosh Asghar Vahedi Grad Dip Midwifery
Associate Lecturer, Midwifery
School of Nursing and Midwifery
Western Sydney University
Parramatta NSW Australia

Acknowledgements

The authors of *Pharmacology for Midwifery* wish to acknowledge and thank the authors of the sixth edition of the Elsevier text *Pharmacology for Health Professionals* – Kathleen Knights, Shaunagh Darroch, Andrew Rowland and Mary Bushell – along with contributors to previous editions, for giving their permission to draw on work from that text. This invaluable support provided the strong foundation that allowed us to create this inaugural pharmacology textbook for midwives practising in Australia and New Zealand.

We wish to thank Libby Houston and all staff and associates of Elsevier for the opportunity to undertake this project, including their guidance, confidence, and patience, especially when we wavered in meeting our ambitions and our deadlines. Shubham Dixit has effectively 'midwifed' a very busy team of people, keeping all authors coordinated, connected, and communicating as we advanced the work for this book. For this we thank him. We extend our sincere appreciation also to those who provided valuable critical review of our writing, informally and formally, including their suggestions for improvement. Claire Linsdell and Melinda McEvoy have provided ongoing valuable advice, guidance and editing to advance our chapters to their final stages – thank you.

To my esteemed and talented co-authors, Maryam, Clare, Michelle, and Kirsten, I am indebted for your commitment to embark on this journey, and thank you for your steadfastness, cooperative effort, and rigour in seeing it through.

Finally, to our readers, we apologise in advance for any errors and welcome your feedback and comments on this first edition so it can be improved and enhanced for the next edition. Our goal is to provide a customised, useful, and robust pharmacological resource for midwives who practise across the continuum of antenatal, intrapartum, and postpartum services, so you are well equipped to provide knowledgeable, safe, and quality care for women and their babies across a diversity of contexts, wherever you may work. We hope you enjoy this book and that it makes a positive contribution to your ongoing learning.

Roslyn Donnellan-Fernandez

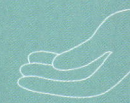

There is currently no other pharmacology textbook dedicated specifically to the Australian and New Zealand midwifery contexts of midwifery practice. This first edition of *Pharmacology for Midwifery* addresses this gap, serving as both an essential foundation pharmacology reference for midwifery students, and a resource for experienced midwife clinicians seeking to refresh or augment their pharmacological knowledge and develop their skills as prescribers.

Midwives require a customised text, with targeted pharmacological content, and knowledge relevant to the comprehensive care of women across the childbearing continuum. Here, both the foundational knowledge essential for safe medication management in midwifery practice, and complex key concepts on pharmacokinetics and pharmacodynamics, are provided in an accessible and easy-to-understand format. Ethical considerations, as well as professional practice standards, competencies, and regulations relevant to midwifery scope of practice in medication management (e.g. administration, supply, and prescribing) is related to the Australian and New Zealand contexts of practice.

There is a consistent focus on quality use of medicines and rational prescribing practice aligned to the National Prescribing Competencies Framework for health professionals, including real-world case studies to enhance applied knowledge. The book is clearly structured and presented in four parts: Part 1 Introduction to pharmacology; Part 2 Principles of pharmacology; Part 3 Pharmacology across the childbearing continuum; and Part 4 Pharmacology for special considerations. Foundational concepts are complemented by additional specialised content. The final chapter, Role of the midwife, focuses on the professional requirements and additional knowledge required for those developing their skills as midwife prescribers.

Hot topics include adverse drug reactions and interactions, and specific chapters cover pregnancy, labour and birth, the postpartum period, lactation and the newborn, and vaccination. In addition, other chapters focus on areas such as diabetes, thyroid, mental health, epilepsy, drugs of addiction and substance dependence.

To enhance learning, chapters begin with a case study that lays the foundation for applying the key physiological, biochemical, and pathological processes that underpin the subsequent discussions of pharmacology. The case studies and accompanying review questions provide interesting real-life scenarios where the midwife is required to apply critical thinking, clinical judgement, and decision making in the systematic assessment, planning, implementation, monitoring, and review of medication management in partnership with the woman, and collaboratively with other members of the healthcare team.

We consider that this integrated approach facilitates an understanding of the cellular and molecular aspects of drug action, the rationales for the clinical use of drugs in particular disease processes, and their therapeutic and adverse effects – including drug interactions. Throughout each chapter, snapshots of key information are provided in the Key Points boxes, and application to the clinical situation is enhanced through Clinical Focus boxes.

In some chapters the information is based on drug groups – detailing when they may be indicated for use in ongoing treatment of chronic health conditions, or discussing complexities experienced by childbearing women – whereas in others the flow of information starts with the relevant stage of the childbirth continuum and leads on to a discussion of the drug groups and complementary alternative medicines (CAMs) relevant to supporting healthy mothers and babies.

Drug Monographs throughout the text provide detailed information on commonly used drugs. It should be noted that specific pharmacokinetic data, drug dosage and formulation, individual adverse effects and drug interactions vary between drugs in the same group; current evidence-based drug information resources should always be consulted before administering any drug, and quality prescribing sources should always be consulted by authorised prescribers.

Case studies and review questions are supported by chapter content that is focused and related to the holistic midwifery assessment and clinical care that takes place during pregnancy, birth and the postpartum period, in partnership with the woman and her family.

This first edition of *Pharmacology for Midwifery* features:

- Key terms and abbreviations
- Critical thinking exercises
- Clinical case studies and review questions
- Key Points boxes that provide a snapshot of important information
- Drug Monographs using either the prototype of a drug group or the most commonly prescribed drug of a group, or drugs that have gained 'drug of first choice' status

- Tables containing detailed information of drug interactions occurring with major drug groups
- Clinical Focus boxes
- Information on the use of CAMs modalities and on interactions between drugs and these therapies
- Key resources, including online resources and additional online case studies.

With advances in drug development, drugs in clinical use continue to have a high rate of obsolescence. The facts learned for a particular drug may therefore become irrelevant when each year brings new drugs with differing modes of action. Similarly, new information on existing drugs may result in a review of current safety categorisation and/or changed recommendations for use and/or recall. With an emphasis on personalised or precision medicine, the challenge for midwives is to stay up to date with advances in the field of pharmacology and their impact on the quality use of medicines. We have used both a scientific and a practice-based clinical approach, founded on evidence-based medicine and always emphasising the clinical use and therapeutic/ adverse effects of drugs. Information on the clinical use of drugs is based on data in the Australian Medicines Handbook, combined with current research.

We are confident that this first edition will fulfil the needs of students, academics and clinicians in midwifery and related professions and will make the study of pharmacology relevant, logical, enjoyable, easy, practical and, above all, interesting.

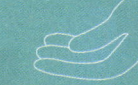

Guide to text

Get the most out of your textbook by familiarising yourself with the key features of *Pharmacology in Midwifery*.

Chapter Opening Features

Chapters have been carefully structured to aid learning. Chapter openings are designed to help you focus and mentally organise content.

KEY ABBREVIATIONS introduces the abbreviations and acronyms that will be used, and provides a quick reference point.

KEY TERMS lists the essential terminology that is bold-faced in the text.

CHAPTER FOCUS highlights what you will learn in the chapter.

KEY DRUG GROUPS lists the drug groups addressed in that chapter.

LEARNING OUTCOMES lists the outlines what you will learn or achieve by the end of the chapter.

CRITICAL THINKING SCENARIO for each chapter allows application of the key physiological, biochemical and pathological processes that underpin the pharmacological use of a particular drug.

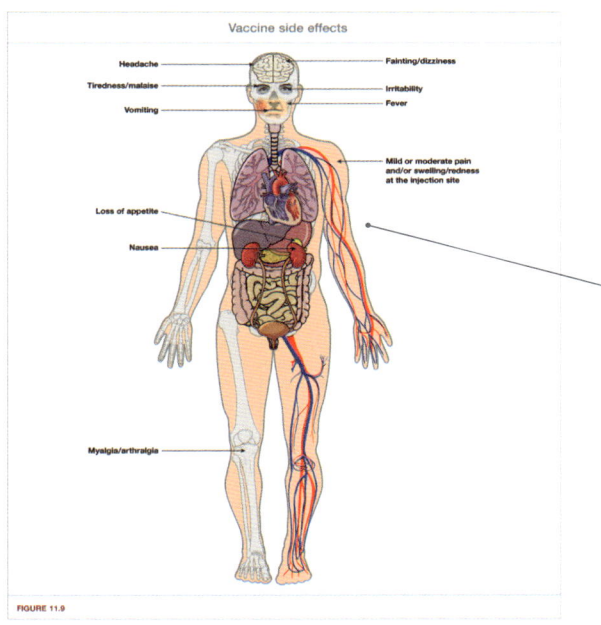

FIGURE 11.9

HUMANOID MODEL use selected organs, tissues, body parts etc. to explain pharmacological/adverse effects of various drugs or drug groups.

Tables and Boxes

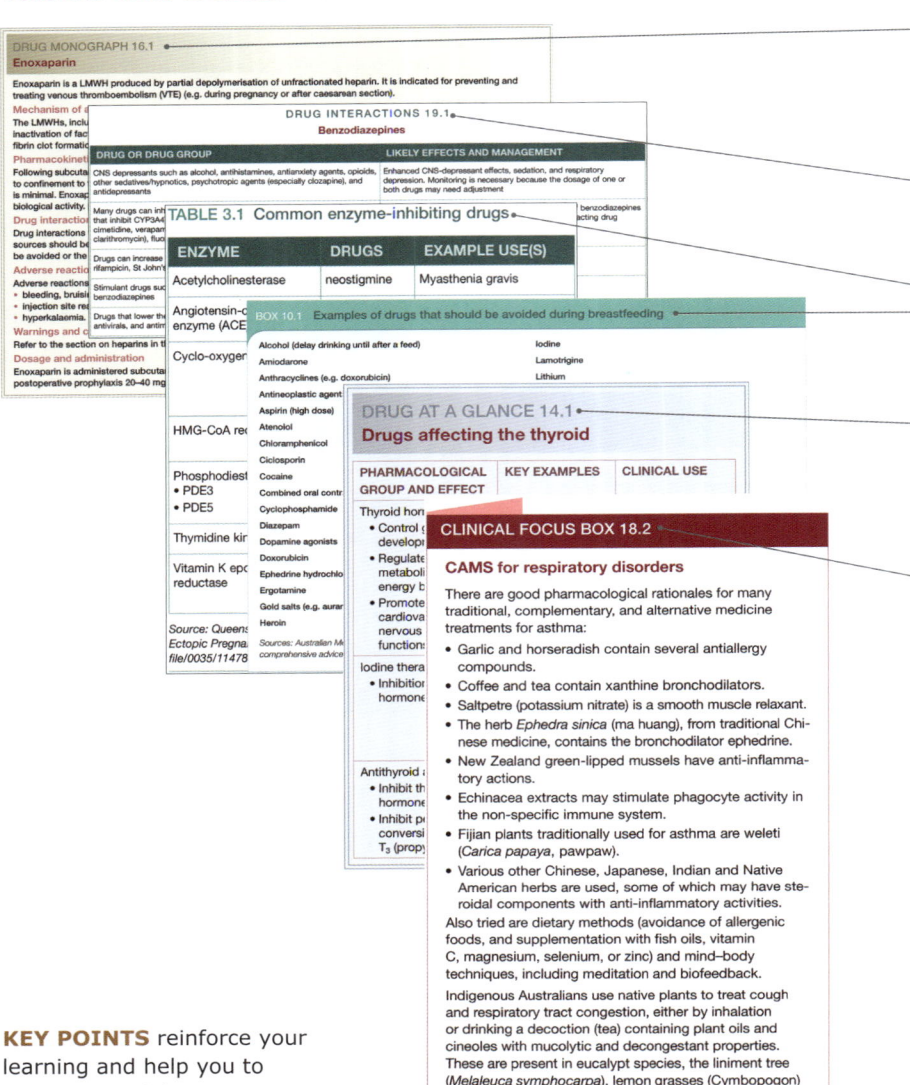

DRUG MONOGRAPHS describe important aspects of either the prototype of a drug group or the most commonly prescribed drug of a group.

DRUG INTERACTIONS TABLES highlight drug interactions of clinical relevance.

TABLES AND BOXES provide additional information and summaries on a range of topics.

DRUGS AT A GLANCE TABLES summarise the main therapeutic groups and effects and give examples of key drugs and their clinical use.

CLINICAL FOCUS BOXES provide descriptions of items of special relevance to Australasia and details of evidence-based pharmacological management of common diseases and conditions.

KEY POINTS reinforce your learning and help you to review material.

KEY POINTS
Female infertility
- Infertility is defined as the absence of conception by a couple after more than 1 year of regular sexual intercourse without contraception.
- Effective treatment requires careful assessment of possible causes in both partners.
- Women who are actively trying to conceive may take pregnancy supplements and vitamins to increase their overall wellbeing.
- It is recommended that women take 400 or 500 micrograms of folic acid per day from 12 weeks prior to conceiving and continuing throughout the first trimester.

REVIEW EXERCISES are given for every chapter to help you master the material in manageable parts.

REVIEW EXERCISES
1 Alison is 8 weeks pregnant and due to hyperemesis is unable to swallow tablets. Alison is required to take her regular medication, drug A, with a bioavailability of 50%, and this must now be administered intravenously. Providing a short justification, estimate the intravenous dose of drug A that would be equivalent to a 100 mg oral dose of this drug.
2 Linda has been using the drug levothyroxine for the past 5 years. She is now 14 weeks pregnant. Discuss the range of factors that could be contributing to variability in her response to the drug.
3 Alex, 5 years old, has been brought to the emergency department of his local hospital with an aspirin digestion. He has accidentally digested aspirin tablets taken by his pregnant mother, who was prescribed them for preeclampsia prevention. A number of management measures have been instituted, including the administration of sodium bicarbonate. Explain why sodium bicarbonate has been administered.

REFERENCES is an up-to-date bibliography at the end of each chapter, with references relevant to all health professionals.

ONLINE RESOURCES lists key websites where you can find additional information. Further web links are also supplied on the Evolve site for this text.

REFERENCES
Australian Medicines Handbook. Adelaide: Australian Medicines Handbook Pty Ltd 2021. 2006;129(Suppl 1):169S-173S.
Gabb GM, Mangoni A, Anderson CS, et al. Guideline for the diagnosis and management of hypertension in adults 2016. Med J Aust. 2016;205(2);85-89. doi:10.5694/mja16.00526
Lowe SA, Bowyer L, Lust K, et al. SOMANZ guidelines for the management of hypertensive disorders of pregnancy 2014. Aust N Z J Obstet Gynaecol. 2015 Oct;55(5):e1-29. doi:10.1111/ajo.12399. Epub 2015 Sep 28. PMID: 26412014.
Rayes B, Ardissino M, Slob EAW, et al. Association of Hypertensive Disorders of Pregnancy With Future Cardiovascular Disease. JAMA Netw Open. 2023;6(2):e230034. doi:10.1001/jamanetworkopen.2023.0034
Salerno E. Pharmacology for health professionals. St Louis: Mosby 1999.
Soma-Pillay P, Nelson-Piercy C, Tolppanen H, et al. Physiological changes in pregnancy. Cardiovasc J Afr. 2016 Mar-Apr;27(2):89-94. doi: 10.5830/CVJA-2016-021. PMID: 27213856; PMCID: PMC4928162.

European Society of Cardiology: https://www.escardio.org/ (accessed 28 February 2022)
National Heart Foundation of Australia – Guideline for the diagnosis and management of hypertension in adults 2016: https://www.heartfoundation.org.au (accessed 28 February 2022)
Safer Care Victoria – Hypertension in pregnancy 2018: https://www.safercare.vic.gov.au/best-practice-improvement/clinical-guidance/maternity/hypertension-in-pregnancy (accessed 16 January 2024)
Society of Obstetric Medicine Australia and New Zealand, Hypertension in pregnancy guideline, Sydney; 2023: https://www.somanz.org/content/uploads/2023/06/SOMANZ_Hypertension_in_Pregnancy_Guideline_2023_Updated_30.6.23.pdf (accessed 19 January 2024)
South Australia Perinatal Practice Guideline – Hypertensive disorders in pregnancy 2024: https://www.sahealth.sa.gov.au/wps/wcm/connect/aa782c004ee49dd483d8f8d150ce4f37/Hypertensive+Disorders+in+Pregnancy_PPG_V5_2.pdf?MOD=AJPERES&CACHEID=ROOTWORKSPACE-aa782c004ee49dd483d8f8d150ce4f37-ocQEdJI (accessed 16 January 2024)

ONLINE RESOURCES
American Heart Association: https://www.heart.org/ (accessed 28 February 2022)
Cardiac Society of Australia and New Zealand: https://www.csanz.edu.au/ (accessed 28 February 2022)

— CHAPTER 1 —

DRUGS AND MEDICINES

Kirsten Small, Roslyn Donnellan-Fernandez

Key Abbreviations

AMH	Australian Medicines Handbook
APF	Australian Pharmaceutical Formulary and Handbook
BP	British Pharmacopoeia
CFB	clinical focus box
CMI	consumer medicine information
DM	drug monograph
INN	international non-proprietary name
NZF	New Zealand Formulary
OTC	over-the-counter
RCCT	randomised controlled clinical trial
TGA	Therapeutic Goods Administration
WHO	World Health Organization

Key Terms

active ingredient 13
approved name 13
assay 2
chemical name 13
clinical trial 11
contraindications 2
dose 2
dose form/
   formulation 2
drug 2
drug development 10
formulary 18
generic name 13
indications 2
medication 2
medicine 2
over-the-counter 2
pharmaceutical 2
pharmaceutics 2
pharmacodynamics 2
pharmacokinetics 2
pharmacy 2

pharmacology/
   pharmacologist 2
pharmacopoeia 2
pharmacy/
   pharmacist 2
potency 2
prescription-only
   medicine 17
proprietary, or trade,
   name 17
prototype drug 17
randomised
   controlled clinical
   trial 11
receptors 3
route 2
selectivity 3
specificity 3
standardisation 10
structure–activity
   studies 9

Chapter Focus

This chapter focuses on the origin, development, and scope of pharmacology. It describes the physical and chemical characteristics of drugs, explains how drugs are named and classified, and how drug information can be sourced. The stages of drug discovery and development, including the phases and important elements in clinical trials of investigational drugs, are outlined. An understanding of basic pharmacology is essential for midwives because of their role in the quality use of medicines, leading to better health outcomes for women and babies.

Learning Outcomes

- Define the terms 'drug', 'medicine', and other commonly used pharmacological terms.
- Describe the ways in which potential candidates for new drugs are discovered or created.
- Outline the steps followed in testing the safety and effectiveness of a new drug.
- Using examples, demonstrate the difference between chemical, generic and trade names for a drug.
- Critique the quality of different sources of pharmacological information for clinical use.

CRITICAL THINKING SCENARIO

Kelly, who is 28 years old and 14 weeks pregnant, was recently diagnosed with depression and prescribed the antidepressant sertraline. Kelly tells her midwife that she does not like taking medicines and would like to learn more about the stages of drug development and the phases of clinical trials that help to promote safe and effective medicines.

1 Explain the stages of drug development.

2 Explain each of the phases of the clinical trial process.

3 Explain how you would report a suspected adverse reaction to a medicine or vaccine.

Kelly has looked at many online resources, blogs, tweets, and relevant Facebook posts to search for information about the safety and effectiveness of sertraline. A lot of information she read is conflicting and, the more she reads, the more confused she gets. Kelly read one online article suggesting 'natural' medicines made from plants are safer than 'unnatural' synthetic medicines, like the one she has been prescribed.

4 List some of the sources Kelly can access for evidence-based information about her new medicine, including information about medication safety in pregnancy and breastfeeding.

5 Discuss whether 'natural' drugs are safer than synthetic drugs.

Introduction

Pharmacology is the study of drugs, including their sources, nature, actions, effects in living systems, and uses. The word '**drug**' is defined by the World Health Organization (2007) as 'any substance or product that is used or intended to be used to modify or explore physiological systems or pathological states for the benefit of the recipient'. The prefix 'pharmaco-' is derived from the Greek word *pharmakon*, meaning 'drug' or 'medicine'. Hence, we have related terms such as '**pharmacy**', '**pharmacodynamics**', '**pharmacokinetics**', '**pharmaceutics**', and '**pharmacopoeia**'.

Pharmacologists study the origins, isolation, purification, chemical structure/synthesis, **assay** (measurement), actions/mechanisms, economics, genetic aspects, and toxicity of drugs, as well as their fate in the body and their medical uses. Pharmacologists work in hospitals, clinics, research institutions, drug companies, government departments of health, medical publishing, and universities. In other words, wherever drugs are developed, studied, and used.

Pharmacology deals with all of the drugs used in society – including legal and illegal drugs, prescription and '**over-the-counter**' (OTC) medications, endogenous substances (those produced within the body), and natural and synthetic products – with beneficial or potentially toxic effects. The pharmacological agents available today have controlled, prevented, cured, diagnosed and, in some instances, eradicated diseases, and have improved the quality of life of billions of people.

However, **medicines** also have the potential to cause harm. To administer a drug safely, one must know the appropriate **dose**, frequency, **route** of administration, **indications**, **contraindications**, significant adverse reactions, major drug interactions, dietary implications (if applicable), and appropriate monitoring approaches, and apply this knowledge to the person and their situation (Table 1.1).

1.1 Drugs and medicines

The word 'drug' has come to have connotations of illicit street drugs. However, it has a much simpler and wider meaning: a drug is a substance with useful effects on living tissues. The terms '**medication**', 'medicine', and '**pharmaceutical**' usually refer to drugs mixed in a **formulation** with other ingredients to improve their stability, taste, or physical form, to allow appropriate administration of the active drug.

Characteristics of drugs

Potency, selectivity and specificity

According to our broad definition of a drug – as a chemical having useful action on living tissue – many substances could be classed as drugs: oxygen, sugar, salt, and water all have a useful effect on the body and can be toxic in overdose. Useful drugs usually have three important attributes: potency, selectivity, and specificity.

Potency relates to the amount of chemical required to produce an effect, and this is an *inverse* relationship – the

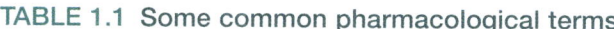

TABLE 1.1 Some common pharmacological terms

TERM	DEFINITION
Adverse drug reaction	An unintended and undesirable response to a drug
Clinical pharmacology	Pharmacology applied to the treatment of humans; the study of drugs in clinical use
Dose	The quantity of a drug to be administered at one time, determined by experience as likely to be safe and effective in most people
Dose form/formulation	The form in which the drug is administered, e.g. as a tablet, injection, eyedrops, or ointment
Drug	A substance used to modify or explore the physiological system or pathological state for the benefit of the person
Indication	An illness or disorder for which a drug has a documented specific usefulness
Medicine	Drug(s) given for therapeutic purposes; possibly a mixture of drug(s) plus other substances to provide stability in the formulation; also, the branch of science devoted to the study, prevention, and treatment of disease
Pharmaceutics	The science of the preparation and dispensing of drugs
Pharmacist	A person licensed to store, prepare, dispense, and provide drugs, and to make up prescriptions
Pharmacodynamics	What drugs do to the body and how they do it; refers to the interaction of drug molecules with their target receptors or cells, and their biochemical, physiological, and possibly adverse effects
Pharmacokinetics	How the body affects a specific drug after administration, i.e. how a drug is altered as it travels through the body (by absorption, distribution, metabolism, and excretion)
Pharmacologist	A person who studies drugs: their source, nature, actions/mechanisms, uses, fate in the body, medical uses, and toxicity
Pharmacology	The study of drugs, including their actions and effects in living systems
Pharmacopoeia	A reference book listing standards for drugs approved in a particular country or jurisdiction; may also include details of standard formulations and prescribing guidelines (a formulary)
Pharmacy	The branch of science dealing with preparing and dispensing drugs; also the place where a pharmacist carries out these roles
Receptor	Protein structure on or within a cell or membrane that is capable of binding to a specific substance (e.g. a transmitter, hormone, or drug), initiating chemical signalling and causing altered function in the cell
Route	The pathway by which a drug is administered to the body, e.g. in the oral route, the drug is taken by mouth and swallowed
Side effect	A drug's effect that is not the intended result for which it was given; side effects may be desirable or undesirable. This term has been generally superseded by the term 'adverse drug reaction'
Toxicology	The study of the nature, properties, identification, effects, and treatment of poisons, including the study of adverse drug reactions

more potent the drug, the lower the dose required for a given effect (see Chapter 4). One of the most potent chemicals known is the natural bacterial product botulinum toxin (commonly known by the trade name Botox), for which the estimated human median lethal dose (LD_{50}) is approximately $1–1.5 \times 10^{-7}$ g IV for a 70 kg adult. It is used to treat spasm of eye muscles and spasticity, as well as in the treatment of neurological disorders and in cosmetic surgery.

Selectivity refers to the narrowness of a drug's range of actions on **receptors**, cellular processes, or tissues. The antidepressant drugs known as selective serotonin reuptake inhibitors SSRIs) – such as fluoxetine (Prozac) (DM 19.2) – have fewer adverse effects than older antidepressants because of their more selective actions.

Similarly to the term 'selectivity', the term **'specificity'** may be used loosely – for example, cardiospecific or cardioselective β-blocking agents. Specificity may also refer to the relationship between the chemical structure of a drug and its pharmacological actions. For example, the effects of salbutamol and similar bronchodilators in asthma are due to their chemical similarity to the neurotransmitter noradrenaline, and hence their specificity for the β-adrenoceptor.

The ideal drug

In designing a new drug, a research pharmacologist might aim for it to be:

- easily administered (preferably orally) and fully absorbed from the gastrointestinal tract

- not highly protein-bound in the blood plasma
- potent
- highly specific
- selective
- rapid onset, and with useful duration of action and a high therapeutic index (no adverse drug reactions, no interference with body functions)
- unlikely to interact with any other drugs or foodstuffs
- spontaneously eliminated
- stable, both chemically and microbiologically
- readily formulated into an easily taken form
- inexpensive.

Unfortunately, there is no *ideal drug*, whether natural product or synthetic. It has been said that any substance powerful enough to be useful is also powerful enough to do harm. The decision to prescribe, administer, or take a drug requires a risk–benefit analysis based on the best information available. The question is: Do the likely therapeutic benefits (efficacy) outweigh the possible harmful effects (toxicity)?

Physical aspects of drugs

In terms of their physical state, drugs may be solids, liquids, or gases. Most are solids at room temperature; but some are liquids in the pure state, such as nicotine, halothane (a general anaesthetic), and ethanol; and some are gases, such as nitrous oxide.

Chemical aspects of drugs: Inorganic/organic

Whether found naturally in plants, animals, minerals, or microorganisms, or synthesised in a laboratory, all drugs are chemicals. They may be inorganic (i.e. do not contain carbon) molecules, such as magnesium salts used to prevent and treat eclamptic seizures, or iodine and iron used to prevent mineral deficiencies. Most drugs are organic molecules, that is, they contain carbon in their structures. All the major classes of organic compounds, including hydrocarbons, proteins, lipids, carbohydrates, nucleic acids, and steroids, are represented in pharmacopoeias. Many drug molecules are acids or bases, which is important not only for their taste and irritant effects but also for how the drugs move across membranes and are affected by metabolism and excretion. This is discussed in detail in Chapter 5.

Chemical aspects of drugs: Molecular size

The size of drug molecules varies enormously, ranging from tiny lithium – the third-lightest element, where a single atom weighs about 7 daltons – through to large proteins such as insulin (molecular mass 5808 daltons) and erythropoietin (34 kilodaltons). Most drugs are in a more intermediate size range, with molecular weights (relative molecular masses) of between 100 and 1000. For example, aspirin has a molecular weight of 180, testosterone (a steroid hormone) 288, digoxin (a cardiac glycoside) 781, and ciclosporin (an immunosuppressant with a cyclic polypeptide structure) 1203. The size and nature of the molecules have important implications for their use. Proteins taken orally are digested in the gut, so they must be administered by injection. In general, large molecules will not readily cross cell membranes and therefore may need to be administered directly to their site of action.

> **KEY POINTS**
>
> **Introduction to pharmacology**
> - Pharmacology is the study of drugs, which are substances used for their beneficial effects on living systems.
> - Drugs may be solids (most commonly), liquids, or gases. Most are organic (carbon-containing) chemicals.

1.2 Drug discovery and development

The goal of the drug discovery process, and its subsequent development, is to produce safe and effective drugs. There are several ways in which the potential therapeutic uses of natural or synthetic chemicals are determined. These can be summarised in the following three steps: (1) understand the science, (2) unravel the story, and (3) apply the technology. Drug discovery has been likened to the processes of evolution: a selection process with a high level of attrition and with many influences affecting survival of the fittest. Recently, drug discovery has become more reliant on computational and artificial intelligence, accelerating the drug discovery process (Hinkson et al 2020).

Where drugs come from

Drugs and biological products are derived from several main sources:

- microorganisms – e.g. fungi used as sources of antibiotics (Fig 1.1A), and bacteria and yeasts genetically engineered to produce drugs such as human insulin
- plants – e.g. *Atropa belladonna* (source of atropine), *Cannabis sativa* (marijuana), *Coffea arabica* (Fig 1.1B; coffee, caffeine), *Digitalis purpurea* (Fig 1.1C; digitalis), *Duboisia* spp. (hyoscine, nornicotine), *Eucalyptus* spp. (eucalyptus oil), and *Papaver somniferum* (Fig 1.1D; opium, morphine)
- humans and other animals, from which drugs such as bovine insulin, human chorionic gonadotrophin, and erythropoietin can be obtained, sometimes by recombinant techniques
- minerals or mineral products – e.g. iron, iodine, and magnesium

Natural sources of important drugs

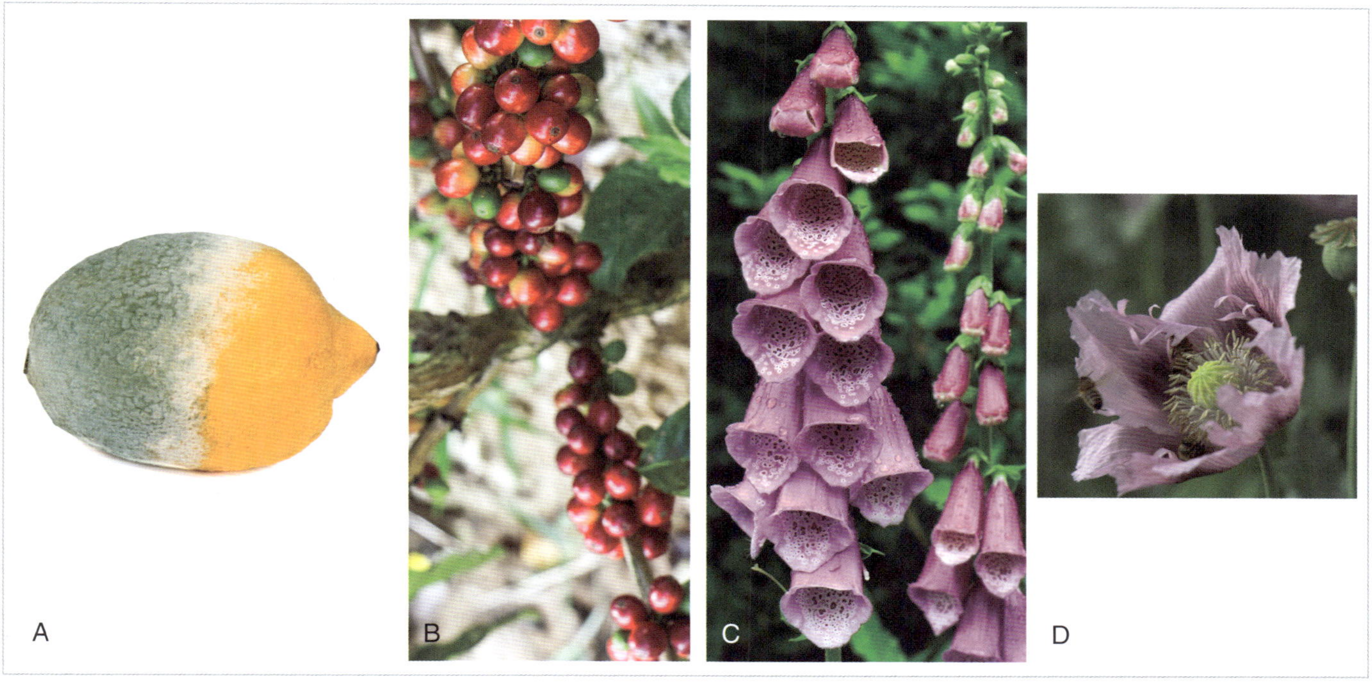

FIGURE 1.1 A *Penicillium notatum* mould, source of penicillin; **B** *Coffea arabica*, source of caffeine (and coffee); **C** *Digitalis purpurea*, source of digoxin; **D** *Papaver somniferum*, source of morphine and codeine.

A–D: iStockphoto/habari1; iStockphoto/kannika2013; iStockphoto/Petegar; iStockphoto/AtWaG

- laboratory-synthesised substances – e.g. sulfonamides, β-blockers, and antidepressants. Drugs are classed as semisynthetic when the starting material is a natural product, such as a plant steroid or microbial metabolite, and is then chemically altered to produce the desired drug molecule.

Drugs sourced from natural or traditional remedies

For thousands of years, people have been trying natural products – animal, vegetable, and mineral – to see if they are useful as foods or in treating disease (Table 1.2). Natural products may be used as crude extracts – such as raw opium, tobacco leaves, or herbal teas – or purified and/or synthesised and then formulated as pharmaceutical preparations, such as tablets, ointments, and injections. Complementary and alternative medicines are sometimes used during pregnancy and breastfeeding, with many of these having plant-based origins, such as red raspberry leaf, traditionally used to make labour easier, and milk thistle used as a galactagogue.

This is called the 'reefs and rainforests' route to new drugs, recognising that there are millions of natural chemicals in the environment to be identified and tested. As biodiversity is lost, we lose chances to discover new drugs in this way. For example, the recent extinction of Australia's gastric-brooding frogs means we will now never know how the frog's eggs avoided digestion in the mother frog's stomach or being moved on into her small intestine – actions that are potentially useful in treating gastrointestinal tract disorders.

'Natural' drugs are not necessarily better

There is a widely held belief that 'natural' drugs are safer than synthetic drugs. A quick scan of naturally occurring substances such as arsenic, botulinum toxin, cocaine, cyanide, deadly nightshade, mercury, methanol, strychnine, thallium, tobacco, and uranium shows that natural is not always good. It would be foolish to expect all natural drugs to be automatically safer than those synthesised in laboratories – or vice versa. Any drug's safety and quality must be tested and proved before approval for clinical use, regardless of its source.

Active constituents of drugs derived from plants

The leaves, roots, seeds, and other parts of some plants may be dried, crushed, boiled, and extracted or otherwise

TABLE 1.2 Some drugs from plants

DRUG	SOURCE	MAIN PHARMACOLOGICAL ACTIONS
Aromatic oils	For example, from eucalyptus, pine, mint	Decongestant, treats the common cold, mild antiseptics
Artemisinins	*Artemisia annua* (sagewort)	Antimalarial
Atropine	*Atropa belladonna* (deadly nightshade)	Antimuscarinic, premedication, treats asthma
Bran	Indigestible vegetable fibre	Laxative, treats constipation
Caffeine	*Coffea arabica* (coffee)	CNS stimulant, diuretic
Cocaine	*Erythroxylum coca*	CNS stimulant, local anaesthetic, addictive
Colchicine	*Colchicum autumnale* (crocus)	Anti-inflammatory, treats gout
Coumarins	Sweet clover	Anticoagulant, prevents thrombosis
Digoxin	*Digitalis lanata* (woolly foxglove)	Cardiac glycoside, treats heart failure
Ephedrine	*Ephedra sinica*	Sympathomimetic, treats asthma
Ergot alkaloids (e.g. ergometrine)	Mould on *Claviceps* spp.	Oxytocic, treats postpartum bleeding
Galantamine	*Galanthus nivalis* (snowdrop)	Anticholinesterase, used in neurological disorders and Alzheimer's disease
Hypericin	*Hypericum perforatum* (St John's wort)	Monoamine reuptake inhibitor, treats depression
Ipecacuanha	Cephaelis root	Expectorant, emetic, treats poisoning
Morphine	*Papaver somniferum* (opium poppy)	Analgesic, sedative, antidiarrhoeal, cough suppressant, addictive
Nicotine	*Nicotiana tabacum* (tobacco)	Vasoconstrictor, CNS stimulant, addictive
Paclitaxel	Yew tree bark	Antineoplastic, treats cancer
Phytoestrogens	Clover, soybeans	Estrogenic, treats menopausal symptoms
Pilocarpine	*Pilocarpus microphyllus*	Muscarinic agonist, treats glaucoma
Quinine, quinidine	Cinchona bark	Antimalarial, treats cardiac arrhythmias
Salicylates, including aspirin	*Salix* spp. (willow)	Anti-inflammatory, analgesic, antipyretic
Strychnine	*Strychnos nux-vomica*	CNS stimulant, convulsant
Vincristine	*Catharanthus roseus* (periwinkle plant)	Antineoplastic, treats cancer

CNS = central nervous system
Source: *Evans 2009*.

processed for use as medicine and, as such, are known as 'crude' drugs or herbal remedies. Their therapeutic effects are produced by the chemical substances they contain. When the pharmacologically active constituents are separated, purified, and quantified, the resulting substances usually have similar pharmacological actions to the crude drugs but are more potent (weight-for-weight), produce effects more reliably, and are less likely to be affected by other constituents or contaminants in the crude preparations. Indeed, the herbal antidepressant St John's wort has been shown to have a similar mechanism of action – and hence similar therapeutic and adverse effects – as the synthetic selective serotonin reuptake inhibitor fluoxetine.

Some types of pharmacologically active molecules found in plants – grouped here according to their chemical properties – are alkaloids, glycosides, steroids, hydrocarbons, alcohols/phenols, proteins, gums, and oils (Table 1.3). Note that the groups are not mutually exclusive – there can be phenolic alkaloids, glycoproteins, and phenolic glycosides. Figure 1.2 shows the chemical formulae of some drugs extracted from plant sources.

TABLE 1.3 Pharmacologically active constituents of plant drugs

CHEMICAL CLASS AND STRUCTURE	CHARACTERISTICS	EXAMPLES
Alkaloids Organic nitrogen-containing compounds that are alkaline and usually bitter-tasting The nitrogen atom is usually in a heterocyclic ring of carbon atoms (Fig 1.2A)	Many alkaloid drugs are amines, so their names often end in the suffix '-ine' Combined as salts to make them more soluble (e.g. morphine sulfate) Plants may have evolved the ability to synthesise bitter alkaloids as a defence against herbivorous animals	Analgesics morphine (Fig 1.2A), cocaine, and codeine Antiasthma drugs ephedrine, theophylline, and atropine Vinca alkaloids (anticancer) Alkaloids used in gout (colchicine), malaria (quinine), and labour (ergot alkaloids) 'Social' drugs: nicotine and caffeine
Carbohydrates Organic compounds of carbon, hydrogen, and oxygen	Sugars are a source of energy Gums and mucilages are carbohydrate plant exudates; when water is added, some will swell and form a gelatinous mass, a useful laxative effect Gums are also used to soothe irritated skin and mucous membranes and may be a rich source of starch	Sugars such as glucose Starches and fibres such as cellulose and inulin, a fructose–furanose polysaccharide (Fig 1.2B) used in kidney function tests Gelling agents such as agar, and gums such as tragacanth and *Aloe vera* products
Glycosides Particular type of carbohydrate that, on hydrolysis, yields a sugar plus one or more additional active substances	The sugar part is believed to increase the solubility, absorption, permeability, and cellular distribution of the glycoside	Digoxin (Fig 1.2C), found in *Digitalis* (foxglove) plants; known as a cardiac glycoside because of its stimulant actions on the heart Glycosides present in oleanders and some other Australian plants are responsible for their poisonous nature Cane toads also contain cardioactive glycosides
Hydrocarbons Organic molecules consisting entirely of hydrogen and carbon May be straight-chain or aromatic (containing benzene rings)	Derivatives such as organic alcohols and esters contribute the fragrances to many plants and perfumes Commonly used by drug companies and pharmacies when preparing topical formulations of drugs, especially creams and ointments	Fats and waxes Oils such as castor, olive, and coconut oil Fatty acids, prostaglandins, and balsams
Oils A subgroup of hydrocarbons May be terpene-type compounds May contain many types of functional groups including ketones, phenols, alcohols, esters, and aldehydes	Viscous liquids high in hydrocarbon content Often flammable and immiscible with water and aqueous solvents Frequently used as flavouring agents, in perfumery, in chemical industries, and as antiseptics A fixed oil dropped onto filter paper will leave a greasy stain, whereas a volatile oil (which evaporates) will not	Eucalyptus, peppermint, and clove oils are volatile oils used in medicine Castor oil (mainly composed of ricinoleic acid, Fig 1.2D) and olive oil are fixed oils Australian Myrtaceae family and *Melaleuca* genus plants contain many fragrant and useful oils, including eucalyptus and tea-tree oils
Phenols Phenols contain a benzene ring with a hydroxyl substituent	Phenols are a specialised type of alcohol, a compound containing a hydroxyl group, –OH	Salicylates, including aspirin-like compounds and flavouring agents (e.g. vanillin) Isoflavones, including phytoestrogens Coumarins, including the anticoagulant dicoumarol (Fig 1.2E) Cannabinols from marijuana Hypericin, from St John's wort, used in depression (Fig 1.2E)
Tannins A specialised type of phenol	Astringent plant phenolics can tan hides (animal skins) by precipitating proteins Common plant constituents, especially in bark, accounting for some of the brown colour in swamps and rivers and in cups of tea	In Australian native medicine, kino, the gum exuded from eucalyptus trees, was an important source of tannins, used to treat diarrhoea, haemorrhage, and throat infections
Isoprenes, terpenes, and steroids Terpenes are 10-carbon molecules built up from small 5-carbon building blocks called isoprenes Plant steroids are also synthesised naturally from isoprene sub-units	Plant steroids, with their characteristic 4-ring structures, are used as the starting material to produce many hormone drugs The plant sterol diosgenin, from the *Dioscorea* species, has been used in the synthesis of estrogenic hormones	Carotenoids such as beta-carotene and vitamin A Salicylate analgesics including aspirin (acetylsalicylic acid) Pyrethrins (insecticides) Menthol (Fig 1.2F), camphor, and thymol, aromatic compounds used in respiratory medicine Gossypol, a male contraceptive agent used in traditional Chinese medicine (Fig 1.2F)

Chemical structures of some active drugs derived from plant sources

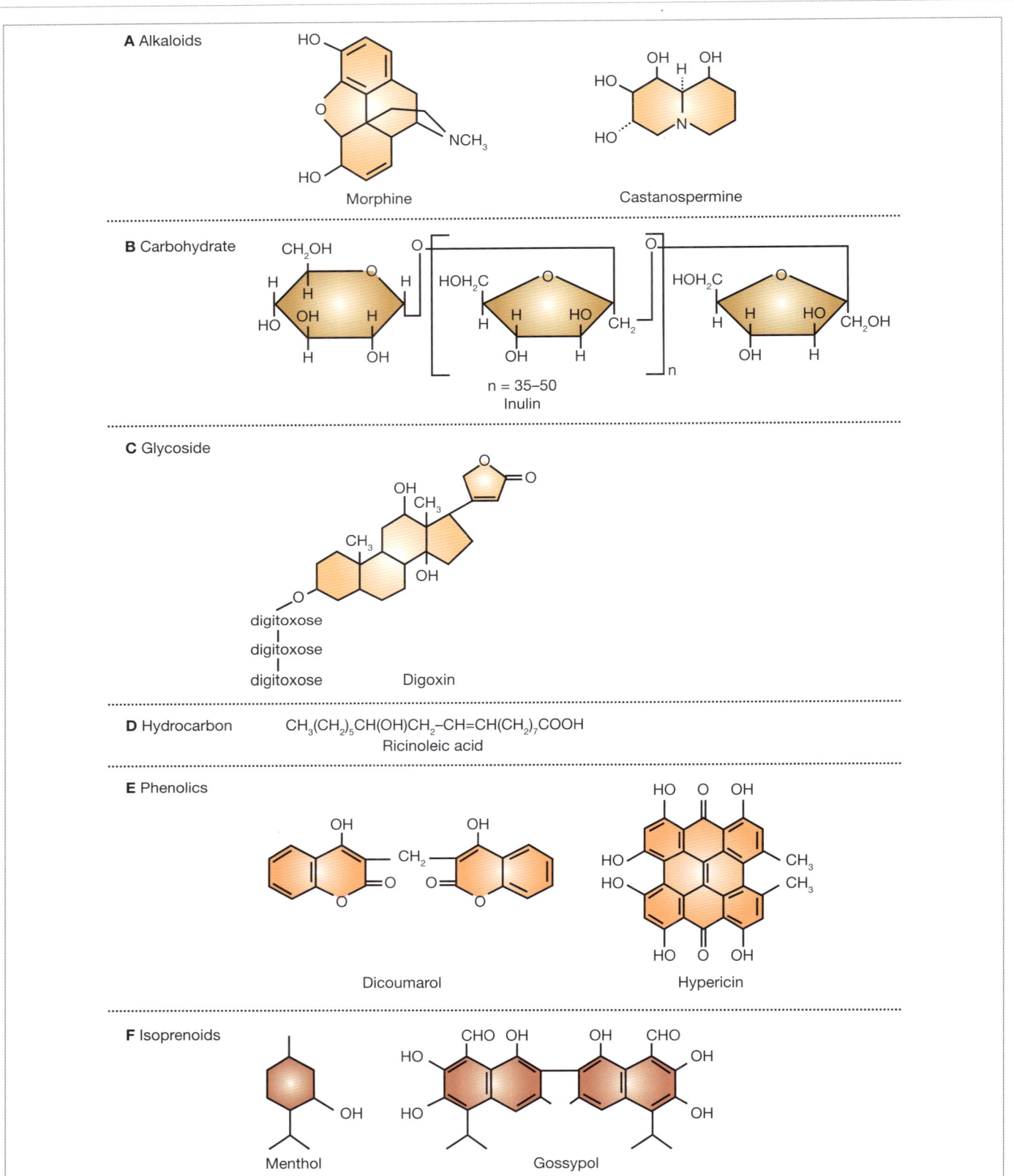

FIGURE 1.2 A Alkaloids: morphine and castanospermine; **B** A carbohydrate: inulin; **C** A glycoside: digoxin; **D** A hydrocarbon: ricinoleic acid; **E** Phenolics: dicoumarol and hypericin; **F** Isoprenoids: menthol and gossypol.

Serendipity

Although sheer good luck plays a part in some drug discoveries – such as Fleming's bacterial culture plate becoming contaminated with a growth of the fungus *Penicillium notatum*, which inhibited bacterial growth – it usually takes lateral thinking (e.g. questioning why bacteria were inhibited near the fungus), intelligence, and years of hard work (extracting the natural antibacterial agent, determining its structure and developing methods of producing enough penicillin to treat people with bacterial infections) to exploit the lucky find.

Other examples of serendipity in pharmacological discovery are the findings that people treated with the first safe synthetic oral antibacterial agents, sulfonamides, had a lowering in their blood glucose levels, which led to sulfonylurea oral hypoglycaemic agents; and men with hypertension treated with the vasodilator minoxidil tended to grow more hair. The drug is now used mainly as a hair restorer.

Chemical plus pharmacological studies

As chemical techniques developed in the 19th and 20th centuries, the structures of pharmacologically active substances could be determined and similar substances synthesised, then tested for activity. These **structure–activity studies** led to many drug groups:

- The second- and third-generation penicillins were modelled on the first penicillin.
- All the sympathomimetic amines were initially noradrenaline 'look-alikes'. Studies of *Ephedra sinica*, long known in traditional Chinese medicine to be useful in respiratory conditions (asthma), led to the purification of the active ingredient ephedrine, then to synthesis of the related β-receptor-activating antiasthma drugs isoprenaline and salbutamol, which result in fewer adverse reactions.
- β-blockers, such as propranolol and atenolol, were designed to act as ligands at the receptor without activating it and proved useful in cardiovascular diseases. (The chemical structures of β-receptor ligands are shown in Figure 1.3.)

Research carried out by pharmacologists, biochemists, and chemists in universities and research institutes may lead to the discovery of new drugs. The pharmaceutical industry monitors such research via the scientific literature, patent applications, and scientific conferences.

Active metabolites of existing drugs

Sometimes drugs are found to be more active after metabolism in the body and so the metabolites are tested. Paracetamol is one of the metabolites of phenacetin, an early antipyretic analgesic agent, and is safer than phenacetin. Many of the benzodiazepine antianxiety agents have pharmacologically active metabolites, some of which are administered therapeutically.

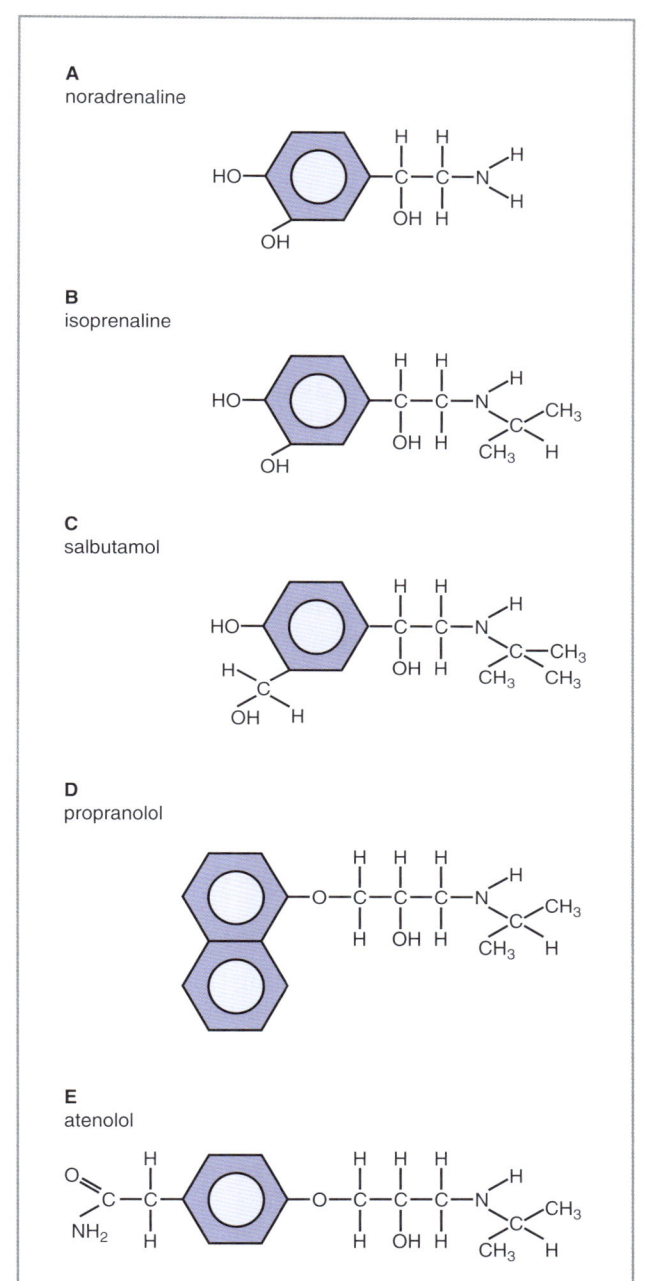

Structure–activity relationships for some drugs binding to adrenoceptors

A noradrenaline

B isoprenaline

C salbutamol

D propranolol

E atenolol

FIGURE 1.3 A Noradrenaline, a sympathetic neurotransmitter; **B** Isoprenaline, a non-selective β-adrenoceptor agonist; **C** Salbutamol, a selective β$_2$-adrenoceptor agonist; **D** Propranolol, a non-selective β-adrenoceptor antagonist; **E** Atenolol, a selective β$_1$-adrenoceptor antagonist with less likelihood of causing asthma. Increasing the 'bulkiness' of the substituents at the catechol end (two adjacent –OH groups) or the amine end (–NH$_2$) may select for ligand-binding affinity or agonist/antagonist activity at specific receptors.

Rational molecular design

Structure–activity studies predict the shape of the active site of a receptor and lead to the design of drugs that may be agonists or antagonists at that receptor. The early antihistamines were modelled on the histamine molecule. Subsequent research led to the discovery of histamine H_2-receptors and the development of specific H_2-antagonists, which revolutionised the treatment of gastric ulcers.

Computer-aided design

Drug receptors, enzymes, ion channels, and transporters are no longer simply 'black boxes' referred to by pharmacologists wishing to explain drug mechanisms. Many are proteins with known amino acid sequences and tertiary structures (three-dimensional shapes) that are able to be cloned. Computer modelling of their active sites allows testing of chemicals for virtual binding affinity. Using such techniques, angiotensin-converting enzyme (ACE) inhibitors were designed for use in hypertension, dopa-decarboxylase inhibitors for administration with levodopa in Parkinson's disease, the anti-flu drug zanamivir to inactivate the flu virus, and potential anticancer drugs to inhibit steps in the pathways of macromolecular synthesis.

Combinatorial chemistry ('combichem') techniques make it possible for millions of new molecules to be synthesised, either actually or virtually. This may involve systematic and repetitive use of commercially available chemical reagents to synthesise 'libraries' of new chemical compounds, preferably small molecules, which are then screened for activities on proteins, receptors, enzymes, and transporters.

Standards and government regulation

The development of new drugs is regulated by government legislation and administered by government authorities such as the Therapeutic Goods Administration (TGA) in Australia, the Ministry of Health and Medsafe in New Zealand, and the Food and Drug Administration (FDA) in the United States (Chapter 2). Regulation protects consumers by ensuring that only safe and effective drugs are approved.

The formulations of drugs vary in strength. In particular, drugs derived from natural sources vary depending on how extracts are harvested and purified. Because accurate dosage and the reliability of drug effects depend on uniformity of strength and purity, **standardisation** (bringing the preparation to a specified concentration or quality) and the publication of standards are necessary.

Drug standards in Australia and New Zealand

The main standards for drugs in Australia are those published in *Martindale: The Complete Drug Reference*, the *British Pharmacopoeia* (BP) and the *Australian Pharmaceutical Formulary* (APF). The BP gives detailed, legally accepted standards for hundreds of drugs and herbal products, with chemical information and the approved formulations containing the substance. It lists criteria for purity, chemical methods for identification and assay (measurement), tests and maximum levels allowed for impurities, and storage conditions. Preparations meeting these standards are referred to as 'the BP preparation'.

The APF is a reference book for **pharmacists** that helps promote quality use of medicines. It contains evidence-based information on medicine and pharmacy-specific topics – for example, dispensing, counselling, and therapeutic management. It also contains key 'recipes' for commonly made formulations by pharmacists. For example, Calamine Lotion APF is one such recipe. It lists the required quantities of individual ingredients (active and excipient), gives the method for preparation of the lotion, and describes the use of the formulation. The *New Zealand Formulary* (NZF) is like the *Australian Medicines Handbook* (AMH), with both providing detailed information about drugs. (For more information about drug standards, see Drug information sources.)

Stages of drug development

Drug development occurs in clearly defined phases involving multidisciplinary teams. These have traditionally been described as the following:

1 *The new idea or hypothesis.* Routes to drug discovery include selection of a target, introduction of a new hypothesis for disease causation, ideas for new molecules, discovery of new natural products, optimisation of lead compounds, and research with new molecular biology, genetic engineering, and formulation technologies.

2 *Design, purification, or synthesis of the new molecule.*

3 *Screening of new compounds for useful pharmacological activities or possible toxic effects.* Screening may be broad, to detect all actions, or specific, for affinity for a particular receptor, transporter, or enzyme. High-throughput screening allows millions of compounds to be run through automated initial screens. These initial three stages may take between two and five years.

4 *Preclinical pharmacology.* This includes in-vitro and in-vivo studies. Pharmacodynamic actions and pharmacokinetic aspects (the fate of the molecule or compound in the body, including susceptibility to phases of metabolism) are usually studied in at least three mammalian species, including non-human primate species.

5 *Toxicology studies (adverse effects).* These include acute toxicity, long-term toxicity (chronic effects and effects on reproduction) and tests for mutagenicity and carcinogenicity. Requirements depend on anticipated exposure and clinical use, whether acute or chronic.

6 *Pharmaceutical formulation and manufacturing.* This involves a scale-up of the synthetic pathway, including stability tests and assay methods. These stages may take one to two years.

7 *An application to drug-regulating authorities for approval to undertake a trial in humans.*

8 *Clinical trials.* If the drug appears to be safe, effective, and worth testing, it will go to **clinical trial** while being closely monitored. Progress must be reported regularly to the national regulatory authority, which may sometimes undertake inspections (the first three phases of a clinical trial may take from five to seven years).

9 *Registration.* Depending on the results of the full clinical trial program, the sponsors may apply for registration of the drug and approval to market it for clinical use.

10 *Ongoing post-marketing studies.* These follow up the drug, monitoring its effects and interactions in the wider community for longer periods.

Clinical trials of drugs

A clinical trial is a prospective study involving human participants that measures the effectiveness and safety of an intervention (e.g. diet, procedure, medical device) or treatment (e.g. drug, vaccine). Clinical trials report data on both safety (adverse reactions) and efficacy. The 'gold standard' of clinical trials is the **randomised controlled clinical trial** (RCCT). In this type of study, participants are randomly allocated so they have an equal chance of being allocated to the treatment undergoing investigation or the control group. The control group will receive the current standard therapy treatment for the condition or a placebo treatment. Placebo treatments contain no active ingredients. The outcomes of interest (e.g. reduction in blood pressure, blood glucose level, or length of labour) are measured in both groups and compared. All clinical studies in humans must be approved by a local human research ethics committee.

Clinical trials are generally required for all new drugs and for new uses (new indications) or new formulations of old drugs. However, there are exceptions:

- Potentially toxic drugs (e.g. anticancer drugs) may go straight to phase II studies in a small number of people with the disease so that volunteers without the disease are not subjected to adverse effects.
- The rules may be bent for orphan drugs (non-patentable) or for rare diseases (see Chapter 2).
- There is public pressure to fast-track drugs that are potentially useful in otherwise fatal diseases such as cancers.

A range of ethical issues and the greater potential for harm to the pregnant woman or the developing fetus mean large-scale clinical trials to test new drugs are not often undertaken in pregnancy. Similar challenges exist with regard to breastfeeding and newborn infants.

The objectives of RCCTs need to be realistic, valid and specific, yet allow for the results to be applied for the population at large. This is known as generalisation. Clinical trials are a staged process, with few participants in the early phases and stepwise decision making so that trials can be stopped if clear differences or toxicities become apparent. It is now customary for a Data Safety Monitoring Board to be appointed for a trial. This board consists of a small number of independent experts who periodically review the emerging safety information.

Phase I: The first tests in humans using healthy volunteers

After extensive testing in vitro and in animals, the drug is administered initially in very low and increasing doses to small numbers of healthy volunteers under close supervision. The objectives are to determine the pharmacological activities, pharmacokinetic parameters including bioavailability, tolerable dosage range, and acute toxicity of the drug.

Phase II: The first administration to people with the condition that the intervention or treatment is designed to treat

In phase II, the first studies on efficacy are conducted. To do this, a small number of people with the condition that the intervention is designed to treat are given either the new drug, a standard drug, or a placebo. There are approximately 50 participants in each treatment group and these participants are closely monitored. The tests may be 'single-blind', where participants do not know which treatment they are getting but the investigators do, or 'double-blind', where neither the participants nor the investigators know. Phase II studies indicate the pharmacokinetic and pharmacodynamic properties, therapeutic range of doses, maximum tolerated dose, and common adverse reactions in people with the disease. They act as pilot studies and serve to optimise the protocol, and determine dosing and sample sizes in the phase III trial.

Phase III: The full-scale randomised controlled clinical trial

This is the clinical trial, as commonly understood, in which the drug is administered to large groups of people, ranging from several hundreds to thousands, to ascertain whether under defined conditions the drug shows clinical benefit for the disease state, and with an acceptably low rate of adverse drug reactions. Important elements of the RCCT are as follows:

- Investigators must believe the new treatment is at least as good as the former treatment.
- Participants must be randomised to ensure groups are initially similar in sex, age range, weight range, and severity of disease.

- Participants must give informed consent after being provided with detailed information about the study, the potential benefits and adverse reactions, and advised that they have the option to withdraw at any stage.
- Double-blinding is usual, with coded packs of drugs so neither investigators nor participants know who received the new drug.
- The institution's ethics committee must have given approval.

If it becomes apparent that one group is benefiting statistically significantly more than the other, or suffering more adverse reactions, the trial is halted. It is important that raw data from clinical trials is published (even negative results) so conclusions can be examined independently.

If the new drug is shown to be safe, efficacious, and cost-effective, it may be approved for market by the government's regulatory body – the TGA in Australia and Medsafe in New Zealand. In both countries, advice is usually taken from the national advisory committee – the Advisory Committee on Medicines in Australia or the Medicines Assessment Advisory Committee in New Zealand.

Phase IV: Post-marketing studies

Research about new drugs does not end once they reach the market. The number of people studied, and the time allotted to the study have been limited (Fig 1.4). Certain types of participants may have been excluded, such as children, pregnant or lactating women, people with multiple disease states, or who are taking other drugs.

Once marketed, the drug is used in many more people and for longer periods. Extended monitoring of safety and efficacy (pharmacovigilance) is then possible. Inevitably, events surface that were not seen during the trial, such as rare adverse reactions, effects in subgroups of the population, and drug interactions. Studies in pregnant women are especially important because rare impacts on development of the embryo or fetus may be detected.

As part of its post-market vigilance, the TGA carries out laboratory investigations of products on the market and ongoing monitoring to ensure compliance with legislation. The TGA publishes details about Australian reports of suspected adverse reactions in an online database call DAEN (Drug Adverse Event Notifications). An example of this in the Australian context, reported in 2021 (TGA 2021), relates to the use of propylthiouracil and carbimazole for the treatment of hyperthyroidism. Propylthiouracil and carbimazole should not be prescribed for women of childbearing age unless the potential benefits outweigh the risks. This relates to a reclassification of the drug to one suspected to have caused, or which may be expected to cause, an increased incidence of human fetal malformations or irreversible damage. In New Zealand, Medsafe regulates clinical trials and carries out similar pharmacovigilance.

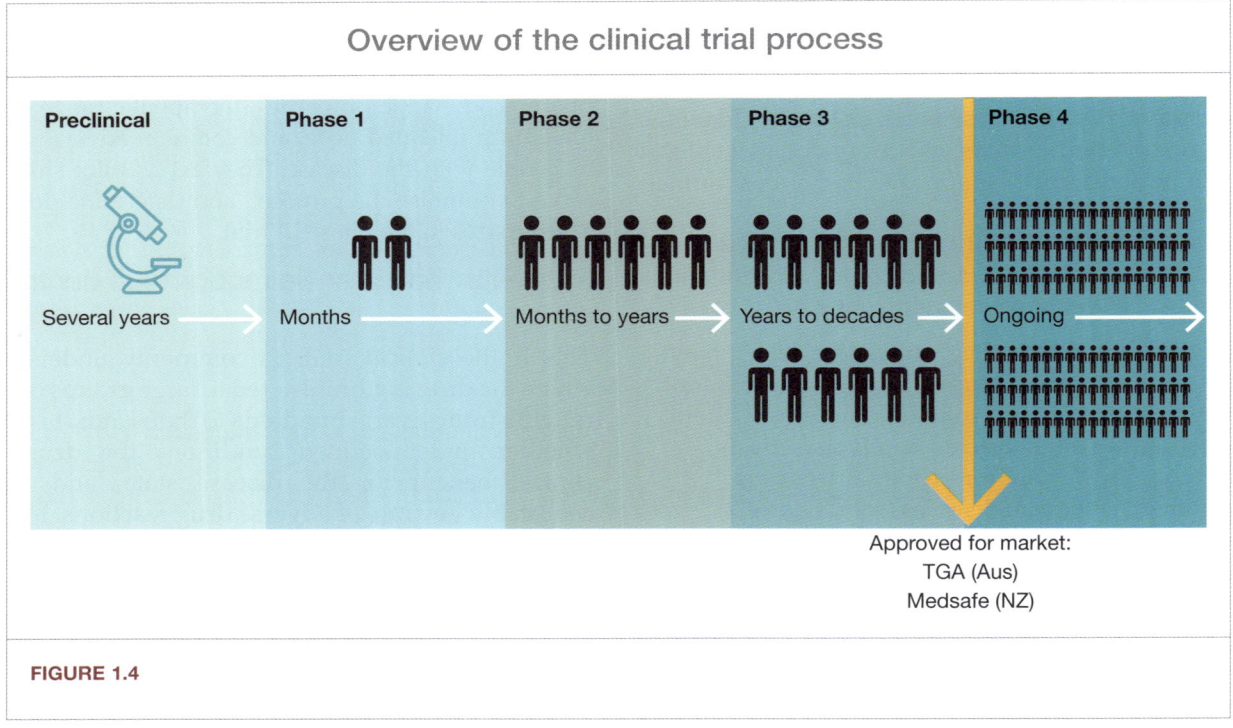

Overview of the clinical trial process

Preclinical	Phase 1	Phase 2	Phase 3	Phase 4
Several years	Months	Months to years	Years to decades	Ongoing

Approved for market:
TGA (Aus)
Medsafe (NZ)

FIGURE 1.4

Pharmacovigilance: The 'blue card'

Through its Advisory Committee on Medicines, the TGA encourages and facilitates the reporting by consumers and health professionals of adverse events they suspect are related to medications and medical devices. Historically, reporting has been by use of a one-page form – the 'blue card' (Fig 1.5). Online reporting is now also possible. Confidentiality is maintained. Consumers can also report adverse reactions via the Adverse Medicine Events Line (1300 134 237).

Reports of adverse reactions are reviewed, entered into DAEN, and analysed for patterns. The Advisory Committee on Medicines informs health professionals about adverse events and can recommend actions ranging from no action required, to change of aspects of prescribing or dispensing, through to withdrawal of a drug from the market. For example, the COX-2 inhibitor lumiracoxib was included in the Pharmaceutical Benefits Scheme in 2006 and became widely used. However, by late 2007 the TGA had received eight reports of serious liver damage, including two deaths, so the drug was deregistered. Since 2010, the TGA has published Medicines Safety Updates.

KEY POINTS

How drugs are discovered and developed

Drugs and biological products are derived from several main sources:

- microorganisms (e.g. antibiotics from fungi)
- plants (e.g. morphine from the poppy *Papaver somniferum*; active plant constituents include alkaloids, carbohydrates, hydrocarbons, phenols, and isoprenoid structures)
- humans and other animals (e.g. human chorionic gonadotrophin)
- minerals or mineral products (e.g. iron and iodine)
- laboratories, in which substances such as β-blockers and antidepressants are chemically synthesised, or made by genetically engineered microorganisms (e.g. human insulin).

Drug development takes place in various stages over many years:

1 Design and synthesis of a new molecule.
2 Screening for useful and adverse biological activities.
3 Pharmaceutical formulation and manufacturing scale-up.
4 Clinical trials:
   i. phase I: first in-human tests, for pharmacokinetics and adverse effects
   ii. phase II: efficacy studies in a small cohort of people, for dose range
   iii. phase III: the randomised controlled clinical trial, double-blinded, statistically valid.
5 If approved and marketed, ongoing post-marketing studies and pharmacovigilance.

1.3 Drug names and classifications

Drug names

Each drug possesses three different types of name: the **chemical name**, the approved (or generic or non-proprietary) name, and the proprietary (or brand or trade) name or names. For example, the chemical name of amoxicillin, a commonly prescribed antibiotic, is actually (2S,5R,6R)-6-{[(2R)-2-amino-2-(4-hydroxyphenyl)-acetyl]amino}-3,3-dimethyl-7-oxo-4-thia-1-azabicyclo-[3.2.0] heptane-24-carboxylic acid, abbreviated to D(−)-α-**am**ino-p-hydr**ox**ybenzylpen**icillin**. Its approved generic name, amoxicillin, is clearly derived from parts of its chemical name. It is marketed under several proprietary names including Alphamox, Amoxil, Bgramin, Cilamox, Fisamox, GenRx Amoxycillin, Maxamox, Ranmoxy, and Yomax; in various formulations such as injections, capsules, tablets, syrups, suspensions, and paediatric drops, and in combinations with other antibacterials and proton pump inhibitors.

It would be helpful if every drug had a name related to other drugs in the same class (Table 1.4); however, this tends to be true only of the more recent drug groups. Thus, we refer to 'the statins', 'gliptins' and 'the glitazones'. Names can be deceiving. The names of most β-blockers end in '-olol', but stanozolol is an anabolic steroid, not a β-blocker. Nystatin is an antifungal agent and somatostatin is a growth hormone release inhibitory factor, and neither is a 'statin'. We cannot assume that drugs whose names sound similar always have similar effects and uses. And note that Table 1.4 cannot be read backwards; that is, while the suffix '-vir' implies the drug is probably an antiviral, not all antiviral drugs end in -vir (think zidovudine and ribavirin).

Chemical names

The **chemical name** is a unique, precise description of the drug's chemical composition and molecular structure. It is particularly meaningful to medicinal chemists – who should be able to draw the chemical structure if given the chemical name – but may be unintelligible to others. Because chemical names are too complicated to remember, or fit on a prescription pad or bottle label, a drug likely to reach the market and be used medically is allocated a name that is simpler and easier to spell.

Active ingredient names

The **active ingredient** name (sometimes referred to as the approved or generic name) is usually suggested by the manufacturer and approved by a drug-regulating authority; it becomes the official or international non-proprietary (INN) name. It is shorter, is often derived from the chemical name, and is the name listed in official

The 'blue card', used by health professionals to report suspected adverse reactions to drugs and vaccines

Australian Government
Department of Health
Therapeutic Goods Administration

TGA use only

Report of suspected adverse reaction to medicines or vaccines
See statement about the collection and use of personal information overleaf, and please attach any additional data to this form

Patient initials or medical record number:	Sex: M ☐ F ☐	Date of birth or age:
	Weight (kg):	

Suspected medicine(s)/vaccine(s)

Medicine/vaccine (please use trade names; include batch number and AUST R or AUST L number if known)	Dosage (Dose number for vaccines eg 1st DTP)	Date begun	Date stopped	Reason for use

Other medicine(s)/vaccine(s) taken at the time of the reaction

Medicine/vaccine	Dosage	Date begun	Date stopped	Reason for use

Reaction(s):   Date of onset of reaction (for vaccines time after administration):   /   /

Describe: (please provide as much detail as possible and include any results of relevant laboratory data and other investigations)

Seriousness: Life threatening ☐   Hospitalised ☐   Required a visit to doctor ☐

Treatment of reaction:

Outcome: Recovered ☐ ▶ Date: / /   Not yet recovered ☐ Fatal ☐ ▶ Date: / /   Unknown ☐

Sequelae?   No ☐   Yes ☐ ▶ Describe:

Reporting: Doctor ☐   Pharmacist ☐   Other ☐   Contact details (email or phone)

Name:

Address:

Postcode: Signature: Date: / /

Thank you for taking the time to complete this form   PTO

FIGURE 1.5

Source: Adapted from Therapeutic Goods Administration https://www.tga.gov.au/sites/default/files/blue-card-adverse-reaction-reporting-form.pdf

Report of suspected reaction to medicines or vaccines ("Blue card")

Privacy statement

For general privacy information, go to <www.tga.gov.au/privacy>.

Information in this report is collected to assist in the post market monitoring of the safety of therapeutic goods under the *Therapeutic Goods Act 1989* (the Act). All reports are entered into the Therapeutic Goods Administration's (TGA's) Adverse Event Management System (AEMS). Further information about how the TGA uses adverse event information that is reported to it is available at <www.tga.gov.au/reporting-adverse-events>.

The TGA collects personal information in this report to:
• monitor the safety of medicines and vaccines under the Act
• contact the reporter of the adverse event if further information is required
• contact representatives of entities that supply therapeutic goods, to discuss reported adverse events
• check that the same information has not been received multiple times for the same adverse event.

At times, this information is collected from someone other than the individual to whom the personal information relates. This can occur when an adverse event is reported to a person or an entity other than the TGA (such as a health professional, a hospital or a sponsor), and that person or entity passes the information on to the TGA. In those cases, ordinarily the TGA will not collect the name and contact details of patients. However, the TGA may collect other information relating to patients, including the date of birth or age, gender, weight, initials and information about the relevant adverse event.

Personal information collected in this report may be disclosed as permitted under the Privacy Act 1988, including by consent or where the disclosure is required by, or authorised under, a law (for example, under section 61 of the Act). Where a report relates to vaccine events, personal information about the reporter or the patient may be disclosed to State and Territory health agencies under subsection 61(3) of the Act.

Fold here first (Please do not use staples on this form)

www.tga.gov.au/reporting-problems   Email: adr.reports@tga.gov.au   Fax: 02 6232 8392

What to report
You do not need to be certain, just suspicious!
Any information related to the reporter and patient identifiers is kept strictly confidential.
Adverse drug reaction reports should be submitted for prescription medicines, vaccines, over-the-counter medicines (medicines purchased without a prescription), and complementary medicines (herbal medicines, naturopathic and/or homoeopathic medicines, and nutritional supplements such as vitamins and minerals). Please include timing of reactions relative to medicine administration where relevant.
The TGA particularly requests reports of:
•   All suspected reactions to new medicines and vaccines
•   All suspected drug interactions
•   Unexpected reactions, that is not consistent with product information or labelling
•   Serious reactions which are suspected of significantly affecting a patient's management, including reactions suspected of causing death, danger to life, admission to hospital, prolongation of hospitalisation, absence from productive activity, increased investigational or treatment costs, and birth defects.

Fold here second   D1073 June 2018

Delivery Address:
PO Box 100
WODEN ACT 2606

No stamp required
if posted in Australia

Medicines Safety Monitoring
Pharmacovigilance and Special Access Branch
Reply Paid 100
WODEN ACT 2606

FIGURE 1.5, cont'd

compendia such as the AMH or the BP. The active ingredient name needs to be distinct in sound and spelling so it is not easily confused with other drugs. Overly fanciful or optimistic names, or those that refer to medical conditions or body parts, are (supposed to be) rejected.

Active ingredient (generic) prescribing and bioequivalence

Because numerous brand names may exist for the same drug, prescribers are mandated to use the active ingredient name (CFB 1.1). This helps avoid confusion between drugs with similar brand names and reduces errors and costs.

TABLE 1.4 Drug classes

PREFIX OR SUFFIX	DRUG GROUP	EXAMPLE GENERIC NAME	PREFIX OR SUFFIX	DRUG GROUP	EXAMPLE GENERIC NAME
cefa/o-	Cefalosporins	cefalexin	-mab	Monoclonal antibodies	rituximab
gli-	Sulfonylureas	glibenclamide	-olol (most)	Beta-blockers	metoprolol
-afil	Phosphodiesterase 5 inhibitors	sildenafil	-onidine	Alpha$_2$-adrenoceptor agonists (α_2-agonists)	clonidine
-a/oquine	Quinine antimalarials	mefloquine	-oxifen(e)	Selective estrogen receptor modulators	tamoxifen
-artan	Angiotensin-II-receptor antagonists (sartans)	candesartan	-prazole	Proton pump inhibitors	omeprazole
-a/ovir	Antivirals	aciclovir	-pril	ACE inhibitors	captopril
-azepam	Benzodiazepines	diazepam	-pristone	Progesterone receptor antagonists	mifepristone
-azole	Azole antifungal agents	fluconazole	-prost	Prostaglandin analogues	latanoprost
-caine	Local anaesthetics	lidocaine	-rubicin	Anthracycline antineoplastic agents	doxorubicin
-cillin	Penicillins	ampicillin	-setron	5HT$_3$ antagonists	ondansetron
-coxib	Cyclo-oxygenase-2 inhibitors (coxibs)	celecoxib	-statin (some)	HMG-coa reductase inhibitors (statins)	simvastatin
-cycline	Tetracycline antibiotics	doxycycline	-stim	Colony-stimulating factors	filgrastim
-dipine	Calcium channel blockers (dihydropyridine-type)	nifedipine	-tidine	Histamine H$_2$-receptor antagonists (H$_2$-receptor antagonists)	cimetidine
-dronate	Bisphosphonates	alendronate	-tinib	Tyrosine kinase inhibitors	imatinib
-eplase	Thrombolytics	alteplase	-triptan	5HT$_1$ agonists (triptans)	sumatriptan
-floxacin	Quinolone antibiotics	ciprofloxacin	-zolamide	Carbonic anhydrase inhibitors	acetazolamide
-glitazone	Thiazolidinediones (glitazones)	pioglitazone			
-i/ythromycin	Macrolide antibiotics	azithromycin			
-lutamide	Antiandrogens	flutamide			

ACE = angiotensin-converting enzyme (converts angiotensin I to angiotensin II, which is a vasoconstrictor and hence raises blood pressure); HMG-CoA = 3-hydroxy-3-methylglutaryl coenzyme A (a coenzyme involved in the early stages of cholesterol synthesis); 5HT = 5-hydroxytryptamine or serotonin.

CLINICAL FOCUS BOX 1.1

Communicate the active ingredient name

In Australia, from February 2021, it became a legal requirement for all prescribers to use the name of a medicine's active ingredient. For example, instead of writing a script for Voltaren 50 mg, a brand (proprietary) name, the script should be written for diclofenac 50 mg (the active ingredient). Prior to this, prescribers used a mix of brand and active ingredient names when prescribing, which was confusing for people using medications and led to medication errors.

It is not uncommon for there to be many brand names for the one active ingredient. To continue using the diclofenac

example, there are many diclofenac brands such as Clonac, Fenac, Viclofen, and Cambia. In Australia and New Zealand, generic brands must show bioequivalence to the original brand before being available to the public. Bioequivalence is when two active ingredients result in similar blood concentration levels that lead to the same physiological effect.

Prior to the legislation, unless brand substitution was not permitted by the prescriber, a prescription written using a brand name could be substituted with another bioequivalent brand. For example, a script written for Clonac 50 mg, could be substituted to Fenac 50 mg. Because it would be impossible for hospital and community pharmacies to stock all the different brands of a medicine, it was routine for substitution to occur. It is hoped that active ingredient prescribing will reduce medication errors and simplify the language around medications. For example, Annette will get used to calling her pain medication 'diclofenac' and look for the active ingredient names on her medicines. Improvement in health literacy surrounding medication use can improve safety and the quality use of medicine as per the National Medicines Policy.

Another step you should take to improve medicine safety is to use the active ingredient name when communicating with users of medications and other health professionals. You will also note that this textbook does not often refer to brand names but instead uses active ingredient names.

Proprietary (trade or brand) names

When a drug company markets a particular drug product, it selects and copyrights a **proprietary, or trade, name** for its drug, thereby restricting use of the name to that individual drug company and to that formulation of the drug. Drug companies carry out extensive advertising to encourage prescribers to choose their version of the drug and to promote sales of trade name drugs. This expense is eventually borne by the consumer, or by government (i.e. taxpayers) if the drug is subsidised.

In this text, we will always use generic (approved) names for drugs but may sometimes add a trade name if it is sufficiently well known (e.g. Valium, Prozac, Viagra) to help readers identify a particular drug. *Note that we do not imply thereby any preference for that brand of the drug.* Approved / generic names use lower-case letters, whereas a trade name always begins with an upper-case letter.

Drug classifications

Drug classification can be approached from many perspectives. Using the example of amoxicillin again, this could be classified by:

- source – where the drug comes from. (*Semisynthetic antibiotic from* Penicillium *spp.*)
- chemical formula or structure. (*B-lactam, penicillanic acid derivative*)
- pharmacokinetic parameters – how the drug is absorbed or metabolised in the body. (*Acid-resistant, β-lactamase-sensitive*)
- activity – the effects of the drug. (*Wide-spectrum antibacterial agent*)
- mechanism of action – how the drug works. (*Inhibitor of bacterial cell wall synthesis*)
- clinical use – conditions for which the drug is prescribed. (*Indicated for treatment of infections by sensitive Gram-positive and Gram-negative organisms*)
- body systems affected by the drug. (*For infections of the respiratory system; ear, nose, and throat; genitourinary tract, etc.*)
- drug schedule – the group into which the drug is classified for legal purposes. (*S4 Prescription-Only medicine*)
- pregnancy safety schedule – grouping drugs depending on their safety for use in pregnancy. (*A: considered safe*)
- popularity. (*One of the most prescribed drugs in the world*)
- whether its use is allowed in sporting competitions. (*Yes, approved by the World Anti-Doping Agency*).

Not surprisingly, students are often confused by drug classification. Sometimes the same drug is classified into different groups depending on the clinical use. For example, aspirin-like drugs may be classified as analgesics, antipyretics, anti-inflammatory agents, or anti-thrombotics. This book uses various approaches where appropriate. For example, antidepressants are grouped as 'tricyclic antidepressants' (a chemical class), or by mechanism of action: 'monoamine oxidase inhibitors' or 'selective serotonin reuptake inhibitors'. Such drug classifications can simplify understanding about individual drugs.

Prototype drugs

Pharmacology is easier to understand and learn when **prototype drugs** are studied – that is, the most important drug in a class, to which other drugs in the class can be compared. In this text, many prototype drugs are described in detail in a consistent format called a drug monograph (DM). When a new, similar drug becomes available, inferences can be made about its basic pharmacodynamic qualities before focusing on specific properties (usually pharmacokinetic) to differentiate it from the prototype.

KEY POINTS

How drugs are named and classified

- A drug may have three main names:
  1 its unique chemical name
  2 an approved (generic) name, allocated by a regulating authority. In Australia and New Zealand, this should be the official INN
  3 a trade or brand name, given by the marketing company.

- Generic prescribing is encouraged and dispensing of substituted products considered bioequivalent is sometimes permitted.

- Drugs are classified by any of several criteria – e.g. by source, chemical group, pharmacokinetic parameters, pharmacological activity, mechanism of action, clinical use, body systems affected, legal drug schedule, pregnancy safety category, popularity, whether allowed in sporting competitions, or whether considered 'essential'.

- Drug classifications help facilitate understanding of pharmacology by comparing the common characteristics of an example of a drug group or classification (the prototype drug) with those of other drugs in the same category.

1.4 Drug information

Important drug information

Drug monographs summarise important basic information about prototype drugs including the:

- group or category
- approved/generic name
- pharmacodynamic effects (what the drug does to the body)
- mechanisms of action
- indications for clinical use
- pharmacokinetic parameters (what the body does to this drug)
- common adverse effects (adverse drug reactions)
- **contraindications** (the conditions in which a drug should *not* be prescribed) and precautions
- significant drug interactions
- dosage and administration guidelines, optimum therapeutic plasma levels, and monitoring techniques.

Information about potential toxic effects and treatment of poisoning may also be relevant, as is safety of use in particular cohorts of people, such as infants or lactating women. The Australian Drug Evaluation Committee's Pregnancy Safety Category indicates the likely safety or risks with the use of a drug during pregnancy (see Online resources).

What users of medications want to know

There is a huge amount of information available on most drugs, especially on the internet, where its accuracy and bias cannot easily be judged. What people most want to know is:

- What is the drug for?
- What will it do to me, i.e. what are the risks and benefits?
- How do I take it?
- What other treatment options are there?
- What might happen if I *don't* take it?

These are questions health professionals – including midwives – prescribing, recommending, or administering drugs should be ready to answer.

The publication of data on new drugs and new information on old drugs is an ongoing process – in scientific journals, news releases, drug information brochures, reference books, and textbooks. Much information (some of dubious quality) is found on the internet (Ioannidis et al 2017). No single source will meet the varied and specialised needs of all professionals and healthcare users. It is important to read critically, beware of bias or selectivity of information, and consider the credibility of the author and the publication, particularly with information found on the internet.

An excellent overview, 'Where to find information about drugs' (Day & Snowden 2016) can be found via the Australian Prescriber website.

Official sources, pharmacopoeias and formularies

Official sources of drug information containing legally or medically accepted standards for drugs are published by government bodies, such as departments of health and hospitals, and by pharmaceutical societies and medical colleges. Pharmacopoeias are reference texts collecting drug information relevant to a particular country, including descriptions, formulae, strengths, standards of purity, and dosage forms.

Formularies are similar but may also include information on drug actions, adverse effects, general medical information, guidelines for pharmacists dispensing medicines, and the 'recipes' for formulation or production of different medicines such as tablets, injections, ointments, and eyedrops. A national **formulary** may also be used by government to limit drugs available or subsidised, to encourage rational, cost-efficient prescribing, and enhance the quality use of medicine (QUM) (see Chapter 2).

The Australian Pharmaceutical Formulary and Handbook

The *Australian Pharmaceutical Formulary and Handbook: A Guide to Best Practice* (APF) is published by the Pharmaceutical Society of Australia. The APF contains formulae for medicines, principles of drug therapy, therapeutic management of common conditions (e.g. cough, fever, tinea), monographs on complementary medicines, counselling guides, health information, physicochemical data on drugs, codes of ethics for pharmacists, and Australian standards. It aims to underpin the expanding roles of pharmacists and encourage 'best practice' pharmacy (Pharmaceutical Society of Australia 2021).

Australian Medicines Handbook

In the years since the *Australian Medicines Handbook* (AMH) was first published in 1998 it has become one of the most trusted sources of peer-reviewed, independent, authoritative information on therapeutic drugs and clinical practice in Australia. It is published by three national bodies concerned with drug therapy: ASCEPT (the Australasian Society of Clinical and Experimental Pharmacologists and Toxicologists), the PSA (Pharmaceutical Society of Australia), and the RACGP (Royal Australian College of General Practitioners). The AMH aims to fulfil a need for 'an evidence-based resource that is concise and easy to use for busy practitioners, but which contains the key information required for better drug treatment and prescribing choices', and contains three main types of information:

- treatment considerations for common diseases, with comparisons between classes of drugs
- statements about classes of drugs, with comparisons between individual drugs in the class; and
- monographs on individual drugs, with some trade names and formulation types.

Preliminary sections provide general prescribing information as well as details on prescribing for specific groups. Appendices provide invaluable reference information, especially on significant drug interactions (see Online resources).

New Zealand drug information

Medsafe is the New Zealand Government's Medicines and Medical Devices Safety Authority. This authority is responsible for ensuring the regulation and safety of medicines and medical devices in New Zealand. The Medsafe website is a great source of independent information for health professionals, students, and consumers. There are prescriber update articles, medicine data sheets, reporting of adverse reactions, drug information leaflets, and media releases as well as information about the classification and regulation of medicines, medical devices, drug abuse, support groups, clinical trials, and complementary medicines.

The New Zealand Ministry of Health and various organisations interested in medicines have developed a *New Zealand Formulary*, which provides point-of-care advice for health professionals and has a companion *New Zealand Formulary for Children*. It includes the New Zealand Universal List of Medicines, a list of all prescription medicines in New Zealand. It is continuously updated and integrated with electronic prescribing and dispensing software packages and provides four main components:

1 preliminary general notes on use of drugs (medicines)
2 practical notes on specific therapeutic categories
3 datasheets (monographs) on individual drugs
4 details of preparations available and the relevant subsidy information.

The NZF therefore parallels much of the AMH, with the advantage that it is freely available and accessible online in New Zealand. This is where it differs from the AMH, which is published annually at a cost to purchasers of approximately A$295 *(at time of publication)*.

Other official sources

Some other examples of official drug information sources are:

- *Martindale: The Complete Drug Reference*: monographs on drugs classified under therapeutic groups, such

as analgesics, anthelmintics, vaccines. It includes details of preparations, and lists of manufacturers and pharmaceutical terms (Buckingham 2020).
- *British Pharmacopoeia* (British Pharmacopoeia Commission): with official standards and monographs on thousands of drugs, formulated medicines, herbal drugs, blood products, and surgical materials
- *United States Pharmacopeia* and the National Formulary (US Pharmacopeial Convention)
- *Handbook of Non-prescription Drugs: An Interactive Approach to Self-Care* (American Pharmaceutical Association): an authoritative source on 'non-prescription drug pharmacotherapy, nutritional supplements, medical foods, non-drug and preventive measures, and complementary therapies'.

Semi-official sources

Semi-official sources of drug information may be published by government bodies or other groups, such as medical and pharmacology societies, and may include drug bulletins, reference books and updates, but not drug advertisements. While not official standards, they attempt to provide up-to-date, independent, and unbiased information on drugs. Information such as lists of food additives, support organisations for specific conditions, poisons information centres, and prescribing guidelines may be included.

Therapeutic Guidelines series

Therapeutic Guidelines Limited is an independent not-for-profit organisation based in Melbourne. It started with a very small booklet called *Antibiotic Guidelines* published more than 20 years ago in a determined bid to encourage rational prescribing of antibiotics at the Royal Melbourne Hospital.

There is now (2023) a series of 19 guidelines, each dedicated to a branch of medicine or major drug therapy – for example, antibiotics, cardiovascular medicine, and palliative care. The guidelines, each written by an 'Expert Group', are intended principally to provide prescribers with clear, practical, succinct, and up-to-date therapeutic information, categorised according to diagnosis and updated every few years. They are published in print and electronic formats suitable for computers and mobile devices (see Online resources).

Cochrane

Cochrane is an international organisation publishing systematic reviews and meta-analyses of evidence from research on healthcare interventions, with the aim of helping people make well-informed healthcare decisions. It aims to avoid duplication of studies, minimise bias, and provide relevant, up-to-date, easily accessible information. There are Cochrane databases for reviews, clinical trials, methodologies, and economic evaluations, among others (see Online resources).

Other semi-official sources

Other examples include:

- *National Prescribing Service (NPS) MedicineWise.* An independent, not-for-profit, Australian organisation working to improve the way health technologies, medicines, and medical tests are prescribed and used. The NPS provides newsletters, websites, fact sheets, apps, and public campaigns to 'deliver meaningful information for health consumers, health professionals, government, research and other businesses to enable the best decisions about medicines and health technologies' (see Online resources).
- *Australian Prescriber.* A free bi-monthly independent review journal, published by the NPS, that provides critical commentary on drugs and therapeutics for health professionals, including Medicines Safety Updates. It has been freely available online since 1996, and articles are now included in the PubMed Central database.
- *Reference books.* These include the *Australian Prescription Products Guide* ('PP Guide'), the *Merck Index*, *Drug Interactions: Analysis and Management* and journals such as *Current Therapeutics*, *Annals of Pharmacotherapy*, and *Drugs*.

Drug or poisons information centres and pharmacists

Drug information centres, usually located in the pharmacy departments of major teaching hospitals, aim to disseminate information about drugs, adverse reactions, drug interactions, treatment of drug overdoses and other related information, to maximise safety, efficacy, and economy in drug use (see AMH, Appendix, 'Drug Information Centres'). They are excellent sources of information for the public and health professionals. Community and hospital pharmacists, as medicines experts, are usually available and willing to provide drug information as part of their professional role.

Other drug information sources

- *Textbooks and drug guides.* An up-to-date pharmacology textbook is a valuable source of drug information for inclusion in the health professional's library. Various drug guides also exist, acting as quick reference sources of summarised information on drugs and most are now available online. Examples are the *MIMS Abbreviated* drug reference guides, which are published and updated four times per year. Drug Names, an app that is easily accessed on a smartphone, provides concise information on a drug's class, mechanism of action, uses, and dosage.
- *Reference books.* For example, *MIMS Annual* provides photographs to assist in identifying an unknown tablet or capsule. MIMS is now also published in various electronic formats (eMIMS) for android and Apple platforms and is suitable for desktops and laptops. It can be integrated into popular dispensing programs, and is available as MIMSonline.
- *Drug company information.* Companies applying for registration of their products must supply information to health authorities on all aspects of the drug to prove its safety, efficacy, and cost-effectiveness. A summary of this information is available in publications such as *MIMS Annual* and the PP Guide, and in consumer medicine information sheets, advertisements, and promotions. Material supplied by drug companies is likely to be less objective than information in independent sources such as the AMH or *Australian Prescriber*. (The ethical aspects of drug advertising are discussed in Chapter 2.)
- *Consumer medicine information (CMI) pamphlets.* These help improve people's understanding and use of prescribed drugs. They are particularly important when a drug is first provided, when the dose or formulation is changed, or the information is revised. Previously, all products had to have CMI handouts but many manufacturers now rely on consumers accessing information on their website.

The internet

With the proliferation of medical sites on the internet, many search engines (e.g. PubMed, Embase, eMedicine, Medline, Ovid, AusDI, Up-To-Date, and the American Society of Health-System Pharmacists' drug information site) and directories are available to provide both general and specialised drug information for health professionals and consumers. Some professional journals, databases, indexes, and abstracting services also provide current drug information on the internet. Examples include LactMed (Drugs and Lactation Database), and Hales Medications and Mothers' Milk.

It is essential to read internet sites critically when seeking drug information because there is no screening system to determine the accuracy of internet information, and incorrect, commercial, or biased information may be posted (Ioannidis et al 2017).*

---

*Students tempted to use Wikipedia as a quick source of drug information for assignments or revision purposes should beware. A comparison study looking at the accuracy and completeness of Wikipedia and Micromedex compared with FDA-approved production information found that Wikipedia was less complete and accurate. The authors concluded that Wikipedia should not be used by health professionals as a reference source (Reilly et al 2017).

monographs. J Am Pharm Assoc (2003). 2017;Mar 1;57(2): 193-196. doi: 10.1016/j.japh.2016.10.007

Therapeutic Goods Administration. Medicines Safety Update: Propylthiouracil and carbimazole – use in pregnancy. https://www.tga.gov.au/news/safety-updates/propylthiouracil-and-carbimazole-use-pregnancy. Published 15/9/2021. Accessed 10/4/2024. Canberra: Commonwealth of Australia, 2021.

World Health Organization. A model quality assurance system for procurement agencies: Recommendations for quality assurance systems focusing on prequalification of products and manufacturers, purchasing, storage and distribution of pharmaceutical products. Geneva: WHO, 2007.

KEY POINTS

Drug information sources

- Information about drugs is available from a wide variety of sources, ranging from official government publications through semi-official sources to drug company information and websites.

- Internet sources can be evaluated on the following criteria: accuracy, appearance, authority, currency, and objectivity.

REVIEW EXERCISES

1 Gillian is prescribed two new drugs, one to manage pregnancy nausea and vomiting and one to reduce the risk of preterm birth. Gillian does not like taking medicines and wants to know they are safe. She asks you, her midwife, to outline and describe the process from preclinical testing to post-marketing surveillance.

2 A doctor prescribes an investigational drug that is new to you. Before you administer the medication, which drug information source would you select to find evidence-based information on this drug? What credibility could you give the information?

3 Compare the advantages and disadvantages of prescribing and using active ingredient (approved or generic) names rather than brand (or trade) names when communicating with people who might use the medication.

ONLINE RESOURCES

Advisory Committee on the Safety of Medicines: https://www.tga.gov.au/ (follow links to Committees) (accessed 17 May 2021)

Australian Government Dept of Health and Aged Care, National Medicines Policy. https://www.health.gov.au/resources/publications/national-medicines-policy?language=en (accessed 10 April 2024)

Australian Medicines Handbook: https://shop.amh.net.au (accessed 17 May 2021)

Australian Pharmaceutical Formulary: https://www.psa.org.au/apf (accessed 17 May 2021)

Australian Prescriber: https://www.nps.org.au/australian-prescriber/ (accessed 17 May 2021)

British Pharmacopoeia: https://www.pharmacopoeia.com (accessed 17 May 2021)

Cochrane: https://www.cochrane.org/ (accessed 17 May 2021)

European Forum for Good Clinical Practice: https://efgcp.eu/ (accessed 17 May 2021)

Hales Medications and Mothers' Milk: https://www.halesmeds.com/ (accessed 4 July 2022)

LactMed [Drugs and Lactation Database – National Library of Medicine US]: https://www.ncbi.nlm.nih.gov/books/NBK501922/ (accessed 4 July 2022)

Martindale: The Complete Drug Reference: https://www.pharmpress.com/Martindale-The-Complete-Drug-Reference (accessed 17 May 2021)

Médecins Sans Frontières, Essential drugs list: http://refbooks.msf.org/msf_docs/en/essential_drugs/ed_en.pdf (accessed 17 May 2021)

Medsafe (New Zealand): https://www.medsafe.govt.nz/ (accessed 17 May 2021)

Medsafe (New Zealand), Centre for Adverse Reactions Monitoring (CARM): https://www.medsafe.govt.nz/safety/report-a-problem.asp (accessed 17 May 2021)

MIMS Annual: https://www.mims.com.au/index.php/products/mims-annual (accessed 17 May 2021)

Prescribing Service (NPS) MedicineWise: https://www.nps.org.au/ (accessed 17 May 2021)

REFERENCES

Buckingham R, ed. Martindale: The Complete Drug Reference. 40th ed. London, UK: Pharmaceutical Press, 2020.

Day RO, Snowden L. Where to find information about drugs. Aust Prescr. 2016;39(3):88-95. doi.org/10.18773/austprescr.2016.075

Evans WC. Trease and Evans' Pharmacognosy. 16th ed. Edinburgh, UK: Elsevier, 2009.

Hinkson IV, Madej B, Stahlberg EA. Accelerating therapeutics for opportunities in medicine: a paradigm shift in drug discovery. Front Pharmacol. 2020;11:770. doi: 10.3389/fphar.2020.00770

Ioannidis JP, Stuart M, Brownless S, et al. How to survive the medical misinformation mess. Eur J Clin Invest. 2017;47(11):795-802. doi: 10.1111/eci.12834

Pharmaceutical Society of Australia. Sansom LN, ed. Australian pharmaceutical formulary and handbook. 25th ed. Canberra: Pharmaceutical Society of Australia; 2021.

Reilly T, Jackson W, Berger V, et al. Accuracy and completeness of drug information in Wikipedia medication

New Zealand Formulary (NZF): http://nzformulary.org (accessed 17 May 2021)

Pharmaceutical Management Agency, New Zealand (Pharmac): https://pharmac.govt.nz/

Therapeutic Goods Administration, Pregnancy safety categories: https://www.tga.gov.au/prescribing-medicines-pregnancy-database (accessed 17 May 2021)

Therapeutic Goods Administration, Reporting adverse events: https://www.tga.gov.au/reporting-adverse-events (accessed 17 May 2021)

Therapeutic Goods Administration, Blue card adverse reaction reporting form: https://www.tga.gov.au/form/blue-card-adverse-reaction-reporting-form (accessed 17 May 2021)

Therapeutic Goods Administration, Clinical trials guidelines: https://www.tga.gov.au/clinical-trials (accessed 17 May 2021)

Therapeutic Guidelines: https://www.tg.org.au (accessed 17 May 2021)

Traditional Healing and Medicine: https://healthinfonet.ecu.edu.au/learn/cultural-ways/traditional-healing-and-medicine/ (accessed 4 July 2022)

United States Pharmacopeia (USP): https://www.uspnf.com/ (accessed 17 May 2021)

World Health Organization, General principles used by WHO in devising and approving INNs: www.who.int/medicines/services/inn/GeneralprinciplesEn.pdf?ua=1 (accessed 17 May 2021)

World Health Organization, Model List of Essential Medicines: https://www.who.int/publications/i/item/WHOMVPEMPIAU2019.06 (accessed 17 May 2021)

CHAPTER 2

CLINICAL, ETHICAL AND LEGAL FOUNDATIONS OF PHARMACOTHERAPY

Roslyn Donnellan-Fernandez, Kirsten Small

Key Abbreviations

ADR	adverse drug reaction
AHPRA	Australian Health Practitioners Regulation Agency
CMI	consumer medicine information
Cth	Commonwealth
DUE	drug use evaluation
EBM/P	evidence-based medicine/practice
EM	endorsed midwife
FDA	US Food and Drug Administration
ICM	International Confederation of Midwives
MBS	Medicare Benefits Schedule
Medsafe	Medicines and Medical Devices Safety Authority (NZ)
NP	nurse practitioner
NPS	National Prescribing Service
OOP	out of pocket
OTC	over the counter
PBAC	Pharmaceutical Benefits Advisory Committee (Aust)
PBS	Pharmaceutical Benefits Scheme (Aust)
PHARMAC	Pharmaceutical Management Agency (NZ)
QUM	quality use of medicines
RCCT	randomised controlled clinical trial
RM	registered midwife
SUSMP	Standard for the Uniform Scheduling of Medicines and Poisons
TGA	Therapeutic Goods Administration

Key Terms

adherence 28
clinical pharmacology 36
controlled drug 42
drug schedule 23
drug use evaluation 31
evidence-based medicine 24
medical ethics 37
Medsafe 25
narcotic 30
National Prescribing Service 25
pharmacovigilance 25
prescription 31
proscribed drug 40
quality use of medicines 24
side effects 31
six rights 33
Therapeutic Goods Administration 25

Chapter Focus

'Pharmacotherapy' refers to the use of drugs for diagnosing, treating, or preventing disease. This is distinguished from theoretical or experimental pharmacology, where drugs are studied to understand their mechanisms of action and effects. This chapter focuses on laws regulating prescription and over-the-counter (OTC) drugs, poisons, controlled substances, proscribed substances, and investigational drugs. The regulation and scheduling of drugs and controlled substances in Australia and New Zealand are compared.

Health professionals who prescribe, formulate, dispense, or administer drugs are legally accountable for their actions related to drug therapy. This chapter reviews the roles of midwives and other health professionals in relation to the use of medicines, and how quality use of medicines and drug use evaluations help optimise pharmacotherapy for childbearing women and their babies.

Many ethical principles apply to drug use, based on human rights and bioethics. These principles underlie decision making related to pharmacology research and clinical practice. Controversy may arise as to how ethical principles are applied in clinical situations.

Learning Outcomes

- Understand the clinical, ethical, and legal foundations of pharmacotherapy related to the professional practice standards and role of the midwife in maternal and newborn care.
- Demonstrate knowledge of the international, national, and state/territory legislation, and common law applicable to the regulation of drugs and prescribing.
- Describe the role and function of Australian therapeutics agencies (Therapeutic Goods Administration and the Pharmaceutical Benefits Scheme) in the regulation of medicine, including the use of **drug schedules**.
- Identify your responsibilities as they relate to the National Medicines Policy and the quality use of medicines, including:
  - the National Prescribing Competencies Framework
  - principles of rational prescribing
  - use of quality prescribing sources
  - if you are a midwife who is also an authorised prescriber – clinical decision making.

CRITICAL THINKING SCENARIO

Georgina, a 30-year-old female, is 14 weeks into her fourth pregnancy. She is experiencing symptoms consistent with a urinary tract infection. While awaiting the microscopy and culture result from a midstream urine specimen, Georgina's primary midwife (an endorsed prescriber), prescribes a course of nitrofurantoin capsules – 100 mg orally, 6-hourly for 5 days.

1　Discuss how we know the medicine that Georgina has been prescribed is safe and effective.

2　Describe the role of the Poisons Standard (the SUSMP). Discuss the access, supply/provision, labelling, storage, records, and advertising for Georgina's prescribed drug as related to its Schedule. Georgina elects to have an electronic prescription, and her prescriber sends her a QR code via a text message to her phone. Georgina then forwards this QR code to her local pharmacy to be dispensed. The pharmacy has Georgina's Medicare and Commonwealth concession card details on file.

3　Outline the requirements for:

(a) a legal prescription

(b) a valid Pharmaceutical Benefits Scheme prescription.

4　Consistent with the National Health (Pharmaceutical Benefits) Amendment (Active Ingredient Prescribing) Regulations, Georgina's endorsed midwife uses active ingredient prescribing. Discuss what active ingredient prescribing is and describe its benefits.

5　Outline several benefits of electronic prescribing over paper-based prescribing.

2.1 Clinical aspects of pharmacotherapy

To optimise the use of drugs in a rational, clinically effective, and cost-effective way, midwives need to understand:

- the evidence on which clinical decisions are based
- the necessary decision-making processes to be followed before drugs are chosen, prescribed, or advised
- how prescriptions are written and dispensed
- the types of formulations in which drugs are administered
- the factors affecting drug responses.

Quality use of medicines

The foundation and chief purpose of pharmacotherapy is **quality use of medicines** (QUM), described in Australia's National Medicines Policy (see Online resources) as the judicious, appropriate, safe, and effective use of medicines. Specifically, QUM means:

- selecting the right management options whether this includes drug therapy or not
- selecting any medicine, taking into consideration the person and their clinical condition, the benefits and

harms of the medicine, the dosage and length of treatment, other medical conditions, other medicines the person is taking, and cost (to the individual, community, and the healthcare system)
- using medicines safely and effectively, i.e. monitoring outcomes and minimising inappropriate use.

Evidence-based healthcare

Evidence-based medicine (EBM) has been defined as 'the conscientious, explicit, and judicious use of current best evidence in making decisions about the medical care of individual patients' (Sackett et al 1996). EBM – or more appropriately, evidence-based practice (EBP) – applies to all therapy, whether with drugs or with interventions such as physiotherapy techniques or approaches to midwifery care.

Integrating EBP improves healthcare outcomes, including quality of life. EBP can also improve health professionals' productivity and reduce healthcare costs. Despite this, studies show that as many as 4 in 10 adults receive care that is not based on current evidence, including ineffective, unnecessary, and even harmful treatments (e.g. antibiotics for the common cold) (Victorian Government Department of Health 2021).

Levels of evidence

Not all evidence is considered equal. When using evidence to inform care, midwives should critically appraise the evidence for its internal and external validity. Internal validity is the rigour with which the study was conducted. External validity is the applicability of the research findings to the real-life healthcare user.

Drug information in objective databases such as PubMed, EMBASE (Excerpta Medica Database), the Cochrane Library, and the Cumulative Index to Nursing and Allied Health Literature (CINAHL) can be consulted. The Australian Prescriber website (2023), Medsafe NZ (2023), the *Australian Medicines Handbook* (2023) and Therapeutic Guidelines (2023) are all based on quality evidence (see Online resources).

Australian medicines policies

In 1985, the World Health Organization (WHO) held a conference on the rational use of drugs, calling on all governments to implement a national medicinal drug policy. In June 1996, the former Council of Australian Governments agreed on the central objectives of the National Medicines Policy:

- timely access to the medicines that Australians need, at a cost that individuals and the community can afford
- medicines meeting appropriate standards of quality, safety, and efficacy
- QUM
- maintaining a responsible and viable medicines industry (see Online resources, National Medicines Policy 2022).

QUM is implemented by health professionals, interested consumer groups, the **Therapeutic Goods Administration** (TGA), the Australian Government's Pharmaceutical Benefits Advisory Committee (PBAC), agencies of government health departments, and many other professional bodies. Examples of programs in QUM include nominating a priority list of medicines commonly required for paediatric use; setting up a system for recalling therapeutic goods; and programs for recommending non-pharmacological therapies such as diet, smoking cessation, and exercise. Further, population-specific programs are also in place, for example Aboriginal and Torres Strait Islander-specific programs, targeted programs and services aimed to support quality use of medicines and culturally appropriate services for Aboriginal and Torres Strait Islander peoples. These include initiatives such as the Indigenous Health Services Pharmacy Support Program, Indigenous Dose Administration Aids, the Aboriginal and Torres Strait Islander Pharmacy Scholarship Scheme, and the Aboriginal and Torres Strait Islander Pharmacy Assistant Traineeship Scheme.

The National Prescribing Service

The Australian **National Prescribing Service** (NPS) was an independent, not-for-profit organisation, established in 1998 to improve the way health technologies, medicines, and medical tests are prescribed and used. Through educational activities targeted to health practitioners, consumers, and the pharmaceutical industry, the NPS has achieved significant savings in drug costs.

NPS MedicineWise programs included Choosing Wisely Australia, Medicine Insight, and Good Medicine Better Health. In January 2023, the Australian Commission on Safety and Quality in Health Care (ACSQHC) assumed responsibility for several quality functions formerly delivered by NPS MedicineWise.

Medicines Australia

Medicines Australia 'leads the research-based medicines industry of Australia. Our members discover, develop and manufacture prescription pharmaceutical products, biotherapeutic products, and vaccines that bring health, social, and economic benefits to Australia. Our members invest in Australian medical research and take local discoveries and developments to the world' (Medicines Australia 2022). It is involved in developing health and industry policies, ensuring viable continuation of the industry, and administering the Code of Conduct for ethical marketing of prescription drugs. The industry body has QUM roles in developing medicines, providing evidence-based information, and partnering with consumer organisations (see Online resources).

The New Zealand Medicines Strategy

The New Zealand Ministry of Health/Manatū Hauora has several programs aimed at achieving QUM. The roles of the Pharmaceutical Management Agency (Pharmac) and the Pharmacology and Therapeutics Advisory Committee (PTAC) are described below, while those of SCOTT, **Medsafe**, and the *New Zealand Formulary* were covered in Chapter 1 in relation to clinical trials and drug information.

The three main goals of the New Zealand medicines strategy are:

- access – to ensure that New Zealanders have access to the medicines they need, regardless of ethnicity, location, or wealth
- optimal use – to ensure that medicines are used to their best effect
- quality – to ensure that medicines are safe and effective.

The system includes several agencies with diverse responsibilities, including:

- QUM and **pharmacovigilance** (e.g. Medsafe, District Health Boards and centres)
- programs for monitoring/implementing adverse drug reactions (ADRs), vaccines, best practice, and quality improvement
- primary health organisations
- the *New Zealand Formulary*
- the *Universal List of Medicines*.

Modifying drug usage over time

Pharmacopoeias, formularies, and pharmacology textbooks are in a constant state of change, and health professionals need to keep up to date. Some influences on evolving drug use relevant to perinatal care and midwifery are described below, with examples.

Why new drugs appear

1 *New technologies.* Until the early 20th century, most drugs were derived from natural sources: plants (morphine, cocaine), minerals (iodine, iron), and animals (vaccines, tissue extracts). As chemical industries and pharmacological techniques developed, drugs such as antibiotics, oral contraceptives, antihypertensives, antipsychotic agents, human insulin, and monoclonal antibodies became available (see Table 1.2 in Chapter 1).

2 *New uses for old drugs.* Drugs are sometimes found to have uses additional to their original indications. Misoprostol, a prostaglandin E1 analogue, that was originally intended for use to prevent NSAID-induced gastric ulcers, became used (off-label) in women's health for a variety of indications, including management of miscarriage, induction of labour, cervical ripening before surgical procedures, and the treatment of postpartum haemorrhage (Allen & O'Brien 2009). Oral misoprostol is the second step of MS-2 Step (after mifepristone is

TABLE 2.1 Principal Australian and New Zealand legislation involved in the regulation of drugs

JURISDICTION	DRUG REGULATION LEGISLATION	ADDITIONAL DRUG OFFENCES ACTS
Australian Commonwealth (Cth)	*Therapeutic Goods Act 1989* (Cth) *Therapeutic Goods Regulations 1990* (Cth) *National Health Act 1953* (Cth)	*Customs Act 1901* (Cth) *Crimes (Traffic in Narcotic Drugs and Psychotropic Substances) Act 1990* (Cth) *Narcotic Drugs Act 1967* (Cth) *Criminal Code Act 1995* (Cth)
Australian Capital Territory (ACT)	*Medicines, Poisons and Therapeutic Goods Act 2008* (ACT) *Drugs of Dependence Act 1989* (ACT) *Drugs in Sport Act 1999* (ACT) Drugs of Dependence Regulations 2009 (ACT)	Criminal Code 2002 (ACT)
New South Wales (NSW)	*Poisons and Therapeutic Goods Act 1966* (NSW) Poisons and Therapeutic Goods Regulations 2008 (NSW)	*Drug Misuse and Trafficking Act 1985* (NSW)
Northern Territory (NT)	*Medicines, Poisons and Therapeutic Goods Act 2012* (NT) Medicines, Poisons and Therapeutic Goods Regulations 2014 (NT)	*Misuse of Drugs Act 1990* (NT)
Queensland (Qld)	*Medicines and Poisons Act 2019* (Qld) Therapeutic Goods Regulation 2021 (Qld) Medicines and Poisons (Poisons and Prohibited Substances) Regulation 2021 (Qld)	*Drugs Misuse Act 1986* (Qld)
South Australia (SA)	*Controlled Substances Act 1984* (SA) Controlled Substances (Poisons) Regulations 2011 (SA) Controlled Substances (Controlled Drugs, Precursors and Plants) Regulations 2014 (SA)	*Criminal Law Consolidation Act 1935* (SA)
Tasmania (Tas)	*Poisons Act 1971* (Tas) Poisons Regulations 2018 (Tas) *Therapeutic Goods Act 2001* (Tas) Poisons (Declared Restricted Substances) Order 2017 (Tas)	*Misuse of Drugs Act 2001* (Tas) *Alcohol and Drug Dependency Act 1968* (Tas)
Victoria (Vic)	*Therapeutic Goods (Victoria) Act 2010* (Vic) *Drugs, Poisons and Controlled Substances Act 1981* (Vic) Drugs, Poisons and Controlled Substances Regulations 2006 (Vic)	*Crimes Act 1958* (Vic)
Western Australia (WA)	*Medicines and Poisons Act 2014* (WA) Medicines and Poisons Regulations 2016 (WA)	*Misuse of Drugs Act 1981* (WA)
New Zealand	*Medicines Act 1981* Medicines Regulations 1984 Medicines (Standing Order) Amendment Regulations 2016 Medicines (Designated Prescriber: Nurse Practitioners) Regulations 2016 Medicines (Designated Pharmacist Prescribers) Regulations 2013 Misuse of Drugs Regulations 1977	*Misuse of Drugs Act 1975*

taken), used to achieve early medical abortion (see Online resources).

3 *Better understanding of mechanisms.* The discovery of the mechanism of action of aspirin (inhibiting synthesis of prostaglandins) and its antiplatelet actions led to its now widespread prophylactic use against thromboembolism, and for preventing fetal growth restriction and preeclampsia (Cadavid 2017).

4 *Better understanding of the aetiology of disease.* Studies of the causes of preeclampsia have increased our understanding of the role of pro-inflammatory factors and those inhibiting the growth of new blood vessels and the resultant damage and dysfunction of blood vessels. These new understandings have prompted researchers to trial new drug therapies to prevent or manage preeclampsia, such as proton-pump inhibitors, metformin, statins, and sildenafil citrate (Fig 2.1).

5 *Changes in popularity of drugs.* There is a recognised cycle in popularity of new drugs, just as there is for new gadgets and devices, for example mobile phones. As a drug is developed and marketed it rapidly surges in popularity. Adverse drug reactions (ADRs) may become apparent, its expense is noted, and replica drugs compete, so its use wanes. Then, as the benefits and risks are evaluated rationally, the drug regains a medium but more stable position in usage. ADRs are covered in depth in Chapter 6.

6 *Changes in cost and availability of drugs.* There may be a major change in the use of a drug as it is moved between Poisons Schedules and becomes either more or less readily available or expensive. When new COX-2 inhibitors (e.g. celecoxib, rofecoxib) and statins (e.g. atorvastatin, simvastatin) were introduced, they were very expensive. Public and drug company pressure in Australia led to their

Schematic showing the development and progression of preeclampsia, including sites of action of several repurposed therapeutics

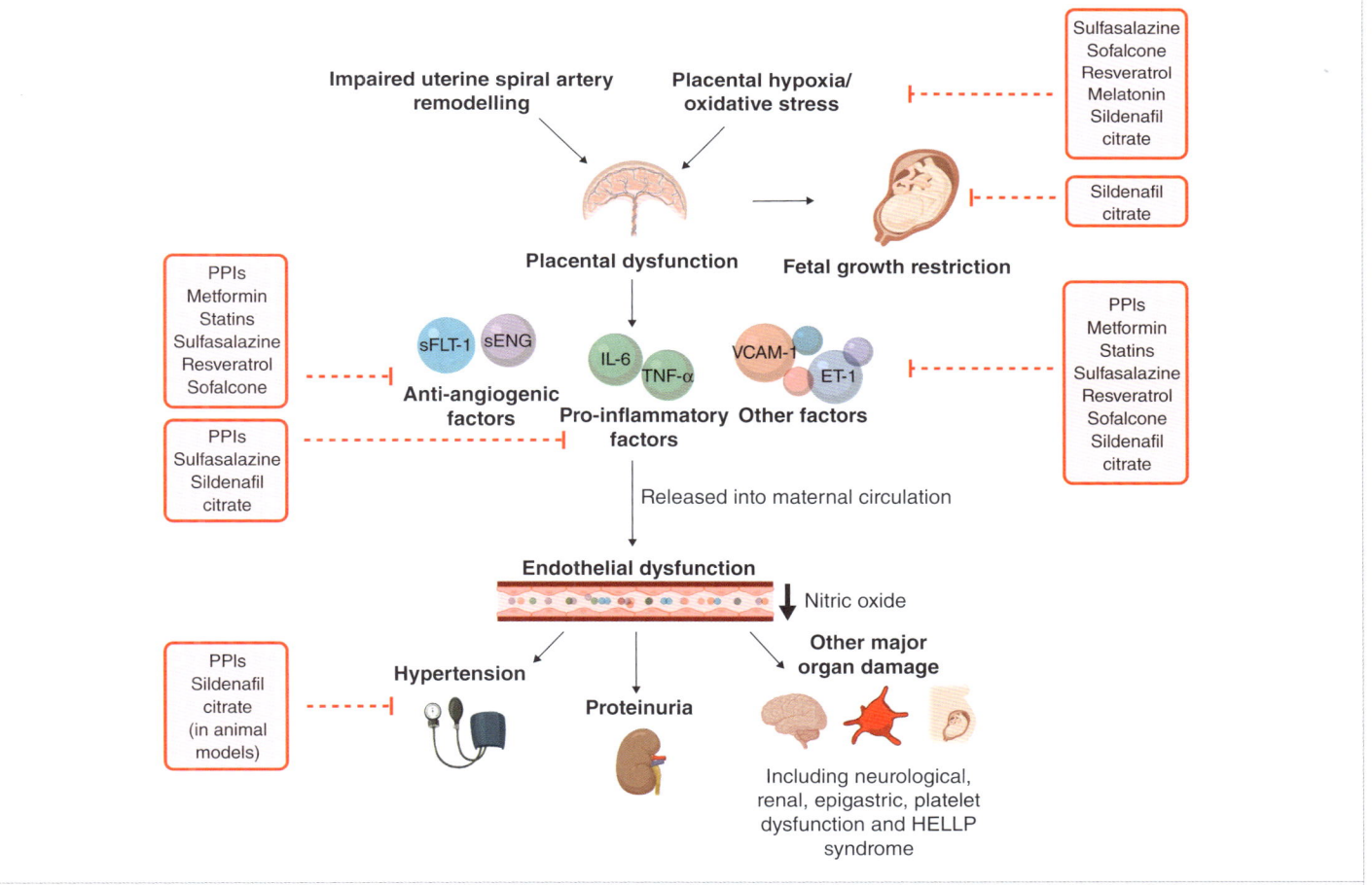

FIGURE 2.1

being subsidised and listed on the PBS. As a result their use skyrocketed, at great expense to governments (i.e. taxpayers). Statins are still the most frequently prescribed medicines in Australia. However, when patent protection for new drug molecules expires, other companies can legally manufacture and market the drug, so competition from 'generics' reduces the price.

Why drugs disappear

1 *No longer optimal therapy.* As better drugs are developed, many less effective and less safe drugs become obsolete. For centuries, syphilis was treated with toxic arsenic- or mercury-containing compounds, because the aetiology was unknown. Once effective treatment was available in the form of safe oral antibacterials, these older treatments fell out of use.

2 *Medicine recalls.* A medicine can be recalled when a deficiency is identified in its quality, safety, or efficacy; when a disease becomes less prevalent; or when company mergers bring competitor products into the market. The manufacturer will notify wholesalers to cease distribution and pharmacists to return stock. Prescribers must then switch to an alternative drug.

3 *Adverse effects become apparent.* ADRs appearing in post-marketing studies (phase IV trials; see Chapter 1) may lead to withdrawal of the product. Thalidomide, for example, was marketed as a safe sedative and antinausea drug in pregnancy until thousands of congenital malformations became evident (CFB 2.1 and McBride 1961).

CLINICAL FOCUS BOX 2.1

Thalidomide

Between 1958 and 1962, thousands of babies across Western countries, including Australia, were born with congenital malformations, including short and absent limbs. The condition was termed phocomelia, meaning 'seal-like limbs', and had previously been incredibly rare. In Germany alone, about 10,000 babies were affected.

Dr Widukind Lenz, of Hamburg, asked mothers of affected babies to list all the drugs they had taken during pregnancy. Contergan, previously considered a safe sedative, appeared in about 30% of the lists. Meanwhile, in Sydney, Dr William McBride had been consulted about several babies with phocomelia. All the mothers had taken Distaval, a mild sedative and antiemetic, during pregnancy. In 1961, Dr McBride wrote to the journal *The Lancet* asking if similar cases had been reported. Lenz replied, and it became apparent the same drug, thalidomide, was implicated.

Case reports flooded in, and the drug was withdrawn. However, cases kept appearing for many years because the drug was marketed under numerous trade names, warnings went unheeded, and bottles of tablets remained available. The critical risk period was so short (between the 37th and 54th days of pregnancy); effects were not observed until many months later; and many mothers forgot having taken drugs in early pregnancy.

Files published for the first time in 2013 revealed that many Australian women were used as 'human guinea pigs' by the Distillers Company in 1960, before tests in pregnant animals had been carried out, and the German manufacturer suppressed warnings about fetal effects. Lawsuits and damages claims against the drug companies continued to be pursued decades later.

The thalidomide disaster led to tighter regulation of medicines and medical devices in Australia. It also saw the establishment of the Australian Drug Evaluation Committee (ADEC). Today thalidomide is used to treat multiple myeloma. It is contraindicated in women of childbearing age who are not using contraception.

Source: McBride 1961.

Drug combinations shown to be unjustified

From the time of the ancient Greeks until the mid-20th century, doctors often wrote prescriptions for complex mixtures 'for nerves' or as 'tonics'. More recently, combinations of antimicrobials, antiasthma drugs, or antihypertensives may be formulated together. **Adherence** with therapy is enhanced when people need only take one 'polypill'. However, it is usually better to prescribe drugs individually, as pharmacokinetic properties of components vary, and doses cannot be individually adjusted.

Pharmacoeconomics

Because of the blowout in demand for and costs of drugs, no country can provide all desirable drugs. Hence, pharmacoeconomic rationalisation is essential, while balanced against the risk of compromising good healthcare. Health economists evaluate and balance the costs of developing and providing drugs, the need for drugs for new conditions (such as antiviral agents for COVID), and indirect aspects, such as savings from shorter hospital admissions, improved quality of life, and surgery avoided. A statistic called the incremental cost-effectiveness ratio can be used to compare a new medicine with its comparator. Overall, policies such as generic substitution (dispensing the cheapest alternative among bioequivalent medicines), rationalisation of drug policies, and QUM help optimise access to essential drugs.

To be listed by the Australian Pharmaceutical Benefits Scheme (PBS) as a subsidised drug, a medication must be safe, effective, and cost-effective. Listing as a 'restricted benefit' or as 'authority required to prescribe' limits the use of expensive medications to those in whom it will be most effective. Whether a prescription is subsidised by the PBS or not is a Commonwealth decision.

Roles of health professionals in QUM

Traditionally, the health professionals most involved with drugs were the doctors who prescribed them, pharmacists who dispensed them, and nurses and midwives who administered them. During the period when medicine was developing as a profession in England, physicians were allowed to prescribe 'physic' (medicine) compounded by apothecaries (pharmacists). Now many more health professionals, including midwives, are involved with medicines and prescribing. The roles of several health professionals, including the midwife, are summarily described below. Specialised aspects of practice encompassing the midwife's role in administration, supply, dispensing, and authorisation to prescribe medication are detailed further in Chapter 22.

National registration guidelines have been developed by many professional boards, now under the auspices of the Australian Health Practitioner Regulation Agency (AHPRA). These outline the role and scope of practice of health professionals in relation to medication management. In Australia, while the Commonwealth regulates therapeutic goods, each state has its own laws determining access to drugs. These laws are not currently harmonised across jurisdictions.

Who can prescribe medicines in Australia and New Zealand?

An increasing number of health professionals can prescribe scheduled medicines, improving public access to medicines in a timely manner. In Australia, medical doctors can prescribe, as can endorsed dentists, nurse practitioners, veterinary surgeons, endorsed midwives, optometrists, and podiatrists.

There are two categories of prescriber in Aotearoa New Zealand:

- authorised prescribers can independently prescribe any medicine that relates to their area of practice. This group includes nurse practitioners, optometrists, dentists, medical practitioners, and registered midwives, as authorised by the *Health Practitioners Competence Assurance Act 2003*
- other health professionals, who can train to be supplementary prescribers.

Midwives and QUM

A midwife is a person who:

- has successfully completed a midwifery education program based on the ICM Essential Competencies for Midwifery Practice and the framework of the ICM Global Standards for Midwifery Education and

which is recognised in the country where they are located
- has acquired the requisite qualifications to be registered and/or legally licensed to practise midwifery and use the title 'midwife'
- demonstrates competency in the practice of midwifery (ICM 2023).

The midwifery scope of practice, as defined by ICM, recognises the midwife as 'a responsible and accountable professional who works in partnership with women to give the necessary support, care and advice during pregnancy, birth and the postpartum period, to conduct births on the midwife's own responsibility and to provide care for the newborn and the infant. This care includes preventative measures, the promotion of normal birth, the detection of complications in mother and child, the accessing of medical care or other appropriate assistance and the carrying out of emergency measures. The midwife has an important task in health counselling and education, not only for the woman, but also within the family and the community. This work should involve antenatal education and preparation for parenthood and may extend to women's health, sexual or reproductive health and childcare. A midwife may practise in any setting including the home, community, hospitals, clinics or health units' (ICM 2023).

In Australia, professional midwifery registration is regulated by the Nursing and Midwifery Board of Australia (NMBA) and underpinned by the Health Practitioner Regulation National Law which is in force in each state and territory. The National Registration and Accreditation Scheme, established in 2010, covers 16 health professions, including nursing and midwifery, each with its own regulatory board. The AHPRA works in partnership with the national boards to ensure that Australia's registered health practitioners are suitably trained, qualified, and safe to practise. Under the National Law, the NMBA has regulatory responsibility for standards of midwifery practice.

In Aotearoa New Zealand, midwifery practice is regulated under the *Health Practitioners Competence Assurance Act 2003* and the responsible authority is Te Tatau o te Whare Kahu/Midwifery Council of New Zealand. In New Zealand, the Medicines Amendment Regulations 2011 allow midwives to prescribe for women and their newborn(s) under their care, in accordance with their scope of practice as defined by the Midwifery Council, at point of graduation.

New Zealand midwives work as the lead maternity carer for women with low-risk pregnancies, during labour and up to 6 weeks postpartum. Midwives are Authorised Prescribers under the 1990 amendments to the *Medicines Act 1984* and Medicines Regulations (Table 2.1 and Midwifery Council of New Zealand under Online resources); The New Zealand College of Midwives sets and reviews professional standards and provides continuing education. While there is no defined list of medicines a midwife can prescribe in New Zealand, amendments to Regulation 39 of the Medicines Regulations 1984 outline some limits. These are detailed in the professional Consensus Statement on Midwife Prescribing in New Zealand (see Online resources). Midwives are permitted to prescribe the controlled drugs pethidine, morphine, and fentanyl for use during birth. The Midwifery Council further regulated the scope of practice (2014) in relation to opioid prescribing and restricts its prescribing for intrapartum use only. The College expects midwives prescribing **narcotics** for intrapartum care to be fully conversant with the New Zealand College of Midwives Consensus statement 'Prescribing and administration of opioid analgesia in labour'.

In contrast, prescriptive authority for midwives in Australia currently requires registered midwives to undertake an additional postgraduate qualification. These qualified midwives then apply to the NMBA for Endorsement for Scheduled Medicines for Midwives to prescribe, supply, and administer some Schedule 2, 3, 4 and 8 drugs for 'women and their infants in the prenatal, intrapartum and postnatal stages of pregnancy and birth' (Department of Health 2022). The medicines that midwives can prescribe are determined by state and territory legislation (Table 2.1) resulting in variations from one place to another. This can be problematic for midwives proving care across a state border.

In most jurisdictions a phone order by a medical prescriber, or clinical 'standing orders', enable midwives without prescribing authority to administer specified prescription medications to women. Where phone orders and medication 'standing orders' apply, this must be followed up with a written doctor's prescription within 24 hours.

The PBS Midwife Items List sets out those medications that are subsidised when prescribed by a midwife (see Online resources). Currently, the PBS listing for midwife prescribing in Australia is limited to 32 items (21 different medications), and not all prescription medications issued by authorised midwife prescribers are included on the PBS, meaning the woman will pay the full cost of these non-PBS-listed medications.

Doctors and QUM

Medical practitioners are responsible for advising on health issues, diagnosing disease, and initiating and monitoring therapy, including prescribing scheduled drugs. Doctors require extensive knowledge of applied clinical pharmacology relevant to their field of practice – for example, general practitioners use a different range of medications to obstetricians. In Australia, the PBS also lists medications eligible for subsidy when prescribed by a doctor. The list is significantly larger than for midwives,

reflecting the broader and varied scope of practices of medical prescribers. Prescribing authority is enabled on graduation from medical school.

Pharmacists and QUM

Pharmacists are medicines experts, generally working in hospital or retail pharmacies. Their main role is to prepare and distribute medicines to those who are to use them. In New Zealand, suitably qualified, trained, and experienced pharmacists may apply to be a Pharmacist Prescriber. In Australia there is movement towards this being achieved. Momentum for change, aligned to the national review of primary care workforce regulations investigating ways to increase Australians' access to quality healthcare, sees trials currently underway in most Australian states and territories for limited pharmacist prescribing. For example, Queensland and Western Australia allow pharmacists to prescribe for urinary tract infections (UTIs). A 2023 Victorian trial allows pharmacists to prescribe repeat scripts for oral contraceptive pills, as well as treatments for some mild skin conditions and UTIs, with a similar trial underway in NSW (Victorian Government Department of Health 2024).

Pharmacists can dispense medications on Schedule 3. These do not require prescriptive authority but can only be dispensed to a named user after consultation with a pharmacist to ensure they are appropriately used.

Other roles of pharmacists include:

- detecting and preventing inappropriate doses, ADRs, drug interactions, or misuse
- compounding of medicines – i.e. the preparation from several ingredients of a product, such as an oral mixture supplied for immediate use by a specific consumer
- monitoring sales of Schedule 2 and 3 medicines
- supervising staff, students, and dispensary assistants
- ensuring the pharmacy is managed according to law and standards of good pharmaceutical practice
- providing professional services, e.g. administering vaccinations, blood pressure monitoring, baby weight assessment, and pregnancy testing
- ordering, safe storage, and disposal of drug supplies
- maintaining all required equipment and reference materials
- collaborating with other health professionals to improve medicine safety
- participating in research and educational activities
- business and professional competencies
- providing drug information services, therapeutic monitoring, pharmacovigilance, and public health programs.

In hospitals, pharmacists carry out many roles such as: filling and maintaining ward stocks of drugs (imprest cabinets and drug trolleys); preparing sterile parenteral solutions, parenteral nutrition solutions and oncology drugs; participating in ward rounds, medication management plans, **drug use evaluations** and therapeutic drug monitoring; and providing advice on drug therapy and other drug information.

Drug prescriptions and formulations

Prescribing drugs

A **prescription** ('script') is a written direction for the preparation and administration of a specified amount of active drug for a specified person. The prescription sign – sometimes shown in typeface as 'Rx' – may derive from the Egyptian character for the Eye of Horus, the symbol of good fortune and healing, or relate to the Roman god Jupiter, or it may be short for the Latin word '*recipe*'. Regardless, the meaning is the same – it means 'take …', instructing the pharmacist to take the ingredients and compound them.

'Prescribing' is defined by the NPS as 'an iterative process involving information gathering, clinical decision-making, communication, and evaluation that results in the initiation, continuation, or cessation of a medicine'. It involves much more than simply writing a prescription. Prescribing includes communicating a recommendation to use or cease a medication that does not require a legal prescription, such as iron supplements. All midwives 'prescribe', even if only some with appropriate qualifications are endorsed to write legal prescriptions.

Decisions to make before prescribing

Any therapeutic intervention – whether administering a drug, implementing a physiotherapy program, carrying out a surgical procedure, altering a person's diet, or administering a complementary and/or alternative therapy such as acupuncture or herbal remedy – will modify the person's body systems. The priority must follow the advice of Hippocrates: FIRST DO NO HARM. There are many questions that should be answered before intervening (Fig 2.2). See Table 2.2 and sections on prescribing in the 'Preliminary information' pages in the current *Australian Medicines Handbook*.

In the context of holistic care for a pregnant woman and her baby, assessment before prescribing includes a comprehensive medical and obstetric health history and assessment to consider factors such as preexisting chronic health conditions with or without current prescription or non-prescription medication use, gestational age, breastfeeding status, consideration of the possibility of differing responses, effects, and potential **side effects** for woman and baby, and the potential for interaction with other treatments or therapies.

Prescription orders

A prescription written by a licensed prescriber can be on a prescription form, an institutional order sheet, or using prescription software (Figs 2.3A and B). Prescriptions must comply with legal formats – for example, as laid down in the Australian *Drugs, Poisons and Controlled Substances Act 1981* and Regulations. Prescriptions are then dispensed by a registered pharmacist.

Prescriptions

A prescription must be clear, concise, and correct. It requires the person's name and address (right person); date written; generic or proprietary drug name (right drug); drug dose, strength, dosage form, and quantity (right dose); route of administration (right route); dosage instructions or frequency of administration (right time); and must bear the signature, name, address, and contact number of the prescriber. The number of times the prescription can be repeated should be specified, with clear instructions to the pharmacist and the person using the medication. This should include clear instructions on how to take the medication, for example, with or without food.

Prescriptions can be paper-based or electronic (with a QR code token). The potential benefits of electronic prescribing include that it:

- reduces some prescribing and dispensing errors (electronic prescriptions are sent directly from the prescriber to the pharmacist supplying the medicine)
- improves prescribing and dispensing efficiency
- supports electronic medication charts in hospitals and other maternity services contexts
- reduces paper wastage and is environmentally friendly
- results in fewer lost prescriptions
- supports digital health services to optimise continuity of care and medicines safety
- reduces exposure to infectious diseases (e.g. COVID-19) by reducing the need to see health professionals face to face on multiple occasions
- supports privacy.

When typing or writing prescriptions, only accepted abbreviations should be used (Appendix 3). If any confusion or doubt about any aspect of the prescription exists, the prescriber is contacted for clarification before dispensing.

Standing orders

Standing orders are in place in Australia and New Zealand to improve access to medicines. A standing order is 'a written instruction issued: by a medical practitioner … it authorises a specified person or class of people (e.g. registered midwives) who do not have prescribing rights to administer and/or supply specified medicines and some controlled drugs. The intention is for standing orders to be used to improve persons' timely access to medicines' (Taylor et al 2017). Standing

Questions to ask and answer when prescribing a drug

1 *What is the problem?*

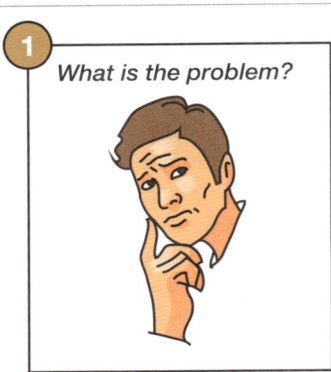

2 *Is there a solution?*

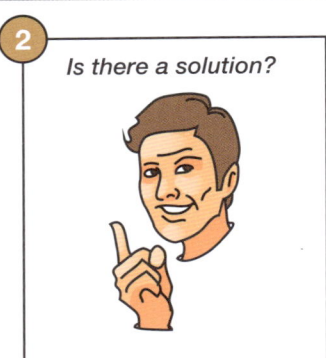

3 *What sort of therapy?*

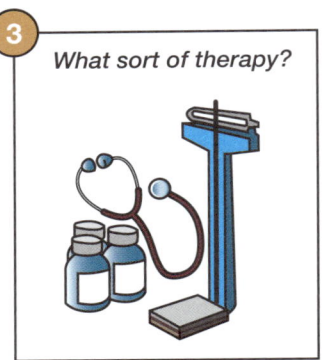

4 *How would your drug act?*

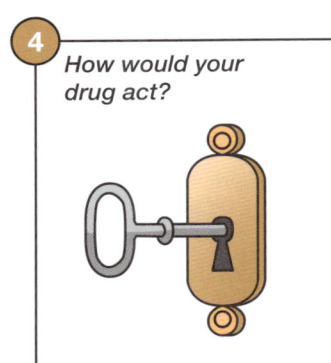

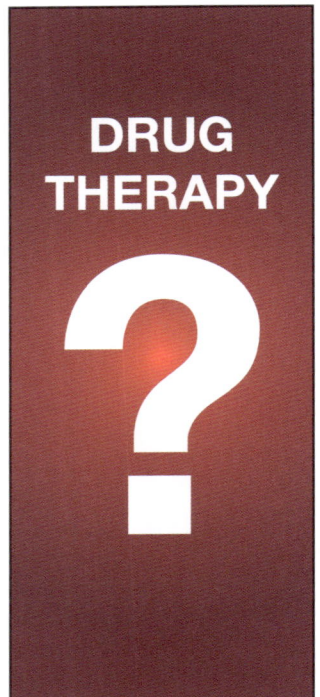

5 *For how long will you treat?*

6 *How will you monitor drug action?*

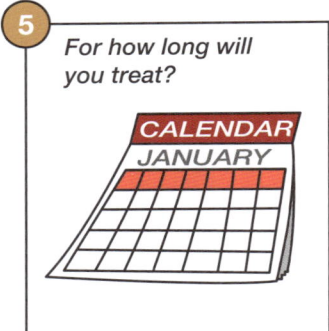

7 *How much drug will you give?*

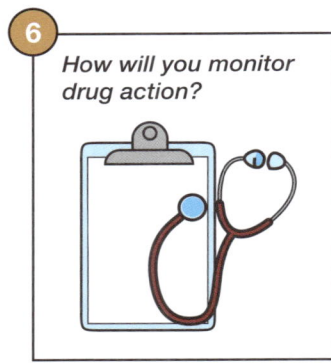

8 *What's special about your patient?*

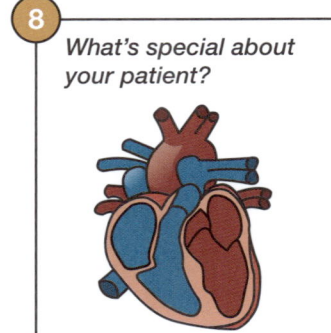

9 *Can you write the prescription?*

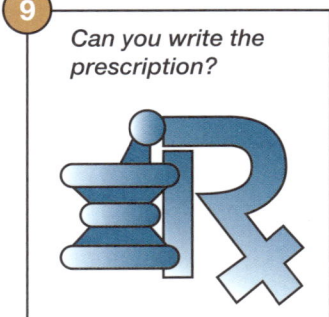

10 *Any warning for patient or staff?*

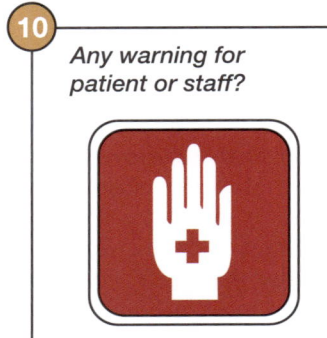

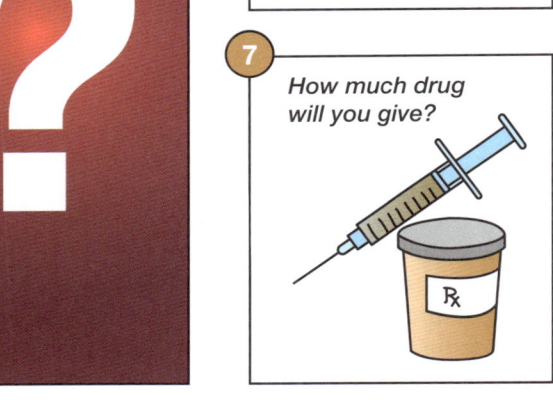

FIGURE 2.2

Source: Adapted from Sweeney 1990; used with permission.

TABLE 2.2 Questions to ask and answer when prescribing a drug

1. WHAT IS THE PROBLEM?	2. IS THERE A (DRUG-BASED) SOLUTION?
The question is: 'What is going wrong here?' A full health history should list the current problems, relevant family history, past and current medications, allergies, ADRs and interactions, social drugs, and all treatment modalities being used.	Not all problems benefit from drug therapy. Practitioners should keep an open mind and consider all modalities – surgery, social support, physiotherapy, podiatry, lifestyle changes (e.g. diet, exercise), psychotherapy and CAM methods, as well as drug treatment.
3. WHAT SORT OF THERAPY?	**4. HOW WOULD YOUR DRUG ACT? AND WHAT DOES IT DO?**
Assuming there are suitable safe, effective drugs to treat the problem, consider: • What class of drugs is appropriate? • Which drug should be selected from this class? • What do QUM guidelines recommend about this drug? • What experience do you have with the drug? • Is more than one drug required? • Are there any cost factors to consider?	• What is known about the pharmacodynamics of the drug? • What is its mechanism and actions? • Does it affect receptors, enzymes, ion channels, transport processes? • How will it help the person's problems? • What do we *not* know that could be important? What are the common ADRs and potential drug interactions? (Checking a data sheet for the drug is helpful here.)
5. HOW LONG WILL YOU TREAT?	**6. HOW WILL YOU MONITOR THERAPY?**
• What is the usual course of the condition and prognosis: will the person get better after short treatment, might there be ongoing relapses and remissions, or will the condition progress? • Are long-term effects of the drug different from immediate effects? • When will you stop or change the therapy?	The person's progress must be monitored to evaluate the effects of the therapy – for example, by measuring: • improvement in the problem • adverse reactions to the drug • plasma levels of the drug (e.g. for drugs with a low therapeutic index).
7. HOW MUCH DRUG WILL YOU GIVE?	**8. WHAT IS SPECIAL ABOUT THIS PERSON?**
• What dose is appropriate? Doses need to be individualised so, if necessary, look it up! Pharmacokinetic principles determine frequency of dosing and appropriate route. The therapeutic index of the drug will determine how critical the exact dose is. The route may determine the formulation, or there may be choices: if oral, will it be tablets, capsules, a mixture, a sustained-release form?	• What is their age and weight? • Are they pregnant and/or breastfeeding? • Are there concurrent conditions or susceptibility to adverse effects? • How are liver and kidney functions? • What might affect adherence or responses? • What significant drug interactions are likely? • What is the woman's preference and what does the person want from this prescribing? • Do they have an experience with this medication/treatment?
9. CAN YOU WRITE (OR DISPENSE, OR ADMINISTER) THE PRESCRIPTION?	**10. ADVICE AND WARNINGS FOR THE PERSON OR STAFF?**
• Are the **'six rights'** (person, drug, dose, route, time, clinical situation) right? • Does the prescription seem appropriate? • Does it conform with legal and institutional requirements and QUM guidelines? • Are the instructions to the person adequate and correct?	People deserve as much medical information as they want about their condition, drugs being prescribed, how and when to take them, possible significant ADRs, drug and food (and alcohol) interactions and what to do if they miss a dose. Printed information should be included, but if not accessible, or if health literacy is challenged, then other resources for service users and consumers such as the TGA site. Finding information about a medicine can be useful for women and people's carers, family, and health professionals who may need information too. Other concerns regarding medication can be addressed by calling 1300 MEDICINE on 1300 633 424 or searching online in Health Direct's medicine section, or NPS MedicineWise Medicines finder, or CMI site medsinfo.com.au (see Online resources). Locally, many tertiary maternity hospitals have dedicated Drug Hotlines available for direct inquiries re medication information in pregnancy.

Source: Prescribing guidelines predominantly adapted from the Australian Medicines Handbook (2023).

orders have no legal validity unless properly written, dated, and signed. Examples of medications commonly used in midwifery practice administered from standing orders include metoclopramide, paracetamol, and oxytocin.

Hospital drug charts

Prescriptions in hospitals are usually written on a drug chart. This may be paper or electronic (Fig 2.3B). The chart has sections for regularly administered medications, medications for anticoagulation or thromboprophylaxis,

Typical prescriptions

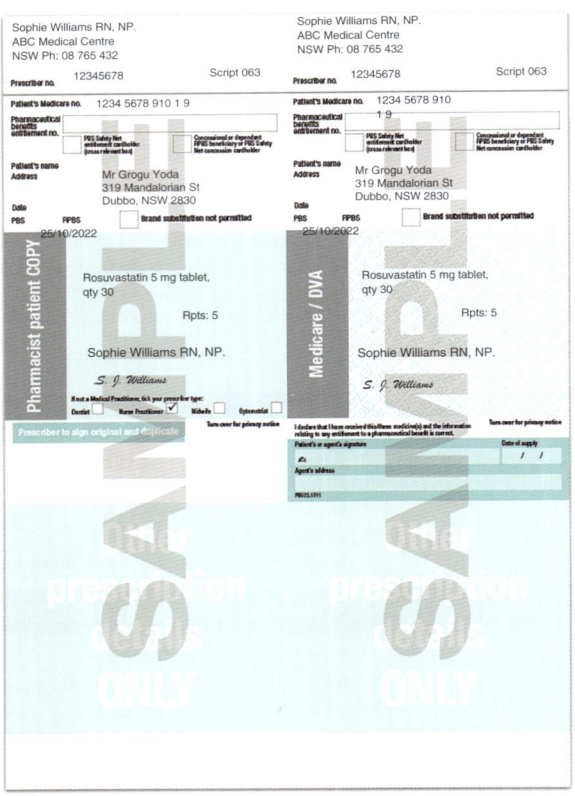

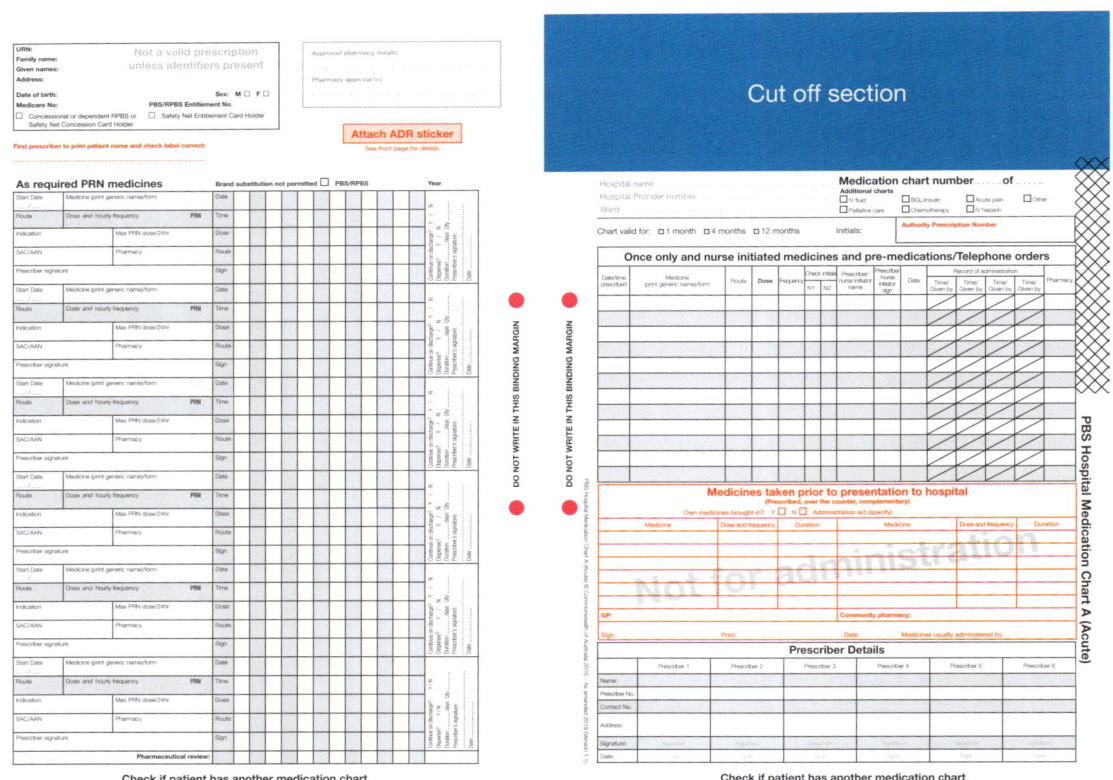

A

FIGURE 2.3 A A typical current Pharmaceutical Benefits Scheme prescription (names and details have been changed).

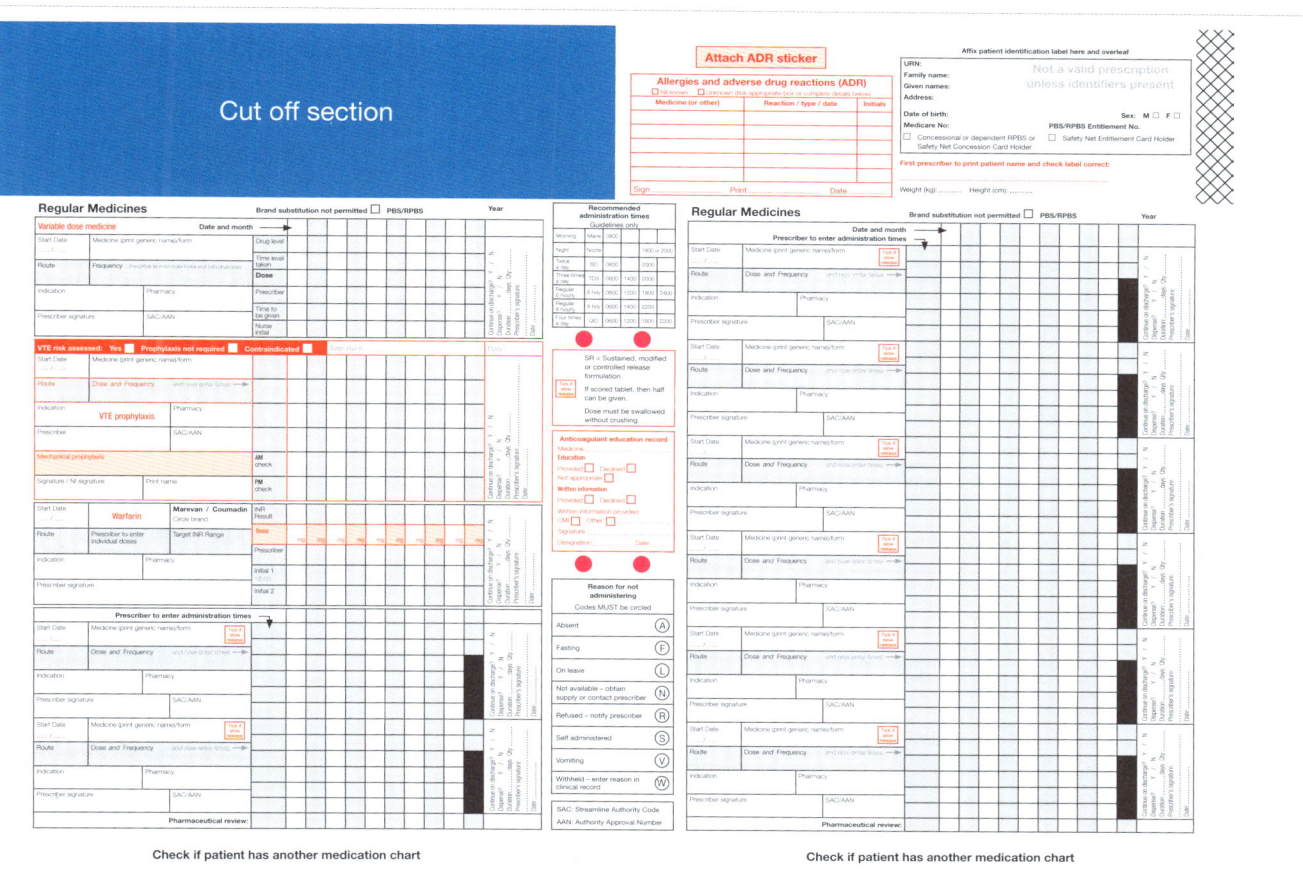

FIGURE 2.3, cont'd **B** Part of a typical medication therapy chart from a hospital record (also known as a drug chart).

Source: Services Australia 2021; reproduced with permission.

midwife- or nurse-initiated therapy (e.g. mild analgesics, laxatives, antacids), telephone orders, 'as required' medications, and for admission drugs and a discharge prescription. The ACSQHC has developed a standardised National Inpatient Medication Chart with both an adult and a paediatric version (see Online resources, and CFB 2.2).

CLINICAL FOCUS BOX 2.2

Instructions and abbreviations in prescriptions

Abbreviations and symbols used in prescriptions can lead to potentially serious errors in administration, requiring an agreed approach to reduce this risk. The ACSQHC provides a document, *Recommendations for Terminology, Abbreviations and Symbols Used in Medicines Documentation*, establishing consistent prescribing terminology, setting recommended terms and abbreviations, and listing those to be avoided as they frequently cause errors.

Some of the principles are:

1. Use plain English – avoid jargon, Latin terms, and Roman numerals.
2. Avoid abbreviations wherever possible.
3. Print all text rather than using cursive writing, especially drug names.
4. Use generic drug names and *never* abbreviate drug names.
5. Express dose frequency unambiguously (e.g. 3 times a week, not 3 times weekly, and write clearly in full, e.g. once daily, or once weekly, rather than using confusing numerical abbreviations such as 1/7).
6. Avoid acronyms and abbreviations for medical terms and drug combinations.
7. Avoid a trailing 0 after a decimal point (e.g. 1.0 mg may be read as 10 mg).
8. Use 0 before a decimal point (e.g. 0.5 mL).
9. Use commas in large numbers (e.g. 10,000 units).
10. When a dose is to be taken only once per week, specify the day (e.g. 'on Tuesdays').
11. Avoid error-prone and ambiguous abbreviations.

Some of the problematic abbreviations include:

- µg. This may be read as mg, resulting in a 1000× overdose. Instead 'microgram' should be written in full.
- D/C. This could be read as either discharge or discontinue.
- IU. This is often misread as IV.
- qd/QD. This stands for *quaque die* in Latin which means 'once a day' whereas qid means 4 times a day. It can either be read correctly as 'every day', or misread as qid, which means '4 times a day'.
- T.i.d. When handwritten this may be misread as bd.
- 6/24. This may be read as either every 6 hours or 6 times per day.
- SC and SL are sometimes confused when handwritten.

Some common abbreviations are shown in Appendix 3. Those shown asterisked are recommended in the *Australian Medicines Handbook*. If there is any possibility of confusion, words should be written in full.

Substitution of drug brands: active ingredient prescribing

In February 2021, it became mandatory for Australian prescribers to include the active ingredient on prescriptions. If a prescriber would like to include the brand name, it must appear after its active ingredient. While there is a cost saving associated with supplying the generic over the brand, there may be clinical and practical reasons why someone should stay with a specific brand.

Off-label prescribing

When a drug is prescribed for an indication, for a group of people, or by a route that is not included in the approved Product Information for that drug, the prescribing is described as 'off-label'. The term does not apply to prescribing for a condition for which the drug is approved but not subsidised by government. 'Off-label' prescribing is not uncommon in maternity care as drug manufacturers may be reluctant to undertake expensive safety testing in pregnant and lactating women. Drugs used 'off-label' in maternity care include misoprostol when prescribed for induction of labour or management of postpartum haemorrhage; metoclopramide or ondansetron for hyperemesis gravidarum; or terbutaline for tocolysis. Off-label prescribing is not illegal but may be unethical if not disclosed to the person for whom the medication is prescribed. It may be costly if the medication is not subsidised. The onus is on the prescriber to act in the person's best interest and be able to defend their prescribing on high-level evidence. The person the prescription is for should give informed consent and be warned their situation may not be listed in the consumer medicine information sheet for the drug.

Teaching prescribing

Healthcare students often say that insufficient time is devoted to teaching **clinical pharmacology** and prescribing in pre-registration courses, resulting in anxiety when they are subsequently required to administer medications and/or write prescriptions. The Australian NPS recognises that all health professionals who prescribe should meet prescribing competencies. NPS has produced a National Prescribing Curriculum, a series of interactive case-based modules that encourage confident and rational prescribing. The modules follow a stepwise approach as outlined in the WHO's *Guide to Good Prescribing*.

KEY POINTS

Clinical aspects of pharmacotherapy

- National drug policies in Australia and New Zealand encourage evidence-based practice and QUM. This is enhanced by educational bodies disseminating objective information about drugs and by studies of drug use in hospitals.

- Many health professionals are involved with pharmacotherapy, whether prescribing, dispensing, administering, or monitoring drugs.

- The range of drugs available for prescribing (or recommending) is very wide. Individual practitioners usually prescribe from a limited list of preferred drugs.

- The list of drugs that are subsidised on the Australian PBS depends on the profession and authorisation status of the prescriber.

- Before a drug is prescribed or advised, factors relating to the person, the drug, and the clinical situation must be considered.

- Prescriptions are legally regulated documents, with specific requirements for format. Abbreviations in prescriptions should be used only cautiously.

2.2 Ethical aspects of pharmacotherapy

The practice of formulating, prescribing, administering, and monitoring drugs needs to be clinically and legally appropriate and carried out in an ethical manner. Ethics can be defined as the science of morals in human conduct, or moral principles. The consideration of ethical principles is to answer the question, '*What should I do in this situation?*'

Human rights, the basis for bioethics

The basic human rights, acknowledged by the United Nations (UN) and accepted by most countries, are the rights to life, security, health, dignity, privacy, autonomy, marriage and procreation, and freedom of thought and religion. Codes of bioethics are based on these human rights and date back as far as the Hippocratic Oath (5th century BCE). Both the Australian and New Zealand Colleges of Midwives have codes relating to ethics that are informed by the International Confederation of Midwives Code of Ethics, which underpins professional midwifery practice internationally (see Online resources).

Medical ethics

Medical ethics are the principles and values that guide the decisions of medical practitioners and, by extension, apply to all health practitioners. They are usually listed as:

- *non-maleficence* – not doing harm
- *beneficence* – doing good
- *justice* – whereby all persons have equal access to healthcare
- *veracity* – the truth will be told to all persons about their condition and treatment
- *confidentiality* of personal and health records – principles set out in Australian privacy legislation relate to the collection, use, and correction of information; data quality and security; openness of policies; assignment of identifiers to individuals; and data flow across borders
- *autonomy* – the healthcare user always retains the right to choose or refuse treatment or participation, and the right to have sufficient information to give 'informed consent'.

Responsibilities of health practitioners

All health practitioners have responsibilities to practise ethically. This requires practitioners to use all appropriate resources in the best interests of the person they are providing care for; to remain competent and up to date in their practice; and to accord healthcare users all basic human rights. What constitutes unethical conduct can sometimes be hard to determine. In the healthcare context, it can mean serious deviation from practices that would reasonably be expected by a general body of colleagues.

Ethical dilemmas: current issues in bioethics

Ethical issues arise frequently and are often hard to resolve. Typically, they involve professional secrecy, consent to treatment, and procedures with legal implications (sterilisation, abortion, assisted conception, euthanasia, and experimentation). This section does not cover all ethical dilemmas relevant to pharmacology, but aspects of some current issues are summarised below, including examples relevant to pharmacotherapy for pregnant and breastfeeding women.

Warnings of risks

Withholding information from persons receiving treatment, including medication, cannot be justified on any grounds. However, it is often challenging to explain every possible adverse event or drug interaction. The High Court of Australia has said that the healthcare users must be informed about 'material' (i.e. significant) risks.

Animal rights

It is recognised that in the testing of drugs, medical devices, or procedures, animals should be used only when necessary. Although results from animal tests cannot automatically be extrapolated to humans, such tests do protect humans. The Australian and New Zealand Council for the Care of Animals in Research and Teaching works diligently to protect animal rights and promote 'the three Rs': **R**eplacement of animals wherever possible, **R**eduction in the numbers of animals used, and **R**efinement of techniques to minimise harm.

Equal access to drugs and medical care

In 2000, the UN launched the Millennium Development Goals to address underlying inequalities in health, including: reducing child mortality; improving maternal health; and combating HIV/AIDS, malaria, and other diseases. Replaced by the Sustainable Development Goals (SDGs) in 2016, 'ensuring good health for all' (SDG 3) is challenged by the increasing costs of medical technologies and new drugs; the demands of ageing populations; healthcare users' expectations; prescribers' fear of litigation; the commercial demands of the pharmaceutical industry; and governments' need for tight budget controls. This makes the rationing of healthcare a difficult ethical issue. The principles of equity and fairness need to be applied, otherwise high-quality care will only be available to the wealthy, those in cities, or those in manufacturer-subsidised trials.

The TGA's Pharmaceutical Benefits Advisory Committee (PBAC) weighs demands from the public for subsidised access to all (safe) drugs and demands from drug companies wanting subsidies for their products, against demands from other interests competing for scarce government health funds. The decision by the PBS to fund a new class of drugs to treat people with hepatitis C cost over a billion dollars, effectively curing many but leading to opportunity cost against wider public health programs. Adding drugs to the PBS-subsidised list should be justifiable and transparent.

Examples of inequitable access to healthcare

Some groups are excluded from participation in clinical trials – for example, children, pregnant women, elderly patients or people with concurrent conditions. The results of trials will not necessarily be applicable to them, and safe treatments may not therefore be developed for these groups.

Children – Children have been described as 'therapeutic orphans' because they can be denied access to new medications, and drugs may not be marketed in dose forms suitable for children. Some authorities now require that drugs likely to be used in children, be trialled in children.

Pregnant women and infants – There is increasing consideration given to ethical issues in therapeutic use and research in pregnant women with respect to inclusion in trials of new medications (Weld et al 2022). There is also recognition that knowledge deficits on drugs in pregnancy and lactation exist – especially a lack of evidence-based information on which to fully describe the dosing and safety of medications to either mother or infant. Drug development research impacts women and infants, and non-participation may confer disadvantage to these groups. Examples include the case of retroviral medications developed to treat Ebola, repurposing of pravastatin to treat preeclampsia, and the disproportionate impact of preexisting autoimmune conditions in women of reproductive age, including how these conditions contribute to complex pregnancy, co-morbidities and poorer outcomes in the absence of further knowledge focused on pharmacological developments and clinical trials (Weld et al 2022).

Elderly patients or people with concurrent conditions – These groups are excluded from clinical trials due to age and underlying medical or age-related conditions that may place them at greater risk for medication-related side effects and/or adverse events.

Aboriginal and Torres Strait Islander peoples have greater morbidity and mortality than other Australians but lower access to healthcare, which limits access to drugs under the PBS. Access to essential medications is critical to improve perinatal outcomes for First Nations mothers and their babies, particularly for the disproportionate numbers managing preexisting chronic illness states. Programs such as the National Agreement on Closing the Gap (2020), the Aboriginal and Torres Strait Islander Health Performance Framework (2023) and the Commonwealth Closing the Gap Implementation Plan (2023) (see Online resources) are all focused towards embedding key priority reforms that improve the population health status of First Nations peoples. Targeted initiatives within health services include improved access to essential PBS-listed medications at low cost or no cost. Similarly, in New Zealand, findings that Māori, Pacific peoples, Indian populations, those aged under 20 years, and those living in areas of high deprivation experience worse perinatal outcomes than those of New Zealand European ethnicity make access to medication an important priority for these groups (Women's Health Strategy 2023).

Clinical trials that would not be approved in countries with strong regulations may be carried out in underdeveloped countries putting vulnerable participants at risk. People in developing countries are often denied drugs due to prohibitive costs and lack of government subsidies. Allowing the production of generic drugs can be lifesaving and reduce suffering.

Promotion of medicines

The World Health Organization has a code of 'ethical criteria for medical drug promotion'. Drug companies obviously consider that advertising drugs to prescribers is effective, otherwise it would not be carried out. However, advertising adds to the cost of bringing new drugs to market. In Australia, 'detailing' of drugs to prescribers is regulated by TGA legislation, guidelines, the Code of Conduct of Medicines Australia, and by complaints from consumers and 'watchdogs'. Breaches of the Code can require withdrawal of promotional material and heavy fines.

Advertising of prescription medicines to the public is not permitted in Australia, but advertising of OTC drugs is allowed. 'Direct-to-consumer' prescription drug advertising is legal in New Zealand and the United States, and increases demand for medicines. Drug companies can boost demand for their products by defining common mild problems as diseases requiring drug treatment, adding to drug costs for governments and, ultimately, taxpayers.

Relationships between health practitioners and the pharmaceutical industry

Prescribers are often 'courted' by drug company representatives to increase their prescribing of a particular drug. Incentives may range from 'starter packs' of drugs, equipment for the desk, and lunches after seminars, to subsidisation of trips to overseas conferences or funding for research. Accepting even a small gift is a conflict of interest for a prescriber. Although prescribers maintain that they can resist such pressures, studies have shown that even subconsciously, their prescribing patterns are affected by donations from drug company 'reps'.

Most biomedical journals now require that authors declare all conflicts of interest, including sponsorship from drug companies. Institutions and professional colleges expect there will be minimal acceptance of gifts or support, that research and publication will be guided by scientific and ethical values, and that Australian clinicians and researchers will make full public disclosure of all financial and other ties with commercial interests.

Ethical aspects of clinical trials

The WHO's Declaration of Helsinki, which was declared in 1964 and recognised internationally, outlines the ethical considerations related to medical research involving human subjects:

> Every biomedical research project involving human subjects should be preceded by careful assessment of predictable risks in comparison with foreseeable benefits to the subject or to others. Concern for the interests of the subject must always prevail over the interests of science and society (WHO – see Online resources).

Currently, pregnant and lactating women are excluded from pharmaceutical clinical trials, based on concerns regarding teratogenicity and toxicity of therapeutic agents due to altered pharmacokinetics and pharmacodynamics. However, there is increasing debate on this topic. Excluding pregnant and lactating women from clinical trials results in drug use based on limited information about the benefits and risks specific to pregnancy and lactation (van der Graaf et al 2018; Sportiello & Capuano 2023).

Many of the general issues in medical ethics discussed above also apply to the situation of a clinical trial. Particularly relevant are:

- personal autonomy and the subject's right to withdraw at any stage (individual rights versus welfare rights)
- the researcher being in a position of potential conflict (the healer vs the investigator)
- randomisation into groups, denying the control group access to the test drug, and the test group access to the current best treatment
- the extent to which subjects should be paid or compensated for expenses
- appropriate makeup of ethics committees
- special guidelines necessary for testing of reproductive technologies or for people who cannot give consent (e.g. minors, or those who have dementia, are aggressive or unconscious)
- trials being subsidised by the manufacturer company, and participating clinicians having conflicts of interest if accepting emoluments.

KEY POINTS

Ethical aspects of pharmacotherapy

- The ethical principles on which clinical practice is based are underpinned by basic human rights and international Declarations.
- Application of medical ethics principles can be controversial in many situations. It is important for health professionals to consider and discuss issues.
- During drug development, drugs need to be tested in animals and humans before being approved as safe and effective. Many ethical issues arise relating to this, including the current exclusion of pregnant and lactating women.

2.3 Legal aspects of pharmacotherapy

Before the 20th century there were few controls on the use of drugs, most of which were natural products with low efficacy. However, as the chemical industries themselves were developed, more potent and efficacious drugs were synthesised (Table 1.2). As a result, the trade in drugs of dependence (addictive drugs) increased in the early 20th century, and the need for controls on drugs was recognised.

International law

Controls on narcotic drugs

The control of drugs in international law began in 1912 when the first Opium Conference was held at The Hague, Netherlands. International treaties were drawn up, calling on governments to:

- limit the manufacturing of, and trade in, medicinal opium to medical and scientific needs
- control the production and distribution of raw opium
- establish a system of governmental licensing to control the manufacture of, and trade in, drugs covered by the treaties.

In 1961, government representatives formulated the *United Nations Single Convention on Narcotic Drugs*, which became effective in 1964. The Convention needs to be ratified and signed by a country before it is binding, then appropriate legislation must be enacted. The Convention consolidated all existing treaties into one document for the control of all **narcotic** substances, except for medical treatment and research.

The Convention, which comes under the auspices of the UN Office on Drugs and Crime (UNODC), lists drugs in schedules depending on their liability for abuse and production of adverse effects.

Australia has signed the following international treaties about drugs:

- Single Convention on Narcotic Drugs 1961 (described above)
- Convention on Psychotropic Substances 1971
- UN Convention Against Illicit Traffic in Narcotic Drugs and Psychotropic Substances 1988.

While it is impossible to prevent illicit drug trafficking, UNDOC acknowledges that many countries face high rates of crime related to this, and endorses a two-pronged approach: to integrate programs to reduce illicit drug supply and demand; and to focus on prevention, treatment, alternative development, and protection of fundamental human rights (see UNODC in Online resources).

Controls on therapeutic drugs

Drugs used therapeutically are controlled because most people assume, but cannot assess, their safety and efficacy. When 'patent medicines' first flooded markets in developed countries early in the 20th century, there were few controls. The birth of thousands of babies with deformities in the 1960s after use of thalidomide led to more rigorous testing and controls of drugs (CFB 2.1 and McBride 1961). More recently, post-marketing studies and meta-analyses of risks/benefits have led to worldwide recalls of drugs such as rofecoxib.

Most governments take a risk assessment role and require the drugs available in their country be assessed for safety, efficacy, quality of manufacture, and cost-effectiveness. This provides protection not only for the public but also for drug manufacturers (and governments). As world trade and health practices globalise, requirements for drug registration and licensing should become uniform in all developed countries.

Regulation of drugs in Australia

The regulation of drugs in Australia via the *Therapeutic Goods Act 1989* has three primary aims: to control the supply of drugs prone to abuse, to regulate the availability of substances for therapeutic use (to ensure safety and quality), and to include certain products on government-sponsored assistance schemes.

Australian laws related to drug regulation can be broadly divided into two types: laws that regulate drugs used for medicinal purposes in humans (discussed in this section) and laws that prohibit the possession, production, and supply of **proscribed drugs** (i.e. prohibited drugs). Legal non-medicinal drugs such as alcohol and tobacco are also subject to regulation. Drug availability can also be controlled at state and local levels – for example, by a hospital's drug committee.

Underpinning all healthcare-related laws are the fundamental principles of human rights and ethics. Some aspects of common law are also relevant: health professionals, including midwives, are considered to have a 'duty of care' and are expected to carry out their roles with people's best interests as the priority.

Commonwealth and state laws

In Australia, drugs are controlled by extensive complex and overlapping pieces of Commonwealth, state, and territory legislation (Table 2.1). Commonwealth legislation cannot apply in all situations, for constitutional reasons, and recent attempts to harmonise the criminal laws of states and territories have not yet succeeded.

Broadly, state and territory laws control 'poisons', and Commonwealth legislation controls 'therapeutic goods'. The role of the Commonwealth is increasing steadily. (Note the term 'poison' is used broadly to cover drugs used clinically, as well as veterinary, agricultural, and domestic chemicals.) Offences related to international drug trafficking are set out in Commonwealth legislation, while the state and territory criminal laws cover the production, possession, use, and distribution of proscribed drugs within those jurisdictions. A substance may be subject to both Commonwealth and state regulation. For example, states and territories have their own guidelines on prescribing and dispensing of drugs with the potential for dependence, with the scheduling and policing of these addictive drugs remaining a Commonwealth responsibility.

Therapeutic Goods Administration

The *Therapeutic Goods Act 1989* regulates 'therapeutic goods' for use in humans for preventing, treating, or diagnosing a disease or pregnancy – for example, drugs, medical devices, diagnostic devices, and biological entities, excluding foods and cosmetics. Before a therapeutic good can be marketed in Australia it must be approved and registered by the TGA, a division of the Commonwealth Department of Health, which evaluates the product before it is marketed, for quality, safety, efficacy, cost-effectiveness, and access for the public (Fig 2.4).

In the case of a new drug, the sponsor, which is usually a drug company, submits material to the TGA, including chemical and manufacturing data and results from pharmacological testing in vitro, in vivo, and in clinical trials (Therapeutic Goods Administration 2021). Experienced evaluators in the relevant advisory committee examine the material closely and the TGA makes the final decision on registering the drug for therapeutic use in Australia, including into which schedule it should be classified. The process also applies to non-prescription drugs, some complementary and alternative remedies, and to medical devices such as breast implants, diagnostic test kits, prostheses, dental materials, contact lenses, and tampons. The TGA also regulates therapeutic goods post-marketing, enforces standards of practice, licenses manufacturers, and verifies compliance.

The six rights of medication administration

The six rights of medicine administration
1. Right patient
2. Right medicine
3. Right dose
4. Right time
5. Right route
6. Right documentation

FIGURE 2.4

Classification into schedules: Standard for the Uniform Scheduling of Medicines and Poisons

Historically, regulation of drug availability in Australia was a state responsibility, which led to anomalies such as a drug being available over the counter in one state – for example, in Albury, NSW – whereas a prescription might be required in Albury's sister town, Wodonga, on the opposite bank of the Murray River in Victoria (or vice versa). In the late 20th century, a review strongly supported a uniform regulatory scheme across states and territories.

The Australian Advisory Committee on Medicines Scheduling (ACMS), which was established under the *Therapeutic Goods Act 1989*, recommends the classification of most drugs and many chemicals into schedules, in the *Standard for the Uniform Scheduling of Medicines and Poisons* (SUSMP). The Standard is published by the Australian Government under Commonwealth law and is registered on the Federal Register of Legislation as the Poisons Standard. The SUSMP is updated at least annually, so it is important to refer to the most recent version. Decisions in relation to the Standard have no force in Commonwealth law, but most states and territories have adopted the Standard in their legislation and regulations that determine how people access a particular drug, and how it is to be packaged and labelled. More information on state/territory scheduling, including contact details for drugs and poisons units, is available on the TGA website (see Online resources).

Trans-Tasman harmonisation

The SUSMP also attempts to unify the scheduling and control of drugs and poisons between Australia and New Zealand. This trans-Tasman scheduling harmonisation has been largely effective, with a few minor discrepancies (see below under 'Regulation of Drugs in New Zealand,').

The drug schedules

The Poisons Standard contains 10 schedules of 'poisons' (i.e. drugs and other chemicals) that are subject to varying levels of controls on labels, containers, storage, disposal, record-keeping, sale, supply, possession and use, and advertising of the scheduled substances. First aid instructions, warning statements and labelling requirements are given in appendices. Drugs are labelled with the 'signal words' of the classification – for example, 'Pharmacy-Only' medicine. This change was made to counteract the false perception in the community that higher S numbers necessarily meant higher toxicity. In fact, the schedules listed in order from greatest to least restrictions are 9, 10, 8, 4, 7, 3, 2, 6, 5.

The decision to classify a substance into a particular schedule depends not only on the potential toxicity of the drug but also on the purposes for which it is used, the dose in the preparation, its potential for abuse, other ingredients present, the formulation (e.g. oral tablet, parenteral injection, or topical ointment), and the need for access to the drug.

Most drugs for therapeutic use are in Schedule 2, 3, 4, or 8. A drug may appear in more than one schedule. For example, aspirin appears in various schedules (2, 4, 5, and 6) depending on the strength and type of the formulation, the route of administration, the quantity of doses in the package, whether other drugs are present, and whether it is intended for human or veterinary use. Where a preparation contains two or more substances (such as paracetamol and codeine), the preparation is in the schedule that is the most restrictive. A few human medicines are included in Schedule 5 and 6 such as head lice preparations and some essential oils.

There may be varying provisions within a schedule; for example, isotretinoin is an S4 Prescription-Only medicine used to treat severe acne (tretinoin cream; DM 41.2) but is teratogenic (causes congenital malformations), so there are strict requirements relating to prescribing and labelling it for women of childbearing age. Drugs may be moved around between schedules as clinical experience and drug usage patterns change. In general, there is a trend to down schedule medicines, improving access to the public in line with one of the central objectives of the National Medicines Policy.

Unscheduled substances

If a substance does not appear in a schedule or appendix of the SUSMP (i.e. is unscheduled), it is not a poison by definition and can be supplied to the public (unless it is subject to other legislative controls).

Includes: laxatives, contact lens products, infant formulae, vitamins (including vitamin K injections), sunscreens, many topical antiseptics, herbal remedies, and small packs of some drugs with high safety margins – for example, non-sedating antihistamines for the short-term treatment of hay fever.

Pharmaceutical substances

Schedule 2 Pharmacy Medicine
Available to the public only from pharmacies, where a pharmacist's advice is available if required, or – where a pharmacy service is unavailable – from persons licensed to sell Schedule 2 poisons.
Includes: some cough and cold preparations, oral antihistamines in larger packs or in combination preparations, mild analgesics, worm tablets, anti-inflammatory agents, topical antifungal preparations, histamine H_2-receptor antagonists (in small packs, for relief of heartburn), topical local anaesthetics (not eyedrops), corticosteroids in some topical formulations, decongestant eyedrops, and some herbal preparations.

Schedule 3 Pharmacist-Only Medicine

Available to the public only from a pharmacist or from medical, dental, or veterinary practitioners but without need for a prescription. Safe use of these substances requires professional advice. Storage of these medications for sale must not be accessible to the public.

Includes: some metered-dose bronchodilator asthma aerosols, topical corticosteroids (some low-strength preparations in small packs), glucagon, antivirals for cold sores, adrenaline (epinephrine) injections for anaphylaxis, serotonin receptor agonists for migraine treatment, and hormones for emergency contraception.

Schedule 4 Prescription-Only Medicine

May be used or supplied only under prescription from an authorised prescriber, including endorsed midwives. Must be stored in a dispensary.

Includes: most drugs – for example, antibiotics, antidepressants, hormones including insulins and hormonal contraceptives (except for emergency contraception), most cardiovascular and central nervous system drugs, antineoplastic agents, and most injections.

Schedule 5 Caution

Substances with a low potential for causing harm, supplied with simple warnings and safety directions on the label. For sale by a pharmacist, Poisons Licence holder, or general dealer. Must not be stored or supplied in a drink or food container.

Includes: some veterinary medicines, household poisons, ether, naphthalene, petrol, and some head lice lotions.

Schedule 6 Poison

More dangerous chemicals than those in Schedule 5, with moderate potential for harm. Extra storage and packaging controls and strong warning labels required.

Includes: many household and garden pesticides and solvents, some iodine tinctures.

Schedule 7 Dangerous Poison

Substances with a high potential for causing harm at low exposure, which require special precautions. A permit is required to buy these chemicals and the purchaser must be over 18 years of age. Special regulations may restrict their availability, possession, storage, or use.

Includes: varying strengths of chemicals such as arsenic, azo dyes, strychnine, cyanide, and commercial pesticides.

Controlled drugs and prohibited substances

Schedule 8 Controlled Drug

Controlled drugs are substances that may produce addiction or dependence. Possession without authority is illegal. Tight controls are applied to reduce abuse and dependence. Drugs must be stored in a locked cabinet and records kept for 2 years in most states, and for 5 years in WA.

Includes: opioids such as morphine, methadone, fentanyl, and high-dose codeine alone; CNS stimulants such as dexamphetamine; cocaine, ketamine, and some cannabis extracts.

Schedule 9 Prohibited Substances

Substances of which the manufacture, possession, sale, or use is prohibited except in special circumstances. Drugs that may be abused or drugs possibly required for teaching, research, or analytical purposes, but which are too toxic for therapeutic use.

Includes: heroin and most recreational drugs such as amphetamine derivatives and LSD.

Schedule 10 Substances of such danger to health as to warrant prohibition of sale, supply and use

Substances (other than those in Schedule 9) so dangerous that sale, supply, and use are prohibited. Included in this schedule are many poisonous plants, herbs and chemicals, poisons such as amygdalin, cinchophen and aristolochia derivatives, and many dyes.

Legal aspects of concern to midwives

As health professionals who administer and/or prescribe Schedule 4 and Schedule 8 drugs, midwives are responsible for adhering to professional standards of practice, to state and territory Acts and regulations, and to NMBA guidelines covering aspects such as the training, education and registration of midwives, and safe medication administration and prescribing practices (CFB 2.3). Other concerns relate to safe storage, possession, and supply of drugs, including adequate record-keeping. Additional professional responsibilities entail requirements for safe management and handling of drugs (e.g. ensuring cold chain maintenance for vaccinations); monitoring controlled drugs of dependence; maintenance of prescription pad safety; mandatory notification or reporting obligations re loss or theft of drugs and/or prescription pads, suspicion of prescription forgery and/or clients who may 'shop' for excessive prescriptions; reporting unprofessional conduct of colleagues involving misuse of scheduled medication or self-prescribing; and other workplace health and safety matters, for example appropriate disposal of unused/expired drugs and/or other equipment, for example administration sharps.

CLINICAL FOCUS BOX 2.3

Fake pharmaceuticals and pharmacies

In Australia, drug regulation and customs surveillance make prevalence of fake or substandard medicines very low (estimated by the World Health Organization as less than 1% of market value). However, the increasing number of drugs purchased online from illegal pharmacies poses a risk. There are at least 36,000 active internet pharmacies globally, of which fewer than 5% are legitimate (i.e. staffed by qualified pharmacists and selling drugs according to regulations). Illegal online pharmacies pose a risk to public safety because they often sell counterfeit and contaminated drugs (with unknown safety profiles), and illicit substances. In some cases, drugs have been ineffective, for example leading to travellers contracting malaria, or toxic, for example causing death due to contamination with diethylene glycol. Illegal online pharmacies encourage people to self-diagnose and remove the opportunity for drug monitoring and the provision of pharmaceutical care.

Health professionals play a vital role in improving medicines safety by educating individuals and the public about the harms of purchasing medicines from illegal internet pharmacies.

Source: Hensey & Gwee 2016.

The Pharmaceutical Benefits Scheme

The PBS began as a limited scheme in 1948, as a list of 139 'life-saving and disease preventing' medicines provided free of charge for Australians. By June 2022, 925 medicines (and 5178 brands) deemed to be essential to the community but too expensive for individual purchase were partially subsidised by the government. (Australian Government Department of Health and Aged Care 2022). Most PBS-listed medicines are dispensed by pharmacists and used by people at home. Some medicines, such as chemotherapy drugs and potent hormones, need medical supervision or can only be prescribed by authorised doctors (the S100 items).

There is a separate section, the Repatriation Pharmaceutical Benefits Scheme, which subsidises a wider range of medications to armed forces veterans and eligible dependants.

Cost of the PBS and access to drugs outside it

In the financial year 2021–22, total PBS government expenditure was A$14.7 billion, compared with A$13.8 billion the previous year, an increase of 6.7%. The number of PBS prescriptions was 215 million, a 0.7% increase from the previous year. Most government expenditure was directed towards concessional card holders. The average dispensed price per prescription of PBS medicines increased to $74.63 compared to $70.65 in 2020–21. The costs increase every year, causing blow-outs in the health budget (Australian Government Department of Health and Aged Care 2022).

The Pharmaceutical Benefits Advisory Committee evaluates the efficacy, safety, and cost-effectiveness of a drug compared with current therapies, then may recommend the drug for subsidy and a price is negotiated. When a drug is listed on the PBS it is affordable for the individual (because part of the cost is subsidised by the government). Members of the committee, government, and doctors are under pressure from drug companies to ensure PBS listing.

Drugs that are not subsidised by the PBS may be obtained by other means – via private prescriptions (where the user pays the full price), or available over the counter in pharmacies, health shops, and supermarkets. In Australia, the limited Midwife List of PBS medications approved for endorsed midwife prescribers can therefore result in costs for consumers where the drug is obtained through private prescription.

Medicines in pregnancy

The TGA, through its Advisory Committee on Prescription Medicines, maintains an 'Australian categorisation of risk of drug use in pregnancy'. The categories are: A (drugs taken by many pregnant women without harmful effects on the fetus); B (drugs taken by a limited number of pregnant women, further categorised as B1, B2, and B3 depending on evidence of safety or harm from animal studies); C (drugs with harmful but probably reversible fetal or neonatal effects); D (drugs suspected to cause malformations or permanent damage); and X (drugs with a high risk of permanent fetal damage that should not be used in pregnancy). The classification is a guide for users and prescribers, rather than a legally enforceable regulation).

KEY POINTS

Definitions of the Australian categories for prescribing medicines in pregnancy

Please refer to the below source for more information:

https://www.tga.gov.au/australian-categorisation-system-prescribing-medicines-pregnancy

---

Regulation of drugs in New Zealand

In New Zealand, legislation relevant to drugs is contained in the *Medicines Act 1981* and Regulations (1984), plus in the *Medicines Amendment Act 2013*, and various subsequent notices and regulations relating to medical devices, approved laboratories, hazardous substances, and to Designated Prescribers, including some NPs, midwives, pharmacists, and optometrists (see Online resources: New Zealand Drug Regulatory Information). The four key elements of the regulatory framework administered by the Medicines and Medical Devices Safety Authority (Medsafe) are: availability, quality, access, and information. Medsafe's mission is 'to enhance the health of New Zealanders by regulating medicines and medical devices to maximise safety and benefit' (see Online resources).

Scheduling and prescribing of drugs

In New Zealand, scheduled medicines are classified into three main categories unless the Minister of Health has gazetted departures from the SUSMP listings:

- prescription medicine (like S4 of the SUSMP)
- restricted medicine (also known as pharmacist-only medicine – S3 of the SUSMP)
- pharmacy-only medicine (S2 of the SUSMP).

These are listed in the First Schedule to the Medicines Regulations 1984 and Amendments.

All other products (other than controlled drugs, see below) are deemed unclassified and are 'general sale medicines'. New Zealand follows Australian guidelines and categories for safety of drugs in pregnancy.

Pharmac

Pharmac is a government body responsible for managing the pharmaceutical budget and funding of medicines, vaccines, and some medical devices. It tenders for subsidised drugs, and its committees set access criteria. Pharmac publishes its Pharmaceutical Schedule (not to be confused with the SUSMP schedules) under two sections. These are Section B: Community Pharmaceuticals, and Section H: Hospital Pharmaceuticals, showing drugs (and brands) subsidised by the government.

The New Zealand Universal List of Medicines is provided under the auspices of the Ministry of Health, with input from Medsafe, Pharmac, and the Pharmacy Guild. It is a 'dictionary of trusted, standardised information about medicines covering medicines approved for supply in New Zealand as well as products listed in Pharmac's Pharmaceutical Schedule' (see Online resources).

Pharmacology and Therapeutics Advisory Committee

The Pharmacology and Therapeutics Advisory Committee is Pharmac's primary clinical advisory committee. It considers and makes recommendations on applications for funding medicines, management of and amendments to the Pharmaceutical Schedule, and need for reviews of drugs. Generally, New Zealanders pay much lower co-payment prices for drugs than do Australians (apart from those on a special scheme). Many more drugs within a class are subsidised in Australia, whereas New Zealand limits the number of bioequivalent 'me-too' drugs subsidised.

Drugs of dependence

The New Zealand *Dangerous Drugs Act 1927* dealt with the controls required by the League of Nations for opium and non-opiate drugs. Before this, opium was readily available. The *Narcotics Act 1965* added controls on mescaline, cocaine, and LSD, as well as opiates. The *United Nations Single Convention on Narcotic Drugs* (1961, 1972) imposed wider controls on drugs, including marijuana. Countries signatory to this Convention are constrained to abide by its agreements.

The *Misuse of Drugs Act 1975* and subsequent regulations (1977) classified controlled drugs into schedules to allow penalties depending on the severity of the abuse, and contain the requirements for the manufacture, sale, supply, prescribing, and labelling of controlled drugs. Alcohol and tobacco are excluded from the Acts. Alcohol is subject to the *Sale of Liquor Act 1989* and amendments.

KEY POINTS

Legal aspects of pharmacotherapy

- Drugs are controlled at many levels: international, national, state, and local institutions regulate access to medicines.

- Laws apply to the classification and control of chemicals, poisons, drugs, and other therapeutic goods. Some chemicals are proscribed, and criminal law relates to offences under relevant Acts.

- Drugs are classified into various Poisons Schedules to control access, supply and provision, labelling, storage, records, and advertising.

- The trans-Tasman harmonisation policy attempts to maintain similar regulations between New Zealand and Australia.

- Governments determine which drugs will be subsidised. Local institutions may determine which can be prescribed.

REVIEW EXERCISES

1 In Australia and New Zealand there are a number of different prescribers. As a health professional it is important you know who can prescribe what. Discuss the different types of prescribers and what they can prescribe in the country in which you (will) practise. Discuss where you would find the legislation outlining the different types of prescribers and which prescribers can prescribe medicines that are subsidised via the Pharmaceutical Benefits Scheme.

2 Jacqueline, a 32-year-old primigravid woman who is at 36 weeks gestation, presents to her local pharmacy requesting medication to alleviate the signs and symptoms of her common cold. The pharmacist asks if she is taking any other medicines, including those purchased over the counter and complementary therapies.

 a. Why does the pharmacist ask if Jacqueline is taking any other medicines?

  Jacqueline says she takes labetalol 100 mg (a medicine to reduce blood pressure) 3 times a day. The pharmacist recommends paracetamol 500 mg two tablets every 4–6 hours for her fever. Jacqueline also requests pseudoephedrine tablets to relieve her nasal congestion. The pharmacist is reluctant to provide the pseudoephedrine, advising caution and recommends Jacqueline consult with her treating health professional prior to use of pseudoephedrine.

 b. List the Poisons Schedule in which paracetamol, pseudoephedrine and labetalol are found. Are these drugs subsidised by your government (i.e. via the PBS in Australia or the New Zealand Pharmaceutical Schedule)?

3 As a health professional you want to determine if a new drug is safe and effective. To do this you read the related peer-reviewed research. Discuss what databases you might search to obtain relevant primary and secondary studies. What challenges currently exist in relation to identifying the safety and efficacy of new drugs in the treatment of pregnant and lactating women?

REFERENCES

Allen R, O'Brien BM. Uses of misoprostol in obstetrics and gynecology. Rev Obstet Gynecol. 2009 Summer;2(3):159-168. PMID: 19826573; PMCID: PMC2760893.

Australian Government Department of Health and Aged Care. Pharmaceutical Benefits Scheme 2023. PBS expenditure and prescriptions report 1 July 2021 to 30 June 2022. https://www.pbs.gov.au/info/statistics/expenditure-prescriptions/pbs-expenditure-and-prescriptions-report-1-july-2021-to-30-june-2022

Australian Medicines Handbook. Australian Medicines Handbook 2023. Adelaide: AMH, 2023.

Cadavid AP. Aspirin: the mechanism of action revisited in the context of pregnancy complications. Front Immunol. 2017 Mar 15;8:261. doi:10.3389/fimmu.2017.00261. PMID: 28360907; PMCID: PMC5350130.

Hensey CC, Gwee A. Counterfeit drugs: an Australian perspective. Med J Aust. 2016;204(9):344.

McBride WG. Thalidomide and congenital abnormalities. Lancet. 1961;278(7216):1358.

Medicines Australia. Who we are (2022). https://www.medicinesaustralia.com.au/about-us/who-we-are/

New Zealand Ministry of Health. Women's Health Strategy 2023. Wellington, New Zealand. https://www.health.govt.nz/system/files/documents/publications/womens-health-strategy-oct23.pdf

Sackett DL, Rosenberg WM, Gray JA et al. Evidence based medicine: what it is and what it isn't. BMJ. 1996 Jan 13;312(7023):71-2. doi: 10.1136/bmj.312.7023.71. PMID: 8555924; PMCID: PMC2349778.

Sportiello L, Capuano A. It is the time to change the paradigms of pregnant and breastfeeding women in clinical research! Front Pharmacol. 2023;14:1113557. doi:10.3389/fphar.2023.1113557

Sweeney GD. Clinical pharmacology: a conceptual approach. New York: Churchill Livingstone, 1990.

Taylor R, McKinlay E, Morris C. Standing order use in general practice: the views of medicine, nursing and pharmacy stakeholder organisations. J Prim Health Care. 2017;9(1):47-55.

Therapeutic Goods Administration. The Australian clinical trial handbook. Department of Health, Ed. Canberra: Commonwealth of Australia, 2021.

van der Graaf R, van der Zande ISE, den Ruijter HM, et al. Fair inclusion of pregnant women in clinical trials: an integrated scientific and ethical approach. Trials. 2018;19:78. https://doi.org/10.1186/s13063-017-2402-9

Victorian Government Department of Health. Authorised midwives – legislative requirements (2022). https://www.health.vic.gov.au/drugs-and-poisons/authorised-midwives-legislative-requirements

Victorian Government Department of Health. Implementing evidence-based practice (2021). https://www.health.vic.gov.au/patient-care/implementing-evidence-based-practice

Victorian Government Department of Health. Victorian community pharmacists statewide pilot – a 12-month statewide pilot aimed at testing an expanded role for community pharmacists (2024). https://www.health.vic.gov.au/primary-care/victorian-community-pharmacist-statewide-pilot

Weld ED, Bailey TC, Waitt C. Ethical issues in therapeutic use and research in pregnant and breastfeeding women. Br J Clin Pharmacol. 2022;88(1):7-21. https://doi.org/10.1111/bcp.14914WELDET AL.21

ONLINE RESOURCES

AMH Children's Dosing Companion 2023: https://shop.amh.net.au/cdcbook (accessed 6 October 2023)

Australian categorisation system for prescribing drugs in pregnancy: https://www.tga.gov.au/prescribing-medicinespregnancy-database (accessed 6 October 2023)

Australian College of Midwives: https://www.midwives.org.au/ (accessed 6 October 2023)

Australian College of Nurse Practitioners: https://acnp.org.au (accessed 6 October 2023)

Australian Commission on Safety and Quality in Health Care: https://www.safetyandquality.gov.au/our-work/medication-safety/medication-charts/national-standard-medication-charts (accessed 6 October 2023)

Australian Government. Medicare Services for Eligible Midwives: https://www.servicesaustralia.gov.au/medicare-services-for-eligible-midwives?context=20 (accessed 5 October 2023)

Australian Government Department of Health. Participating Midwives MBS Item Changes: http://www.mbsonline.gov.au/internet/mbsonline/publishing.nsf/Content/F8DFEE057E379A25CA2587CF0077BAF0/$File/Factsheet-Participating-Midwives-Changes-22.03.01v2.pdf (accessed 5 October 2023)

Australian Government Department of Health and Aged Care. 2022 Office of Drug Control – Prescribing unapproved drugs: https://www.odc.gov.au/medicinal-cannabis/prescribing-unapproved-drugs (accessed 6 October 2023)

Australian Government Department of Health and Aged Care. The Pharmaceutical Benefits Scheme – Midwife PBS prescribing – Browse by Midwife Items – Medications which may be prescribed by authorized midwives: https://www.pbs.gov.au/browse/midwife (accessed 5 October 2023)

Australian Government Federal Register of Legislation. Therapeutic Goods Act 1989. Latest Version C2023C00240 (C84) 21 September 2023: https://www.legislation.gov.au/C2004A03952/latest/text (accessed 30 January 2024)

Australian Health Practitioner Regulation Agency (AHPRA): https://www.ahpra.gov.au/ (accessed 6 October 2023)

Australian Institute of Health and Welfare (AIHW). Aboriginal and Torres Strait Islander Health Performance Framework: summary report July 2023: https://www.indigenoushpf.gov.au/getattachment/4a44660b-5db7-48d0-bcec-1e0a49b587fc/2023-july-ihpf-summary-report.pdf (accessed 1 February 2024)

Australian Pharmaceutical Formulary: https://www.psa.org.au/apf (accessed 6 October 2023)

Australian Prescriber: https://www.nps.org.au/australian-prescriber/ (accessed 6 October 2023)

Commonwealth of Australia 2023. Commonwealth Closing the Gap implementation plan: https://www.niaa.gov.au/resource-centre/indigenous-affairs/commonwealth-closing-gap-implementation-plan-2023 (accessed 1 February 2024)

Consumer Medicine Information: https://medsinfo.com.au/ (accessed 1/2/2024)

Declaration of Geneva (1948): https://www.wma.net/what-we-do/medical-ethics/declaration-of-geneva/ (accessed 6 October 2023)

Declaration of Helsinki: https://www.wma.net/policies-post/wma-declaration-of-helsinki-ethical-principles-for-medical-research-involving-human-subjects/ (accessed 6 October 2023)

Health Direct Australia – Medicines information service: https://about.healthdirect.gov.au/medicines-information-service (accessed February 1 2024)

Health Direct MS-2 Step (medical abortion medicine): https://www.healthdirect.gov.au/ms-2-step-medical-abortion-medicine (accessed 27 October 2023)

International Code of Medical Ethics (1949): https://www.wma.net/policies-post/wma-international-code-of-medical-ethics/ (accessed 6 October 2023)

International Confederation of Midwives: https://www.internationalmidwives.org/our-work/policy-and-practice/icm-definitions.html#;,:text=A%20midwife%20is%20a%20person,who%20has%20acquired%20the%20requisite (accessed 5 October 2023)

Medicines Australia: http:// https://medicinesaustralia.com.au (accessed 2 November 2021)

Medicine Finder – NPS MedicineWise: https://www.nps.org.au/medicine-finder (accessed 1 February 2024)

Medsafe NZ: https://www.medsafe.govt.nz/index.asp (accessed 6 October 2023)

Midwifery Council of New Zealand: https://www.midwiferycouncil.health.nz (accessed 6 October 2023)

National Agreement on Closing The Gap 2020: https://www.closingthegap.gov.au/sites/default/files/2021-05/ctg-national-agreement_apr-21.pdf (accessed 1 February 2024)

National Medicines Policy (Australia): https://www.health.gov.au/resources/publications/national-medicines-policy?language=en (accessed 6 October 2023)

NPS MedicineWise 2020 Prescribing competencies framework – embedding quality use of medicines into practice: https://www.nps.org.au/assets/NPS/pdf/NPS2321_Prescribing_Competencies_Framework_DRAFT.pdf (accessed 6 October 2023)

National Prescribing Service (NPS): https://www.nps.org.au/ (accessed 6 October 2023)

New Zealand College of Midwives: https://www.midwife.org.nz/ (accessed 6 October 2023)

New Zealand College of Midwives: Consensus Statement Midwife Prescribing https://www.midwife.org.nz/wp-content/uploads/2019/05/Midwife-Prescribing.pdf (accessed 5 October 2023)

New Zealand Drug Regulatory Information: https://www.medsafe.govt.nz/regulatory/Guideline/GRTPNZ/overview-of-therapeutic-product-regulation.pdf (accessed 6 October 2023)

New Zealand Formulary: https://www.nzformulary.org/ (accessed 6 October 2023)

New Zealand Midwifery Council/Pharmacy Council: Midwives and pharmacists – Collaborative roles and responsibilities. https://pharmacycouncil.org.nz/wp-content/uploads/2021/03/Joint-Midwifery-Council-statement-May-2019-1.pdf (accessed 5 October 2023)

New Zealand Ministry of Health/Manatū Hauora: https://www.health.govt.nz/ (accessed 6 October 2023)

New Zealand Ministry of Health: https://www.health.govt.nz/our-work/primary-health-care/about-primary-health-organisations (accessed 6 October 2023)

New Zealand Universal List of Medicines: https://www.nzulm.org.nz/ (accessed 6 October 2023)

Nursing and Midwifery Board of Australia: https://www.nursingmidwiferyboard.gov.au/ (accessed 6 October 2023)

Pharmac (NZ): https://www.pharmac.govt.nz/ (accessed 6 October 2023)

Pharmaceutical Benefits Scheme: https://www.pbs.gov.au/pbs/home (accessed 6 October 2023)

Pharmaceutical Benefits Scheme. Medicines which may be prescribed by authorised midwives: https://www.pbs.gov.au/browse/midwife (accessed 12 October 2023)

Queensland Government 2023. Medicines and Poisons Act 2019. Extended Practice Authority 'Midwives' V2. March 2023: https://www.health.qld.gov.au/__data/assets/pdf_file/0026/1108943/epa-midwives.pdf (accessed 12 October 2023)

Therapeutic Goods Administration (TGA), Australian categorisation system for prescribing drugs in pregnancy: https://www.tga.gov.au/prescribing-medicinespregnancy-database (accessed 6 October 2023)

Therapeutic Goods Administration (TGA), .2023 Advisory Committee on Medicines Scheduling (ACMS): https://www.tga.gov.au/about-tga/advisorybodies-and-committees/advisory-committee-medicinesscheduling-acms (accessed 30 January 2024)

Therapeutic Goods Administration (TGA), Find information about a medicine: https://www.tga.gov.au/products/medicines/find-information-about-medicine (accessed 1 February 2024)

— CHAPTER 3 —

MOLECULAR DRUG TARGETS AND PHARMACODYNAMICS

Maryam Bazargan, Kirsten Small, Roslyn Donnellan-Fernandez

Key Abbreviations

ATP	adenosine triphosphate
cAMP	cyclic adenosine monophosphate
cGMP	cyclic guanosine monophosphate
DNA	deoxyribonucleic acid
GDP	guanosine diphosphate
GPCR	G-protein-coupled receptors
GTP	guanosine triphosphate
HMG-CoA	3-hydroxy-3-methylglutaryl coenzyme A

Key Terms

affinity 49
agonists 54
allosteric
    modulators 56
antagonists 54
efficacy 54

potency 57
receptors 50
selectivity 49
specificity 49
substrate 51

Chapter Focus

Drugs have been a mainstay in the treatment of disease for centuries. Belief in their 'magical' powers has been replaced by scientific understanding of the basis of drug action. Scientific knowledge enabled health professionals to use drugs more effectively and safely, and pharmaceutical companies and scientists to develop new drugs producing targeted therapeutic effects with diminished adverse effects. An understanding of the molecular targets for drug action and the relationship between exposure to a drug and the pharmacological response it produces underpins many aspects of the use of drugs.

Learning Outcomes

- Understand different types of drug targets
- Understand how drugs interact with their target's pharmacodynamics
- Understand the different types of drug-target interactions including agonist and antagonist
- Understand drug potency and efficacy
- Critically apply knowledge of pharmacodynamics in the pharmacological management and care of a woman and her fetus/newborn/breastfeeding baby

CRITICAL THINKING SCENARIO

Samantha is a 35-year-old woman who is 35 weeks pregnant. At 30 weeks she was diagnosed with gestational hypertension and was prescribed methyldopa (a centrally acting α2-adrenergic agonist). She has now been admitted to hospital for preeclampsia, and nifedipine (a calcium channel antagonist) has been added to her hypertension management. One of these drugs is an agonist and the other an antagonist.

1   What do these terms mean?

2   Both of these drugs act at different targets, and there is a lot of overlap in how and why they are used. How can these apparently opposing approaches to treatment work together to produce better control of blood pressure than either could if used alone?

3   What education is important for Samantha in relation to the use of these medications, including some of the side effects she may experience?

Introduction

Drugs do not confer new functions on a tissue or organ. Instead, drugs modify existing physiological, biochemical, or biophysical processes to change the existing functions of a tissue or organ to achieve a therapeutic outcome. For example, when a hypoglycaemic drug is prescribed for a person with diabetes, the effectiveness of the drug can be monitored by repeated measurements of the person's blood glucose concentration. Drugs can act by interacting with endogenous small molecules (e.g. antacids neutralise gastric acid), altering the activity of a cell membrane (e.g. local anaesthetics), or interaction with protein (e.g. adrenaline increases the heart rate by interacting with receptors in the heart). The site at which a drug binds is called the molecular target, or site of action. In most cases the molecular target is a protein, but there are exceptions such as antimicrobials and cytotoxic chemotherapy drugs that bind to deoxyribonucleic acid (DNA).

3.1 Drug specificity, selectivity, and affinity

The **specificity** of a drug describes the number of effects the drug produces, while **selectivity** describes the number of molecular targets the drug interacts with. An ideal drug would interact with a single molecular target, at a single site, and cause only one effect. Such a drug would be described as having complete specificity. Unfortunately, no drugs can lay claim to that title. Most drugs show some degree of selectivity – that is, a preference for a molecular target – but may lack specificity either because they act on more than one molecular target or because they act on a molecular target located in multiple organs or tissues throughout the body. For example, isoprenaline is non-selective because it interacts with β1 adrenoceptors in the heart, causing an increase in heart rate and force of contraction, and with β2 adrenoceptors in the lungs, causing bronchodilation. In contrast, salbutamol is selective for β2 adrenoceptors, and greater site (in this case, tissue) selectivity is achieved when the drug is inhaled. At higher doses, salbutamol causes muscle tremor by interacting with β2 adrenoceptors in skeletal muscle. Although selectivity for β2 adrenoceptors is retained at higher doses, tissue selectivity is lost, leading to a loss of specificity and multiple effects. Another example is aspirin, an irreversible inhibitor of cyclooxygenase (COX)-1. It also modifies COX-2 enzymes. Aspirin is useful as an anticoagulant and anti-inflammatory agent. Aspirin is being used in prevention of fetal growth restriction (FGR) since it stops platelet clots developing in the placenta.

To understand how drugs act, we need to understand the site on the molecular target at which they bind, the molecular mechanisms by which an extracellular signal alters an intracellular pathway and causes a functional change in a cell, and why under some circumstances the response to drugs decreases with time. The strength of the interaction between a drug and its molecular target – that is, the avidity with which a drug binds – is defined as the **affinity** of a drug for its molecular target. A drug's selectivity and affinity for a target can be determined in a laboratory by spraying the drug over a surface coated with the target of interest and measuring the scattering of light caused as the drug binds to the target and changes the structure of the surface. The selectivity and affinity of a drug depend on its chemical structure, molecular size, and electrical charge. Changes in any of these parameters can dramatically increase or decrease the binding of a drug to its molecular target, altering its therapeutic efficacy, and/or toxicity.

Drug specificity, selectivity and affinity

- Except for drugs that target cancer and infection by acting on nucleic acids, most drugs act by binding to proteins, which are referred to as molecular targets.
- An ideal drug would interact with only one molecular target, at one site, and have only one effect. That is, it would be specific. Most drugs show selectivity, as they display a preference for a molecular target.

3.2 Molecular drug targets

Most drugs cause their effect by acting on one of four types of protein targets. These are called regulatory proteins because they mediate the actions of hormones, neurotransmitters, and other chemical messengers. The four types of regulatory proteins are:

1 transporters
2 ion channels
3 enzymes
4 receptors.

Transporters

The integrity of the cell membrane is essential for maintaining homeostasis. Many small molecules and ions are too polar to passively diffuse across membranes and so must be transported. In some cases, transport across a cell membrane can be passive (e.g. carrier-mediated or facilitated diffusion), but more commonly it is an active process. In many cases, active transport uses adenosine triphosphate (ATP) as an energy source to actively pump a substance across the membrane against an electrochemical gradient. Transporters that facilitate this type of passage across a membrane contain a distinct ATP-binding site and are called ABC (ATP-binding cassette) transporters. In other cases, transport of an organic molecule is coupled to transport of an ion, such as sodium, through a process of secondary active transport. If the movement of both molecules across the membrane is in the same direction, the transporter is called a symporter (e.g. the transport of sodium/potassium/chloride in the Loop of Henle). If the molecules are moved across the membrane in opposite directions, the transporter is called an antiporter (e.g. the exchange of sodium and potassium in the proximal convoluted tubule). Other important transporters that function this way include those involved in the uptake of neurotransmitters such as noradrenaline/norepinephrine, serotonin, and glutamate. These specific transporters are often targets for drugs. Fluoxetine, an antidepressant, is an example of a drug that acts on a transport system. Fluoxetine blocks presynaptic serotonin (5HT1A) receptors,

and in doing so inhibits transporter-mediated uptake of serotonin, an important neurotransmitter in the central nervous system. The role of transporters in the uptake and efflux of drugs and in drug–drug interactions is becoming increasingly recognised as important in the clinical use of drugs.

Ion channels

Ion channels are proteins embedded within the cell membrane that control the flow of ions into and out of the cell, thereby maintaining an electrochemical gradient between the interior and exterior of the cell. Ion channels are present in the membranes of all cells and represent one of the two classes of ion transporting proteins, the other being ion transporters. Ion channels have two distinct features that differentiate them from other transporters:

- The rate of flow through the channel is very high (millions of ions can flow through a channel every second)
- Ions can only pass through an ion channel down their electrochemical gradient from a compartment containing a higher concentration of ions to a compartment containing a lower concentration.

A variety of drugs target ion channels. These include the diuretic amiloride, which blocks entry of sodium into renal tubular cells; benzodiazepines used as anticonvulsants and sleep induction such as diazepam, which enhances the entry of chloride into neurons; and various calcium channel-blocking drugs such as verapamil, nifedipine, and diltiazem used for their impact on the cardiovascular system.

Enzymes

Enzymes are biological catalysts that control biochemical reactions within the cell. Although it is possible for a drug to either activate or inhibit an enzyme, in clinical practice almost every drug that acts on an enzyme works by inhibiting the enzyme. For example, the anticoagulant drug warfarin inhibits the enzyme vitamin K epoxide reductase, preventing activation of vitamin K1 and blocking production of vitamin K1–dependent clotting factors. This drug is used to reduce the risk of future events in people that have previously experienced blood clots. Another example are the nonsteroidal anti-inflammatory drugs (NSAIDs) that inhibit the enzyme cyclooxygenase (COX) and methotrexate which is currently used as a treatment for ectopic pregnancy as an alternative to surgery. Common drugs that act on enzymes are listed in Table 3.1.

Receptors

Receptors are signalling proteins that recognise and respond to chemical messengers, including hormones, neurotransmitters, and other mediators, to change function

TABLE 3.1 Common enzyme-inhibiting drugs

ENZYME	DRUGS	EXAMPLE USE(S)
Acetylcholinesterase	neostigmine	Myasthenia gravis
Angiotensin-converting enzyme (ACE)	captopril lisinopril	Hypertension Heart failure
Cyclo-oxygenase (COX)	aspirin celecoxib ibuprofen	Inflammation Postnatal pain Antiplatelet (prevention of preeclampsia)
HMG-CoA reductase	atorvastatin simvastatin	Hypercholesterolemia
Phosphodiesterase • PDE3 • PDE5	milrinone sildenafil	Heart failure (milrinone) Prevention of FGR
Thymidine kinase	acyclovir	Herpes simplex virus
Vitamin K epoxide reductase	warfarin	Deep vein thrombosis Pulmonary embolism Stroke prevention

Source: Queensland Government, 2022. Methotrexate Treatment for Ectopic Pregnancy https://www.health.qld.gov.au/__data/assets/pdf_file/0035/1147895/Methotrexate-treatment-for-ectopic-pregnancy_v1.0.pdf.

within a cell. Receptors are the largest and most diverse type of molecular drug target.

Families of receptors

Receptors respond to a variety of signals and control many different functions within a cell. In some cases, such as synaptic transmission, receptor-mediated effects occur very rapidly – usually over a millisecond time scale. In other cases, such as steroid hormone signalling, the effects occur much more slowly – over hours to days. Differences in time scale are due to different coupling (signal transduction) mechanisms that link the occupation of the receptor by a ligand (drug or endogenous chemical) to the ensuing response. Receptors are divided into four types (superfamilies) based on differences in their structure and coupling mechanisms:

Type 1: Ligand-gated ion channels are membrane-bound channels that are activated when a ligand binds to a specific site (orthosteric site) on the protein. Nifedipine and verapamil produce their clinical effects by binding to the beta-subunit of L-type calcium channels and blocking them.

Type 2: G-protein-coupled receptors (GPCRs) are discussed further in the following section. GPCRs have a slightly slower response than the type 1 receptors, usually in the order of seconds because of the associated signal transduction mechanisms. Prostaglandin receptors are heptahelical (seven membrane-spanning helices) transmembrane GPCRs located in cytoplasmic membranes.

Type 3: Kinase receptors are similar in structure to GPCRs but with different signal transduction mechanisms. Response is typically measured in hours because these receptors are linked to processes that alter gene transcription and therefore protein synthesis, which does not occur rapidly. Receptors of this type include tyrosine kinase receptors acted on by epidermal growth factor, atrial natriuretic peptide, vascular endothelial growth factor, nerve growth factor, and many more trophic hormones. Drugs that inhibit kinase receptors are increasingly used to treat cancers.

Type 4: Nuclear receptors regulate gene transcription and include the peroxisome proliferator activated receptor that binds some hypolipidemic drugs, the retinoic and retinoid X receptors, and the steroid hormone receptors. Although called nuclear, they are often located in the cytosol and require binding of various other molecules before translocating to the nucleus where they interact with specific response elements located on genes – for example, steroid hormone receptors. Response time for nuclear receptor activation, like to the type 3 receptors, usually occurring hours later because of the time taken to alter cell processes such as gene transcription.

Type 1, 2 and 3 receptors are all located in the cell membrane and have an orthosteric site (ligand binding site) that faces outwards to respond to extracellular messengers. Type 4 receptors affect gene transcription (e.g. the glucocorticoid receptor) and are located in the cytosol, migrating into the cell nucleus when activated by binding with a **substrate** or drug.

G-protein-coupled receptors

GPCRs are the largest family of plasma membrane receptors. GPCRs mediate responses to most of our hormones and neurotransmitters, as well as our sense of smell, taste, and sight. These receptors are often familiar to health professionals. They include muscarinic acetylcholine receptors, receptors for epinephrine and norepinephrine (adrenoceptors), dopamine receptors, adenosine receptors, histamine receptors, and opioid and opioid-like receptors. GPCRs are therefore important targets exploited in pharmacotherapy.

There are many different types of G-proteins and, through a series of reactions, the activated G-protein changes the activity of a second messenger specific to the type of G-protein. A simplified schema is shown in Figure 3.1.

Second messengers

For a cell to respond to an external stimulus (e.g. binding of a drug or hormone to a receptor), the signal has to be communicated from the exterior of the cell to the

Schematic representation of activation of G-protein-coupled receptors by drugs

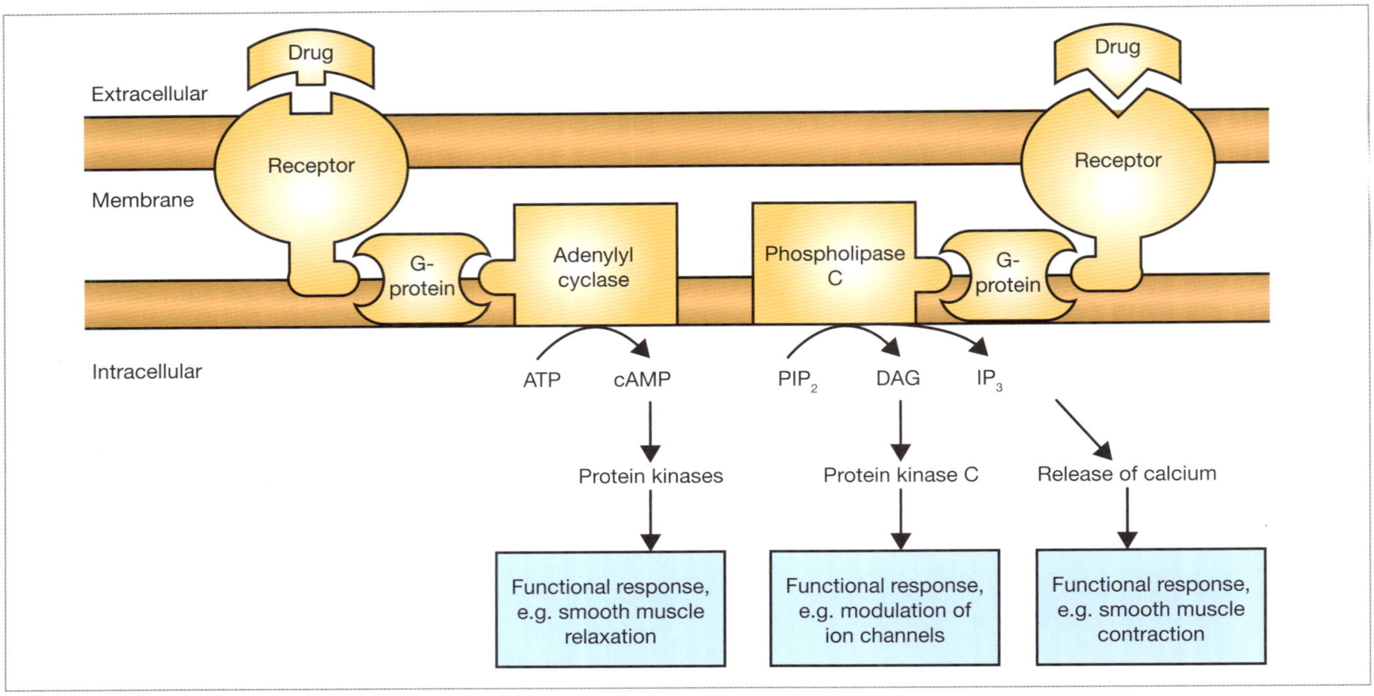

FIGURE 3.1 The second messenger systems involved include: (1) cAMP, which activates various protein kinases linked to cellular functions (e.g. smooth muscle relaxation); and (2) activation of phospholipase C, which cleaves phosphatidylinositol-4,5-bisphosphate (PIP2) to form diacylglycerol (DAG), which activates protein kinase C, and inositol triphosphate (IP3), which releases intracellular calcium. ATP = adenosine triphosphate.

respective response elements within the cell. This mechanism of communication often involves a second messenger system, which initiates signalling within the cell through a specific biochemical pathway. The signal and the response are highly coordinated within the cell and this often involves multiple highly integrated pathways.

cAMP and cGMP

One of the most studied second messengers is cyclic adenosine monophosphate (cAMP), which is synthesised by membrane-bound adenylyl cyclase under the control of a number of GPCRs. cAMP mediates effects such as the breakdown of fat, conservation of water by the kidney, and the rate and force of contraction of the heart. It exerts most of its effects through a series of protein kinases that control cell function by phosphorylating proteins (adding phosphate groups to the protein) (Fig 3.3).

The breakdown of cAMP by phosphodiesterase enzymes terminates its action. Inhibition of phosphodiesterase, which results in an increase in the intracellular concentration of cAMP and hence calcium, is one of the mechanisms by which caffeine and theophylline are thought to produce cardiac effects. The cAMP second messenger system is linked to the action of β-adrenoceptors and many other receptors (Fig 3.2).

Another important second messenger is cyclic guanosine monophosphate (cGMP), which is involved in controlling the function of smooth muscle and nerve cells and monocytes and platelets. cGMP is formed by two distinct forms of guanylyl cyclase. The soluble form is activated to cGMP by nitric oxide. Nitric oxide is important in cardiovascular health and plays a role in both the autonomic and central nervous systems. The second form of guanylyl cyclase is membrane-bound and is activated by natriuretic peptides. Similar to cAMP, the effects of cGMP are terminated by the phosphodiesterase enzymes.

Phosphoinositides and calcium

Another well-studied second messenger system involves hydrolysis of a minor component of cell membranes, splitting it into two second messengers: diacylglycerol and inositol triphosphate (Fig 3.1). Diacylglycerol is confined to the cell membrane where it activates protein kinase C, in turn changing the activity of other enzymes that ultimately produce the functional response (e.g.

Cyclic AMP pathways in myometrial tissue

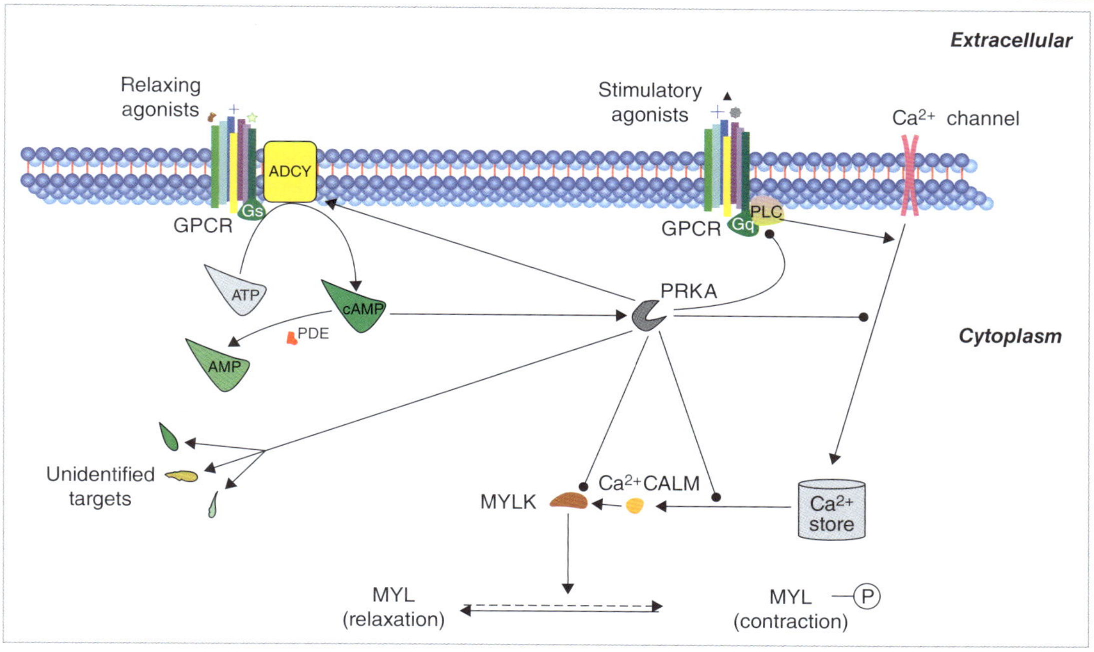

FIGURE 3.2 Activation of membrane receptors (GPCR) coupled to Gs activates adenylyl cyclase (ADCY) which converts ATP to cAMP. The levels of cAMP are tightly regulated by phosphodiesterases (PDE), especially PDE4 isoforms. It is thought that cAMP induces uterine relaxation via activation of a specific protein kinase (PRKA) which phosphorylates and inhibits myosin light chain kinase (MYLK). PRKA may also oppose the effect of stimulatory receptors which operate through the phospholipase C (PLC)/calcium pathway. However, the precise targets for PRKA phosphorylation in human myometrium are under investigation (→ stimulation, ⊸ inhibition).

Source: Yuan, W., López Bernal, A. Cyclic AMP signalling pathways in the regulation of uterine relaxation. BMC Pregnancy Childbirth 7 (Suppl 1), S10 (2007). https://doi.org/10.1186/1471-2393-7-S1-S10.

increased glandular secretions). Inositol triphosphate diffuses through the cytoplasm and causes the release of calcium from storage sites. Increased intracellular calcium regulates the activity of other enzymes, producing a response such as increased contractility. These particular second messengers are important for producing the effects mediated by α-adrenoceptors and muscarinic receptors.

Desensitisation and receptor turnover

Receptor populations are not static. Receptors may undergo several changes over time, including loss of responsiveness at the individual receptor level or a change in the number of receptors.

Desensitisation (also referred to as adaptation or refractoriness) refers specifically to decreased responsiveness of the receptor–second messenger system and is a common feature of many receptors. The mechanisms underlying receptor desensitisation are complex and include: (i) an uncoupling of the receptor from its second messenger system, (ii) altered binding of the drug to the receptor, or (iii) a decrease in the total number of receptors.

The total number of receptors in the cell membrane at any one time can also change. A decrease in receptor number is called downregulation and can contribute to desensitisation and loss of response. An increase in receptor number is referred to as upregulation and can cause receptor hypersensitivity. An example of upregulation is the increase in oxytocin receptors as pregnancy progresses (Uvnäs-Moberg et al 2019; Prevost et al 2014).

KEY POINTS

Molecular drug targets

- There are four main types of regulatory proteins that drugs act on. These are: transporters, enzymes, ion channels, and receptors.

- Receptors are cellular protein macromolecules directly concerned with chemical signalling that initiates a change in cell function. They are common targets for drug action.

- Receptors can lose responsiveness (tachyphylaxis), become desensitised, or be downregulated or upregulated.

3.3 Pharmacodynamics

Pharmacodynamics is the study of the interaction between a drug and its molecular target, and of the pharmacological response: what the drug does to the body (Fig 3.3). The magnitude of a pharmacological effect of a drug depends on the nature of the interaction with the target, the affinity of the drug for the target, and the concentration of a drug at the site of action.

Drug target interactions

The interaction of a drug with its target is classified differently depending on the type of molecular target (i.e. receptor, channel, enzyme, or transporter). In general terms, the binding of a drug with its target will either make something happen ('switch the target on') or stop something from happening ('switch the target off'). Drugs acting on enzymes, transporters, and channels elicit their effect by switching the target off. These drugs are called inhibitors when they act on an enzyme (e.g. aspirin is a COX inhibitor) or transporter (e.g. fluoxetine is a serotonin reuptake transporter inhibitor), and are called blockers when they act on a channel (e.g. nifedipine is a calcium channel blocker). Drugs that act on receptors can either 'switch on' or 'switch off' the target and are classified according to what they do, and how they do it.

Receptor agonists

Binding of a drug to a receptor causes a functional response, which is governed initially by the affinity of the drug for the receptor as determined by the chemical forces that cause the drug to bind. Once bound, the ability to activate the receptor (i.e. to produce an effect or response) is determined by the **efficacy** of the drug. Defining the response caused by a drug binding to a receptor can be complex. At the least complex level, drugs that bind to a receptor are simply termed **agonists** (because they produce a response) or **antagonists** (because they prevent a response). A drug that functions as an agonist binds and activates the receptor producing the same response as the endogenous (natural) ligand (Fig 3.4). Depending on where on the receptor binding occurs, a drug may be a direct agonist or an allosteric agonist. Examples of endogenous ligands include hormones (e.g. oestrogen), neurotransmitters (e.g. dopamine), and catecholamines (e.g. epinephrine). An agonist may be a full agonist or a partial agonist, depending on the capacity of the drug to cause the same response as an endogenous ligand.

Partial agonists

Partial agonists bind to and activate a receptor but cannot elicit the same response as the endogenous ligand for that

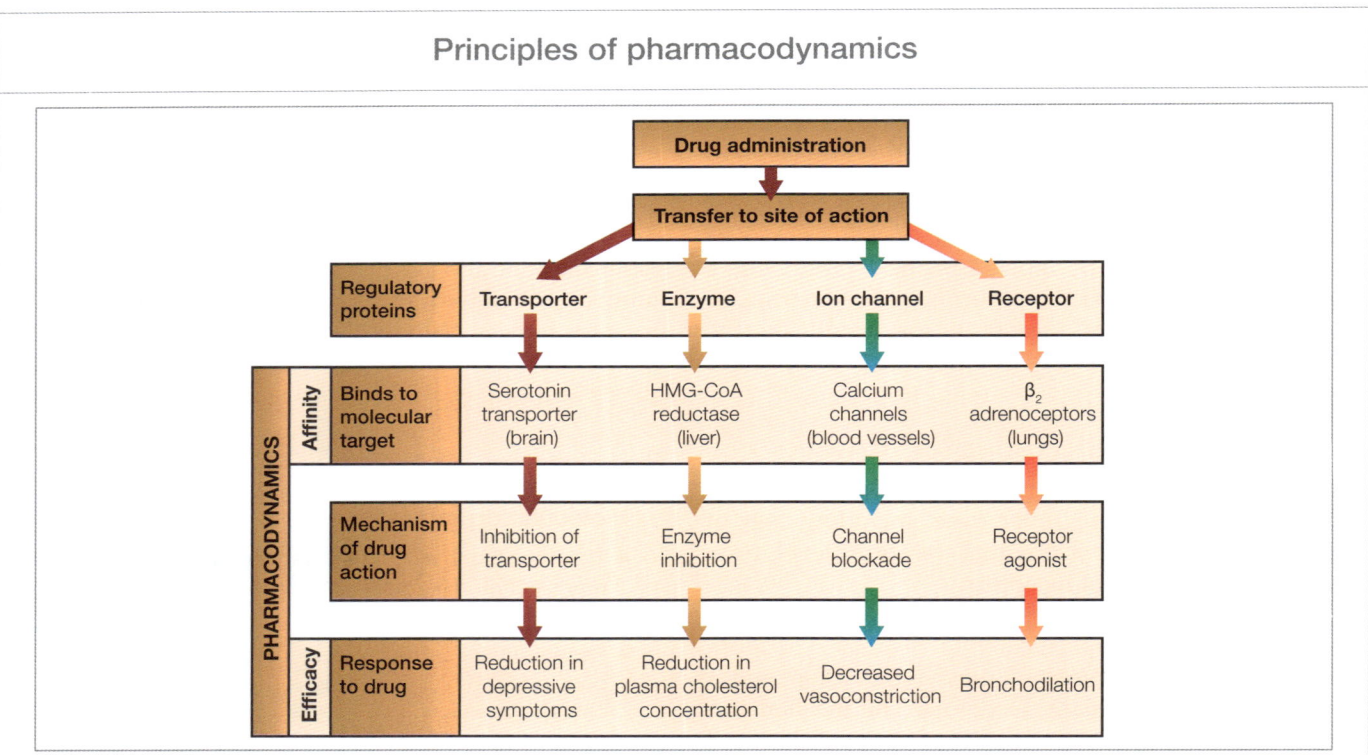

FIGURE 3.3 The figure shows the four main types of regulatory proteins and illustrates the concept of pharmacodynamics by using an example of each type of protein. Note the interrelationships between the affinity of a drug and drug efficacy (response). This illustration does not consider the effects of absorption, distribution, metabolism, and excretion, which all affect the concentration of drug reaching the molecular target.

Illustration of drug–receptor interactions

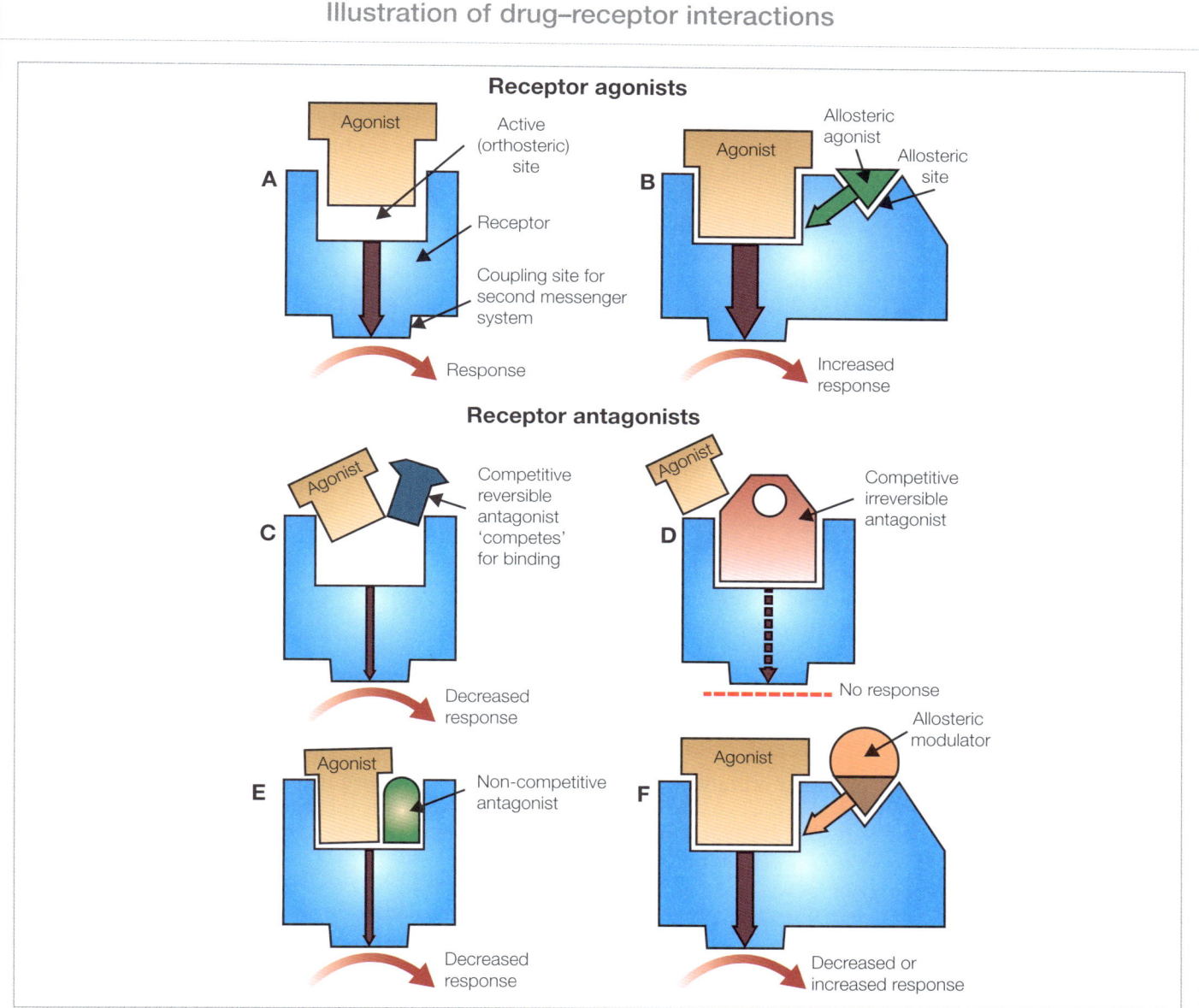

FIGURE 3.4 A An agonist drug binds to the active site of the receptor and produces a response; **B** An allosteric agonist binds at a site distinct to the active site and in this case increases the response elicited by the agonist; **C** A competitive inhibitor 'competes' with the agonist for binding, ultimately causing a decreased response; **D** A competitive irreversible antagonist binds to the receptor, irreversibly preventing agonist binding – hence, no response; **E** A non-competitive antagonist binds independently, blocking the response to the agonist at some point within the receptor-coupling cascade and causes a decreased response; **F** An allosteric modulator binds to the allosteric site producing a change in the protein, either causing reduced affinity of the primary agonist (antagonism) and hence reducing the response or potentiating (facilitating) the effect of the primary agonist and hence increasing the response.

receptor, even when all receptors are occupied. An example of this type of drug are the selective oestrogen receptor modulators like tamoxifen and raloxifene. These are used to treat breast cancers that express oestrogen receptors. They block the effect of oestrogen in the breast but activate oestrogen receptors in other tissues such as bone (providing prevention for osteoporosis) and the endometrium (increasing endometrial cancer risk).

Antagonists

Receptor antagonists bind to the orthosteric site of the receptor (they retain affinity for the receptor) without eliciting a response (they have no efficacy). In doing so, the antagonist prevents the binding of an agonist to the receptor and so prevents activation of the receptor (Fig 3.4). An example of a receptor antagonist is naloxone.

Naloxone is a μ-opioid receptor antagonist used to reverse harmful effects caused by the administration of opioid agonists (e.g. morphine, heroin). Antagonists are classified based on how and where they bind to the receptor. The two defining characteristics that are of greatest clinical importance are reversibility and competitiveness.

Reversible competitive antagonists

Reversible competitive antagonists interfere with the binding of the endogenous agonist to the orthosteric site by competing for binding sites on the receptor. Their action can be overcome by increasing the concentration of the agonist. When there is a higher concentration of an agonist, this out-competes the antagonist and the tissue responds once again to the agonist. For example, higher concentrations of epinephrine are used to overcome the competitive blockade of β-adrenoceptors by propranolol. Competitive antagonists reduce the potency of the receptor agonist, but they do not alter the efficacy of the agonist. That is, they shift the agonist concentration–response curve to the right (there is need for a higher dose of the drug) but do not alter the slope or maxima (the same relationship between drug dose and effect will be achieved, but at a higher dose).

Irreversible competitive antagonists

Irreversible competitive antagonists make the target receptor permanently unavailable for binding of the endogenous agonist. They have a high affinity for the receptor and dissociate from the receptor so slowly they are in essence an 'irreversible' antagonist. Their action is usually prolonged and it is not terminated until the receptors 'die' and are replaced by new receptors. This limits their use in clinical practice, but they are experimentally useful to investigate receptor function. Examples of chemicals in this class include some inhibitors of acetylcholinesterase and chemicals such as nerve gases (see Chapter 9). Therapeutically used drugs of this class include aspirin, which irreversibly inhibits an enzyme in platelets and therefore prevents platelet aggregation. This explains the long duration of impact of aspirin as an anticoagulant. New platelets must replace those blocked by aspirin before platelet function returns to normal. Irreversible competitive antagonists permanently occupy the receptor and effectively remove them from the system; they reduce both the potency and efficacy of the receptor agonist. That is, they cause the agonist concentration–response curve to shift to the right and reduce the slope and maxima.

Non-competitive antagonists

Non-competitive antagonists block the response to an agonist at some point within the cascade of intracellular events. Both the antagonist and the agonist bind independently of each other, and the antagonist drug may dissociate so slowly from the receptor that its action is very prolonged. In general, non-competitive antagonists reduce both the maximal response and the slope of the agonist concentration–response curve. An example of a drug in this category is buprenorphine, which is a partial agonist at the μ-opioid receptor but that acts as a non-competitive antagonist in the presence of an opioid receptor agonist because it occupies and dissociates slowly from the receptor.

Allosteric effects

Allosteric modulators indirectly alter the function of a receptor in either a positive (allosteric agonist) or negative (allosteric antagonist) way. These drugs bind to a distinct (allosteric) site on the receptor that is separate from the orthosteric site (Fig 3.4). Allosteric modulators can alter the function of receptors and produce a pharmacological response by:

- activating the receptor, causing a different biological response to the agonist
- altering the binding affinity of the receptor agonist
- changing the efficacy of receptor activation by the agonist.

The most prominent example of allosteric modulators is a class of drugs called benzodiazepines that includes diazepam and temazepam (see Chapter 20). Binding of benzodiazepines to an allosteric site on the GABAA receptor increases the affinity of the receptor for the endogenous inhibitory neurotransmitter GABA, thus inhibiting neurotransmission and leading to a range of sedative effects.

Concentration–response relationship

When making decisions about the use of a drug, it is important to know how big an effect the drug will have and how much drug is required to have an effect. These considerations are addressed by the concentration–response relationship, which is commonly depicted as a drug concentration–response curve.

How does knowledge of the concentration–response relationship for a drug serve a useful purpose? When an agonist drug is administered, the response usually increases in proportion to the dose until the receptors are saturated. Increasing the dose further at this stage does not produce any further increase in response. The sigmoidal shape of the concentration–response curve on a logarithmic plot includes a linear portion that occurs between 20% and 80% of the maximal response. This section 'most often applies to drugs at therapeutic concentrations and increasing drug concentration above 80% maximal response achieves very little in terms of extra therapeutic effects, but increases the risk of adverse effects' (Birkett 1995) (Fig 3.5).

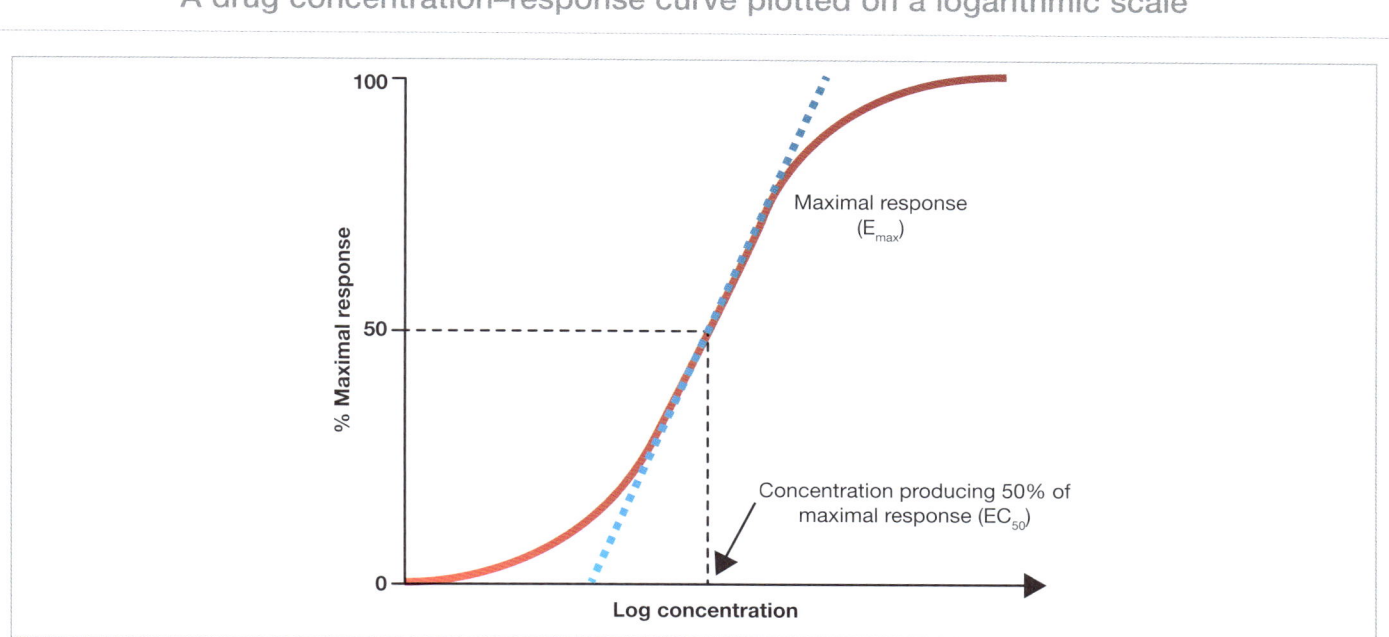

A drug concentration–response curve plotted on a logarithmic scale

FIGURE 3.5 The EC50 is the drug concentration at which 50% of the maximal response is observed. Emax is the maximal response when all the receptors are occupied.

Potency

Drugs are often referred to as being 'potent' or 'very potent', but what does this mean and how is it calculated? If we think about the concentration–response relationship, **potency** is the measure of how much drug is required to have an effect. For example, fentanyl and oxycodone are two opioid analgesics that relieve pain by activating μ-opioid receptors. As a highly potent drug, fentanyl elicits a response at a very low concentration. Oxycodone, a less potent drug, is able to elicit the same response but requires a much higher concentration to do so. The more potent a drug, the lower the dose that is required (i.e. a lower dose of fentanyl compared with oxycodone to achieve the same analgesic effect). Potency is measured as the EC50, which can reflect either the concentration that causes half the maximal effect (graded relationship) or the concentration that causes an effect in half the population (quantal relationship). Plotting the concentration–response data for several drugs using a semi-logarithmic scale allows us easily to visualise the relative potencies of the drugs (Fig 3.6).

Efficacy

Another term that is commonly used to describe drugs is maximal efficacy. Often simply called efficacy, this is a measure of 'how big an effect the drug will have' when all targets are occupied. Again, the concentration–response curves allow us to visualise the efficacy of a drug – that is, the maximum response a drug can produce (Emax). Several drugs can have the same potency but differ in their efficacy (Fig 3.7). Conversely, as shown in Figure 3.6, drugs may differ in potency but have the same efficacy. This is important clinically, because the maximal effectiveness of a drug depends on its efficacy and not on its potency. To illustrate this point, let us assume that the three drugs in Figure 3.8 are used as analgesics to manage the pain of a woman following ceasarean section. The question could be asked: Does it matter which drug is used if they are equipotent (possessing the same potency) analgesics? Knowing the concentration–response curves for the various drugs would provide the answer. Drugs A and B would provide a greater clinical response (better analgesia) than drug C because they have greater efficacy.

Let us now consider the effect on the concentration–response curve of an agonist in the presence of a competitive antagonist. The curve is shifted to the right. How far it is shifted to the right depends on the concentration of the competitive antagonist in displacing the agonist and the affinity of the antagonist for the receptor. This indicates that a much higher concentration of agonist is needed to produce 50% of the maximal response (EC_{50}), but in this situation maximal efficacy of the agonist is unchanged (Fig 3.8).

For health professionals, understanding drug efficacy is clinically very important. For example, consider two

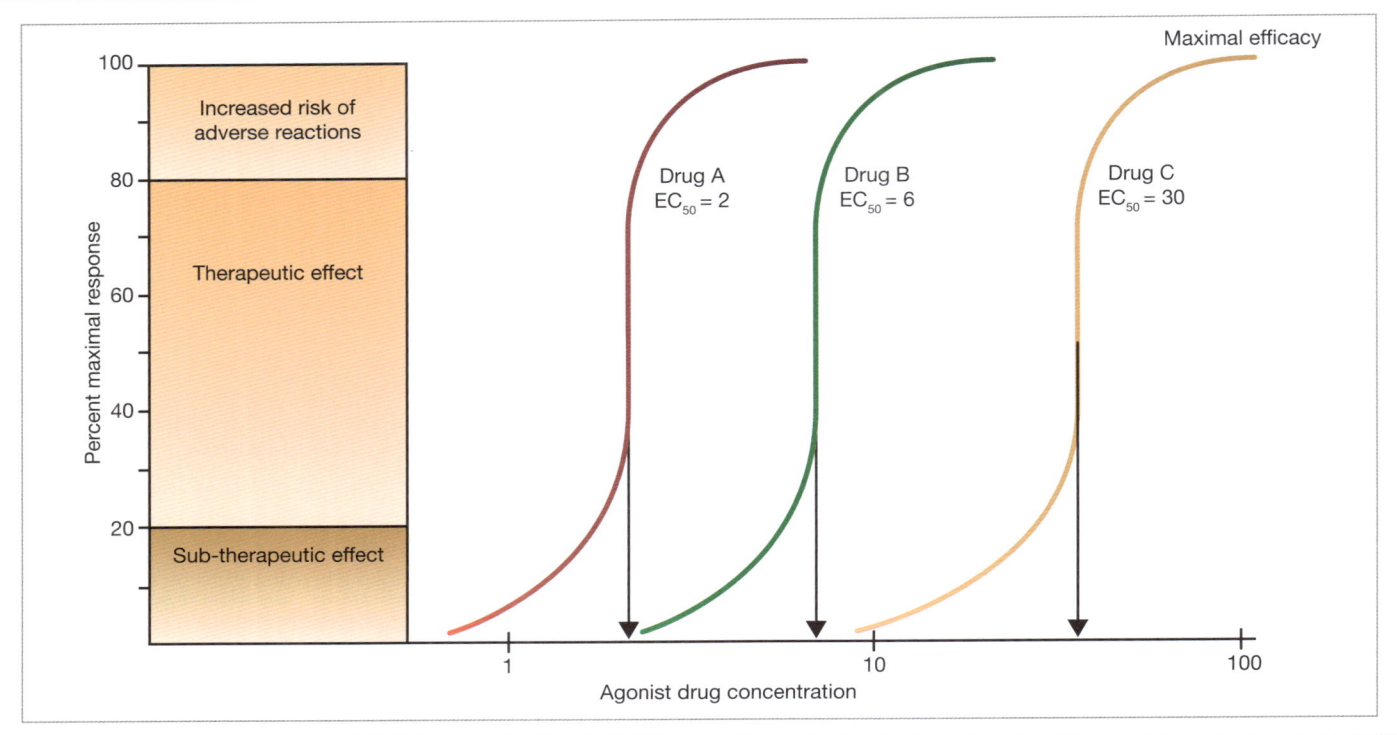

Theoretical concentration–response curves on a logarithmic scale for drugs A, B and C

FIGURE 3.6 The drugs are all agonists acting on the same receptor and eliciting the same response. Drug A (EC50 = 2) is three times more potent than is B (EC50 = 6), which is five times more potent than C (EC50 = 30). Drugs A, B and C all differ in their potency but have the same maximal efficacy.

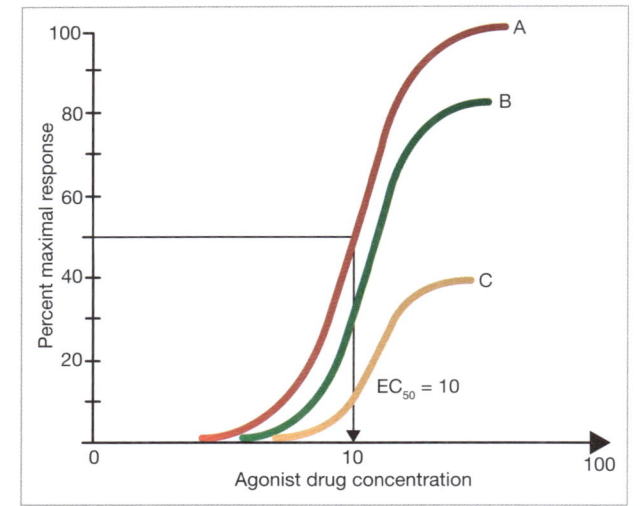

Concentration–response curves for drugs A, B and C, all with the same potency (EC50 = 10) but different maximal response.

FIGURE 3.7 In this example, drugs B and C are classed as partial agonists as they produce less than the maximal effect achieved with the full agonist drug A.

drugs that have the same affinity for opioid receptors, which mediates analgesia and constipation. Drug A is an agonist and drug B is an antagonist. If you administer drug A, it will produce analgesia but cause constipation as a side effect. If you administer drug B, it will result in reversal of both the analgesic effect and constipation. Understanding other aspects of the pharmacokinetics of both drugs opens opportunities to make use of the benefits of both. For example, naloxone, an opioid antagonist, is poorly absorbed orally but effective in the gut. When combined with the opioid agonist oxycodone which is well absorbed from the gut, the combination produces good analgesia but avoids much of the constipation seen when oxycodone is used in isolation.

KEY POINTS

Pharmacodynamics

- An agonist binds to the orthosteric site of the receptor (governed by affinity) and activates the receptor (governed by efficacy) to produce the same response as the endogenous ligand.

Competitive antagonism of the response produced by drug A (curve 1) by increasing concentrations (curves 2 and 3) of the competitive antagonist drug B

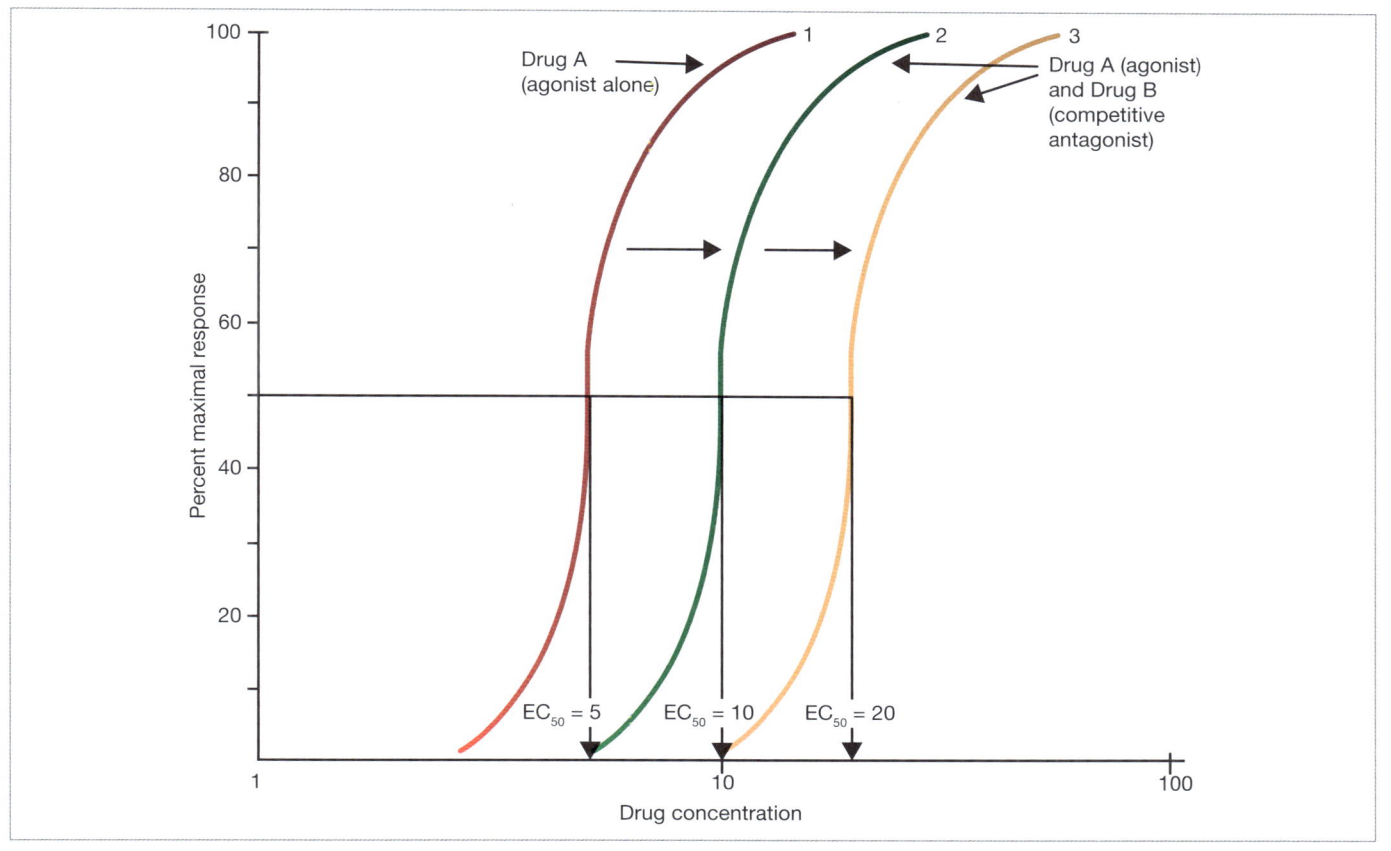

FIGURE 3.8 Note the shift of the concentration–response curve to the right without a change in the maximal efficacy of drug A.

- Partial agonists produce less than the maximal effect caused by the endogenous ligand, even when all receptors are occupied.

- An antagonist binds to a receptor and blocks access of the endogenous ligand, diminishing the normal response.

- When a drug is administered, the response usually increases in proportion to the dose until the receptors are saturated. Increasing the dose further does not produce any further increase in response.

- Potency is measured as the EC50, which is the concentration at which a drug produces 50% of its maximal response.

- Efficacy refers to the ability of a drug to elicit a response once it is bound to the molecular target. The maximal efficacy of a drug is the maximum response a drug can produce.

- The clinical effectiveness of a drug depends on its efficacy, not on its potency.

REVIEW EXERCISES

1 Ella is admitted to the antenatal ward. She is 35 weeks pregnant. She is diagnosed with gestational hypertension and receives a stat dose of labetalol, a β-adrenoceptor antagonist, to decrease her blood pressure. She is also prescribed methyldopa, a centrally acting α2-adrenergic agonist. Considering the pathways that these two drugs work on, explain how a receptor agonist and a receptor antagonist could both be used to treat the same disease state.

2 Suzy has been prescribed norethisterone 350 micrograms daily as a safe contraceptive alternative to use during breastfeeding. The pharmacy has run out, but has another equally effective progestogen-based contraceptive available – levonorgestrel. Only 30 micrograms of levonorgestrel are in each dose. Using

your knowledge of drug potency, explain why two drugs in the same drug class can have the same clinical effect but require different doses.

3 Emma has had a caesarean section and needs postoperative pain management. There are many drug options that are available for managing pain. As a health professional, discuss the practical importance of maximal drug efficacy in managing pain.

REFERENCES

Birkett DJ. Pharmacokinetics made easy 10 Pharmacodynamics – the concentration–effect relationship. Aust Prescr. 1995;18: 102-104. doi.org/10.18773/austprescr.1995.088

Prevost M, Zelkowitz P, Tulandi T, et al. Oxytocin in pregnancy and the postpartum: relations to labor and its management. Front Public Health. 2014;2:1. doi: 10.3389/fpubh.2014.00001

State of Queensland (Queensland Health) 2022. Queensland Clinical Guidelines – Methotrexate treatment for ectopic pregnancy. https://www.health.qld.gov.au/__data/assets/pdf_file/0038/1189595/c-epl-methotrexate.pdf

Uvnäs-Moberg K, Ekström-Bergström A, Berg M et al. Maternal plasma levels of oxytocin during physiological childbirth – a systematic review with implications for uterine contractions and central actions of oxytocin. BMC Pregnancy Childbirth. 2019 Aug 9;19(1):285. https://doi.org/10.1186/s12884-019-2365-9

DRUG ABSORPTION, DISTRIBUTION, METABOLISM AND EXCRETION

Maryam Bazargan, Kirsten Small

Key Abbreviations

ABC	ATP binding cassette
ATP	adenosine triphosphate
CYP	cytochrome P450
GIT	gastrointestinal tract
MRP	multidrug resistance protein
SLC	solute carrier
UGT	UDP-glucuronosyltransferase

Key Terms

Chapter Focus

The duration and extent of exposure by an individual to a drug is a key determinant of its therapeutic efficacy and tolerability. Inadequate exposure results in a lack of efficacy ('therapeutic failure'), while excessive exposure increases the risk of toxicity and reduces tolerability. Drug exposure is determined by the processes of absorption, distribution, metabolism, and excretion. Understanding these processes provides a theoretical framework for inter-individual variability in exposure and the design of drug dosing regimens.

Learning Outcomes

- Understand drug absorption and how different routes of administration impact the rate and extent of drug absorption and the 'bioavailability' of drugs.
- Explain drug distribution and elimination, and how clinical factors can modify these.
- Understand the impact of ionisation and protein binding on drug distribution.
- Understand elimination of drugs – metabolism and excretion.
- Understand drug disposition between mother and fetus through the placenta 'fetal exposure to drugs'.
- Understand the pharmacokinetics of drugs in the fetus.
- Critically apply pharmacokinetic knowledge in the pharmacological management of a pregnant woman.

CRITICAL THINKING SCENARIO

Michelle is 30 weeks pregnant and has undergone emergency surgery for a fractured arm due to a fall. While in hospital she was receiving 10 mg of intramuscular morphine twice daily. As part of her hospital discharge, she is given a prescription for oral morphine. The prescription is for ten 30 mg morphine tablets and the instructions say to take one tablet every 12 hours for the next 5 days.

1 Is this a medication error?

2 If not, what is the reason for Michelle being given an oral dose of morphine that is three times greater than the intramuscular dose she was taking while in hospital?

3 Does morphine cross the placenta and is it safe for the fetus?

Introduction

For a drug to produce an effect, it must interact with a molecular target. The concentration of drug that interacts with the target is influenced by pharmacokinetics, or how the drug passes through the body via the processes of **absorption**, **distribution**, **metabolism**, and **excretion** (known as **ADME phases**). Absorption, distribution, metabolism, and excretion are predicated on two main mechanisms that relate to the movement of drugs: passive diffusion and carrier-mediated transport.

The relationship between these four processes is shown in Figure 4.1. The study of the passage of a drug through the body via these processes is collectively described by the term **pharmacokinetics**, or simply 'what the body does to the drug'.

Many physiological changes that occur during pregnancy and the early postpartum period affect the pharmacokinetics of drugs. These changes affect the woman's responses to any drug during pregnancy and lactation, and impact on the potential drug exposure of the developing fetus and child.

4.1 Drug absorption

Absorption is an important factor for all routes of drug administration with the exception of the intravenous route, where the drug is administered directly into the systemic circulation and does not require absorption from the site of administration.

Before a drug can be distributed to its site of action, it must be absorbed from the point of application into the systemic circulation. An oral drug may be in a solid form (tablet, capsule, or powder) or in liquid form (solution or suspension). Disintegration of solid dosage forms must occur before dissolution, a process by which a drug goes into solution and becomes available for absorption (Fig 4.2). To be absorbed, a drug must be in solution. The more soluble the drug, the more rapidly it will be presented for

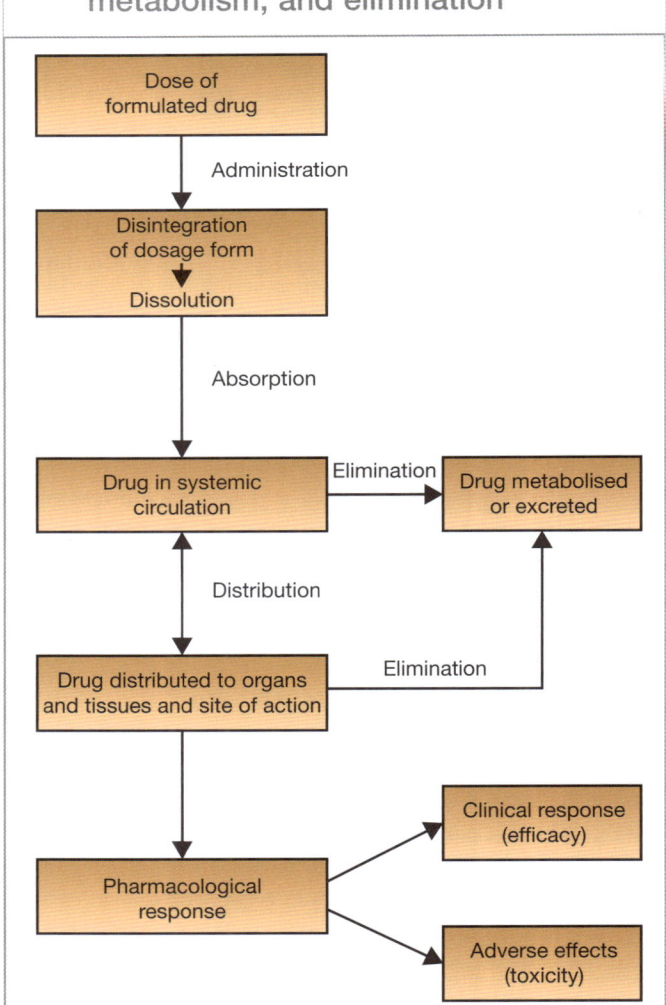

Interrelationship between drug absorption, distribution, metabolism, and elimination

FIGURE 4.1 Note: For some drugs the site of action is the vascular system.

The processes of tablet disintegration, dissolution, and drug absorption

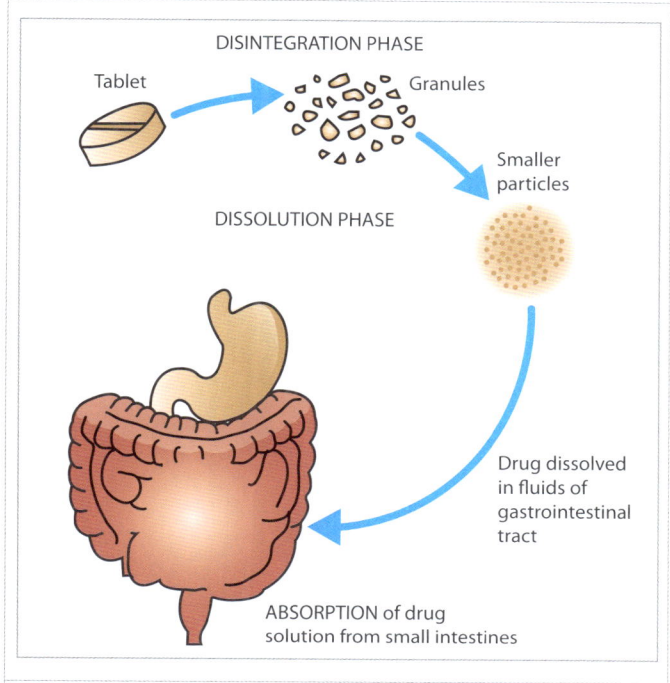

DISINTEGRATION PHASE

Tablet

Granules

Smaller particles

DISSOLUTION PHASE

Drug dissolved in fluids of gastrointestinal tract

ABSORPTION of drug solution from small intestines

FIGURE 4.2

Source: Salerno 1999, Figure 4-2; used with permission.

absorption. For orally administered drugs, absorption is as follows, from fastest to slowest: liquids, elixirs, and syrups > suspensions > powders > capsules > tablets > coated tablets > enteric-coated tablets and sustained (or controlled or 'slow' release) formulations.

Absorption across biological membranes

For absorption to occur, it is necessary for a drug to cross cell membranes in the gut and vascular system. The cell membrane typically consists of a lipid bilayer that contains protein molecules irregularly dispersed throughout it. Lipid-soluble drugs readily pass through the lipid membrane, while ionised (charged) drugs have difficulty crossing cell membranes. The membrane also contains narrow-diameter aqueous channels called aquaporins, which permit the passage of small uncharged water-soluble substances such as urea as well as water itself, but not the passage of drugs given their larger size. Absorption of drugs occurs by two main processes: **passive diffusion** and **carrier-mediated transport** (Fig 4.3).

Passive diffusion

Most drugs cross membranes by passive diffusion, which is the transfer of the drug across the membrane from a region of higher concentration to a region of lower concentration until equilibrium is established (Fig 4.3). Passive diffusion is influenced by the surface area of the membrane exposed to the drug, the concentration gradient of the drug, and its lipid–water partition coefficient. For acidic and basic drugs, diffusion is also influenced by the ionisation state.

Carrier-mediated transport

In contrast to passive diffusion, carrier-mediated transport requires the involvement of a membrane protein. Carrier-mediated transport may be active (requiring energy) or facilitated (not requiring energy – Fig 4.3). Active transport processes permit the movement of a compound against a concentration gradient (from an area of low concentration to an area of high concentration) or, in the case of ions, against the electrochemical gradient (e.g. the sodium–potassium 'pump'). The role of transporters in drug disposition is complex, and this is an ongoing area of research. It is now clear, however, that they play important roles in drug absorption from the gastrointestinal tract (GIT).

Variables affecting drug absorption

The rate and extent to which a drug is absorbed are influenced by the physicochemical properties of the drug and the physiological characteristics of the absorption site.

Nature of the cell membrane that the drug must traverse

The surface area of the absorbing site is an important determinant of drug absorption. Larger absorbing surfaces ease greater drug absorption and the more rapid effects. Gaseous anaesthetics are absorbed immediately from the pulmonary epithelium because of the large surface area of the lung. The small intestine, which also offers a large surface area, is another site from which drugs are efficiently absorbed.

Blood flow

Blood circulation to the site of administration is a significant determinant of the rate and extent of drug absorption. A rich blood supply (e.g. the sublingual route) enhances absorption, whereas a poor vascular site (e.g. the subcutaneous route) delays it. This is because removal of the drug in blood following absorption maintains the concentration gradient necessary for passive diffusion. An individual in shock, for example, may not respond to intramuscularly administered drugs because of poor peripheral circulation. Drugs injected intravenously, on the other hand, are placed directly into the systemic circulation and are immediately available to exert an effect. Food increases splanchnic blood flow and can enhance absorption of orally administered drugs.

Movement of drugs across biological membranes by passive diffusion, facilitated transport, and active transport. Aquaporins allow passage of water and urea, but not drugs

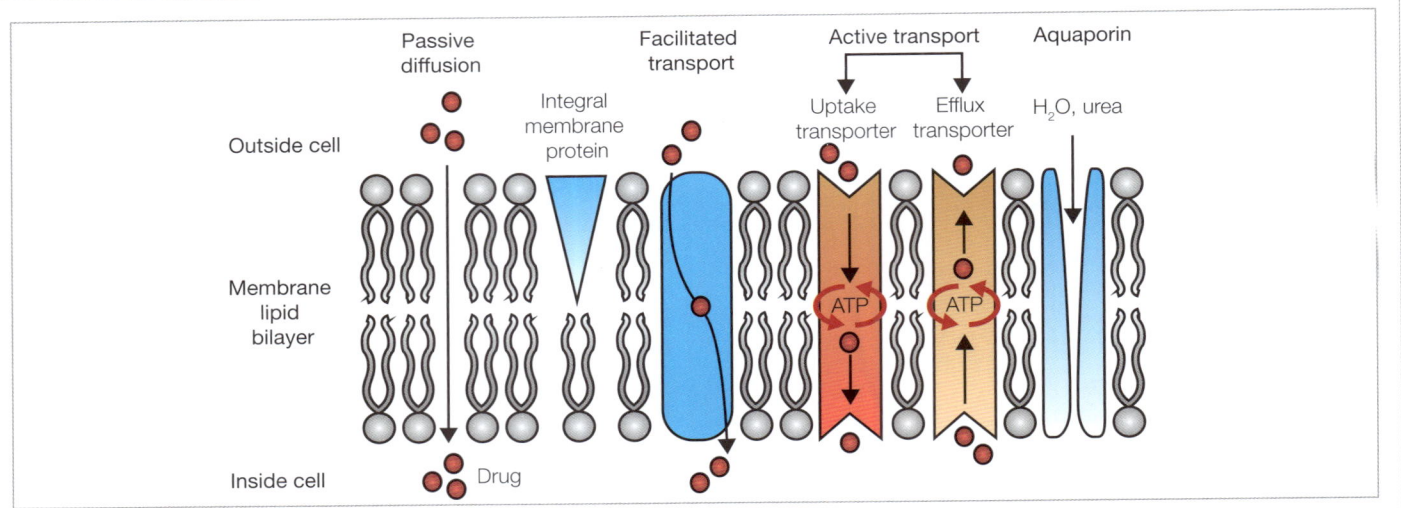

FIGURE 4.3

Solubility

Because cell membranes are composed of a lipid bilayer, lipid solubility is an essential attribute of drugs absorbed from certain areas (e.g. the GIT). Chemicals and minerals that form insoluble precipitates in the GIT, such as barium salts, drugs that are resins (e.g. the bile acid-binding resin cholestyramine), and drugs that are not soluble in water or lipids are not absorbed.

Ionisation

Many drugs are weak acids or weak bases that are present in body fluids as either ionised or un-ionised forms. The ionised (charged polar) form is usually water-soluble (lipid-insoluble) and does not diffuse readily through the cell membranes of the body. In contrast, the un-ionised (neutral, non-polar) form of a drug is more lipid-soluble (less water-soluble) and is more capable of crossing cell membranes. In general, an acidic drug is relatively un-ionised in an acid environment such as the stomach, but a basic drug tends to ionise in the same acid environment. In contrast, a basic drug is less ionised in a less acidic site such as the small intestine, while the acidic drug tends to be more ionised. Despite the varying states of ionisation, negligible drug absorption occurs in the stomach (because of the small surface area, the thick lining of mucus and tight intracellular junctions), whereas most drugs are absorbed in the small intestine (duodenum, jejunum, and ileum).

The extent of ionisation is determined by the pH of the environment. To illustrate how a change in pH affects ionisation, consider the following example. Drug X is a weak acid with a pKa of 5. In an acidic environment of pH 2, pH − pKa = −3 and drug X will be ~0.1% ionised. In this situation the majority of drug X is un-ionised and hence available to diffuse across cell membranes. However, in a more basic environment (pH 8), pH − pKa = 3 and drug X will be ~99.9% ionised. Conversely, if a drug is a weak base (pKa ~8), in an acidic environment of pH 3, pH − pKa = −5 and hence a basic drug will be over 99.9% ionised and only the 0.1% of the drug that is un-ionised will diffuse across cell membranes.

Formulation

Drug formulations can be manipulated to achieve desirable absorption characteristics. A drug can be coated with a resin or contained in a matrix from which it is slowly released. Sustained (or controlled) release formulations are useful for drugs that have a short elimination half-life (see Chapter 5). Drugs may also be prepared with a coating that offers relative resistance to the acidic environment of the stomach (e.g. enteric coating). Enteric coatings on drugs are used to:

- prevent decomposition of chemically sensitive drugs by gastric acid (e.g. penicillin G and erythromycin are unstable at an acidic pH), thus improving bioavailability
- prevent dilution of the drug before it reaches the intestine
- prevent nausea and vomiting induced by the effect of the drug in the stomach
- provide delayed release of the drug.

Routes of drug administration

The route of drug administration can affect both the rate of onset of action and the magnitude of the therapeutic response that results. When a drug is given for a systemic effect, absorption is an essential first step before the drug enters the systemic circulation and is distributed to a location distant from the site of administration.

A drug may enter the circulation either by being injected there directly (intravenously) or by absorption from other extravascular sites. The traditional or standard routes of drug administration fall into the following major categories:

- oral (also called enteral)
- parenteral – includes subcutaneous, intramuscular, intravenous, intrathecal, or epidermal
- inhalation
- topical
- rectal.

New technologies continue to emerge, with drugs delivered by drug-eluting stents in cardiology, the application of nanoparticles targeting brain tumours, administration of antibody–drug conjugates in cancer chemotherapy, the use of nanocarriers for transdermal vaccine administration, and miniature micro-electromechanical devices for passive and active drug delivery.

Oral route

Oral, or enteral, ingestion is the most common route for drug administration. It is a safe, convenient, and economical route of administration. However, the frequent changes in the GIT environment produced by food, emotion, physical activity, and other medications may at times make absorption of drugs unreliable and slow. Drugs may be absorbed from several sites along the GIT and they may also be metabolised by enzymes in the gastrointestinal mucosa before they are absorbed and enter the systemic circulation.

Absorption from the oral cavity

Although the oral cavity possesses a thin lining, a rich blood supply, and a slightly acidic pH, little absorption occurs in the mouth. However, despite its small surface area, the oral mucosa is capable of absorbing certain drugs as long as they dissolve rapidly in the salivary secretions (i.e. drugs given by sublingual or buccal routes). In sublingual administration the drug is placed under the tongue to permit tablet dissolution in salivary secretions. Misoprostol, used to induce labour, can be administered in this manner, and the person is advised to refrain as long as possible from swallowing saliva containing the tablet form of the drug. Misoprostol has a rapid sublingual absorption and therefore the shortest time to peak serum concentration. Drugs absorbed sublingually enter the systemic circulation directly without entering the portal system, thus bypassing the liver and escaping first-pass metabolism. Accordingly, absorption is rapid, and the effects of the drug may become apparent within 2 minutes. With buccal administration the drug (tablet) is placed between the teeth and the mucous membrane of the cheek. Glucose gel administration for managing transient neonatal hypoglycaemia uses this route as it is achieving a rapid onset of action.

Absorption from the stomach

Although the stomach has a rich blood supply, it has a thick layer of mucus, tight intracellular junctions, and a relatively small surface area. It is therefore not a major site of drug absorption. The length of time a drug remains in the stomach is a significant variable in determining the rate of gastrointestinal absorption. Generally, a slow gastric emptying rate decreases the rate of drug absorption in the small intestine. This is why many drugs are administered on an empty stomach, with sufficient water to ensure dissolution of the drug and rapid passage into the small intestine. (Drugs that cause gastric irritation are usually given with food.) After solid-dose drug administration the recipient should be encouraged to sit upright for at least 30 minutes to shorten gastric emptying time (the time required for the drug to reach the small intestine) and to reduce the potential for tablets or capsules to lodge in the oesophageal area.

Absorption from the small intestine

The small intestine is highly vascularised and, with its many villi, presents a significantly larger and more permeable absorption surface compared with the stomach. It is the major site for absorbing orally administered drugs that pass from the stomach into this region, and drugs are absorbed primarily in the upper part of the small intestine. The pH of the intestinal fluid, which is close to neutral (ranging from 5.5 to 7 in the duodenum to 7.5 in the ileum), influences the extent of ionisation of a drug within the lumen of the GIT. It should be noted, however, that ionisation of a weak acid or a weak base does not prevent absorption from the small intestine.

Weak acids and weak bases exist in biological fluids in a dynamic equilibrium between the more lipid-soluble un-ionised form and the more water-soluble ionised forms (Fig 4.4). The un-ionised (lipid-soluble) form of the drug is readily absorbed across the small intestinal membrane. Because of the dynamic nature of the equilibrium, more ionised drug is then converted to the un-ionised form to compensate for the amount absorbed, and the un-ionised drug then in turn becomes available for absorption. Consequently, most weak acids and weak bases are well absorbed after oral administration. By contrast, strongly acidic (e.g. the H1 receptor antagonist proxicromil) and basic drugs (e.g. gentamicin) are not

Weak acids and weak bases exist in biological fluids in a dynamic equilibrium between the more lipid-soluble un-ionised form (HA) and the more water-soluble ionised form (A− + H+). The un-ionised form of the drug (HA) is readily absorbed across the small intestinal membrane into the bloodstream where it dissociates, re-establishing the dynamic equilibrium between HA and A− + H+. In the lumen of the small intestine, because of the dynamic nature of the equilibrium, more ionised drug is then converted to the un-ionised form to compensate for the amount absorbed; the un-ionised drug then in turn becomes available for absorption

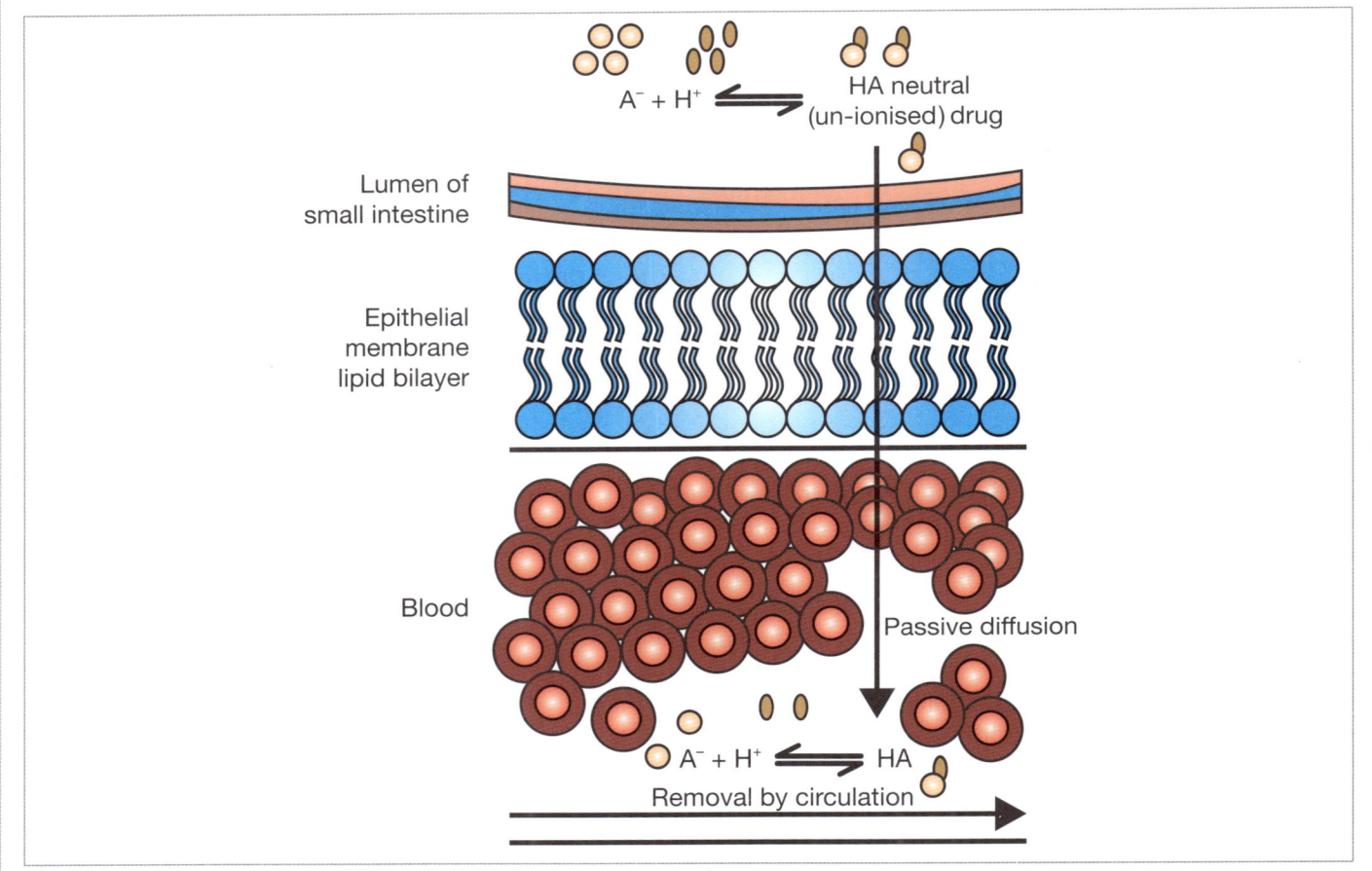

FIGURE 4.4

absorbed when given orally because essentially all drug present in the small intestine will be ionised.

Although passive diffusion is the dominant process involved in the absorption of most drugs, uptake transporters have been identified on the apical (luminal) membrane of enterocytes and possibly contribute to drug absorption. Efflux transporters that move drugs into rather than out of the intestinal lumen are also expressed on the apical membrane of enterocytes. These limit the absorption of some drugs since, following oral absorption, the drug may be actively transported back into the lumen of the small intestine. Efflux transporters are also expressed in placental tissue, especially in the first trimester, and are believed to reduce fetal exposure to some drugs and exogenous compounds (Fig 4.5) (Blackburn 2017).

Absorption from the rectum

The surface area of the rectum is not very large, but drug absorption does occur because of extensive vascularity. The veins of the rectum include the superior, middle, and inferior veins. Only the superior rectal veins unite to

Transport across the placental barrier

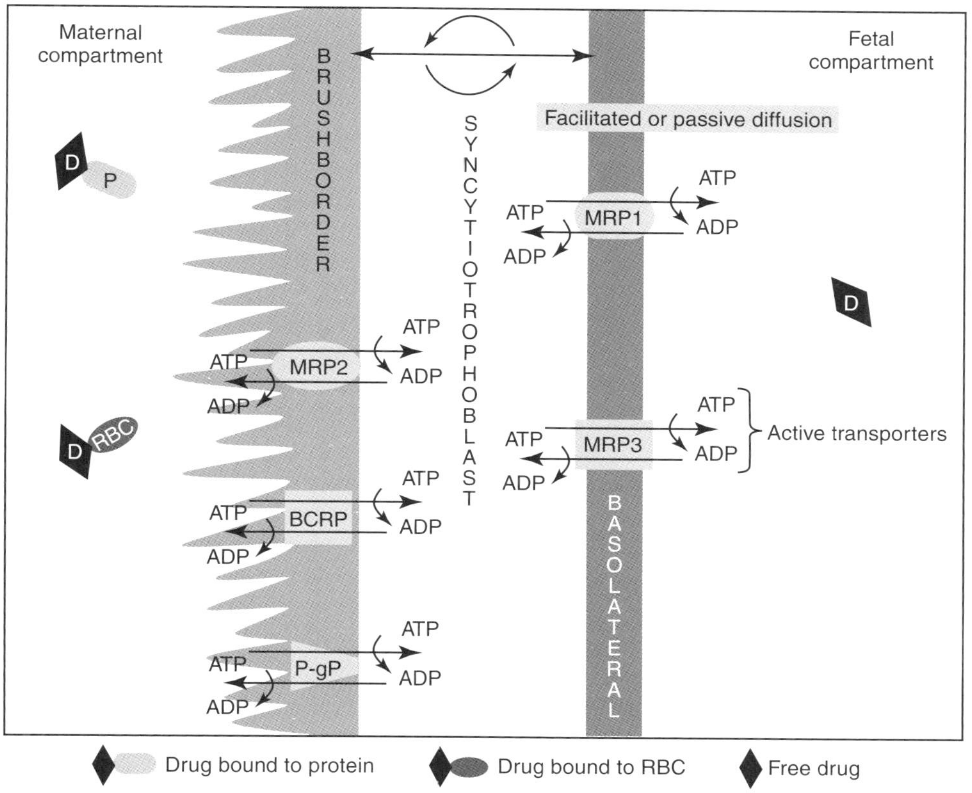

FIGURE 4.5

Source: Adapted from Gedeon C, Koren G. Designing pregnancy centered medications: drugs which do not cross the human placenta. Placenta. 2006; 27(8):861-868. ISSN 0143-4004, https://doi.org/10.1016/j.placenta.2005.09.001.

form the inferior mesenteric vein, which is a tributary of the portal vein. A drug absorbed via the superior rectal veins flows to the liver via the portal vein and is metabolised, while the remainder of the drug that is absorbed (approximately 50%) escapes first-pass metabolism as it bypasses the liver. Rectal drug administration may be used for both local and systemic effects. This route is often used in unconscious individuals, in fasting patients, in those unable to swallow or when severe vomiting is present. Disadvantages to rectal drug administration include erratic absorption because of rectal contents, interruption of drug absorption resulting from defecation, local drug irritation with some medications, uncertainty of drug retention, and acceptability to the medication user.

Parenteral route

'Parenteral administration' commonly refers to the administration of drugs by injection. Intravenous administration is the most rapidly effective route of drug administration, with high concentrations achieved quickly in the systemic circulation. The **bioavailability** of a drug administered intravenously is 100% because the entire dose is delivered directly into the systemic circulation. Absorption from subcutaneous or intramuscular injection sites is faster than via the oral route but is less reliable because local blood flow and diffusion through the tissue influences the pattern of absorption.

1 *Subcutaneous:* A subcutaneous injection of a drug is given beneath the skin into the connective tissue or fat immediately underlying the dermis. This site can be used only for drugs that are not irritating to the tissue, otherwise severe pain, necrosis, and sloughing of tissue may occur. The rate of absorption is slow and can provide a sustained effect.

2 *Intramuscular:* 'Intramuscular administration' refers to the injection of a drug solution into muscle. Most often the drug is fully soluble in an aqueous solution and absorption occurs more rapidly than with subcutaneous injection because of greater tissue blood flow. However, not all drugs are formulated as aqueous solutions. Procaine penicillin is poorly

soluble and is injected as an aqueous suspension that is slowly absorbed and hence has a prolonged duration of action. Some steroid hormones are synthesised as chemical esters, which increases their solubility in oil and slows the rate of absorption. Drug absorption via this route may occur at different rates in obese or emaciated people because of differences in subcutaneous fat distribution.

3 *Intravenous:* This route of drug administration has both advantages and disadvantages. The intravenous route produces an immediate pharmacological response because the desired amount of drug is injected directly into the bloodstream, thereby circumventing the absorption process. However, adverse effects may occur because of the rapid attainment of a high plasma concentration. Intravenous drugs may be given as a bolus dose or by constant infusion, which should generally be administered slowly to prevent adverse effects.

4 *Intrathecal:* 'Intrathecal drug administration' means the drug is injected directly into the spinal subarachnoid space, bypassing the blood–brain barrier. Many compounds cannot enter the cerebrospinal fluid or are absorbed in this region only very slowly. When rapid central nervous system effects of drugs are desired – for example, with spinal anaesthesia or in treatment of acute infection of the central nervous system – this route may be used.

5 *Epidural:* 'Epidural drug administration' refers to the injection of a drug within the spinal canal on or outside the dura mater that surrounds the spinal column.

6 *Inhalation:* The lungs provide a large surface area for absorption and the alveolar membrane is thin. The rich capillary network adjacent to the alveolar membrane promotes ready entry of drugs into the bloodstream. Drug delivery via the lungs avoids first-pass extraction by the liver. Drugs such as bronchodilators are administered by various metered-dose inhalation devices (nebulisers, 'puffers'), delivering the drug during inhalation into the airway, producing primarily a local effect with reduced systemic adverse effects compared with oral administration.

Topical route

Depending on the site of application, absorption of drugs applied topically to the skin and mucous membranes is generally rapid. Examples include cutaneous application, nasal sprays, vaginal creams/gels, and eyedrops.

1 *Skin*: Drugs applied to the skin are used to produce either a local or a systemic effect through the use of ointments or transdermal patches. Passage across the stratum corneum, the outer hard layer of skin, is rate-limiting. However, following passage through the stratum corneum, lipophilic drugs diffuse freely through the remainder of the epidermis and dermis. The dermis is perfused by capillaries, which aids dermal drug absorption by maintaining a concentration gradient. Absorption occurs more readily through abraded or burnt skin, and factors that enhance cutaneous blood flow or hydrate the skin also increase absorption – for example, massaging, warming the skin, or covering with an occlusive dressing.

2 *Eyes:* Topical administration of ophthalmic drugs produces a local effect on the conjunctiva or anterior chamber. Systemic absorption can occur through drainage from the naso-lacrimal canal and, as this route bypasses the liver (no first-pass metabolism), adverse systemic effects may occur (e.g. unwanted effects due to the use of corticosteroid eyedrops). Suspensions and ointments are also used and eye/lid movements may promote the distribution of drug over the surface of the eye.

3 *Ears:* Otic administration of drops into the auditory canal may be chosen to treat local infection, inflammatory conditions, or to help remove wax in the external ear.

4 *Nose:* Nasal drops or sprays containing medications may be applied or sprayed directly onto the nasal mucosa. This route is commonly used for treatment of sinus conditions resulting from viral infection or hay fever.

5 *Vagina:* Vaginal medications are used for local and systemic effects. For treatment of vaginal infections, creams, tablets, or gels are used. Progesterone pessaries are used as prophylaxis for preterm birth prevention. Induction of labour with prostaglandin gel or pessaries uses the vaginal route of administration.

Bioavailability

After a drug crosses the membranes of the GIT, it enters the portal vein. The portal vein then carries the blood containing the drug to the liver, which is the main site of drug metabolism. The drug may pass through the liver and enter the systemic circulation as intact parent drug (unmetabolised) or may undergo metabolism in the liver. The extent to which a drug is metabolised (extracted) by the liver is highly variable. The fraction of the drug dose absorbed from the GIT and the fraction of absorbed drug that escapes first-pass metabolism by the liver, determine the amount of intact drug reaching the systemic circulation.

First-pass metabolism

After absorption, orally administered drugs travel first through the portal system and the liver before entering the systemic circulation. Depending on whether the drug is metabolised or not, a variable amount of drug can be extracted (EH) by the liver before the drug ever reaches the systemic circulation. In the example shown in Figure 4.5, 80 mg of the drug reaches the liver and 60 mg is extracted in the first pass through the liver. Consequently, the bioavailability of that drug is 20% and hence only 20 mg (a small fraction of the original 100 mg dose) is available for distribution and to produce a pharmacological effect. For such medications the oral drug dose is calculated to compensate for **first-pass effect**. For example, morphine undergoes significant first-pass metabolism – 30 mg oral morphine is equivalent to 10 mg morphine administered intramuscularly, intravenously, or subcutaneously.

Absorption of drugs during pregnancy

Pregnancy delays gastric emptying and decreases motility, which can increase or decrease drug absorption. For example, drugs that require an acidic environment for absorption such as iron tablets may have a delayed absorption pattern because of lower production of hydrochloric acid in the stomach during pregnancy. In addition, frequent vomiting may prevent normal oral drug administration and also alter the plasma concentration of a drug because of unpredictable absorption.

KEY POINTS

Absorption

- Absorption is defined as the process by which unchanged drug proceeds from the site of administration into the blood. It is an important factor for all routes of administration except intravenous administration.

- Variables that affect drug absorption include the nature of the absorbing membrane, blood flow, the solubility of the drug, the degree of ionisation, and formulation characteristics.

- Bioavailability of a drug is defined as the proportion of the administered dose that reaches the systemic circulation intact.

- Two factors determining bioavailability are the amount of drug absorbed from the GIT and the amount of drug escaping hepatic extraction.

- Physiological changes during pregnancy can affect the absorption of drugs.

4.2 Distribution

After a drug reaches the systemic circulation, it can be distributed to various body compartments within the body. Distribution is defined as the process of reversible transfer of a drug between one location and another (one of which is usually blood) in the body (Fig 4.1). Some drugs remain almost exclusively in blood. These include penicillin and warfarin. Other drugs are distributed to well-perfused organs (e.g. heart, liver, and kidneys), and the drug concentration in these organs may be high initially. Drugs are distributed more slowly to organs with poor blood supply, which include skeletal muscles and fat. Eventually, the concentration of drug equalises in all body organs. An example of a drug that is widely distributed in the body is morphine.

The rate and extent to which a drug enters the different compartments of the body depends on the properties of the drug and the tissue. This includes the permeability of the capillaries, perfusion, the presence of drug transporters, and the partitioning of the drug between the vascular and tissue compartment (e.g. the blood–brain barrier, or the placental barrier). As already discussed, lipid-soluble (un-ionised) drugs can readily cross capillary membranes to enter most tissues and fluid compartments, whereas ionised (lipid-insoluble) drugs do not diffuse readily across membranes.

Plasma protein binding

On entry into the systemic circulation, a proportion of free drug molecules binds reversibly to proteins and lipoproteins to form drug–protein complexes. Plasma protein binding is commonly expressed as a percentage, which represents the proportion of the total drug bound, or as the fraction unbound (e.g. 75% bound corresponds to a fraction unbound of 0.25). The extent of drug binding depends on the affinity or attraction of the drug for the protein, the relative concentrations of the drug and the protein, and the number of drug binding sites on the protein. Drugs with a high affinity for the binding protein will be more 'tightly' but still reversibly bound and the fraction of unbound drug will be low (i.e. the percentage bound is higher). Although plasma protein binding is a saturable process, the concentrations of most drugs in blood following therapeutic doses are generally lower than that required to saturate the binding sites on these proteins. However, there are exceptions. For example, the high plasma concentrations of salicylate achieved with anti-inflammatory doses as used in the treatment of rheumatoid arthritis can result in non-linear binding to albumin. Non-linear binding occurs when the concentration of the drug saturates the protein binding sites and adding more drug disproportionately increases the unbound concentration of the drug in plasma and can cause drug toxicity. Protein binding is a reversible and dynamic process, with bound and unbound drug in equilibrium.

Drug–protein complexes cannot cross membranes as the drug–protein molecule is too large to diffuse through the blood vessel membrane. Only free or unbound drug can cross membranes. As free drug is removed from the circulation (e.g. by distribution, metabolism, excretion), the drug–protein complex dissociates so more 'free' drug is released to replace what is 'lost'. This is important, as it is only the free or unbound drug that exerts a pharmacological effect. This is illustrated below. In this example, the initial plasma drug concentration is 100 mg/L, the fraction of drug that is bound to plasma proteins is 0.8 (80%) and the unbound fraction is 0.2 (20%).

Hypoalbuminaemia

Albumin is a common site for drug binding. Hypoalbuminaemia, or low levels of albumin in the blood, may be caused by hepatic dysfunction such as in severe preeclampsia. A relative fall in albumin concentration occurs in pregnancy due to a combination of haemodilution and renal loss. Lower albumin concentration results in an increase in free drug available for distribution to tissue sites. When a person is given the usual dosage of a drug in the presence of decreased plasma protein binding, more of the free (unbound) drug is available to exert a pharmacological effect. This may result in toxicity, and the drug dosage should be reduced.

Tissue binding

Adipose tissue

Lipid-soluble drugs have a high affinity for adipose tissue, which is where these drugs are stored. Moreover, the relatively low blood flow in adipose tissue makes it a stable reservoir for a limited number of drugs. Accumulation in adipose tissue is one reason for a drug having a prolonged half-life.

Bone

Some drugs have an unusual affinity for bone. For example, the tetracycline antibiotics accumulate in bone after being absorbed onto the bone-crystal surface. This serves as a storage site for tetracycline antibiotics, which can depress bone growth in premature infants. Distribution of tetracycline to the teeth in a young child causes discolouration, due to formation of a tetracycline–calcium–orthophosphate complex. Brownish pigmentation of permanent teeth may result if this drug is given during the prenatal period or early childhood.

Tissue-specific barriers to drug distribution

A number of tissues and organs are 'protected' by barriers, which typically involve specific characteristics of the capillary membranes (e.g. tighter junctions between cells and thicker basement membrane), reinforcement by secondary cell types (e.g. astrocytes in the brain), and high levels of expression of efflux transporters. Examples of organ-specific barriers include the blood–brain and placental barriers.

Blood–brain barrier

The blood–brain barrier comprises the endothelial cells of brain capillaries, which are joined to each other by tight junctions. The capillary structure is further reinforced by astrocytic end-feet that project from astrocytes to form a near continuous layer over the thick basement membrane that underlies the endothelial cells. Although the barrier does allow penetration of lipid-soluble drugs into the brain and cerebrospinal fluid, further protection of the brain is provided by transporters. On the luminal membrane of brain capillary endothelial cells, a number of drug transporters are expressed, including efflux transporters. In some circumstances, such as meningitis, the blood–brain barrier can become 'leaky', and this allows access of drugs that would not normally be able to penetrate the brain. Using penicillin systemically to treat bacterial meningitis is an example of taking advantage of the inflammatory disruption of the blood–brain barrier.

Placental barrier

The placenta separates the blood vessels of the woman from the fetus, but does not afford complete protection to the fetus from substances in the maternal circulation. Like the blood–brain barrier, lipophilic drugs readily diffuse across the placenta while the passage of more polar compounds is generally impeded. The main processes involved in transplacental transfer of nutrients and drugs is passive diffusion, with facilitated diffusion and active transport having lesser roles. Consequently, some drugs intended to produce a therapeutic response in the woman may cross the placental barrier and some exert harmful effects on the fetus.

Drug distribution in pregnancy

In addition to the substantial physiological change of essentially rapidly developing an additional organ (the placenta), more subtle changes in the woman's body mass and fluid distribution change the volume of distribution of drugs during pregnancy. There is an increase in plasma volume (30–50%) and a 25% increase in body fat. The latter may affect the distribution of drugs that are deposited in fatty tissues and can result in a fall in their plasma concentrations. Albumin concentration decreases from the second trimester through to the time of birth by approximately 20%. This affects the protein binding of drugs such as phenytoin and valproate where dosage adjustment is difficult. This remains important as the likelihood of fetal abnormalities is dose-dependent with both these drugs.

Transplacental drug distribution

Distribution of drugs to the fetus via the placenta is the only route of drug exposure in the fetus (unless there has been direct administration of a drug to the fetal compartment for diagnostic or treatment purposes).

Distribution of a drug across the placenta places the fetus at risk for pharmacological and teratogenic effects of the drug. During the first 10 weeks of embryonic development (week 12 of gestation) fetal–placental–maternal circulation is not fully developed, with drugs reaching the fetus via diffusion through extracellular fluid. Drug transfer into the fetal circulation via the placenta depends on the maternal plasma concentration of the drug and physicochemical properties of the drug. The polarity, protein binding, and lipid solubility of a drug are important factors in transfer of a drug across the placenta via passive diffusion. For example, low-molecular-mass drugs (250–500 Da) freely cross the placenta, while drugs of molecular mass over 1000 Da (e.g. heparin) do not. Additionally, lipid-soluble drugs easily cross the placenta while diffusion of hydrophilic drugs is poor.

Eventually the concentration of free drug on either side of the placenta will equalise; that is, the fetal plasma drug concentrations will equal the maternal drug concentration.

With advancing gestation, there is enhanced utero–placental blood flow and thinning of the membranes that separate maternal blood flow and placental capillaries.

This results in increased placental transfer of un-ionised, lipophilic unbound drugs by passive diffusion. Drug transporters, including efflux transporters, are found in the maternal-facing apical membrane and in the fetal-facing basolateral membrane of the placenta. Table 4.1 summarises some factors that influence the distribution of drugs in the fetal compartment.

Drug distribution in the fetus

The factors that influence drug distribution through the placenta (Table 4.1) may influence drug distribution in the fetus; however, information about fetal drug disposition is scarce.

KEY POINTS

Distribution

- Distribution is defined as the process of reversible transfer of a drug between one location and another (one of which is usually blood) in the body.

- On entry into the systemic circulation, free drug molecules bind reversibly to proteins to form drug–protein complexes. Protein binding decreases the free drug concentration and

---

TABLE 4.1 Factors influencing drug distribution through the placenta and in the fetal compartment

FACTOR	POSSIBLE INFLUENCES
Type of drug	Factors that increase transfer include lipid solubility, low molecular weight (less than 500 to 600 daltons for lipid-soluble and less than 100 daltons for polar substances), non-ioinised, and unbound.
Amount of drug	Transfer is increased by greater maternal-to-fetal gradient, especially for drugs transferred by diffusion.
Membrane permeability	Diffusion of substances increases with increasing gestation and greater placental efficiency. Some drugs have greater affinity for specific fetal tissues (e.g. tetracycline in teeth, warfarin in bones, phenytoin in the fetal heart [because this is a highly lipid organ in the fetus, whereas in adults the central nervous system has a high lipid content owing to myelin sheaths], streptomycin in the optic nerve).
Fetal body water compartment	Drug distribution and dilution change as the total body water compartment decreases with increasing gestation. With an increased volume of distribution, peak volumes of drugs are reduced and excretion may be delayed.
Fetal circulation	Maternal and fetal blood flow rates will influence transfer. Upon reaching the fetal circulation, drugs may be shunted by the ductus venosus past the liver (thus missing an opportunity for detoxification), with the highest concentrations of these substances in blood going to the heart and upper body.
Serum protein binding	Protein binding of a drug in the maternal system limits the amount of free drug available for transfer to the fetus. Binding of drugs to macromolecules in the fetal circulation may increase the maternal-to-fetal transfer by maintaining a concentration gradient from the mother to the fetus.
Receptor function	Functional ability of receptors on cell membranes increases with gestation, leading to increased specificity to respond to or exclude certain drugs.
Placental enzymes	Enzymes produced by the placenta (e.g. insulinase) may detoxify drugs and reduce transfer to the fetus.
Gestational age	Many of the factors identified above are altered with advancing gestation and maturity of the fetus and placenta. The size and efficiency of the placental exchange area increase with increasing gestational age.
Fetal pH during labour	The fetal pH is usually 0.1 to 0.15 units below that of the mother. A decrease in the fetal pH may increase the transfer of acidophilic agents from the mother to fetus. Hypoxia alters blood flow and thus drug distribution, metabolism, and excretion. For example, with hypoxia, blood flow to the liver and kidneys may be reduced with preferential flow to the brain. Albumin binding of drugs may also be reduced, resulting in more free drug in the fetal circulation.

limits tissue distribution. As free drug is removed from the circulation, the protein–drug complex dissociates so more free drug is released.

- Only free or unbound drug exerts a pharmacological effect.
- While barriers to free drug movement are present in certain areas of the body (such as the blood–brain and placental barriers), movement of some drugs across these is still possible.
- Physiological changes during pregnancy can affect the distribution of drugs.

4.3 Drug elimination (metabolism and excretion)

Drug **elimination** is irreversible removal of drugs from the systemic circulation. It occurs through the processes of metabolism and extraction.

Drug metabolism

Drug metabolism is the process of chemical modification of a drug and is almost invariably carried out by enzymes. The liver is the primary site of drug metabolism but, with certain drugs, other organs (e.g. kidneys, lungs, and intestine) may also be involved to a limited degree. Most drugs (around 70%) undergo metabolism to some extent, and in most (but not all) cases, the products of metabolism have less biological activity than the parent drug. An exception to this is the use of prodrugs, which are drugs that require activation (often in the liver) to elicit a therapeutic action. The commonly used analgesic codeine is a prodrug, requiring metabolism to morphine to produce an analgesic effect. For most therapeutic drugs, metabolism results in the formation of a more water-soluble compound or metabolite, which can be more readily excreted. Metabolism clears the drug from the systemic circulation and promotes urinary excretion.

Classification of drug metabolism reactions

Most drugs are metabolised in the liver by either functionalisation (known as phase I metabolism) and/or conjugation reactions (known as phase II metabolism). It is important to recognise that a drug may:

- not be metabolised, being excreted unchanged (e.g. gentamicin)
- undergo functionalisation and be directly excreted (e.g. caffeine)
- undergo conjugation and be directly excreted (e.g. paracetamol)
- undergo both functionalisation then conjugation prior to excretion (e.g. phenytoin).

These processes are not necessarily sequential and can occur simultaneously (e.g. the metabolism of codeine by oxidation to morphine and by glucuronidation to codeine-6-glucuronide).

Functionalisation reactions

These reactions generally involve introducing or unmasking a polar functional group into the molecule, thereby producing a more water-soluble metabolite. Common functionalisation reactions include dealkylation (de-ethylation or demethylation), hydrolysis, hydroxylation, and oxidation. In some cases, metabolites are more pharmacologically active than the parent compound and, uncommonly, may be more toxic. For example, N-acetyl-p-benzoquinone imine (NAPQI) is the toxic metabolite of paracetamol responsible for the severe liver damage associated with overdose of this drug. Cytochrome P450 is the major family of enzymes associated with these reactions. Other functionalisation enzymes include esterases, alcohol dehydrogenase, flavin-containing mono-oxygenases, and xanthine oxidase.

Cytochromes P450

The enzymes of greatest importance in functionalisation reactions are the superfamily of cytochrome P450 (CYP) enzymes. CYP are found in the smooth endoplasmic reticulum of cells and are particularly abundant in hepatocytes. CYP are involved not only in drug metabolism but also in the metabolism of environmental pollutants and dietary chemicals, and in the synthesis and metabolism of bile acids, steroids, hormones, and fatty acids. There are more than 50 individual human CYP enzymes, classified on amino-acid sequence identity into families and sub-families. Of these, approximately 18 enzymes in families 1, 2, and 3 can metabolise drugs. In naming them, the suffix 'CYP' is followed by a number designating the family, which is followed by a letter denoting the sub-family and then another number in order of their discovery. For example, CYP3A4 is the fourth member of CYP family 3, sub-family A. The human CYPs of greatest importance in hepatic drug metabolism are CYP1A2, CYP2C8, CYP2C9, CYP2C19, CYP2D6, CYP2E1, and CYP3A4. Table 4.2 lists some common therapeutic drugs that are substrates for these CYPs.

Conjugation reactions

Conjugation reactions join a functional group present in the drug molecule with the polar group of an endogenous substance in the body (e.g. glucuronic acid, sulfate, acetyl-coenzyme A or glutathione). The conjugated drug molecule is generally more polar or more water-soluble, which enhances urinary excretion. The relationship between drug metabolism and renal excretion is illustrated in Figure 4.6. along with the enzymes and co-factors that are involved in their catalysis.

TABLE 4.2 Representative drugs metabolised by CYP enzymes

CYP	DRUGS METABOLISED
CYP1A2	Amitriptyline, caffeine, clozapine, haloperidol, lidocaine (lignocaine), olanzapine, ondansetron, tamoxifen, thalidomide
CYP2C8	Cerivastatin, chloroquine, montelukast, paclitaxel, repaglinide
CYP2C9	Diclofenac, gliclazide, irbesartan, losartan, naproxen, phenytoin, sildenafil, sulfonylurea, S-warfarin, fluoxetine
CYP2C19	Citalopram, clopidogrel, diazepam, esomeprazole, omeprazole, pantoprazole, sertraline, TCAs (tricyclic antidepressants)
CYP2D6	Amitriptyline, codeine, dexamfetamine, dextromethorphan, fluoxetine, fluvoxamine, haloperidol, metoprolol, mirtazapine, perhexiline, quetiapine, risperidone, timolol, venlafaxine
CYP2E1	Ethanol, enflurane, halothane, methoxyflurane, acetaminophen (paracetamol), nicotine (tobacco)
CYP3A4	Amiodarone, aprepitant, atorvastatin, carbamazepine, ciclosporin, erythromycin, felodipine, hydrocortisone, HIV protease inhibitors (e.g. saquinavir), simvastatin, tacrolimus, tyrosine kinase inhibitors (e.g. axitinib), verapamil, zolpidem, acetaminophen (paracetamol), diazepam, codeine

Relationship between drug metabolism and renal excretion. Metabolism via functionalisation and conjugation reactions results in decreasing lipid solubility, increasing water solubility and progressive enhancement of urinary excretion

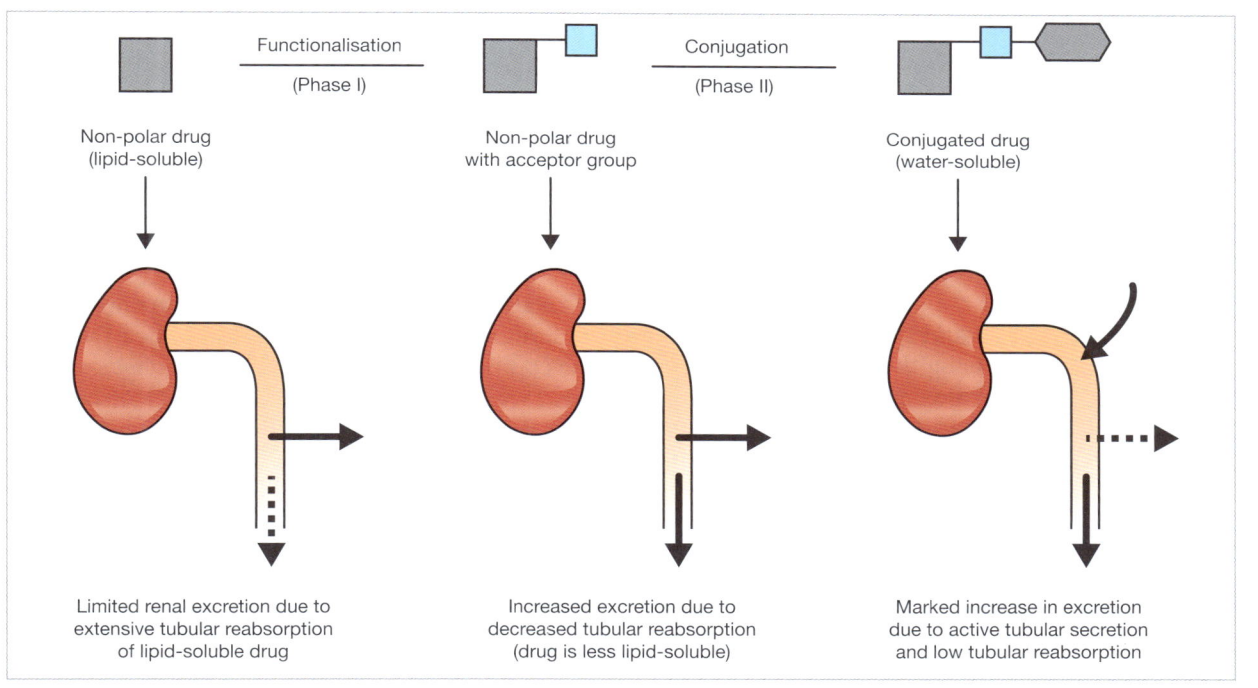

FIGURE 4.6

Source: Birkett et al 1979, Figure 2; reproduced with permission.

Variability in drug metabolism

There are differences between individuals in the extent and rate of metabolism of many drugs. Metabolism is important in determining the therapeutic and toxic effects of many drugs. This variability can be due to:

- genetics
- environmental factors – e.g. co-administered drugs, diet, alcohol, smoking
- age and gender
- disease states – e.g. hepatic, cardiovascular
- hormonal changes – e.g. pregnancy.

Drug interactions

Metabolic drug interactions can occur when two or more chemicals (drugs, herbs, or environmental chemicals) are present in the body at the same time. In this situation, one chemical (the interaction perpetrator) alters the activity of the enzyme involved in eliminating the other chemical (the interaction victim). Metabolic drug interactions are typically caused by the co-administration of two drugs (drug–drug interactions) but may also occur when a chemical present in a herbal preparation (herb–drug interaction) or food item (diet–drug interaction) alters the metabolism of a drug. Such reactions result from either induction or inhibition of enzyme activity. Induction of drug metabolism usually arises from increased synthesis of more of the enzyme protein via an effect on the genes that encode the specific drug-metabolising enzyme. The clinical impact of enzyme induction depends on the extent to which the plasma drug concentration is decreased (suboptimal) over the course of treatment with normal dosing. For example, cigarette smoke induces expression of CYP1A2 and therefore increases the metabolism of clozapine and olanzapine; this can result in a substantially higher dose requirement for some people.

Inhibition of drug metabolism typically occurs when two drugs compete for metabolism by the same enzyme. This results in reduced metabolism of one or both of the drugs. The clinical consequences of inhibition of drug metabolism include a decreased rate of elimination from the body, resulting in an increased plasma concentration and risk of toxicity. Examples include:

- inhibition of warfarin metabolism by amiodarone or fluconazole, increasing the risk of bleeding
- inhibition of oxycodone metabolism by erythromycin and clarithromycin, increasing the risk of increased plasma concentration of oxycodone and risk of CNS depression
- inhibition of ciclosporin and tacrolimus metabolism by erythromycin, increasing the risk of nephrotoxicity and neurotoxicity
- inhibition of diazepam metabolism by cimetidine, prolonging central nervous system depression.

Disease states

In people with cardiac failure, liver perfusion and oxygenation may be decreased, and this can reduce the activity of drug-metabolising enzymes. In liver disease, the effects are harder to predict because they depend on the disease type and severity, both of which can influence drug metabolism. In general, in severe cirrhosis and viral hepatitis the clearance of drugs metabolised by CYP enzymes is decreased.

Female sex and pregnancy

Although sex-related differences have been observed for drug-metabolising enzymes in animal species, differences in humans are often minor and clinically insignificant. However, pregnancy can have important effects on drug metabolism, particularly during the third trimester when increased activity of many metabolic enzymes occurs. For example, it is well established that doses of the anticonvulsant drugs carbamazepine (metabolised by CYP3A4) and phenytoin (metabolised by CYP2C9) should be increased during pregnancy to maintain therapeutic plasma concentrations. Following birth, doses decline to pre-pregnancy requirements. In contrast, there is evidence suggesting that the metabolism of caffeine declines during pregnancy. Thus, although induction occurs more commonly than inhibition, the impact of pregnancy on drug metabolism is not always predictable. Table 4.3 demonstrates pregnancy-induced changes in hepatic drug-metabolising enzyme activity.

Drug metabolism in the placenta

Our knowledge of drug metabolism in the human placenta is limited; however, it is well established that the placenta has both phase I and phase II metabolising enzymes. It is also well established that the activity of placental drug-metabolising enzymes is altered in women who either use drugs, smoke, or consume alcohol. The primary CYP450

TABLE 4.3 Pregnancy-induced changes in hepatic drug-metabolising enzyme activity

ENZYME	EFFECT ON CLEARANCE	TRIMESTER	EXAMPLES OF DRUGS AFFECTED
CYP1A2	Decrease	1st, 2nd and 3rd	Caffeine
CYP2A6	Increase	2nd and 3rd	Nicotine
CYP2C9	Increase	3rd	Phenytoin
CYP2C19	Decrease	2nd and 3rd	Proguanil
CYP2D6	Increase	3rd	Dextromethorphan, metoprolol, fluoxetine, nortriptyline
CYP3A4	Increase	3rd	Nifedipine, saquinavir, ritonavir, indinavir, lopinavir
UGT1A4	Increase	1st, 2nd and 3rd	Lamotrigine
UGT2B7	Increase	3rd	Morphine, zidovudine, oxazepam

isoforms seen to date include CYP1A1, which is present in the placenta throughout pregnancy, while CYP1A2 is present in the first trimester. The activity of CYP1A1 is increased by smoking, and the extent of induction depends on the stage of pregnancy. Importantly, CYP1A1 activates polycyclic aromatic hydrocarbons found in tobacco, which can lead to detrimental effects on the fetus. CYP2E1, which metabolises ethanol, is present in the placenta from the first trimester, but the levels of this enzyme vary enormously, possibly reflecting variable alcohol consumption in pregnant women. Other reported isoforms of CYP450 enzymes in the human placenta are CYP3A4, CYP3A7, and CYP4B1, although with low activity. UGT1A and UGT2B enzymes are present in the placenta throughout pregnancy but, like the CYP enzymes, UGT enzyme activity is highly variable. It is thought that placental UGT enzymes play a role in placental metabolism through formation of polar metabolites that are then more easily eliminated from the fetal compartment. Drug metabolism enzyme activities of the placenta may influence transfer of specific substances from woman to fetus; however, to date, there is no information on the clinical importance of metabolism of drugs in the placenta.

Drug metabolism in the fetus

Maternally administered drugs enter the fetal circulation via the umbilical vein. Between 40–60% of umbilical venous blood enters the fetal liver, with the remainder entering directly into the fetal systemic circulation, bypassing the first-pass effect, if there is any. Drug effects in the fetus can be more significant and prolonged than in the woman because the fetus has immature liver drug-metabolising enzymes and thus metabolises drugs differently from adults. Fetal harm from a drug or its metabolites can occur if the metabolite is toxic and binds to fetal plasma proteins, or if metabolism by the fetal liver results in the formation of a water-soluble metabolite that does not readily cross the placenta. Under these circumstances, drugs and metabolites are renally excreted and accumulate in amniotic fluid, where they can be reabsorbed after fetal swallowing of amniotic fluid. This results in prolongation of the duration of exposure and higher fetal plasma concentration.

KEY POINTS

Metabolism

- Drug metabolism, or biotransformation, is the process of chemical modification of a drug and is almost invariably carried out by enzymes.

- Most drugs are metabolised in the liver by functionalisation and/or conjugation reactions.

- Large differences may occur between individuals in the rate of metabolism of drugs. This variability may be due to genetic, environmental, age, or disease-related factors.

- Pregnancy-induced changes in hepatic drug-metabolising enzyme activity may have significant clinical implications for dose adjustment of some drugs during pregnancy.

4.4 Excretion of drugs and drug metabolites

In pharmacokinetic terms, elimination refers to the irreversible loss of drug from the site of measurement and occurs by the processes of metabolism and excretion. For example, after administration, a drug may be metabolised by the liver and its metabolites remain in the body. For example, pethidine has a much shorter half-life than its metabolite, norpethidine. In this case, the parent drug is considered to have been eliminated. The terms 'elimination' and 'excretion' are often used interchangeably, but excretion applies solely to the loss of (chemically) unchanged drug or metabolites in, for example, urine or bile. The term 'unchanged' in this context may appear confusing, but it refers to the immediate chemical species that is being excreted, which can be either a parent molecule or a metabolite. In this regard, the liver, being the major site of drug metabolism, is the main organ of elimination, while the kidneys are the main organs of excretion.

Hepatic uptake and biliary excretion

Although lipophilic drugs freely diffuse across the membrane of hepatocytes, the presence of uptake transporters facilitates the uptake of drugs that are organic anions and cations as well as other polar compounds. Once in the hepatocyte, the drug becomes available for metabolism by enzymes such as CYP and UGT or for excretion into bile by the efflux transporters located on the canalicular membrane. Metabolites formed within the hepatocyte may (1) diffuse, or (2) be transported across the apical membrane back into blood for subsequent excretion in urine, or (3) be transported into the bile (by the transporters present on the canalicular membrane), passed into the duodenum and excreted in faeces.

Drugs and drug metabolites excreted into bile become available for reabsorption once the bile is released into the small intestine. In the small intestine, the drug may be reabsorbed and returned to the liver via the portal vein, a process referred to as enterohepatic recycling. Since many drugs (e.g. atorvastatin, digoxin, ethinylestradiol, indometacin, morphine, rifampicin, kinase inhibitors and many antimicrobials) are excreted in bile to some extent, they are likely to undergo some enterohepatic cycling. Glucuronide metabolites excreted into the bile can be hydrolysed by bacterial enzymes in the GIT to re-form the parent drug, which can subsequently undergo enterohepatic recycling.

Renal excretion

Renal excretion of drugs and drug metabolites is influenced by the processes of glomerular filtration, tubular secretion, and reabsorption (Fig 4.7). Glomerular filtration and tubular secretion facilitate the transfer of drugs and metabolites from blood into urine, while reabsorption counters these processes. Free unbound drugs and water-soluble metabolites are filtered by the glomeruli, whereas protein-bound substances are not filtered. Since there are no drugs that circulate in blood completely bound to protein or erythrocytes, all drugs and metabolites will undergo some degree of glomerular filtration. Drug transporters in the proximal tubule transfer drugs and metabolites that are organic acids and bases from the interstitial fluid into the tubule cell. However, once in the urine, lipophilic drugs can transfer back into the tubule cell and interstitial fluid (reabsorption). Most of the approximately 120 mL of water from the plasma filtered at the glomerulus per minute is reabsorbed during its passage through the renal tubule, and only about 1–2 mL finally appears as urine. As the water is reabsorbed, a concentration gradient is established between the drug in the tubular fluid and the unbound drug in the blood. (That is, the drug in the urine is concentrated relative to that in the blood.) If the drug is lipid-soluble enough to pass through the membranes, it will be reabsorbed from the tubular fluid back into the systemic circulation. If the urine flow rate is high, there is less of a concentration gradient and less drug is reabsorbed. Conversely, if the urine is more concentrated due to a low urine flow rate, there is more of a concentration gradient and more drug is reabsorbed. In contrast to lipophilic drugs, polar, water-soluble compounds such as acids, bases and polar drug metabolites (e.g. glucuronides) are not reabsorbed and are excreted in the urine (Fig 4.6).

The proximal tubule is the main site of transporter-mediated secretion of drugs and/or their metabolites into the lumen of the nephron. Both acidic and basic drugs are taken up from the interstitial fluid into tubular cells via the basolateral uptake 'acid' and 'base' transporters. At times it may be clinically useful to reduce the renal excretion of a drug. One way of doing this is to competitively inhibit tubular secretion. For example, probenecid, which is used to treat gout, reduces the renal excretion of penicillin. It does this by inhibiting transporters that shift penicillin from the tubular cell into the lumen of the nephron and hence reduces excretion of penicillin in urine. Clinically, this prolongs the effect of the antibiotic by maintaining a therapeutic plasma concentration for a longer period.

Pulmonary excretion

Gases and volatile drugs (e.g. general anaesthetics such as halothane) are inhaled and excreted (exhaled) via the lungs. On inspiration, these agents enter the bloodstream and, after crossing the alveolar membrane, access the systemic circulation. Excretion from the lungs depends on the rate of respiration. Volatile chemicals, such as ethanol, that are highly soluble in blood, may be excreted in limited amounts by the lungs. Approximately one part in 2000 of the ethanol in blood is in the gaseous state, and pulmonary excretion is the basis of the alcohol breath test.

The drug excretion process, illustrating:
1 glomerular filtration, 2 tubular reabsorption and, 3 secretion

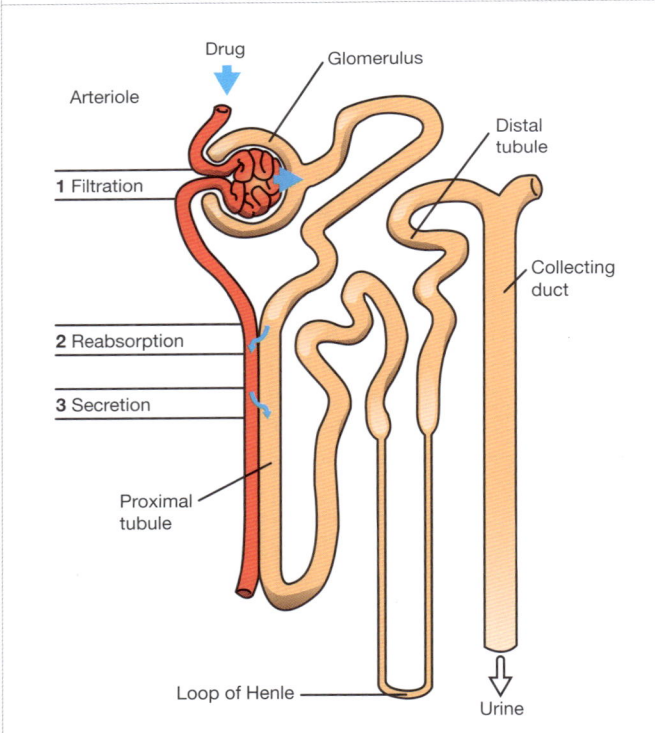

FIGURE 4.7

Source: Salerno 1999, Figure 4-6; used with permission.

KEY POINTS

Excretion

- The major organs for the excretion of unchanged drugs and drug metabolites are the kidneys.

- The process of renal excretion of drugs is influenced by glomerular filtration, tubular secretion, and reabsorption.

- During pregnancy, increases in renal blood flow and GFR increase the elimination rate of drugs excreted predominantly unchanged by the kidneys. This may lead to the need for dosage adjustment.

- Activities of placental drug-metabolising enzymes are altered in pregnant women who either use drugs, smoke, or consume alcohol.

4.5 Pharmacokinetics during pregnancy and early life

Renal excretion during pregnancy

During pregnancy, renal blood flow and the GFR increase by 50–80%, increasing the elimination rate of drugs excreted predominantly unchanged by the kidney. This may lead to the need for dosage adjustment. This increase in renal blood flow starts shortly after conception and persists until the last few weeks of pregnancy when a reduction in GFR may be observed. To date there is very little information on whether pregnancy has any effect on the secretion or reabsorption of drugs in the renal tubule. Drugs shown to have increased renal clearance during pregnancy include the antibiotics, ampicillin, cefuroxime, ceftazidime, and piperacillin, and lithium. The blood concentration of lithium in second trimester of pregnancy decreased by 36% (Wesseloo, 2017). Elimination of lithium is via renal excretion as unchanged drug. Lithium excretion in pregnancy decreased. Other drugs include lithium, sotalol, dalteparin, and enoxaparin sodium (Anderson, 2005). Drugs continued into and during pregnancy should be titrated to the desired clinical response, with therapeutic monitoring of serum concentrations advised for drugs with increased potential for maternal or fetal toxicity, such as lithium and phenytoin or gentamicin.

Pharmacokinetic development during early life

Neonates

Drug use in neonates requires special consideration because they lack many of the protective mechanisms of older children and adults. Their skin is thin and permeable, their stomachs have lower levels of acid, and their lungs are yet to acquire a thick mucous barrier. Neonates regulate body temperature poorly and become dehydrated easily. After the transition from fetal status, neonates are no longer able to make use of maternal metabolic processes, and are dependent on their own drug-metabolising enzymes to metabolise drugs and chemicals. The time taken to achieve maturation of hepatic drug functionalisation and conjugation enzymes may account for the toxicity of some drugs in the newborn. Expression of CYPs changes markedly during development. Some change within hours of birth, while others mature over 1–3 months. This reduced metabolic capacity results in slower drug clearance and prolonged elimination than in fetal or later life. For example, phenobarbital (phenobarbitone) plasma half-life is 70–500 hours in neonates (younger than 7 days), 20–70 hours in those younger than 1 month, 20–80 hours in children 1–15 years of age, and 60–180 hours in young adults. Another example is pethidine which has been used as analgesic in labour. Pethidine has a plasma half-life of 3–5 hours in the mother and up to 32 hours in the fetus and is responsible for adverse neonatal effects.

Drug exposure from breast milk

Many drugs or their metabolites cross the epithelium of the mammary glands and are excreted in breast milk. The scale of infant exposure to these drugs during breastfeeding depends on maternal plasma drug concentration and the amount of milk ingested by the infant. Breast milk is acidic (pH 6.5). Therefore, basic compounds with low plasma protein binding and high lipid solubility such as narcotics (e.g. morphine and codeine) achieve high concentrations. A major concern arises over the transfer of such drugs from women to their breastfed babies, which can result in adverse effects such as sedation and failure to thrive.

KEY POINTS

Pregnancy and early life

- The amount of drug diffusing across the placenta at any given time depends on the maternal plasma drug concentration. Eventually, the fetal plasma drug concentration will equal the maternal drug concentration.

- The disposition of drugs in neonates differs from that in the fetus and adults because of factors such as growth, concentration of drug-metabolising enzymes, plasma and tissue binding, and physiological maturation of organ systems.

REVIEW EXERCISES

1 Freya is 8 weeks pregnant and due to hyperemesis is unable to swallow tablets. Freya is required to take her regular medication, drug A, with a bioavailability of 50%, and this must now be administered intravenously. Providing a short justification, estimate the intravenous dose of drug A that would be equivalent to a 100 mg oral dose of this drug.

2 Linda has been using the drug levothyroxine for the past 5 years. She is now 14 weeks pregnant. Discuss the range of factors that could be contributing to variability in her response to the drug.

3 Alex, 5 years old, has been brought to the emergency department of his local hospital with an aspirin digestion. He has accidentally digested aspirin tablets taken by his pregnant mother, who was prescribed them for preeclampsia prevention. A number of management measures have been instituted, including the administration of sodium bicarbonate. Explain why sodium bicarbonate has been administered.

REFERENCES

Anderson GD. Pregnancy-induced changes in pharmacokinetics: a mechanistic-based approach. Clin Pharmacokinet. 2005;44(10):989-1008. doi: 10.2165/00003088-200544100-00001

Blackburn ST. Maternal, fetal and neonatal physiology: a clinical perspective. 5th edn. Vol 1. Elsevier: 2017.

Salerno E. Pharmacology for health professionals. Mosby: St Louis, 1999.

Wesseloo R, Wierdsma AI, van Kamp IL, et al. Lithium dosing strategies during pregnancy and the postpartum period. Br J Psychiatry. 2017;211(1):31-36. doi: 10.1192/bjp.bp.116.192799. PMID: 28673946; PMCID: PMC5494438

ADDITIONAL RESOURCES

Anderson GD. Pregnancy-induced changes in pharmacokinetics: a mechanistic-based approach, Clin Pharmacokinet. 2005;44(10):989-1008. doi: 10.2165/00003088-200544100-00001 [Seminal paper describing the changes in drug exposure that occur during pregnancy.]

Birkett DJ. Pharmacokinetics made easy: pocket guide (2nd edn), McGraw Hill: Sydney, 2010.

Birkett DJ, Grygiel JJ, Meffin PJ, et al. Fundamentals of clinical pharmacology; 4 Drug biotransformation. Current Therapeutics. 1979;6:129-138.

Miners JO, Bowalgaha K, Elliot DJ, et al: Characterization of niflumic acid as a selective inhibitor of human liver microsomal UDP-glucuronosyltransferase 1A9: application to the reaction phenotyping of acetaminophen glucuronidation. Drug Metab Dispos. 2011;39(4):644-52. doi: 10.1124/dmd.110.037036

CHAPTER 5

PHARMACOKINETICS AND DOSING REGIMEN

Maryam Bazargan, Kirsten Small

Key Abbreviations

CL	clearance
CL_S	systemic clearance
C_{SS}	steady-state plasma drug concentration
E_H	hepatic extraction ratio
F	bioavailability
$t\frac{1}{2}$	half-life
V_D	volume of distribution

Key Terms

clearance 80
half-life 80
steady state 83

volume of distribution 80

Chapter Focus

Choosing a drug is influenced by many factors, and using the right dose is essential both for achieving the desired effect and for limiting adverse effects. An understanding of pharmacokinetic principles allows selection of the right dose and the prediction of the effects of disease states, drug interactions, and environmental factors on dosing regimens. The importance of the key pharmacokinetic concepts of clearance, volume of distribution, and half-life are illustrated in this chapter using clinically relevant examples.

Learning Outcomes

- Describe the impact of pharmacokinetics on drug and dosage selection.
- Explain how disease state, pregnancy and drug interaction impact on drug pharmacokinetics.
- Critically apply knowledge of changed pharmacokinetics on drug dosage and regimen.

CRITICAL THINKING SCENARIO

Bernadette is a 23-year-old with a history of hypothyroidism and is on regular levothyroxine 100 mcg daily. She is 15 weeks pregnant in her first pregnancy. Consistent with the national pregnancy guidelines, Bernadette recently had her thyroid function tests checked to see if she would benefit from a dose change.

1 Her GP recommended she increase the dosage of her levothyroxine. How does pregnancy impact the pharmacokinetics of levothyroxine?

2 Why would Bernadette be advised to adjust the dosage of the drug?

(Based on Galoiu S, 2016; and Kashi et al 2015.)

Introduction

The rational use of drugs is based on an assumption that a particular concentration of a drug will have the desired therapeutic effect and that adverse effects will be negligible. For many drugs, there is a sufficient relationship between plasma drug concentration and clinical response for dosing regimens to be designed to maintain the concentration within a therapeutic range. Because therapeutic ranges are generally derived from population-level data of healthy male adults they are considered to reflect the range of drug concentrations having a high probability of producing the desired therapeutic effect and a low probability of producing adverse effects, but they cannot reliably predict what will happen for a specific individual. For a limited number of drugs it is possible, and in some cases necessary, to adjust the dosing regimen to achieve the desired plasma concentration for an individual by considering their characteristics (e.g. pregnancy, age, health status, liver and kidney function) and the pharmacokinetics of the drug. This process, which has had many titles, is increasingly known as precision dosing.

5.1 Plasma concentration–time profile of a drug

Usually there is direct correlation between the plasma concentration of a drug at any given time and the therapeutic response or toxicity of that drug. For example, the theoretical drug in Figure 5.1 has been administered as a single oral dose. It has an onset of action of approximately 2 hours, a peak plasma concentration at 5 hours, and a 6-hour duration of action (the length of time the plasma drug concentration remains within the therapeutic range). In this case, the processes of absorption, distribution, and elimination (i.e. metabolism and excretion) influence the plasma concentration–time profile of the drug.

Intravenous (IV) administration of a drug as a single bolus dose followed by an infusion, or as a single bolus dose alone, or as an infusion alone, all give different plasma concentration–time profiles that are influenced by distribution and elimination but not by absorption (Fig 5.2).

How does this knowledge help you to design an appropriate dosing regimen? Buried within these plasma drug concentration–time profiles are the key pharmacokinetic parameters of **clearance**, **volume of distribution** and **half-life**. The clearance of a drug and its volume of distribution are determined by the characteristics of both the person and the drug, whereas the plasma half-life of the drug is a composite parameter that is related directly to the volume of distribution of the drug and inversely to the clearance of the drug.

5.2 Key pharmacokinetic concept: Clearance

Clearance (CL) describes the ability of either an individual organ or the body to eliminate a drug. Clearances by each organ are additive and, hence, total clearance from the systemic circulation – that is, systemic clearance (CL_S) – reflects the total sum of all the clearance processes relevant to the particular drug (Fig 5.3):

$$CL_{Systemic} = CL_{Renal} + CL_{Hepatic} + CL_{Other}$$

In general, for most drugs, clearance is through liver (hepatic clearance) and/or renal clearance. For most drugs, unless indicated otherwise, clearance by other organs (e.g. the lungs) is negligible. For a particular drug and a specific person, providing they remain physiologically stable, clearance is constant. For example,

Plasma concentration–time profile for a theoretical drug administered as a single oral dose

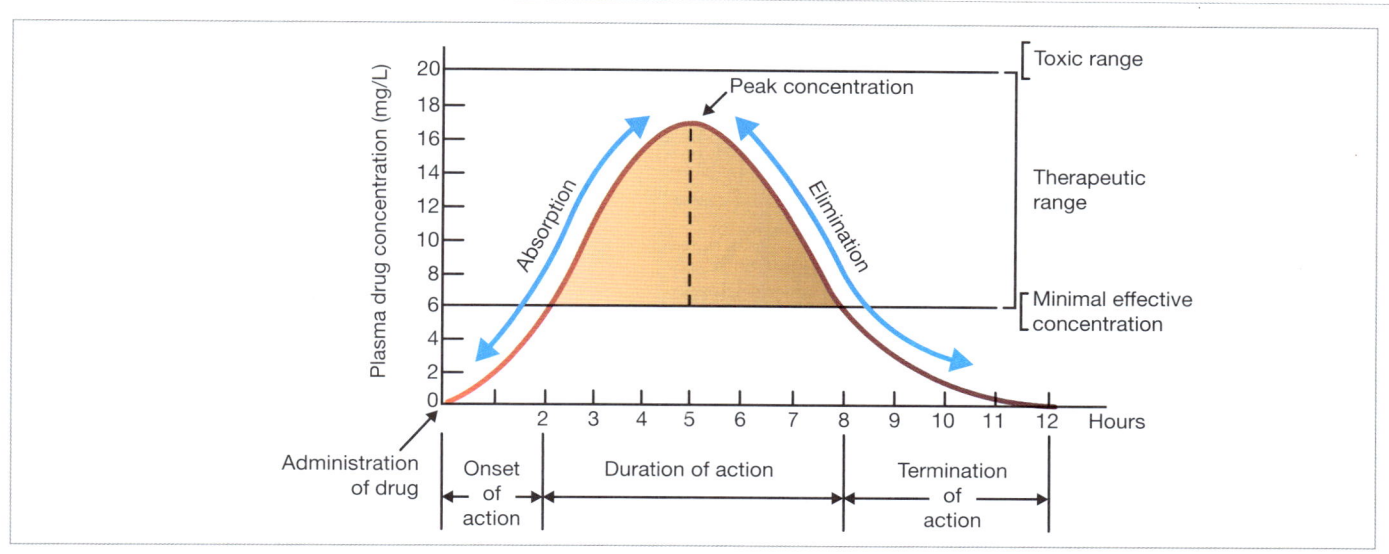

FIGURE 5.1 The correlation between the plasma concentration of a drug at any given time and the therapeutic response.

Source: Adapted from Salerno 1999, Figure 4-7; used with permission.

Plasma concentration–time profiles for a drug administered as (1) Red line: a single IV bolus dose followed by an IV infusion, (2) Green line: an IV infusion only, and (3) Dotted yellow line: a single IV bolus dose

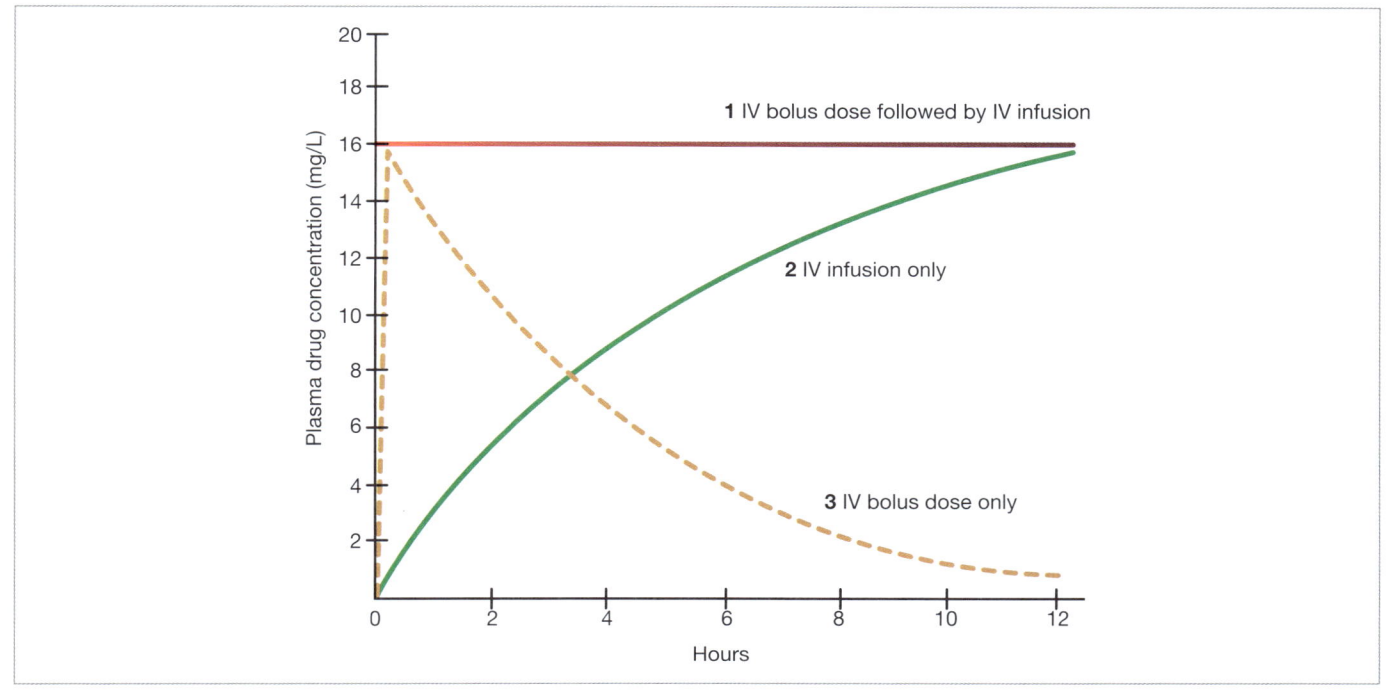

FIGURE 5.2

Concept of systemic (total body) clearance of a drug from plasma

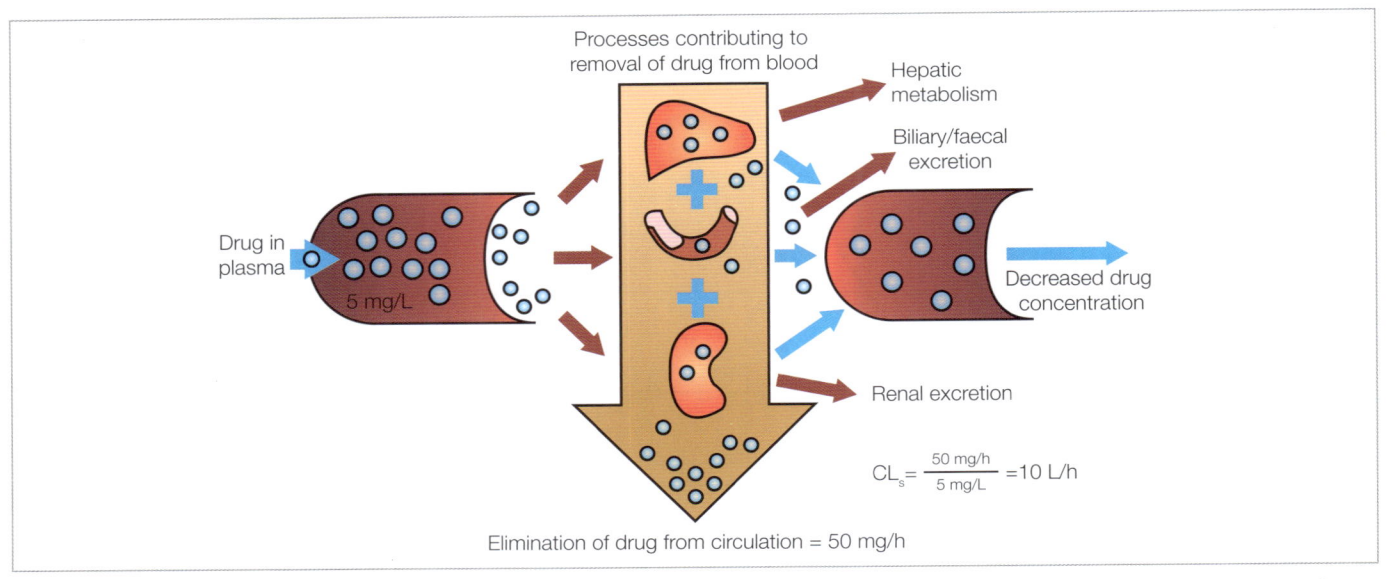

Processes contributing to
removal of drug from blood

Hepatic
metabolism

Biliary/faecal
excretion

Drug in
plasma

5 mg/L

Decreased drug
concentration

Renal excretion

$$CL_s = \frac{50 \text{ mg/h}}{5 \text{ mg/L}} = 10 \text{ L/h}$$

Elimination of drug from circulation = 50 mg/h

FIGURE 5.3 Only some drug molecules are extracted from plasma on each pass of blood through the kidneys, liver or other sites contributing to drug elimination. In this example, the plasma drug concentration is 5 mg/L and the elimination rate is 50 mg/h; hence, systemic clearance is 10 L/h.

if you measured the clearance of paracetamol in yourself, it should not change very much from day to day, provided the activity of your liver enzymes that metabolise paracetamol did not change. However, paracetamol clearance in a population will broadly reflect the inter-individual variability in the activity of drug-metabolising enzymes in that population.

During pregnancy, due to physiological changes in renal and hepatic systems, clearance of some drugs may be altered, both from the pre-pregnant state and during the course of the pregnancy, and may need dosing adjustment to retain efficacy and avoid adverse effects.

Hepatic clearance

A drug will enter the liver in the blood delivered via the portal vein, from the gastrointestinal tract, and via the hepatic artery, from the systemic circulation. The rate of drug entering the liver is determined by liver blood flow (about 90 L/hr) and the concentration of drug in blood entering the liver. A drug will leave the liver in the blood via the hepatic vein and be returned to the systemic circulation. The difference between the concentration of drug entering the liver and the concentration of drug exiting the liver defines the proportion of drug that is extracted by the liver and is called the hepatic extraction ratio. Hepatic clearance (CL_H) is simply the extracted amount of drug by the liver per unit of time.

Drugs cleared by the liver can be classified into three categories – as having either a low, intermediate, or high hepatic clearance – based on the following criteria:

- low hepatic clearance: CLH < 20 L/h
- intermediate hepatic clearance: CLH between 20 and 60 L/h
- high hepatic clearance: CLH ≥ 60 L/h.

Examples of drugs in these categories are shown in Table 5.1. Low hepatic clearance does not mean that the drug is then cleared by the kidneys. It indicates that the capacity of the hepatic enzyme or enzymes to metabolise the drug is low and therefore the drug will simply be cleared more slowly.

TABLE 5.1 Examples of drugs with either a low, intermediate, or high hepatic clearance

LOW CLEARANCE	INTERMEDIATE CLEARANCE	HIGH CLEARANCE
Carbamazepine	Caffeine	Lidocaine (lignocaine)
Diazepam	Fluoxetine	Morphine
Ibuprofen	Midazolam	Propofol
Phenytoin	Omeprazole	Propranolol
Warfarin	Paracetamol	Zidovudine

Effects of enzyme induction and inhibition on hepatic clearance

For an orally administered drug, induction of drug metabolism will typically result in a decrease in drug exposure (a decrease in plasma concentration and half-life), and inhibition will typically result in an increase in drug exposure (an increase in plasma concentration and half-life). However, the impact of metabolic induction impacts drugs with high or low hepatic clearance differently. The induction or inhibition of hepatic metabolising enzymes has a more significant impact on the bioavailability of drugs with high hepatic clearance.

During pregnancy, the induction or inhibition of hepatic metabolising enzymes due to physiological adaptation can impact hepatic clearance of some drugs. This impact on drugs with high hepatic clearance can have a clinical implication and lead to a significant decrease or increase in the plasma concentration of the drug.

The different impacts of induction and inhibition of hepatic drug-metabolising enzyme activity on bioavailability and clearance (and drug exposure) for low- and high-hepatic clearance drugs are summarised in Table 5.2.

Renal clearance

Renal drug clearance is the net effect of glomerular filtration, active secretion, and passive reabsorption. Because only unbound drug (the fraction of drug unbound in plasma) is filtered at the glomerulus, clearance by glomerular filtration will depend both on the glomerular filtration rate (GFR) and the fraction of the drug which is unbound. It is independent of the total concentration of the drug, which is the sum of bound and unbound drug to plasma proteins.

As all drugs must be partially unbound in plasma, they will be filtered to some extent. Hence, for some drugs, there may be a significant component of the drug secreted into the renal tubule and significant reabsorption. For most drugs, changes in renal function do not always necessitate an adjustment in drug dosage. However, during pregnancy, there is a significant increase in GFR as a physiological adaptation of pregnancy. Therefore, the renal clearance of

drugs may increase significantly and lead to sub-therapeutic plasma concentration of the drug during pregnancy. As mentioned above, this can be significant if the drug is more than 50% cleared by the kidneys. In some pregnancy-induced disease states, such as preeclampsia where there can be a reduction in GFR, drug clearance by the kidneys may decrease significantly and lead to drug toxicity. For example, magnesium sulfate levels need to be monitored closely in woman with preeclampsia to avoid toxicity.

The importance of clearance

Clearance refers to the rate at which a drug is removed from the body, typically through metabolism and excretion, such as via the liver, kidneys, or other organs. Continued drug administration eventually leads to a situation where the rate of drug going in equals the rate of drug going out and the plasma drug concentration remains constant.

KEY POINTS

Clearance

- Clearance determines the maintenance dose rate required to achieve the target plasma concentration at **steady state**.

- The impact of the induction and inhibition of drug-metabolising enzyme activity on bioavailability and clearance differs between drugs with high and low hepatic clearance.

5.3 Key pharmacokinetic concept: Volume of distribution

It is important to understand that the term 'volume of distribution' (V_D) of a drug is an abstract term and that it is not referring to a 'real' volume.

For example, if a drug is tightly bound to plasma proteins, most of it will remain within the circulatory

---

TABLE 5.2 Impact of changing enzyme activity on clearance and bioavailability for low- and high-hepatic clearance (CL_H) drugs

EFFECT ON ENZYME ACTIVITY	LOW-CL_H DRUG		HIGH-CL_H DRUG	
	CLEARANCE (CL_H)	BIOAVAILABILITY	CLEARANCE (CL_H)	BIOAVAILABILITY
Induction	Increased (*decreased drug exposure*)	Negligible (*drug exposure essentially unchanged*)	Negligible (*drug exposure essentially unchanged*)	Decreased (*decreased drug exposure*)
Inhibition	Decreased (*increased drug exposure*)	Negligible (*drug exposure essentially unchanged*)	Negligible (*drug exposure essentially unchanged*)	Increased (*increased drug exposure*)

system and it will have a volume of distribution similar to that of the blood volume. If, however, it is distributed out of the circulatory system and binds to tissue components (e.g. protein, fats), less remains in the blood and the drug will appear to be distributed in a larger volume. The larger the volume, the more widespread (tissue-bound) the drug is within the body. This is illustrated in Figure 5.4 using a bucket filled to its maximum capacity of 5 L, which is its actual or real volume. When the drug remains in the 'blood', volume of distribution remains at 5 L. However, when the drug distributes out of the 'blood', even though it is still a 5 L bucket, volume of distribution becomes 50 L.

In this example, the volume of the full bucket is 5 L and the amount of drug placed in each bucket is 100 mg

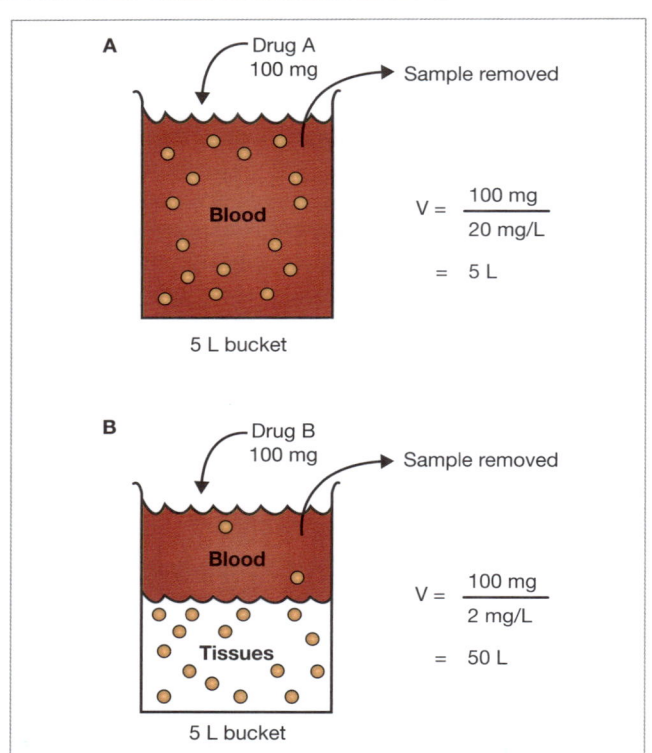

FIGURE 5.4 After the drug has distributed, a 'blood' sample is removed from each bucket and the concentration of the drug is measured. **A** Bucket A is filled with 'blood' to represent the circulatory system. Drug A binds tightly to plasma proteins and remains within the circulation. The concentration of drug measured in the 'blood' sample is 20 mg/L and the calculated volume of distribution of drug A is 5 L, the same as the volume of the bucket. **B** Bucket B is filled with a mixture of 'blood' and 'tissues' to represent the intravascular and extravascular compartments. Drug B moves from the 'blood' and is distributed to the 'tissues', where it binds strongly to tissue proteins. The concentration of drug measured in the 'blood' sample is 2 mg/L, and the calculated volume of distribution of drug B is 50 L, 10 times greater than the volume of the bucket!

If the volume of distribution is 'not a real volume', of what use is it clinically? First, it provides an indication of accumulation of drugs in extravascular (tissue) compartments (e.g. fat, muscle).

Second, volume of distribution is a major determinant of the half-life of a drug. Third, on occasion it is necessary to achieve a high plasma concentration quickly to produce the desired therapeutic response. To do this, a loading dose is administered to 'fill up' the volume of distribution. Because rapid intravenous administration is often undesirable because of the high plasma concentrations achieved before the distribution phase, loading doses may be given over a period of minutes or even hours. For example, in preeclampsia, magnesium sulfate will be given as a loading dose over 20 minutes, and then followed with an infusion to maintain the steady state. In this situation the loading dose is administered to produce a rapid pharmacological effect.

The volume of distribution changes with age, body composition, pregnancy, and disease states, and differs between males and females. For example, in infants under one year of age, volume of distribution is approximately 75–80% of body weight; in adult males, it is approximately 60% of body weight; and in adult females, it is 55% of body weight. As we age, there is also a progressive reduction in total body water and lean body mass with a relative increase in body fat.

KEY POINTS

Volume of distribution

■ The volume of distribution of a drug is defined as the volume in which the amount of drug in the body would need to be uniformly distributed in order to produce the observed concentration in blood.

■ The loading dose is the initial amount of drug required to fill the volume of distribution.

5.4 Key pharmacokinetic concept: Half-life

Half-life (t½) is a useful and commonly used parameter when describing a person's exposure to a drug. Indeed, half-life is the major determinant of:

● The duration of action of a drug after a single dose. If a drug is administered as a single dose, the longer the drug's half-life the longer the plasma drug concentration will remain within the therapeutic range (CFB 5.1).

● The time taken to reach steady state with repeated dosing. In general, it takes three to five half-lives to reach the desired steady-state plasma drug concentration (Fig 5.5).

- The dosing frequency required to avoid massive fluctuations in plasma drug concentration during the dosing interval. Once steady state has been reached, the half-life and the dosing interval determine the extent to which the plasma drug concentration fluctuates. If a drug is given orally every half-life, then the concentration will fall by one-half between doses and the plasma drug concentration will remain within the therapeutic range between doses (Fig 5.5).

Determinants of half-life

The two processes that influence half-life are distribution and clearance. Changes in either of these processes will alter the half-life of a drug. It can be seen from Figure 5.6 that, if two drugs have the same clearance but different volumes of distribution, the half-life will be shorter for the drug with the smaller volume of distribution. Similarly, if the two drugs have the same volume of distribution but different clearances, the half-life will be shorter for the drug with the higher clearance. Changes in half-life may necessitate changes in the dosing regimen.

During pregnancy, due to physiological adaptations, there is an increase in plasma volume, a decrease in plasma albumin concentration, and the possibility of changes in hepatic and renal clearance of some drugs. These changes can impact the half-life of a drug and therefore, the need for adjusting the dosing regimen. However, the clinical implications of physiological adaptations on drug half-life have been poorly studied

Effects of volume of distribution and clearance on half-life

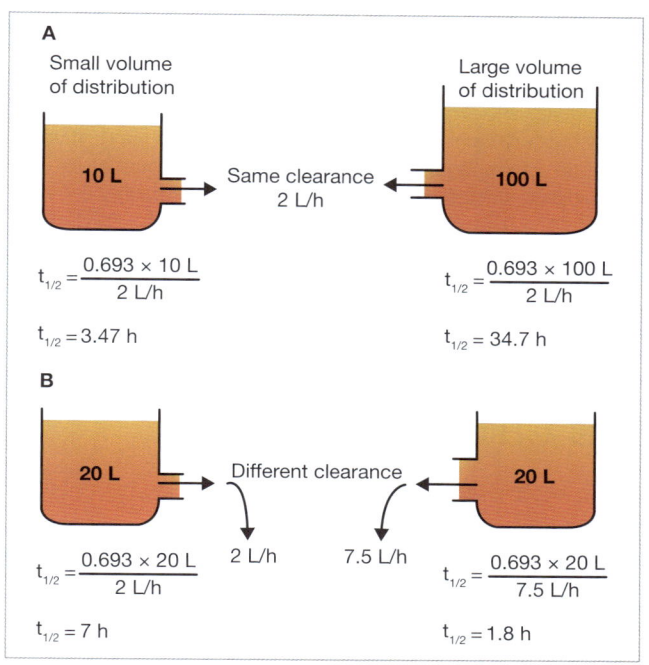

FIGURE 5.6 In **A** the drugs have the same clearance but differing volumes of distribution, and the half-lives differ by about 10-fold. In **B** the drugs have the same volume of distribution, but clearances differ about fourfold. In both examples the half-life alters in relation to the change in volume of distribution or the change in clearance.

In this example, the drug has a half-life of 4 hours and is given orally every 4 hours

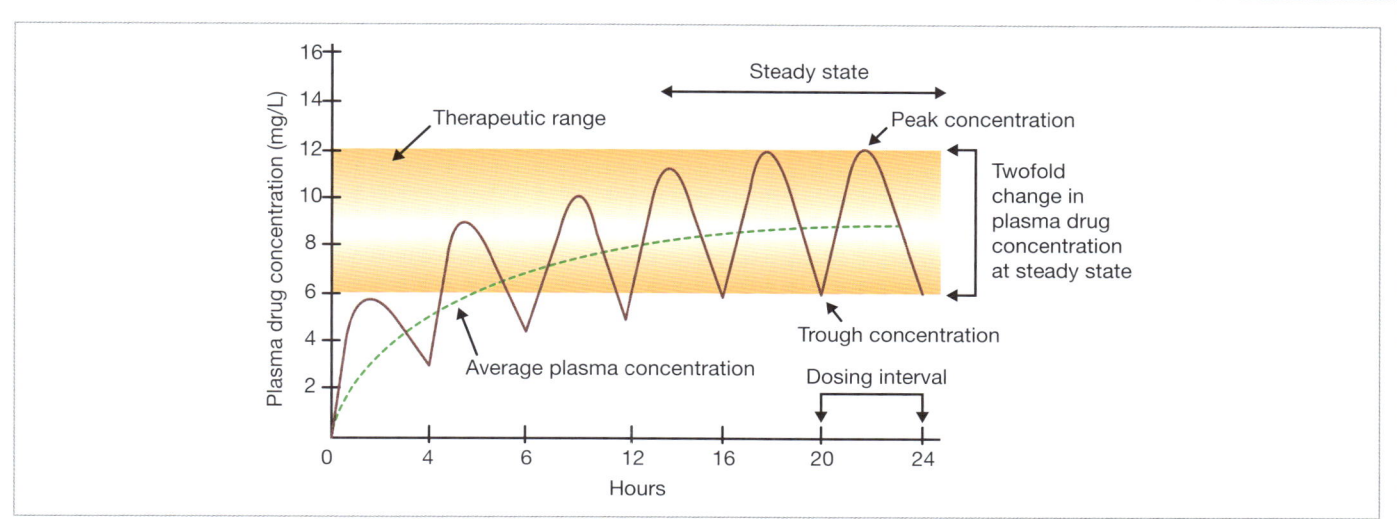

FIGURE 5.5 After one half-life the average plasma concentration is 50% of the eventual steady-state concentration, which is reached after three to five half-lives. Once steady state is reached, the plasma drug concentration will fluctuate twofold between doses if dosing continues on the half-life.

in pregnancy and data in this regard is scarce. Therefore, vigilance and close monitoring for drug toxicity or therapeutic failure during pregnancy are important.

KEY POINTS

Half-life

- Half-life is the major determinant of the duration of action of a drug after a single dose, the time taken to reach steady state with repeated dosing and the dosing frequency to minimise fluctuations in plasma drug concentration.

- The processes influencing half-life are volume of distribution and clearance.

5.5 Dosage measurements and calculations

Measurement systems

The main system of measurement in use for administering drugs is the metric system, based on SI units (Système International d'Unités) – this is the most widely used and the most convenient because units change in multiples of 10. Useful conversion tables to convert between metric measures and imperial ones, such as inches or pints, are included in some reference books, or conversions can be done online.

Metric system

The metric system has several basic units of measure including:

- length, the metre (m)
- time, the second (s)

- mass, the kilogram (kg)
- amount of substance, the mole (mol).

Derived units

Other useful derived units are: for volume, the cubic metre (m^3); for area, the square metre (m^2); for temperature, degrees Celsius (°C); and for mass, the gram (g). Other accepted units are the minute (min), the litre (L; 1 L = 1000 cm^3) and, for mass of atoms or molecules, the atomic mass unit (u), approximately equal to the mass of a hydrogen atom (also sometimes referred to as the dalton, Da).

The mole is the amount of any substance that contains Avogadro's number (about 6.022×1023) of atoms or molecules of the substance, and is equivalent to the molecular weight expressed in grams. The mole is therefore a different weight depending on the substance. For example, 1 mole of sodium chloride (molecular weight 58.5) is present in 58.5 g pure NaCl and 1 mole of water in 18 g pure H_2O. This unit is used mainly in laboratories and research situations, not for dosing drugs.

Metric prefixes

The metric system is a decimal system in which the basic units can be divided or multiplied by 10, 100 or 1000 to form a secondary unit. The names of the secondary units are formed by joining a Greek or Latin prefix to the name of the primary unit (Table 5.3); for example, the gram is the metric unit of weight commonly used in weighing chemicals and various pharmaceutical preparations. A gram is 1/1000 of a kilogram, and 1000 times greater than a milligram. Hence to change milligrams to grams, divide by 1000, and to change metres to centimetres, multiply by 100. When performing dose calculations, the unit micro (μ) should be written out or mc used if there is a possibility of confusion with 'm'. (A mistake, such as

TABLE 5.3 Metric prefixes, meanings and relations

PREFIX	MEANING	POWER OF 10
giga (G)	billions (thousand millions)	10^9, 1 000 000 000
mega (M)	millions	10^6, 1 000 000
kilo (k)	thousands	10^3, 1 000
hecto (h)	hundreds	10^2, 100
deca, deka (da)	tens	10^1, 10
deci (d)	tenths	10^{-1}, 1/10, 0.1
centi (c)	hundredths	10^{-2}, 1/100, 0.01
milli (m)	thousandths	10^{-3}, 1/1000, 0.001
micro (μ or mc)	millionths	10^{-6}, 0.000001
nano (n)	billionths	10^{-9}

dosing someone with 250 mg fentanyl instead of 250 µg, could be fatal.)

Conventional notations

The following is the style of notation as recommended for the International System of Units:

- Units are not capitalised (gram, not Gram).
- No full stop should be used with unit abbreviations (mL, not m.L. or mL.).
- Only decimal notation should be used, not fractions (0.25 kg, not 1/4 kg).
- Quantities less than 1 should have a zero placed to the left of the decimal point (0.75 mg, not .75 mg) to avoid mistakes.
- Abbreviations should not be made plural (10 kg, not kgs).
- There is a space between the numerical value and the unit symbol (100 g, not 100g).

There are some situations in medicine in which SI units are not used. These include:

- Percentage solutions, where the strength of a solution may be expressed as a percentage (e.g. 2% solution) rather than in mol/L or g/L. By convention, in this context '%' means grams of solute per 100 mL solution.
- Drip rates for infusion sets. Commonly, a standard set delivers 20 drops of aqueous liquid per mL (15 drops for blood), whereas a microdrip set delivers 60 drops per mL.
- Electrolyte solutions, which may be expressed in milliequivalents (mEq). For example: 1 L of a 1 mM solution of calcium chloride ($CaCl_2$) contains 1 mEq calcium ions and 2 mEq chloride ions.

CLINICAL FOCUS BOX 5.1

The dilemma of the missed dose

Often the question is raised, 'What do I do if I forget to take my medication?' Inevitably, on one or more occasions, a person will miss a dose of their drug. The simple issue of what to do if this occurs is rarely explained to women, and an unintentionally missed dose is construed too readily as noncompliance. For some drugs (e.g. a lipid-lowering drug), a missed dose is of little consequence, but for others a missed dose can result in a decrease in the therapeutic plasma concentration and subsequent clinical manifestations (e.g. epilepsy). Pregnancy as a result of missing a dose of the oral contraceptive pill is well recognised.

Knowledge of the drug's half-life is useful for making a recommendation if a dose is missed. In general, when the clinical effect of a drug is related to its half-life, a single missed dose is less of a problem for a drug with a long half-life than for a drug with a short half-life, for which the therapeutic effect will be lost rapidly. For some drugs (e.g. the oral contraceptive pill), specific recommendations exist for when a single dose is missed. A double dose should usually not be taken to make up for the dose missed because with many drugs (e.g. warfarin) this can cause adverse effects. The normal dosing regimen should be resumed and the next prescribed dose taken at the normal time.

A missed dose can be a problem with antimicrobial agents, and the recommendation is to take the dose as soon as remembered. For antimicrobial agents, the drug concentration in plasma should be above the minimum inhibitory concentration (MIC) to assure therapeutic response and to decrease the chance of antibacterial resistance.

Source: Gilbert et al 2002.

Dosage calculations

When in doubt, it is advisable to double-check all calculations with another health professional, especially with a pharmacist who will be highly trained in dose and concentration calculations. The examples of dose calculations in Appendix 4 are the types of problems that may be encountered. Each problem is solved in a stepwise manner, in some cases showing alternative possible methods. Where appropriate, helpful hints are included.

Body surface area for paediatric drug dosing

Nomograms for the estimation of body surface area from weight and height can be found in common drug guides. When specific dosage information is not available, specialist information should be sought from the drug information services in major hospitals.

Although rules have been devised for converting adult dosage schedules to those for infants and children, it must be emphasised that no rules or charts are adequate to guarantee safety of dosage at any age, particularly in the neonate. Always take care to check whether the drug doses are expressed either as a mg/kg/dose or on a mg/kg/24 hours basis. No method takes into account all variables, particularly inter-individual differences. The calculated dose is a guide for initiating therapy, but the severity of the primary disorder, the presence of co-existing conditions, clinical response and therapeutic drug monitoring all contribute to ascertaining the optimal dose.

Rounding off

As dosage calculations underpin a physical activity, there are some logistical limitations associated with this activity that need to be accounted for. For example:

- the capacity to administer a fraction of a drop in an infusion (round off to whole number)
- the capacity to administer a small fraction of a mL in a syringe (round off to one decimal place).

Dosage measurements and calculations

- The primary system of measurement for drug administration is the metric system, based on SI units. Understanding these units is fundamental for accurate dosage calculations.

- Dosage calculation errors can lead to serious consequences. Adherence to standardised units minimises mistakes and ensures clarity in communication.

REVIEW EXERCISES

1   Nika is taking labetalol (a high-hepatic clearance drug) for gestational hypertension and is administered a second drug that is known to inhibit the metabolism of labetalol. Should her dose of labetalol be adjusted? If the current dose is maintained, what are the possible clinical consequences?

2   Lara is diagnosed with preeclampsia and commenced on a magnesium sulphate infusion following receiving the loading dose as IM. If the urine output (renal clearance) is decreased, what would need to happen? Explain why it is important to monitor Lara's urine output.

REFERENCES

Gilbert A, Roughead L, Sansom L. I've missed a dose; what should I do? Aust Prescr. 2002;25:16-18.

Galoiu S, First trimester of pregnancy reference ranges for serum TSH and thyroid tumor reclassified as benign. Acta Endocrinol (Buchar). 2016 Apr-Jun;12(2): 242-243. doi: 10.4183/aeb.2016.242

Kashi Z, Bahar A, Akha O, et al. Levothyroxine dosage requirement during pregnancy in well-controlled hypothyroid women: a longitudinal study. Glob J Health Sci. 2016 Apr;8(4):227-233.

ADDITIONAL RESOURCES

Rang HP, Dale MM, Ritter JM, et al. Rang and Dale's pharmacology. Edn 7. Edinburgh: Churchill Livingston, 2012.

CHAPTER 6

ADVERSE DRUG REACTIONS AND DRUG INTERACTIONS

Maryam Bazargan, Kirsten Small

Key Abbreviations

ADR	adverse drug reaction
CAM	complementary and alternative medicine
DDI	drug–drug interaction

Key Terms

adverse drug event 90

adverse drug reaction 90

complementary and alternative medicine 91

drug–drug interaction 91

pseudoallergic reaction 92

Chapter Focus

With the increasing use of multiple concurrent medications, known as polypharmacy, drug interactions are increasingly a cause for concern because they may result in loss of efficacy (decreased benefit) or the development of toxicity (unwanted effects). Additionally, with the widespread use of complementary and alternative medicines (CAMs) such as vitamin, herbal, aromatherapy, and homeopathic products, drug–CAM interactions are adding to the burden. Many studies have confirmed adverse drug reactions and drug interactions are major clinical problems, accounting for a significant number of hospital admissions, extended hospital stays and substantial costs to the healthcare system. Health professionals should be aware of the adverse reaction and drug interaction profiles of drugs and CAMs and be ever-vigilant for the occurrence of adverse outcomes.

Learning Outcomes

- Understand the different types of adverse drug reactions and how to minimise them.
- Understand drug–drug interaction and drug–CAM interaction and how they impact the pharmacology (pharmacokinetic or pharmacokinetic interactions) of the other drug.
- Critically apply knowledge of adverse drug reactions and drug–drug interaction management to the care of a woman and her infant.

CRITICAL THINKING SCENARIO

Abeba is a primiparous woman at 39 weeks of gestation who was induced for preeclampsia. She experienced a post-partum haemorrhage (PPH) of 1.2 L.

1   In the management of her PPH, what considerations regarding medications are important and why?

Introduction

Throughout the centuries, the use of medicinal products has gone hand-in-hand with reports of **adverse drug reactions** (ADRs). Public concern about ADRs arose in the late 19th century because of sudden deaths associated with the use of chloroform. This led to the development of regulatory bodies, such as the Food and Drug Administration (FDA) in the United States, which establish the safety of new drugs. Despite regulatory frameworks, there have been many notable incidences of ADRs that have resulted in withdrawal of the offending drug (Table 6.1). Public interest in the safety of drugs has increased due to better communication between consumers and health professionals.

6.1 Adverse drug reactions

The World Health Organization (WHO) defines an ADR as 'any response to a drug which is noxious, unintended, and which occurs at doses normally (and appropriately) used in man for the prophylaxis, diagnosis, or therapy of disease' (WHO 1984). Clinical responses to an ADR include modifying the dose, discontinuing the drug, hospitalising the person, or providing supportive measures. This definition does not encompass drug overdose, drug withdrawal, drug abuse, or errors in administration. These are included within the definition of an **adverse drug event**.

Risk factors for developing an adverse drug reaction

Risk factors for ADRs are specific to both the person and the drug. Factors relating to the person include:

- age – the elderly and neonates
- sex – women appear to be more susceptible
- kidney or liver disease
- genetic factors
- history of prior drug reactions
- polypharmacy (five drugs or more).

Factors specific to the drug can include:

- chemical characteristics – e.g. large molecules such as heparin can themselves be immunogenic
- class of drug – e.g. anticoagulants
- route of drug administration – topical and oral routes generally involve a lower incidence of drug allergy
- dose – many ADRs are dose-related
- duration and frequency – prolonged and frequent use can increase the risk of an ADR.

TABLE 6.1 Example of notable adverse drug reactions necessitating withdrawal of the drug

YEAR	DRUG	USE	ADVERSE DRUG REACTION
1961	Thalidomide	Sedative	Congenital malformations
1983	Zomepirac	Anti-inflammatory	Anaphylaxis
1992	Temafloxacin	Antibiotic	Blood dyscrasias
1998	Terfenadine	Antihistamine	Ventricular dysrhythmia
2000	Troglitazone	Hypoglycaemic	Liver damage
2008	Rimonabant	Antiobesity	Severe depression and suicide
2011	Sitaxentan	Treatment of pulmonary hypertension	Fatal idiosyncratic hepatic failure
2021	Belviq (lorcaserin)	Weight loss	Increased risk of cancer

Incidence of adverse drug reactions

Adverse drug reactions are a major cause of morbidity and mortality. Taking multiple drugs contributes to the incidence of ADRs. In addition to prescribed medications and those bought over the counter, women may use **complementary and alternative medicines** (CAMs). The trend has been strongest among pregnant women and includes the use of herbal medicines and aromatherapy oils. ADRs occur in people of all ages and are twice as common in women.

Classification of adverse drug reactions

The current classification system is not ideal, and not every ADR fits perfectly into one of the categories. It is generally accepted that there are two main categories of ADR, type A (augmented) and type B (bizarre), and two subordinate categories, type C (chronic) and type D (delayed). A further two classes include end-of-use or withdrawal effects (type E) and unexpected failure of therapy (type F).

Type A (augmented, dose-related) ADRs

Type A ADRs are characterised by:

- predictable reaction based on the pharmacology of the drug (often an exaggeration of effect)
- relationship to dose
- common occurrence (about 80% of ADRs)
- usually mild
- high morbidity and low mortality
- reproducibility in animal models.

Factors predisposing to type A reactions include the dose, pharmaceutical variation in drug formulation, pharmacokinetic variation (e.g. renal failure), pharmaco-dynamic variation (e.g. altered fluid and electrolyte balance, pregnancy) and **drug–drug interactions** (DDIs) (e.g. inhibition of metabolism of one drug by another concomitantly administered drug). Examples include:

- sedation with the use of antihistamines
- bleeding with anticoagulants
- hypoglycaemia from the use of insulin
- hypokalaemia with the use of diuretics.
- constipation and nausea with the use of oxycodone.

Type B (bizarre, non-dose-related) ADRs

Type B ADRs are characterised by:

- unpredictability
- no relationship to dose
- uncommon occurrence (about 20% of ADRs)
- increased severity
- high morbidity and high mortality
- lack of reproducibility in animal models.

These reactions are less common but often cause death. Factors contributing to type B reactions include pharmaceutical variation, receptor abnormalities, unmasking of a biological deficiency (e.g. glucose-6-phosphate dehydrogenase deficiency), abnormalities in drug metabolism (e.g. slow acetylators of the antituberculosis drug isoniazid), drug allergy and DDIs (e.g. rare incidence of hepatitis). Examples include interstitial nephritis with the use of non-steroidal anti-inflammatory drugs, penicillin hypersensitivity, and eosinophilia with the use of anticonvulsants such as carbamazepine and phenytoin.

Type C (chronic, dose-related and time-related) ADRs

Type C ADRs are related to long-term use. Examples include:

- adaptive changes (e.g. development of drug tolerance and physical dependence)
- appearance of tardive dyskinesia in those treated long term with neuroleptic drugs for schizophrenia
- rebound phenomena (e.g. rebound tachycardia after the abrupt discontinuation of beta-blockers and acute adrenal insufficiency after abrupt withdrawal of corticosteroids).

Type D (delayed, time-related) ADRs

Type D ADRs are characterised by the appearance of delayed effects. These may be acceptable if the benefit of drug therapy outweighs the risk, as in the case of irreversible infertility in young people receiving cytotoxic drugs for malignancies. In general, however, they are considered unacceptable. Examples include carcino-genesis (e.g. the association of lymphoma with immunosuppressive drugs) and teratogenesis.

Type E (end-of-use, withdrawal) ADRs

Type E ADRs are uncommon and are related to withdrawal of a drug. They include opiate withdrawal syndrome and myocardial ischaemia after abrupt cessation of beta-blockers. Newborn abstinence syndrome (NAS) is an example of type E ADR, where after birth, a newborn no longer receives maternally ingested opioids via the placenta.

Type F (failure, unexpected failure of therapy) ADRs

Type F ADRs are increasingly common and are often caused by a drug interaction (e.g. inadequate dose of the oral contraceptive when a drug that induces the metabolism of oestrogen is administered concomitantly).

Drug allergy

A drug allergy, or hypersensitivity, is a type B ADR. Drug allergies are characterised by:

- occurrence in a small number of people
- the requirement for previous exposure to either the same or a chemically related drug

- the rapid development of an allergic reaction after re-exposure
- production of clinical manifestations of an allergic reaction.

The diagnosis of a drug allergy is often difficult to establish because there are no reliable laboratory tests that can identify the relevant drug, and in some cases the symptoms can imitate infectious disease symptoms. The situation may be easier if the drug administered is commonly suspected of causing an allergic reaction (e.g. penicillin), but it is difficult if the drug used is seldom reported to produce an allergic reaction.

Some drugs can produce a **pseudoallergic reaction** that resembles an allergic reaction but has no immunological basis. Usually, these reactions occur because of mast cell degranulation and subsequent release of histamine. Clinically, they resemble the type I hypersensitivity reaction, but do not involve drug-specific immunoglobulin E. An example of a pseudoallergic reaction is the release of histamine that occurs with opiates (e.g. morphine), vancomycin, and radiological contrast media. Allergic reactions to drugs generally follow the type I–IV classification. Table 6.2 lists the types of reactions, the main clinical manifestations and examples of drugs commonly implicated.

Immune-modulating drugs and adverse drug reactions

Drugs that modulate the immune system are commonly used to treat diseases such as cancer, rheumatoid arthritis, multiple sclerosis, inflammatory bowel disease, and lupus. Although beneficial in many clinical settings, immune-modulating drugs are associated with a significant number of ADRs. Suppression of the immune response increases the risk of infection and cancer. The potential risk of corticosteroids used in pregnancy for fetal lung maturation can be the increased risk of infection in the mother.

> **KEY POINTS**
>
> ### Adverse drug reactions
>
> - An ADR is defined as any response to a drug that is noxious and unintended, and that occurs at doses normally used for the prophylaxis, diagnosis, or therapy of disease.
> - ADRs occur in people of all ages and are twice as common in women. They are a major cause of morbidity and mortality.
> - There are two main categories of ADR, type A (predictable) and type B (unpredictable), and subordinate categories, type C (chronic use), type D (delayed reactions), type E (end-of-use or withdrawal effects), and type F (unexpected failure of therapy).
> - The diagnosis of a drug allergy can often be difficult to establish because there are no reliable laboratory tests that can identify the relevant drug, and the symptoms can sometimes imitate infectious disease symptoms (e.g. fever).
> - Risk factors for developing an ADR include, but are not limited to, age, sex, presence of concurrent disease, multiple chronic medical problems, drug class, polypharmacy, renal/hepatic impairment, pregnancy, genetics, history of prior drug reaction, the drug dose, and the duration and frequency of drug use.

6.2 Drug interactions

A drug interaction occurs when a drug's pharmacological effect is altered by another drug, food, or CAM: that is, there is an increased therapeutic and/or adverse effect or a decreased therapeutic and/or adverse effect. Drug interactions are often unanticipated and go unrecognised, and the clinical and economic importance is frequently underestimated.

Frequency of drug interactions

The exact frequency of drug interactions is unknown, although anecdotal evidence suggests that they are

TABLE 6.2 Allergic drug reactions

(TYPE)/REACTION	CLINICAL MANIFESTATIONS	EXAMPLES OF DRUGS
(I) Immediate hypersensitivity	Urticaria, anaphylaxis, angio-oedema, bronchospasm	Penicillins, streptomycin, local anaesthetics, neuromuscular blocking drugs, radiological contrast media
(II) Antibody-dependent cytotoxic	Cytopenia, vasculitis, haemolytic anaemia	Quinine, rifampicin, metronidazole
(III) Complex-mediated	Serum sickness, vasculitis, interstitial nephritis	Anticonvulsants, antibiotics, hydralazine, diuretics
(IV) Cell-mediated or delayed hypersensitivity	Contact sensitivity	Local anaesthetic creams

relatively common and result in a significant number of hospital admissions. The possibility of a drug interaction exists whenever two or more medications are prescribed to an individual, and the likelihood of an interaction will increase as the number of medications used increases (polypharmacy). It may be difficult to identify which 'drugs' are involved in a DDI, especially if the person is using over-the-counter drugs, CAMs, and/or dietary/nutritional supplements. Those at greatest risk of a drug interaction are:

- the severely ill, who typically receive multiple drugs
- those receiving chronic therapy, often comprising a cocktail of drugs (e.g. in the treatment of either HIV infection or cancer)
- older adults, who tend to have multiple pathologies and often receive multiple drugs concurrently.

Drug interactions are of greatest concern for drugs with a narrow therapeutic index. Even a small change in the concentration of the drug available in the plasma can lead to a major alteration in response. For example: enhanced anticoagulation (bleeding) with warfarin resulting from concomitant use of the antidysrhythmic drug amiodarone, which inhibits the metabolism of warfarin. Concomitant administration of ondansetron and selective serotonin reuptake inhibitors (SSRIs) can increase the risk of a potentially life-threatening condition called serotonin syndrome.

Interactions involving drugs with a wide therapeutic index (e.g. penicillin antibiotics, beta-adrenoceptor antagonists) cause fewer problems. Knowledge of the mechanisms of drug interactions enables health professionals to prevent interactions occurring (wherever possible) and to systematically analyse potentially new drug interactions. Indeed, analysis of known and potential interactions is critical in the planning of a therapeutic regimen.

Classification of drug interactions

Drug interactions are broadly classified, according to their pharmacological mechanism, into either pharmacodynamic or pharmacokinetic interactions.

Pharmacodynamic drug interactions

Pharmacodynamic drug interactions may be 'direct' or 'indirect'. Direct pharmacodynamic interactions involve additive effects at a common target (and possibly potentiation) or antagonism due to actions at different sites in an organ. An example of antagonism at a common receptor site is the concurrent use of a beta$_2$-adrenoceptor agonist (used to treat asthma, e.g. salbutamol) and a non-selective beta-adrenoceptor antagonist (used to treat hypertension, e.g. propranolol). Both drugs have opposing effects at the same receptor (i.e. the beta$_2$-adrenoceptor). An example of agonist activity at a common receptor site (opioid receptor μ) is concurrent use of oxycodone and tapentadol. Both oxycodone and tapentadol are opioid analgesics that bind to the μ-opioid receptor. When these medications are used together, they have an additive effect on pain relief, as they are both working at the same receptor site to increase the inhibition of pain signals. It is important to note that using multiple opioid medications together also increases the ADRs such as sedation, respiratory depression, and dependence. Unintentional drug interactions of this type should not occur because they are so obvious from the known pharmacology of the drugs.

Examples of direct pharmacodynamic interactions involving drugs with different mechanisms of action include the following:

- monoamine oxidase (MAO) inhibitors – used in the treatment of depression, increase the amount of noradrenaline (norepinephrine) stored in nerve terminals, and interact dangerously (to cause marked hypertension) with 'sympathomimetic' drugs such as ephedrine that cause the release of stored noradrenaline. Tyramine, present in foods such as cheese, yeast extracts and Chianti-type wines, produces a similar response in people treated with MAO inhibitors because it is an indirect-acting sympathomimetic, which displaces noradrenaline from the nerve terminals.
- warfarin – an anticoagulant that inhibits vitamin K–mediated synthesis of clotting factors. The risk of bleeding is increased by co-administration of aspirin, which decreases platelet aggregation by inhibiting the synthesis of thromboxane A2.

An indirect pharmacodynamic interaction occurs when the pharmacological effect of one drug alters the response to another drug, even though the two effects are not themselves directly related. Common examples include certain diuretics (e.g. furosemide [frusemide] or hydrochlorothiazide), which lower the blood potassium concentration. This will enhance the toxic effects of the cardiac glycoside digoxin, which is used to treat atrial fibrillation and cardiac failure, and of type III antidysrhythmic drugs (e.g. amiodarone) that prolong the cardiac action potential.

Pharmacokinetic drug interactions

The plasma concentration of a drug may be altered by interactions occurring during absorption, distribution, metabolism, and excretion.

Absorption

Absorption interactions involve a change in either the rate or the extent of absorption. Drugs that change the rate of gastric emptying (i.e. the time it takes for the contents of the stomach to empty into the small bowel) will alter the rate of absorption of co-administered drugs.

Mu (μ) opioid receptor antagonists (e.g. morphine) delay gastric emptying and gastrointestinal motility. This combination of effects delays drug absorption from the gastrointestinal tract. Many drugs, including tricyclic antidepressants and histamine-1-receptor antagonists that possess antimuscarinic properties, delay the absorption of co-administered drugs. Gastric emptying rate is slowed by opioid drugs, including morphine, oxycodone, and pethidine, and hence the time to reach the peak plasma concentration is generally increased for a drug co-administered with an opioid.

Co-administered drugs may also decrease the extent of drug absorption. Whereas changes in the rate of absorption generally affect only the time to onset of action, changes in extent of absorption can alter response. For example, colestyramine is a bile acid-binding resin used to treat hypercholesterolaemia. Unfortunately, colestyramine also binds other drugs, reducing the amount of drug that is absorbed. Because colestyramine reduces the absorption of corticosteroids, digoxin, thyroxine, and warfarin (and probably other drugs), these drugs should be administered either several hours before or after the colestyramine dose.

Co-administration of drugs with another drug that alters stomach pH may affect the rate and extent of drug absorption. For example, proton pump inhibitors (PPIs) and H2 blockers reduce stomach acid production, or antacids that neutralise stomach acid, can decrease the absorption of medications that require an acidic environment for proper dissolution and absorption, such as absorption of oral iron preparations.

Physiological adaptations of pregnancy, including decreased stomach acidity and decreased GI motility can interact with drugs at absorption phase.

Distribution

Because many drugs circulate in the blood bound (at least in part) to the proteins albumin and α1-acid glycoprotein, they may compete for the same binding sites. Displacement from plasma protein of one drug by another is common, and this leads to an increase in the unbound, pharmacologically active, concentration of the drug in the blood. Although it is widely believed the increase in unbound concentration arising from 'displacement interactions' may precipitate drug toxicity, this is rarely the case. Following a drug displacement interaction, the concentration of unbound drug in the blood does indeed increase. However, the unbound drug is available for distribution into tissues, leading to an increase in the volume of distribution, hepatic clearance, and renal excretion. There is, however, a decrease in total drug concentration (i.e. bound plus unbound drug) because of the higher clearance.

Interaction at distribution phase may be significant for drugs with a small volume of distribution and/or high protein binding. Lithium is a medication with a narrow therapeutic index and is used in the treatment of bipolar disorder. Approximately 80–90% of lithium in the bloodstream is bound to albumin and the remaining 10–20% is free or unbound. Lithium has a very small volume of distribution of about 5 L. Any changes in the fraction unbound or its volume of distribution affect its pharmacokinetics and toxicity.

During pregnancy, there is a significant decrease in plasma albumin concentration and expansion of the plasma and interstitial fluid volumes. These physiological adaptations can modify distribution phase drug interactions.

Metabolism

Administration of some drugs can lead to decreased (inhibited) or increased (induced) activity of drug-metabolising enzymes such as cytochrome P450 (CYP). Many important drug interactions arise from altered metabolism, and the clinical importance of the interaction depends on the change in clearance and the therapeutic index of the altered drug. A 10% change in clearance is unlikely to be important, but a 30% change in the clearance of a narrow therapeutic index drug such as warfarin can have serious implications. Importantly, just as there is considerable inter-individual variability in the clearance of metabolised drugs, there is significant variability in the magnitude of the change in clearance associated with any metabolic drug interaction. Drugs known to cause enzyme induction are generally non-selective in their effects on CYP enzymes. Examples include:

- the antituberculosis drug rifampicin, which appears to induce all CYP and UDP-glucuronosyltransferase (UGT) isoforms, therefore potentially decreasing the blood concentration of all co-administered drugs that are metabolised by these enzymes
- the anticonvulsant drugs phenobarbital (phenobarbitone), phenytoin, and carbamazepine induce CYP2C9 and CYP3A4, and possibly other enzymes of CYP and UGT families. People with epilepsy receiving these drugs are prone to drug interactions and their consequences (e.g. unwanted pregnancy due to enhanced metabolism of oral contraceptive steroids)
- chronic consumption of ethanol (alcohol) induces CYP2E1, although there are relatively few clinically used drugs that are metabolised by this enzyme. The combination of alcohol and paracetamol use can cause liver damage. Oxidation of paracetamol by CYP2E1 produces the toxic metabolite of NAPQI (N-acetyl-p-benzoquinone imine), which can cause liver damage if it accumulates in the liver.

Inhibitory drug interactions are relatively common, and inhibition of metabolism increases the steady-state blood concentration and the likelihood of drug toxicity.

Some drugs, notably the H2 antagonist cimetidine, inhibit the activity of most CYP enzymes (although UGT is unaffected). Conversely, probenecid inhibits most UGT enzymes (without affecting CYP). Most inhibitory interactions are relatively selective for one or a limited number of drug-metabolising enzymes because they most commonly arise from competition for metabolism at the enzyme active site. It is generally not correct to refer to a drug as 'an inhibitor of drug metabolism'. Rather, a drug will normally selectively inhibit the metabolism of other drugs for a limited number of enzymes, and this specificity of interaction is used to predict and interpret metabolic drug interactions. Some selective inhibitors of CYP enzymes are shown in Table 6.3. As an example, fluoxetine causes interactions with many drugs metabolised by CYP2D6 (e.g. other antidepressants and perhexiline), which generally requires a reduction of the dose. The clearances of drugs metabolised by CYP3A4 are similarly decreased by the commonly used antibiotic erythromycin, again generally requiring a dose reduction. The following are examples of CYP metabolic drug interactions:

- Amiodarone and its active metabolite desethylamiodarone inhibit CYP2C9, which metabolises S-warfarin. This interaction increases the risk of major bleeding.
- Paroxetine, a CYP2D6 inhibitor, reduces the plasma concentration of endoxifen, an active metabolite of tamoxifen used in breast cancer treatment.
- Fluoxetine, also a CYP2D6 inhibitor, interferes with the metabolism of oxycodone and beta-blockers, increasing the plasma concentration of these drugs and a higher risk of toxicity.
- Macrolide antibiotics, such as erythromycin and clarithromycin, are known to inhibit the activity of the CYP3A4 enzyme in the liver. This can decrease the metabolism of oxycodone, which is metabolised primarily by CYP3A4.

TABLE 6.3 Examples of clinically significant inhibitors of CYP enzymes

ENZYME	INHIBITORS
CYP1A2	Ciprofloxacin, fluvoxamine
CYP2C8	Gemfibrozil, trimethoprim
CYP2C9	Fluconazole
CYP2C19	Fluconazole, fluvoxamine, moclobemide, ticlopidine
CYP2D6	Cinacalcet, doxepin, fluoxetine, paroxetine, perhexiline, quinine
CYP3A4	Clarithromycin, diltiazem, erythromycin, indinavir, itraconazole, ritonavir, saquinavir, verapamil

- Many azole antifungals inhibit CYP3A, decreasing clearance of some statins, which increases the risk of statin-induced myopathy.

Metabolic drug interactions also occur with other drug-metabolising enzymes. For example, fluconazole appears to inhibit only UGT2B7 (that metabolises morphine and zidovudine). In the case of the fluconazole–morphine drug interaction, a rise in the plasma concentration of morphine may result in respiratory depression. Another example is probenecid, used to treat gout and other conditions. It can inhibit UGT2B7 and can increase the blood levels of drugs that are metabolised by this enzyme, such as morphine and other opioids.

A potentially fatal interaction occurs when azathioprine and allopurinol are co-administered. Allopurinol is an inhibitor of the enzyme xanthine oxidase and is used to treat gout and gouty arthritis. Azathioprine (used mainly in cancer treatment) is converted to an active metabolite, 6-mercaptopurine, which is metabolised by xanthine oxidase. Co-administration of azathioprine and allopurinol leads to accumulation of 6-mercaptopurine, resulting in potentially life-threatening bone marrow suppression.

Excretion

Interactions may occur between drugs that are substrates for secretory and efflux transporters in the kidney. The mechanism of such interactions is simply competition for the same transporter. For example, the plasma concentrations of penicillin, ciprofloxacin, furosemide (frusemide) and tenofovir are increased by co-administration of probenecid, which inhibits an organic anion secretory transporter (OAT1/3) in the basolateral membrane of the proximal tubule, thereby reducing active secretion of the drugs into the renal tubule. As a result, probenecid can decrease the concentration of nitrofurantoin in urine, increases the duration of action of penicillin and ampicillin, and impairs secretion of methotrexate in the urine.

Changing urine pH can impact renal excretion of drugs. For example, penicillin antibiotics and aspirin are both weak acids, so they are excreted more rapidly in alkaline urine. This is because the ionised form of these drugs (in the alkaline environment of urine) is less likely to be reabsorbed in the tubular system of the kidney. To treat methotrexate toxicity and aspirin (salicylate) toxicity alkalinisation of urine by administering sodium bicarbonate is used. Alkalinisation of the urine increases ionisation of these drugs in the urine and enhances their excretion, thereby reducing the toxicity.

Drug interactions with nutrients and CAMs

Although there is wide appreciation of drug interactions, interactions between nutrients and/or food components and CAMs are less often considered and, in fact, may be discounted. Foods may alter the activity of drug-metabolising enzymes. Notable in this regard are chemicals present in grapefruit juice that inhibit the activity of CYP3A4 present in the gastrointestinal tract. The enzyme present in the small bowel appears to contribute significantly to the first-pass metabolism of numerous CYP3A4 substrates. Thus, the bioavailability of certain drugs, such as ciclosporin, felodipine, midazolam, triazolam, and verapamil, increases significantly when they are taken with grapefruit juice, enhancing the potential for toxicity.

There is also interest in the effects of herbal medicines on drug metabolism and the consequences of herb–drug interactions, based on the same pharmacokinetic and pharmacodynamic mechanisms as DDIs. Herbal medicines are used widely, particularly by women, given the perception that 'natural' products are a safe and effective alternative to pharmaceuticals. As plant products, herbal medicines typically contain hundreds of different chemicals. It is not surprising some of these alter the activity of drug-metabolising enzymes. In the United States, the seven top-selling herbal medicines in descending order are: ginkgo, St John's wort, ginseng, kava, saw palmetto, garlic, and echinacea. Interestingly, the top 10 herbal/botanical supplements reported to have the most interactions with individual drugs are (in descending order): St John's wort, ginkgo, kava, digitalis, willow, Asian ginseng, astragalus, licorice, saw palmetto, and garlic; and the drugs involved in the most interactions were warfarin, insulin, aspirin, digoxin, and ticlopidine.

Important in terms of drug interaction is St John's wort, taken to treat depression. St John's wort contains chemicals called hyperforins, which mimic the effects of rifampicin as an inducer of CYP enzymes. Consumption for 2 weeks significantly induces the activity of both hepatic and intestinal CYP3A4 and the intestinal transporter P-glycoprotein. Thus, the clearance of amitriptyline, carbamazepine, ciclosporin, HIV protease inhibitors, warfarin and several other drugs is increased in subjects taking St John's wort, with risk of therapeutic failure. Similarly, the plasma concentrations of alprazolam and midazolam are reduced in healthy volunteers taking St John's wort. Furthermore, oral contraceptives contain ethinylestradiol, which is metabolised by CYP3A4. Concomitant administration of St John's wort increases the metabolism of ethinylestradiol, and unplanned pregnancy has been reported as an issue in women who use oral contraceptive steroids and St John's wort. Not surprisingly given its use in depression, interactions with 'synthetic' antidepressants have been reported. The combination of St John's wort and the serotonin reuptake inhibitors (sertraline, paroxetine, and venlafaxine) may result in headaches, changes in mental state, tremors, autonomic instability, gastrointestinal upset, myalgias and motor restlessness (secondary to central serotonin excess). These symptoms may be explained by inhibition of serotonin reuptake in the brain by St John's wort.

There is evidence to suggest that multiple complementary medicines interact (pharmacodynamically or pharmacokinetically) with 'pharmaceutical' drugs, and studies investigating the mechanisms involved and quantifying the magnitudes of any interactions are ongoing. Interactions between herbal medicines and conventional drugs are increasingly observed, and it is likely that their incidence is more common than anticipated initially. Information on the use of complementary medicines should be obtained from any individual, including pregnant women, prior to prescribing any drug, as it is essential to determine if concomitant use of complementary medicines may exacerbate the potential for drug interactions.

KEY POINTS

Drug interactions

- Drug interactions are broadly classified according to their pharmacological mechanisms, i.e. pharmacodynamic or pharmacokinetic.

- Pharmacodynamic drug interactions may be 'direct' or 'indirect'.

- Direct pharmacodynamic interactions involve additive effects at a common target (and possibly potentiation) or antagonism due to actions at different sites in an organ.

- An indirect pharmacodynamic interaction occurs when the pharmacological effects of one drug alter the response to another drug, even though the two types of effects are not themselves directly related.

- A pharmacokinetic drug interaction can alter the concentration of drug in the systemic circulation through interactions occurring at any stage – i.e. during absorption, distribution, metabolism, or excretion.

- Multiple CAMs (including St John's wort, ginkgo, and kava) are known to interact either pharmacodynamically or pharmacokinetically with prescription drugs.

- Strategies for reducing the incidence of ADRs and drug interactions include careful history-taking, considering non-drug treatment, correct and appropriate dosing, frequent review of therapeutic goals and drug regimens, avoiding polypharmacy, and careful communication with the person or carer.

REVIEW EXERCISES

1 Sarah presents with a rash that occurs days after having taken an antibiotic. Which class of antibiotics is most frequently implicated in causing a rash? Potentially, what type of adverse drug reaction is this? What advice will you give to Sarah in terms of future administration of antibiotics?

2 Linda has been using oral contraceptives for the last 5 years, since the birth of her third child. Recently, she needed to start taking antibiotics and was advised to use additional contraceptive methods to avoid the risk of pregnancy. She is confused about how she could get pregnant while taking her oral contraceptives as usual. She is also curious about how an antibiotic she is taking might reduce the effectiveness of contraception. How would you explain this?

3 Monica has depression and has been using prescribed fluoxetine. She has heard from a friend that St John's wort can help her mood to improve. Why is it important to counsel pregnant women against the consumption of St John's wort?

REFERENCES

World Health Organization. Collaborating centres for international drug monitoring. WHO: Geneva, 1984. (WHO publication DEM/NC/84:153 (E)).

— CHAPTER 7 —

PREGNANCY

Clare Davison, Roslyn Donnellan-Fernandez

Key Abbreviations

CAM	complementary and alternative medicine
COC	combined oral contraceptive
FASD	fetal alcohol spectrum disorder
FSH	follicle-stimulating hormone
hCG	human chorionic gonadotropin
HG	hyperemesis gravidarum
HRT	hormone replacement therapy
IUD	intrauterine device
LH	luteinising hormone
NSAID	non-steroidal anti-inflammatory drug
NVP	nausea and vomiting in pregnancy
OC	oral contraceptive
OTC	over the counter
PG	prostaglandin
SSRI	selective serotonin reuptake inhibitor
TA	tranexamic acid

Key Terms

Chapter Focus

This chapter provides an overview of the female reproductive system. The use of drugs in pregnancy is considered, including discussion of some complementary and alternative medicines (CAM) to manage discomfort and common complaints. Drug therapy in the pregnant woman, as contrasted with the rest of the adult population, is considered regarding the anatomical and physiological adaptations associated with pregnancy. Risks for the developing fetus are discussed (teratogenesis), as well as other possible effects.

Learning Outcomes

- Describe the physiology and normal functioning of the female reproductive system and understand its common complications.
- Understand how the physiological changes of pregnancy and gestation influence drug selection, pharmacodynamics and pharmacokinetics.
- List and discuss the common prescription, non-prescription and complementary and alternative medications, used during pregnancy to manage discomfort, including their side effects.
- Understand and apply the safe use of pharmaceutical medicines in pregnancy and the implications for midwifery practice to optimise maternal and fetal health.

CRITICAL THINKING SCENARIO

Mira is 28 years old and 8 weeks pregnant with her second child. Her first pregnancy, 2 years ago, was with a different partner. In her first pregnancy, Bella experienced debilitating morning sickness during the first and second trimester which required extended periods of hospitalisation. A diagnosis of hyperemesis gravidarum contributed to Bella considering the termination of that pregnancy. Bella is extremely fearful of how she will manage if this situation recurs, especially with an active toddler to care for. She is currently experiencing daily nausea and vomiting for extended periods. Although self-assessed as 'not as severe as during the previous pregnancy', Bella is anxious to manage these symptoms. Her pre-pregnancy weight was 52 kg and she currently weighs 50 kg. She is particularly concerned regarding the possible teratogenic effects of substances on her developing baby, and her diet is high in organically grown fruit and vegetables. As Bella's primary midwife, what advice and recommendations would you provide regarding the current management of her symptoms, including consideration of prescription medication and non-prescription alternatives?

7.1 Overview of the female reproductive system controls and hormones

There are several levels of control in the **female reproductive system** (Fig 7.1), involving factors and hormones that can be used to treat gynaecological disorders and affect reproductive functions:

- The hypothalamus secretes a releasing factor (gonadotrophin-releasing hormone [GnRH, gonadorelin]), which stimulates the anterior pituitary gland. It helps initiate puberty.
- The anterior pituitary gland releases trophic hormones – the gonadotrophins follicle-stimulating hormone (FSH) and luteinising hormone (LH]) – which control ovarian function in the menstrual cycle.
- The target gland (gonadal) hormones are estrogens and progesterone, which control female secondary sex characteristics, the reproductive cycle, and growth and development of accessory reproductive organs. Periodic cycling of hormone levels results in the menstrual cycle, which normally continues throughout reproductive life from menarche until menopause, except during pregnancy.
- Inhibins – glycoproteins produced in the gonads – decrease secretion of FSH and LH.
- Human chorionic gonadotrophin (hCG) and placental lactogen are secreted by the placenta during pregnancy.
- Prolactin and oxytocin, released from the anterior and posterior pituitary gland respectively, are involved in breast tissue proliferation, breastfeeding, and childbirth.

The 'puberty clock'

The prolonged period of childhood in humans allows a long period of learning before the onset of reproductive life. After the age of about 10 years, hormonal changes start to occur in both sexes: increased pulsatile output of GnRH from the hypothalamus in girls stimulates the pituitary gland to increase production of FSH and LH, stimulating the ovaries to produce estrogen and progesterone, and causing ovulation, maturation of female reproductive organs, development of secondary sexual characteristics and accelerated growth, followed by closure of the epiphyses of the long bones. The first menstrual period (**menarche**) is closely correlated with a skeletal age of 13 years but may occur some years earlier or later (range is 8–15 years).

The actual 'clock' that switches on reproductive development and function is unknown; the timing depends mainly (50–80%) on multiple genetic factors, as well as stimuli from the nervous system, metabolic hormones leptin and ghrelin, neurokinin B and kisspeptin peptides, now considered the master regulators of reproductive functions in mammals (Abreu & Kaiser 2016). Puberty is occurring earlier worldwide, possibly associated with increased dietary intake of animal protein and the increasing prevalence of obesity and height gain in childhood.

Delayed puberty (no pubertal changes in girls older than 13 years) may be due to familial late development, hypopituitarism, anorexia, or chronic severe illness. Treatment with the appropriate sex hormone(s) accelerates growth rate, development, and closure of the epiphyses of long bones, potentially leading to short stature.

The menstrual cycle

The changes occurring during the **menstrual cycle** and the actions of pituitary gonadotrophins and ovarian hormones are illustrated in Figure 7.2.

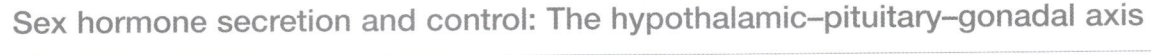

Sex hormone secretion and control: The hypothalamic–pituitary–gonadal axis

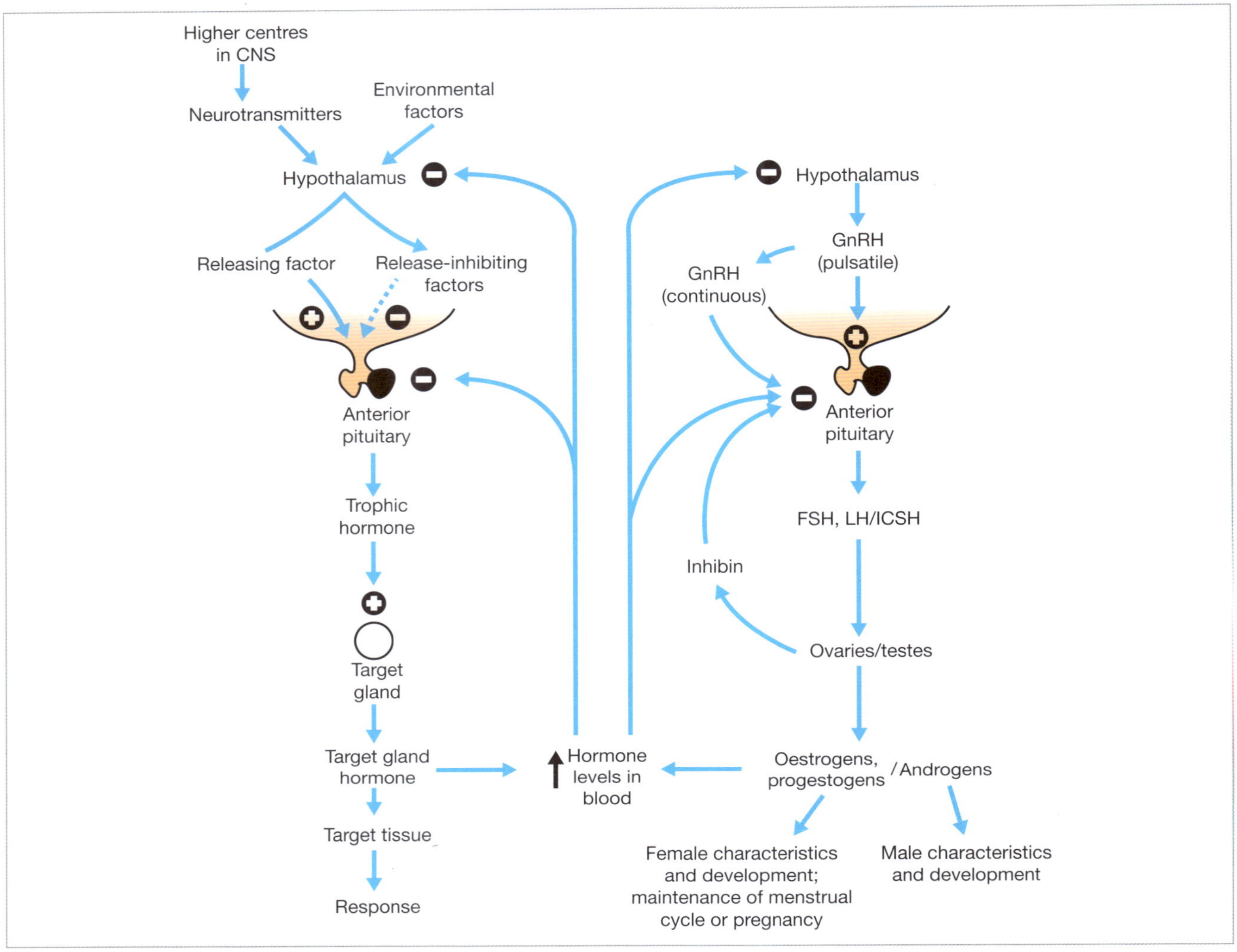

FIGURE 7.1

The physiological processes of a typical 28-day cycle are summarised below:

- Days 1–5, menstruation: Uterine lining is being shed, and FSH is stimulating follicle growth and production of estrogen in the ovary.
- Days 4–14 (roughly), proliferative stage: Rising estrogen levels prepare the uterus for a fertilised ovum and stimulate the pre-ovulatory surge in pituitary LH production (by positive feedback) and, later, the mid-cycle FSH surge.
- About day 14, ovulation: Occurs when the mature follicle ruptures and releases its ovum.
- Days 13–16, fertile period: The ovum travels through the oviduct to the uterus; if fertilised, it implants in the uterine wall and continues to divide and grow (pregnancy).
- Days 15–25, secretory phase: LH causes luteinisation – the ruptured follicle capsule changes into the corpus luteum, which releases estrogen and progesterone. Progesterone maintains the endometrium to facilitate implantation and suppresses further ovulation to prevent subsequent pregnancy. Inhibin from follicle and corpus luteum inhibits secretion of FSH and LH.
- Days 25–28: (a) If fertilisation (pregnancy) occurs, the corpus luteum continues to produce progesterone and maintains endometrium and pregnancy, and secretion of hCG begins. Levels of estrogens and progestogens continue to rise, and all changes of pregnancy begin to occur.

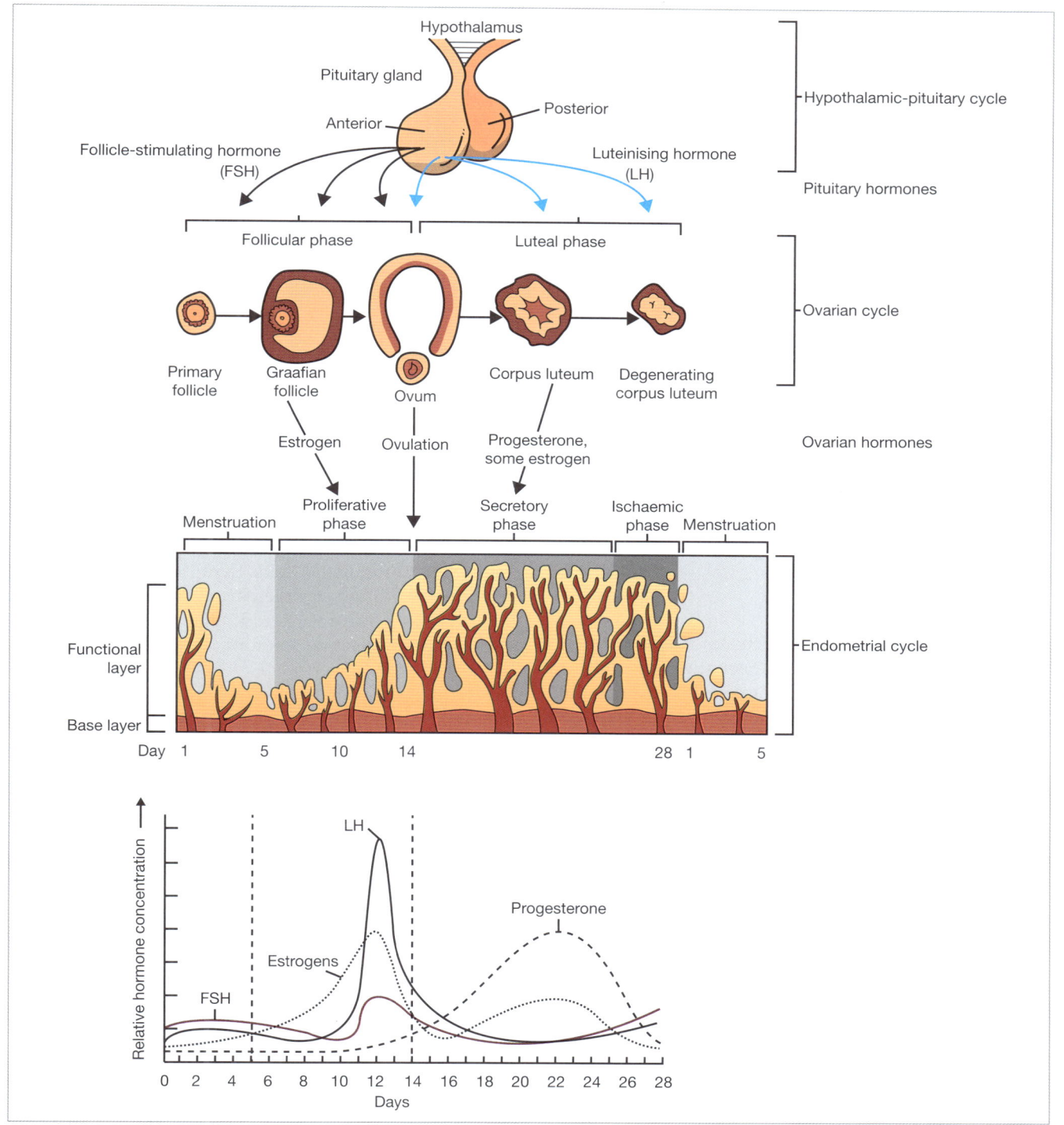

The menstrual cycle (in the absence of fertilisation and pregnancy)

FIGURE 7.2

Source: Adapted from Salerno, 1999. Used with permission.

or

- (b) If fertilisation does not occur, then, in the absence of hCG to 'rescue' the corpus luteum, luteal cells become less responsive to LH, levels of estrogen and progesterone fall, the endometrium degenerates and is sloughed off, resulting in menstruation.

The timing of ovulation and length of cycles vary (25–31 days); therefore, ovulation is not always predictable. The cyclical nature of menstruation is regulated by the ovaries and by the time required for the follicle and functional lifespan of the corpus luteum, rather than by cyclical release of hypothalamic or pituitary hormones. Urine test kits used by women to predict time of ovulation detect the LH surge, which indicates that ovulation is likely to occur within the next 24–36 hours.

Later in life, gonadal (ovarian) function decreases, and women experience menopause, or cessation of menses.

Disorders of menstruation

Uterine smooth muscle undergoes physiological rhythmical contractions, with myometrial cells in the fundus (inner surface of the dome) acting as pacemakers. During the menstrual cycle contractions are weak on days 6–14, become gradually stronger and more prolonged until menstruation (days 1–5), when coordinated contractions can lead to cramping pain.

Dysmenorrhoea

Painful menstruation (dysmenorrhoea) occurs in about 40% of young women and is incapacitating in about 3%. The pain and spasms of uterine muscles are likely due to prostaglandins (PG), for example PGF2a, released from degenerating endometrium. The most effective treatments for excessive uterine bleeding are:

- the levonorgestrel intrauterine contraceptive system
- oral contraceptive (OC) progestogen formulations used in an extended-cycle manner
- combined oral contraceptive (COC) preparations containing at least 35 micrograms of ethinyl estradiol (EE).

Also used are tranexamic acid, an antifibrinolytic drug, and non-steroidal anti-inflammatory agents (NSAIDs), especially naproxen, which also has analgesic actions and decreases contractions, symptoms, and blood loss (Bryant-Smith et al 2018).

Heavy menstrual bleeding

Heavy menstrual bleeding (formerly called menorrhagia) may be ovulatory (earlier in life) or anovulatory (leading up to menopause). Ovulatory bleeding is due to a structural cause such as uterine fibroids; treatment may include anti-anaemic drugs (iron, folic acid), NSAIDs (naproxen) to relieve symptoms, tranexamic acid, the oral contraceptive pill, or depot progestogen; less frequently,

GnRH agonists are used. Anovulatory bleeding is when intervals between periods lengthen and uterine lining builds up, leading to heavier periods (formerly called dysfunctional uterine bleeding). Treatment usually involves balancing progestogen and oestrogen levels with COC or HRT preparations, or a progestogen-only IUD.

Heavy menstrual bleeding occurs in about 5% of menstruating women. It is relatively common around puberty and menopause, and in association with platelet dysfunction, cervical cancer, endocrine disorders, or in women with low body-fat mass or who do excessive exercise. Primary causes should be sought, and anaemia monitored. Surgical treatments include dilation and curettage of the uterus, laser endometrial ablation and, as a last resort, hysterectomy.

Premenstrual syndrome

Premenstrual syndrome refers to the breast tenderness, backache, depression or anxiety, mood swings, headache, bloating, nausea, and oedema suffered by up to 12% of women during the luteal phase, 2–3 days before onset of menstruation, and which impairs daily activities. Symptoms may be due to increased sensitivity to cycling estrogen and progesterone, increased aldosterone and plasma renin activity, and abnormalities of neurotransmitters, especially serotonin (5-HT) and gamma aminobutyric acid. Symptoms resolve shortly after menstruation. Premenstrual dysphoric disorder is a more severe form, suffered by 2–4% of women.

Low-dose selective serotonin reuptake inhibitor SSRI antidepressants (sertraline, escitalopram), a COC preparation, diuretics, dietary modifications, exercise, calcium, vitamin B6 (50–100 mg pyridoxine daily), and cognitive behaviour therapy are useful treatments. Second-line therapies are GnRH **analogues** with combination patches, and/or HRT preparations and surgery (see RCOG guidelines in 'Online resources'; and review by Hofmeister & Bodden 2016).

Other disorders of menstruation

Other menstrual disorders are listed below.

- *Amenorrhoea* – absence of menstruation, which is physiological before menarche, during pregnancy and lactation and after menopause. Pathological causes include stress and endocrine tumours.
- *Irregular bleeding (formerly called metrorrhagia)* – bleeding from the uterus other than during a normal menstrual period. Although strictly speaking not a disorder of menstruation, it is a significant warning sign for cancer of the uterine cervix or endometrium.

Endometriosis

Endometriosis is a chronic condition of endometrial tissue at unusual (ectopic) locations – for example, within oviducts (fallopian tubes), ovaries, myometrium, or pelvis. It occurs in about 10% of women of reproductive age. Aetiology may involve altered estrogen receptors (ERs) or metabolism, leading to hormone imbalances. Ectopic tissue undergoes cyclical changes and produces menstrual fluid that cannot escape the abdominal cavity or other location. This can lead to ovarian cysts, pain, chronic inflammation, scar formation, infertility, dysmenorrhoea, and dyspareunia (painful intercourse). First-line treatment is surgical, to remove ectopic endometrial tissue. Hormonal treatments trialled include levonorgestrel IUD, progestogens such as dienogest, COC preparations, androgens (to inhibit GnRH release and block LH surge) or GnRH analogues (e.g. nafarelin, continuous dose for gonadal suppression). NSAIDs are used to reduce inflammation and pain (Brown & Farquhar 2015).

Polycystic ovary syndrome

Polycystic ovary syndrome is present in approximately 5–10% of women of childbearing age. It commonly causes infertility, menstrual irregularities, hirsutism, acne and pattern alopecia, and may be associated with obesity, metabolic syndrome, diabetes mellitus, ovarian dysfunction and hyperandrogenic anovulation. Adipocytes (increased in obesity) synthesise and release mediators (adipokines), including leptin and tumor necrosis factor alpha (TNF-α) involved in cardiovascular risk and insulin resistance.

The most common therapies are COC tablets, anti-androgens, weight reduction and exercise, and hypoglycaemic agents, especially insulin sensitisers such as metformin and thiazolidinediones. Metformin reduces hyperinsulinaemia, improves cardiovascular risk factors such as high blood pressure and dyslipidaemia, reduces free fatty acids, reduces high androgen levels, promotes weight loss, and overall improves the chance of ovulation and outcome of pregnancy.

In women hoping to conceive, ovulation inducers such as clomifene citrate and aromatase inhibitors are used.

Hirsutism

Hirsutism – excessive growth of coarse pigmented hair in women – can be distressing and require treatment. It may be an inherited trait or a response to drugs, including phenytoin, minoxidil or testosterone-derived progestogens. Androgens from hyperactive ovaries (e.g. polycystic ovaries), from the adrenal cortex or from other virilising endocrine disorders cause relative androgen excess at hair follicles, especially on the lower face and midline of the trunk.

Possible treatments include suppression of ovarian functions with hormonal treatments such as the oral contraceptive pill, suppression of the adrenal cortex – for example, with dexamethasone – or administration of anti-androgens such as cyproterone or spironolactone.

KEY POINTS

The female reproductive system – controls and hormones

- Follicle-stimulating hormone, luteinising hormone, estrogen, and progesterone have major roles in regulating the functions of the female reproductive system.

- The cyclical nature of the menstrual periods is regulated by the ovaries.

- The timing of ovulation and length of the menstrual cycles vary (25–31 days); therefore, ovulation is not always predictable.

- Human chorionic gonadotrophin (hCG) and placental lactogen are secreted by the placenta during pregnancy.

7.2 Female infertility

Fertility in humans requires effective, coordinated and appropriately timed functioning of several reproductive processes and many hormones: production of viable gametes in both woman and man, deposition and motility of sufficient spermatozoa in the female reproductive tract, fertilisation of a mature oocyte, then its implantation and development in the primed uterine mucosa and maintenance of pregnancy. Defects in any step can lead to infertility, defined as the absence of conception by a couple after more than 1 year of regular sexual intercourse without contraception. It affects 10–15% of all cohabiting couples wishing to conceive and can cause great emotional distress. Effective treatment requires careful assessment of possible causes in both partners. Infertility is attributed to male factors in about 40% of cases, female factors in about 40% of cases and couple factors in 20% of cases. In women, cycles may be anovulatory due to hyperprolactinaemia, hypothalamic or pituitary dysfunction or ovarian.

Preconception

Many women who are actively trying to conceive will take pregnancy **supplements** and vitamins to increase their overall wellbeing. (See Table 7.1 Pregnancy supplements and vitamins in pregnancy – Summary of evidence; Table 7.2 Summary of evidence regarding macronutrient and micronutrient intakes during pregnancy.) It is important that midwives take a thorough history of all medicine and supplements.

Folic acid

Folate is a naturally occurring vitamin B found in foods like leafy green vegetables, citrus fruit, legumes, and nuts. Folate is water-soluble and is easily destroyed by cooking, making it difficult for many women to have adequate amounts. Decreased levels of folate are linked

TABLE 7.1 Pregnancy supplements and vitamins in pregnancy – summary of evidence

Folic acid	Dietary supplements of 400 µg folic acid a day, ideally taken from 1 month before conception and throughout the first 3 months of pregnancy, to reduce the risk of a baby having neural tube defect
Vitamins	In the absence of identified deficiency, supplements of vitamins A, C and E are of little or no benefit during pregnancy and excessive amounts may cause harm
	Vitamin B6: insufficient evidence to detect clinical benefits in pregnancy (Salam et al 2015), although it appears to be of benefit in reducing nausea (mean difference in nausea score -3.7; 95% CI -6.9 to -0.5; very low certainty) (Sridharan & Sivaramakrishnan 2018)
	Vitamin B12: insufficient evidence on vitamin B12 supplementation in pregnancy to draw conclusions. May be of benefit for women with vegetarian or vegan diets, as vitamin B12 is generally not present in plant foods (Pawlak et al 2014)
	Vitamin D: vitamin D supplementation may be a consideration for women with vitamin D levels lower than 50 nmol/L
Iron	The recommendation for iron supplementation is assessed through a blood test at 28 weeks. If an iron supplement is necessary, weekly supplementation (80–300 mg elemental iron) is as effective as daily supplementation (30–60 mg elemental iron) in preventing (but not treating) iron-deficiency anaemia, with fewer adverse effects
Calcium	Calcium supplements are recommended for women at high risk of preeclampsia
Iodine	Iodine requirements increase during pregnancy and a supplement of 150 micrograms a day is advised
Omega 3-fatty acids	Supplementation with omega-3 long-chain polyunsaturated fatty acids (800 mg docosahexaenoic acid [DHA] and 100 mg eicosapentaenoic acid [EPA] per day) may reduce the risk of preterm birth among women who are low in omega-3
Herbal preparations	The effectiveness and safety of herbal preparations varies according to the herbal preparation and the condition being treated

Source: Australian Government Department of Health and Aged Care. Pregnancy Guidelines 2021. https://www.health.gov.au/resources/pregnancy-care-guidelines/part-c-lifestyle-considerations

TABLE 7.2 Macronutrient and micronutrient intakes during pregnancy – summary of evidence

NUTRIENT	RECOMMENDATIONS FOR INTERVENTIONS/SUPPLEMENT USE[1]	NON-PREGNANT ADULT FEMALES (19–50 YEARS)[2]	PREGNANT ADULT FEMALES (19–50 YEARS)[2]
Macronutrients			
Energy	Energy restriction reduces GWG but could adversely affect birth weight and is currently not recommended in pregnancy	EER (kcal/day)[3] = 354 − (6.91 × age [year]) + PA × [(9.36 × weight [kg]) + (726 × height [m])]	Non-pregnant EER + 340 and 452 kcal/day in second and third trimesters
Protein	Balanced energy/protein supplements (≤ 25% total energy from protein) are recommended only in undernourished women to prevent stillbirth and SGA	0.8 g/kg/day (46 g/day)	0.8 increasing to 1.1 g/kg/day in second half of pregnancy (71 g/day)
Total fibre[4]	Fibre-rich diet may reduce preeclampsia and GDM but no specific recommendations are currently available; fibre supplements can be used to relieve constipation if diet modification is unsuccessful	14 g/1000 kcal (or 25 g/day)	14 g/1000 kcal or (or ~28 g/day to account for GWG)
Carbohydrates (GI and GL)	Low GL or GI diets may be beneficial for women at risk of GDM or LGA but can increase risk of SGA. No specific recommendations are currently available	130 g/day of carbohydrates	175 g/day of carbohydrates
Essential fatty acids[4] (linoleic acid [*n-6*] and α-linoleic acid [*n-3*])	*n-3* PUFAs may prevent preterm birth but can increase post-term birth and LGA. No specific recommendations are currently available	12 g/day (linoleic) 1.1 g/day (α-linoleic)	13 g/day (linoleic) 1.4 g/day (α-linoleic)
Micronutrients			
Folate/folic acid	Recommended (400 µg/day) from preconception until at least 12 weeks to prevent NTDs	400 µg/day	600 µg/day
Vitamin A	Not recommended except in areas with severe deficiency/night blindness	700 µg/day	770 µg/day

TABLE 7.2 Macronutrient and micronutrient intakes during pregnancy – summary of evidence—cont'd

NUTRIENT	RECOMMENDATIONS FOR INTERVENTIONS/SUPPLEMENT USE[1]	NON-PREGNANT ADULT FEMALES (19–50 YEARS)[2]	PREGNANT ADULT FEMALES (19–50 YEARS)[2]
Thiamine (B_1)	B-complex vitamins are not recommended to improve pregnancy outcomes until further evidence is available	1.1 mg/day	1.4 mg/day
Niacin (B_2)		14 mg/day	18 mg/day
Riboflavin (B_3)		1.1 mg/day	1.4 mg/day
Pyridoxine (B_6)		1.3 mg/day	1.9 mg/day
Cyanocobalamin (B_{12})		2.4 μg/day	2.6 μg/day
Vitamin C	Not recommended until further evidence relating to safety and PROM is available	75 mg/day	85 mg/day
Vitamin E		15 mg/day	15 mg/day
Vitamin D[4]	Not recommended for improving pregnancy outcomes but should be given to women with deficiency (200 IU/day)	5 μg/day	5 μg/day
Calcium[4]	Recommended (1.5–2.0 g/day) to prevent hypertensive disorders in women with low dietary calcium intake or who are at high risk of hypertension	1 g/day	1 g/day
Iodine	Recommended only in women at high risk to prevent IDDs (i.e. in countries where < 20% of households have access to iodised salt)	150 μg/day	220–250 μg/day
Iron	Recommended (30–60 mg/day) to prevent maternal anaemia, puerperal sepsis, LBW and preterm birth	18 mg/day	27–60 mg/day
Zinc	Not recommended for improving pregnancy outcomes until more rigorous research is available	8 mg/day	11 mg/day
Alcohol	Not recommended during pregnancy until safe upper limits are established	NA	None
Caffeine	Reducing intake is recommended in women with high caffeine intake (> 300 mg/day) to prevent pregnancy loss and LBW infants	NA	< 200 mg/day

[1]Based on World Health Organization recommendations; [2]dietary reference intakes derived from Institute of Medicine guidelines and expressed as recommended dietary allowance (RDA) unless otherwise indicated; [3]EER = estimated energy requirement for adult women, reflecting the average energy intake predicted to maintain energy balance in a healthy adult of a defined age, weight, height and level of physical activity; [4]values reflect average intakes (AI) as RDAs are not available. GWG, gestational weight gain; EER, estimated energy requirement; PA, physical activity; SGA/LGA, small-/large-for-gestational-age; GI, glycaemic index; GL, glycaemic load; GDM, gestational diabetes mellitus; PUFAs, polyunsaturated fatty acids; NTDs, neural tube defects; PROM, premature rupture of membranes; IDDs, iodine deficiency disorders; LBW, low birth weight; NA, not applicable.
Source: Reproduced from Mousa et al 2019.

to neural tube abnormalities in the fetus; therefore it is essential that women have adequate levels of folate, preconception, to reduce this risk. Research clearly demonstrates that women who have received **folic acid** supplementation are much less likely to have a fetus with neural tube defects (Mousa et al 2019).

In humans, folate is essential for the production of thymidine, which is a component of DNA. Without it, folate cell division is impaired, affecting the embryo and formation of blood cells.

Due to the difficulty in gaining an adequate level from foods alone, the current recommendation for women who are planning a pregnancy or actively trying to conceive is to commence folic acid supplements. Folic

acid is the synthetic form of folate. The recommended dose is 400 or 500 micrograms of folic acid per day from 12 weeks prior to conceiving and continuing throughout the first trimester.

Women who are at increased risk of a pregnancy with neural tube defects are advised to take a higher dose of folic acid (5 mg) (Table 7.2).

Risk factors include:

- previous history of a giving birth to a child with neural tube defect
- family history that includes a child with neural tube defects
- malabsorption

- diabetes
- epilepsy.

Adverse effects: Adverse effects of folic acid supplementation for most women are extremely rare. Women with epilepsy are advised to discuss their preconception plans with their care provider as there is an increased risk of seizures with folic acid.

Vitamin B12 deficiency has also been reported.

KEY POINTS

Female infertility

- Infertility is defined as the absence of conception by a couple after more than 1 year of regular sexual intercourse without contraception.

- Effective treatment requires careful assessment of possible causes in both partners.

- Women who are actively trying to conceive may take pregnancy supplements and vitamins to increase their overall wellbeing.

- It is recommended that women take 400 or 500 micrograms of folic acid per day from 12 weeks prior to conceiving and continuing throughout the first trimester.

7.3 Pregnancy

The safe and effective prescribing and administration of medications is an essential component of midwifery care. Prescribing medications to pregnant women differs from that for the rest of the adult population and requires additional knowledge and caution due to the potential for **teratogenesis**, altered pharmacokinetics, maternal concerns, and potential for short- and longer-term harm to the fetus. Drugs taken by a pregnant woman may reach the fetus via the maternal circulation and cause birth defects or adverse reactions. Medication use in pregnancy is common, with research showing over 80% of pregnant women in Western countries, including Australia, reporting medication use for short-term or chronic conditions. Excluding vitamin and iron supplements, the range of frequently prescribed and over-the-counter (OTC) medications taken during pregnancy includes antacids, analgesics, antiemetics, and antibiotics (Lupattelli et al 2014).

However, a recent study in the UK found that many practitioners are reluctant to prescribe medications to women during the childbirth continuum, leading to stress, anxiety, and frustration. Fear of fetal harm restricts the prescribing and taking of some advised medications. Although guidelines for prescribing are available for clinicians, disappointingly, research found that this advice was not often followed, or there was conflict in professional opinion, reluctance to prescribe or dispense which resulted in women needing to negotiate complex and distressing pathways to obtain required medications (Sanders et al 2023).

For most women, pregnancy, birth and the puerperium are seen as normal physiological processes. In a small number of cases, pathological situations will arise. Women face difficult decisions about using medication in pregnancy and want specific information from their care providers to assist in their decision making (Lynch et al 2018).

Medicines in pregnancy can be used in three ways:

- *Inadvertently* – e.g. the use of medication, drugs prior to being aware of pregnancy
- *Preventatively* – e.g. Rh(D) immunoglobulin prophylaxis for women with rhesus negative blood type, antibiotic prophylaxis
- *Therapeutically* – e.g. the treatment of preexisting illness, such as SSRI for depression, Ventolin for asthma.

Maternal adaptations

Maternal adaptations to pregnancy include anatomical changes due to fetal growth and weight gain due to fetus, placenta, amniotic fluid and enlarged uterus. Endogenous hormone levels change markedly from the non-pregnant cycling state, with high levels of chorionic gonadotrophin, placental hormones (progesterone, estrogens, chorionic somatomammotropin, growth hormone, adrenocorticotrophic hormone, and thyroid-stimulating hormone), prolactin and relaxin (a peptide hormone produced by corpus luteum and placenta).

Physiological adaptations may affect pharmacokinetic factors or how the woman responds to drugs. Cardiac output, stroke volume, heart rate and blood volume all increase by 15–30%, while blood pressure usually falls due to vasodilation of peripheral vessels in response to progesterone and relaxin, to accommodate the increased cardiovascular circulatory volume leading to dilution in the concentration of medications (Soma-Pillay et al 2016). Pulmonary function increases to meet oxygen demands of the fetus. Decreased GIT motility and increased nausea and vomiting may reduce absorption of nutrients and drugs. Chronic conditions that the woman may have experienced before pregnancy, such as diabetes, epilepsy, asthma, hypertension, arthritis, peptic ulcer, migraine, depression, thyroid disorder, or urinary tract infection need careful monitoring and treatment to optimise the woman's (and fetus's) health.

Drug use in pregnancy

During pregnancy, any substance consumed and absorbed may reach the fetus by way of the maternal circulation. Drug use during pregnancy should be avoided or limited to essential treatment and where the benefit to the woman is considered greater than the risk to the fetus. All pregnant women, and women of childbearing age who are not using contraceptives and who are sexually active, should be counselled to avoid exposure to unnecessary drugs (including CAM) and chemicals, and drugs prescribed carefully, as effects on the embryo may occur before a woman is aware she is pregnant.

With the recent trend towards higher birth rates in the age group of 35–44 years, some women who are pregnant may be taking medications for chronic medical conditions (e.g. allergies, hypertension, diabetes, depression, and epilepsy), increasing the risk of exposure of the fetus to maternal drugs.

'Social drugs' can also affect the infant: alcohol consumption during pregnancy can cause central nervous system (CNS) depression and abnormalities, and babies born to smokers are smaller and have increased incidence of jaundice. Babies born to women dependent on narcotic analgesics such as heroin, or who are on methadone maintenance programs, may suffer a withdrawal syndrome after birth. If it is necessary to administer drug therapy, the most important factors to be considered include:

- the potential for the drug to produce harmful effects in the fetus
- fetal gestational age at the time of drug exposure
- any other drugs or complementary medicines administered concurrently
- the drug dose, dosing intervals and duration of treatment
- risks to the woman and fetus if the woman is not treated with necessary drugs.

Teratogenesis: Causing abnormal fetal development

The first trimester is when the developing embryo is most vulnerable to the teratogenic effects of any chemicals that the woman is exposed to during this time (Fig 7.3). These include prescription and OTC drugs, complementary medicines (which include vitamin, mineral, herbal, aromatherapy, and homeopathic products), social drugs (alcohol and nicotine) and drugs of abuse. Some examples are described below and in Table 7.3.

Diethylstilboestrol

The use of the oestrogen diethylstilboestrol during pregnancy was not initially found to cause any problems;

Schematic illustration of critical periods in human prenatal development

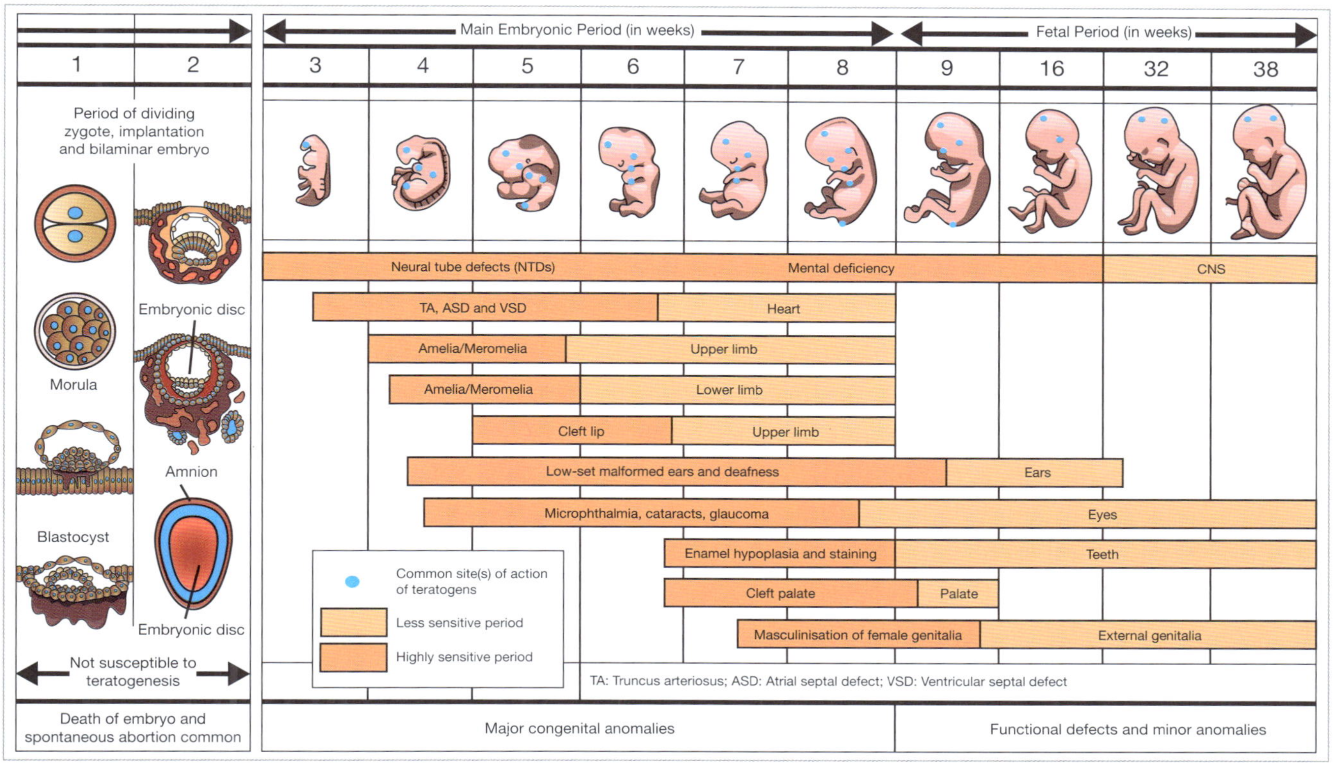

FIGURE 7.3

Source: Keith L. Moore, T. V. N. Persaud, Mark G. Torchia, The developing human: Clinically Oriented Embryology, 10th edition. 2016 Saunders.

TABLE 7.3 Examples of drugs and teratogenic effects in the human fetus

DRUG	CRITICAL TIME PERIOD	POTENTIAL DEFECT
Alcohol (chronic use)	< 12 weeks > 24 weeks	Fetal alcohol spectrum disorder (FASD): heart defects, CNS abnormalities, low birth weight, delay in development
Androgens	> 10 weeks	External female genitalia masculinisation
Angiotensin-converting enzyme (ACE) inhibitors and angiotensin receptor antagonists	1st–3rd trimester	Renal dysgenesis, defects in skull ossification, prolonged renal failure and hypotension in neonates
Carbamazepine	< 30 days after conception	Neural tube defects, craniofacial defects
Clomipramine	3rd trimester	Neonatal lethargy, hypotonia, cyanosis
Cocaine	2nd–3rd trimester 3rd trimester	Abruptio placentae Premature labour and birth, intracranial bleeding
Cyclophosphamide	1st trimester	CNS malformations, secondary cancer
Isotretinoin	> 15 days after conception	Hydrocephalus, CNS abnormalities, fetal death
Lithium	< 2 months	Ebstein's anomaly and other heart defects
Methotrexate	6–9 weeks after conception	Skull ossification defect, limb and craniofacial defects
Phenytoin	1st trimester	Craniofacial defects, underdevelopment of phalanges or nails, impaired neurological development
Tetracycline antibiotics	> 20 weeks	Stained teeth, bone growth defect
Thalidomide	1st trimester	Phocomelia, internal malformations
Valproic acid	< 1 month after conception 1st trimester	Neural tube defects, craniofacial defects
Vitamin A (high doses and parenteral)	1st trimester	Fetal abnormalities including urinary tract malformations, growth retardation
Warfarin	1st–3rd trimester	CNS and skeletal defects, low birth weight (< 10th percentile), hearing loss

Source: Katzung BG: Basic and clinical pharmacology, ed 12, New York, 2012, McGraw-Hill.

however, during the 1970s it was linked to a delayed increased risk of vaginal and cervical cancer in female offspring and to genital abnormalities in both male and female offspring. Diethylstilboestrol taken by the woman during the first trimester of pregnancy presumably accumulated in the fetus, which was unable to metabolise it. The recognition that a drug taken during developmental stages in pregnancy can cause problems in the next generation is still a concern.

Thalidomide

Thalidomide is a well-known example of a drug with teratogenic effects during organogenesis. It was used in Australia and New Zealand as a sedative hypnotic drug to treat morning sickness from the 1950s to the early 1960s (see CFB 2.1, Chapter 2).

Alcohol

Alcohol easily crosses the placenta, entering the fetal bloodstream; consumption during pregnancy therefore substantially increases the risk of fetal abnormalities.

One drink a week is associated with the possibility of mental health problems, and at the severe end of the spectrum are fetal alcohol spectrum disorders (FASD) – congenital abnormalities including small head (microcephaly), low birth weight, intellectual disability and growth restriction, impaired coordination, irritability in infancy, hyperactivity in childhood, cardiac murmurs, cleft lip or palate, and hernias (Sarman 2018). Current guidelines recommend that, for women who are pregnant or planning a pregnancy, or for women who are breastfeeding, not drinking alcohol is the safest option.

Antiepileptic drugs

Antiepileptic drugs are infamous for potentially causing birth defects or developmental problems in infants of women taking antiepileptics during pregnancy (see Table 7.3 [carbamazepine, phenytoin and valproic acid] and Chapter 20). Preconceptual planning can support the woman to transition to monotherapy in a bid to reduce the risk of teratogenicity; however, most people take dual medications. Transition to monotherapy can take time and women should be counselled to transition before conception.

Retinoids

These vitamin A derivatives are used to treat severe acne. They are potentially teratogenic.

Cocaine

The abuse of cocaine during pregnancy can result in spontaneous abortions, fetal hypoxia, premature birth, placental abruption, congenital abnormalities (skull defects, cardiac abnormality) and cerebral infarction or stroke. At birth, the newborn may exhibit symptoms of cocaine drug withdrawal (irritability, increased respiratory and heart rates, diarrhoea, irregular sleeping patterns and poor appetite). Long-term behavioural patterns, such as poor attention span and a decrease in organisational skills, may also occur in the offspring of women who use cocaine.

Part of the midwife's role is to counsel women on the safety and efficacy of medication. For the midwife to be able to make evidence-based decisions and/or recommendations and provide quality information to the woman and her family, an understanding of pharmacology and the physiological changes that occur in pregnancy is essential. Because the research base for decision making around prescribing in pregnancy is not as robust as in other areas of clinical practice – due to ethical issues surrounding researching/testing medications on pregnant women and consequent limitations of the data that form the safety information around prescribing – additional caution is warranted. (See Chapter 1).

Database for prescribing medicines in pregnancy

The Australian Advisory Committee on Prescription Medicines categorises drugs into Pregnancy Categories A–D and X, based on their potential for harmful effects (CFB 7.1), so that the safest effective drug can be prescribed. The Australian categorisation system considers that most medicines cross the placenta. The known harmful effects of medicines on the developing baby include the potential to cause birth defects; unwanted pharmacological effects around the time of birth which may or may not be reversible; and problems in later life.

CLINICAL FOCUS BOX 7.1

Australian categorisation system for prescribing medicines in pregnancy

The **Australian categorisation system for prescribing medicines in pregnancy** has seven categories (A, B1, B2, B3, C, D and X) to indicate the level of risk to the fetus of drugs used at recommended therapeutic doses. Category A drugs are considered the least problematic, whereas drugs in Category X are considered the most dangerous

and should not be used in pregnancy or if there is a possibility of pregnancy. The categorisation of B drugs (B1–B3) is based on animal data or contains drugs which have been taken by only a limited number of pregnant women; Category B drugs should not be considered 'safer' than drugs with a Category C designation. Category D drugs have caused, or are suspected to have caused, human fetal malformations.

The categorisation of a particular drug assumes it will be used at normal therapeutic doses in women; if the therapeutic dose is exceeded, the category assigned is no longer valid. A drug may have two categories; for example, isotretinoin is in Category D when used topically, in which case both the dose of the drug and the likely exposure of the fetus are low; however, it is in Category X when used systemically, when the dose and fetal exposure are greater. The categories do not differentiate between different stages of pregnancy (see Kennedy 2014).

Extensive information on this categorisation system and access to the database is available at the TGA's website, which is updated regularly and allows searching by either generic name/active ingredient or pharmacological classification/action. Note that accessing the website requires the reader to acknowledge a disclaimer that the material is general information and not specific advice.

The database does not contain all medicines approved for use in Australia because certain classes of medicines are generally exempted from categorisation. Few complementary medicines are included; these have little safety data. A full list of exempt medicines can be found on the TGA's website.

As of 2015, the US Food and Drug Administration (FDA) discontinued its pregnancy risk categories system (which had been substantially similar to Australia's), and replaced it with the FDA Pregnancy and Lactation Labeling Rule, requiring narrative text describing risk and other data for each drug.

Source: Therapeutic Goods Administration – see Online resources.

KEY POINTS

Medication use during pregnancy

- Physiological adaptations may affect pharmacokinetic factors or how the woman responds to drugs.
- Drugs taken by the mother pass across into the fetal circulation and may cause adverse pharmacological effects in the fetus.
- Drug use during pregnancy should be avoided or limited to essential treatment and where the benefit to the woman is considered greater than the risk to the fetus.
- The Australian categorisation system for prescribing medicines in pregnancy has seven categories (A, B1, B2, B3, C, D and X) to indicate the level of risk to the fetus of drugs used at the recommended therapeutic doses.
- The midwife's role is to counsel women on the safety and efficacy of medication use during pregnancy.

7.4 Common conditions in pregnancy

Physiological changes in pregnancy have effects on a woman's body that may cause unpleasant symptoms. As these symptoms are physiological and not pathological, women's concerns are often minimised, so it is important that the midwife does not dismiss or minimise these concerns. For some women symptoms will resolve naturally or with changes to lifestyle; however, for others there may be a need for further support and treatment of symptoms with medications or complementary alternatives.

Management of physiological discomforts of pregnancy vary widely. It is important that all treatments, including alternative therapies and herbal preparations, are reviewed to ensure they are safe to use in pregnancy. Midwives should also ensure a thorough assessment is conducted to differentiate between common discomforts of pregnancy and pathological presentations caused by preexisting conditions or changing health status related to pregnancy complexities.

Nausea and vomiting in pregnancy (NVP)

Nausea, retching and vomiting in pregnancy are common and often distressing for women. Referred to as 'morning sickness', symptoms are more prevalent in early pregnancy and usually resolve or improve to a manageable level by the second trimester. Symptoms can occur at any time during the day – for some women a feeling of nausea is experienced, for others frequent vomiting occurs.

Despite its prevalence, the mechanism causing **nausea and vomiting** in pregnancy is largely still unknown. High levels of human chorionic gonadotrophin (hCG) are associated with nausea and vomiting during the first trimester – in pregnancies with no nausea, the risk of miscarriage is higher. NVP is also associated with changes in blood sugar levels and multiple pregnancies. Exciting new research has found a link between GDF15, a hormone acting on the brainstem, and NVP. Recent studies show that levels of GDF15 are higher in pregnant women with NVP and that the feto-placental unit is the major source of that GDF15 in maternal blood (Fejzo et al 2024). This recent development indicates that the severity of nausea and vomiting of pregnancy is the result of the interaction of fetal-derived GDF15 and the mother's sensitivity to this peptide, which is substantially determined by her prior exposure to the hormone (Fejzo et al 2024).

Many treatments are available to women, including drugs and complementary and alternative therapies. Nonpharmacological approaches are usually the first-line management. However, severe vomiting (hyperemesis gravidarum) may require hospitalisation, intravenous (IV) rehydration and drug therapy. Hyperemesis gravidarum is extremely debilitating and can cause serious complications if not managed adequately, including the maternal request for termination of pregnancy (Kametas et al 2008; Nana et al 2022).

Vomiting

Vomiting is often, but not always, accompanied by nausea, which is the 'feeling' or conscious recognition of feeling sick. The vomiting reflex is governed by the autonomic nervous system. Vomiting involves a complex serious of movements that rid the gut of its contents and can have several symptoms such as increased salivation, sweating, dizziness, pallor, hypotension and tachycardia, hyperventilation, and anxiety. During vomiting the lower oesophagus and upper stomach relax and the duodenum and lower stomach contract. The stomach is squeezed between the diaphragm and abdominal wall and the contents of the stomach are expelled. There is always a risk of aspiration during vomiting and women may lose consciousness, so should not be left alone.

As NVP tends to occur more frequently in the first trimester, due to the self-limiting nature of the condition first-line management is usually diet and lifestyle changes. Women are advised to avoid foods, smells, activities, or situations that they find nauseating and to eat small frequent meals of dry, bland foodstuffs. Due to the concern that medicines may adversely affect the development of the fetus, placing the pregnancy at risk, the use of pharmacological medications for NVP is generally approached with caution (Box 7.2).

Research studies have examined the effectiveness of many treatments including acupressure to the P6 point on the wrist, acustimulation, acupuncture, ginger, chamomile, vitamin B6, lemon oil, mint oil, and several drugs that are used to reduce nausea or vomiting (Tan et al 2023). A Cochrane review of 5449 women using a variety of different CAM therapies to resolve NVP in 41 RCTs showed some benefit in improving nausea and vomiting symptoms for women, but generally effects were inconsistent and limited (Matthew et al 2015). Overall, studies had low risk of bias related to blinding and reporting on all participants in the studies. However, some aspects of the studies were reported incompletely in a way that meant how participants were allocated to groups was unclear and not all results were fully and clearly reported. Most studies had different ways of measuring the symptoms of nausea and vomiting and therefore results could not be combined. Few studies reported maternal and fetal adverse outcomes; however, there was little information on the effectiveness of treatments for improving women's quality of life (Matthews et al 2015).

It is essential that women are listened to and that their symptoms are adequately managed to avoid serious complications such as: dehydration, electrolyte imbalance, ketone formation, hypotension, vasovagal episodes, anxiety and distress, persistent vomiting and

BOX 7.1 Assessment, management and treatment of NVP

Several validated scoring systems exist for assessing the severity of NVP, including the Rhodes Score (originally designed for chemotherapy patients) and the Motherisk Pregnancy-Unique Quantification of Emesis and Nausea (PUQE) scoring index. The PUQE system uses three questions relating to symptoms to assess the severity of nausea and vomiting experienced over 24 hours (Ebrahimi et al 2009).

Motherisk Pregnancy-Unique Quantification of Emesis (PUQE) Index

Total score is the sum of replies to each of these three questions:

1. In the last 24 hours, for how long have you felt nauseated or sick to your stomach?

   Not at all (1)

   1 hour (2)

   2–3 hours (3)

   4–6 hours (4)

   More than 6 hours (5)

2. In the last 24 hours how many times have you vomited?

   I did not throw up (1)

   1–2 times (2)

   3–4 times (3)

   5–6 times (4)

   7 or more times (5)

3. In the last 24 hours how many times have you had retching or dry heaves without bringing anything up?

   No time (1)

   1–2 times (2)

   3–4 times (3)

   5–6 times (4)

   7 or more (5)

PUQE-24 score: Mild = ≤ 6; Moderate = 7–12; Severe = 13–15.

How many hours have you slept out of 24 hours? _____ Why?
_____

On a scale of 0 to 10, how would you rate your wellbeing? __
_____

0 = worst possible, 10 = the best you felt before pregnancy

Can you tell me what causes you to feel that way? _____
_____

Source: Adapted from Ebrahimi et al 2009.

BOX 7.2 Commencement and titration of pharmacological treatment for NVP or HG

1 Mild–moderate NVP:

   Start with ginger ±B6

   Add oral antihistamine or dopamine antagonist if needed.

2 Moderate–severe NVP or inadequate response to initial treatment:

   Consider IV/IM antihistamine or dopamine antagonist

   In the event of excessive sedation or inadequate response:

   Add /substitute oral or IV serotonin

   Antagonist, at least during daytime

   Add acid suppression therapy.

3 Refractory NVP or HG:

   Consider corticosteroids in addition to other antiemetics

   Intensify acid suppression

   Manage/prevent constipation with laxatives.

Source: Adapted from SOMANZ 2020 NVP-GUIDELINE-1.2.20-1.pdf (somanz.org)

hypovolemia, malnutrition, vitamin deficiencies (e.g. Wernicke encephalopathy) and extreme weight loss, reduced placental flow and restricted growth to the fetus, gastrointestinal trauma due to vomiting, dental problems and long-term mental health implications (Chiossi et al 2006).

Management and treatment for NVP

Ginger

Zingiber officinale, commonly known as ginger, has been used as a broad-spectrum antiemetic in the various traditional systems of medicine for over 2000 years. Three systematic reviews have addressed the effectiveness of ginger for NVP. One found four RCTs that met the criteria, and all found that oral ginger was more effective than placebo in reducing nausea and vomiting. The first, a review of the effectiveness and safety of ginger for pregnancy-induced nausea and vomiting, reviewed four clinical trials and concluded that oral ginger was more effective than placebo in reducing NVP (Ding et al 2013). The second included a total of 10 RCTs, comparing ginger with placebo (five studies), with vitamin B6 (four studies), and one with dimenhydrinate. Ginger was superior to placebo and equal to vitamin B6 and dimenhydrinate at improving nausea and vomiting (Dante et al 2013). The final systematic review analysed six studies with a total of 508 women randomised to ginger or placebo and concluded that ginger was more effective (Thomson et al 2014). Ginger was superior to placebo but less effective than metoclopramide in a randomised trial including 102 women with NVP. Another group investigated the effect of ginger biscuits and found them to be better than placebo at reducing nausea (Basirat et al 2009).

Despite the research demonstrating the effectiveness of ginger in reducing NVP, caution is recommended as the pharmacological action of ginger is not fully understood. Rather than using ginger as it has been traditionally used in its natural state, such as in ginger tea, fresh ginger or ginger biscuits, in recent times more women are using ginger medication in capsule form and there is no consensus on what type of treatment, dose, frequency, form or duration of treatment is safe or effective. No increased risk of major malformations has been reported with use of ginger; however, some researchers have highlighted concerns regarding potential maternal adverse effects, including an anticoagulant effect, stomach irritation and a potential interaction with beta-blockers and benzodiazepines (Sharifzadeh et al 2018; Tiran 2012).

Pyridoxine (vitamin B6)

Pyridoxine has been used as an antiemetic for over 50 years. Pyridoxine is a water-soluble vitamin. It works as an H1 receptor inhibitor, acting indirectly on the vestibular system, and decreases stimulation of the vomiting centre. The available research into the effectiveness of vitamin B6 is inconclusive. Some studies demonstrate that vitamin B6 reduces nausea; however, in other studies it has been used either as a control or has been taken in addition to other interventions (Mazzotta & Magee 2000; Sheehan 2007; Bsat 2003; Rad 2012; Sharifzadeh 2018).

Multiple studies have demonstrated that 200 mg/day is considered safe. However, it is also reported that a known side effect of vitamin B6 is peripheral neuropathy, which has symptoms of tingling, burning or numbness, usually in the hands or feet. Neuropathy occurs at high doses or following long-term use of products containing vitamin B6. Peripheral neuropathy is not associated with normal dietary intakes of vitamin B6 (see Online resources: TGA).

Recommended dose: pyridoxine 25–50 mg orally, up to 4 times daily (maximum 200 mg/day) A sustained-release tablet combining doxylamine 10 mg and pyridoxine 10 mg has been available for many years in Canada. In 2013, it was also approved in the USA following an RCT which showed it was effective and well tolerated; however, this preparation is not currently available in Australia or New Zealand (Nuangchamnong et al 2014).

Antiemetics

There are many different **antiemetics** available for use during pregnancy, labour and birth. Due to the nature of vomiting, single-medication treatment may not be effective so a combination of therapies may be recommended. A brief overview of the main medications used to treat NVP is provided below. Specific medications and their doses are provided in Tables 7.4a–c and 7.5.

TABLE 7.4a – c Oral antiemetic medications for mild–moderate NVP

TABLE 7.4a Herbal/vitamin

	GINGER	VITAMIN B6 (PYRIDOXINE)
Mechanism of action	Improvement in gastrointestinal motility: weak effect on cholinergic M3 receptors and serotonergic 5-HT3 and 5-HT4 receptors in the gut	Water-soluble vitamin, inhibits H1 receptor, acts indirectly on vestibular system, some inhibition of muscarinic receptors to decrease stimulation of vomiting centre
Evidence for efficacy	↓N but not V Superior to placebo Equal to vitamin B6, dimenhydrinate, metoclopramide, doxylamine, P6 (LOE-II)	↓N but not V Less effective than dimenhydrinate (LOE-I)
Recommended/max dose	Use standardised products rather than foods: up to 1200 mg/day split doses, e.g. 250 mg QID	10–25 mg PO 3–4×/day Up to 200 mg/day Or 37.5 mg combined with ginger 600 mg up to 2×/day
Side effects	Inability to tolerate treatment, sedation and heartburn	Sensory neuropathy has been reported with chronic intake of pyridoxine at doses > 500 mg/day
Risk of teratogenesis	No increase	No increase
Practice points	Theoretical but unproven risk of bleeding risk by decreasing platelet-aggregation May inhibit growth of *Helicobacter pylori*	More effective when used in combination, e.g. with doxylamine or dicyclomine (equivalent to metoclopramide)

Source: Lowe SA, Bowyer L, Beech A, Robinson H, Armstrong G, Marnoch C, Grzeskowiak L, Guideline For The Management Of Nausea And Vomiting In Pregnancy And Hyperemesis Gravidarum, 2019, SOMANZ. (Table 3A, p24).

TABLE 7.4b Histamine/dopamine antagonists

	DOXYLAMINE[S]/DIMENHYDRINATE[S] DIPHENHYDRAMINE[S]/CYCLIZINE[S]/ PROMETHAZINE[S]	METOCLOPRAMIDE
Mechanism of action	Indirectly affect the vestibular system, decreasing stimulation of the vomiting centre	Dopamine and serotonin receptor antagonist which stimulates upper gastrointestinal motility and acts on CNS vomiting centre
Evidence for efficacy	Doxylamine: ↓N compared with placebo, with or without pyridoxine (LOE-II) Dimenhydrinate/diphenhydramine/Cyclizine: (LOE-III)	Equal to ondansetron for N but less effective for V (LOE-II)
Recommended/max dose	Doxylamine*: 6.25–25 mg tds po, max 50 mg/day Diphenhydramine*: 25–50 mg tds, max 150 mg/day Dimenhydrinate*: 25–50 mg tds, max 100 mg/day Cyclizine*: 12.5–50 mg tds, max 150 mg/day Promethazine*: 25 mg TDS, max 75 mg/day	10 mg TDS, max 30 mg/day
Side effects	Sedation, anticholinergic effects	Less sedation, akathisia, depression Rare: tardive dyskinesia with chronic use
Risk of teratogenesis	No increase	No increase
Practice points	Doxylamine and dimenhydrinate are available as non-prescription sleeping tablets or travel sickness tablets. Dimenhydrinate is often combined with caffeine and hyoscine. Safety data on combination indicates no concerns. Best reserved for evening dosing	

Dosing: BD = twice a day; TDS = three times per day; QID = four times per day; max = maximum recommended total daily dose.
*Do not combine these agents with similar mechanism of action and side effects; [S] = sedating, preferably use nocte only.
Source: Lowe SA, Bowyer L, Beech A, Robinson H, Armstrong G, Marnoch C, Grzeskowiak L, Guideline For The Management Of Nausea And Vomiting In Pregnancy And Hyperemesis Gravidarum, 2019, SOMANZ. (Table 3B, p25).

TABLE 7.4c Phenothiazines*

	PROCHLORPERAZINE[S]	CHLORPROMAZINE[S]
Mechanism of action	Central and peripheral dopamine antagonists	
Evidence for efficacy	Superior to placebo for NVP (LOE-I)	(LOE-III)
Recommended dose	5–10 mg TDS, max 30 mg/day	10–25 mg TDS
Side effects	Sedation, akathisia, anticholinergic effects, hypotension Rare: dystonias, tardive dyskinesia with chronic use	
Risk of teratogenesis	No increase	
Practice points	Best reserved for evening dosing	

Dosing: BD = twice a day; TDS = three times per day; QID = four times per day; max = maximum recommended total daily dose.
* Do not combine these agents with similar mechanism of action and side effects
[S] = sedating, preferably use nocte only.
Source: Lowe SA, Bowyer L, Beech A, Robinson H, Armstrong G, Marnoch C, Grzeskowiak L, Guideline For The Management Of Nausea And Vomiting In Pregnancy And Hyperemesis Gravidarum, 2019, SOMANZ. (Table 4, p26)

Antihistamines

Antihistamine medications act on the H1 receptors associated with both the vestibular system and the vomiting centre in the medulla oblongata in the brain. Oral antihistamines are effective within 15–60 minutes, with effects lasting for 3–6 hours. Antihistamines can have a sedating effect so they should be used with caution.

Adverse effects: All H1 receptor antagonists can influence the central nervous system, therefore the main concern is sedative effects. Effects include sedation, reduced alertness and reaction times, confusion, and impaired coordination. In some circumstances the opposite effect is observed and symptoms such as agitation and restlessness are observed. The side effects

TABLE 7.5 Oral antiemetic medications for severe NVP and HG

	ONDANSETRON	CORTICOSTEROIDS
Mechanism of action	Central (medullary vomiting centre) and peripheral (small bowel) serotonin receptor blocker	Antiemetic effect on the chemoreceptor trigger zone in the brainstem
Evidence for efficacy	Superior to combination doxylamine/B6 for reduction in N and V Superior to metoclopramide for reduction of V but not N in HG	Improved sense of wellbeing, appetite and increased weight gain in HG patients No difference in days of hospital admission or readmission rates compared to placebo Equal to promethazine with fewer side effects (LOE-I) Superior to IV metoclopramide (LOE-I)
Recommended dose	4–8 mg up to TDS	Prednisone 40–50 mg/day. (May be commenced as hydrocortisone 100 mg IV BD)
Side effects	Constipation, headache, dizziness	Potential Cushing's syndrome, mood disturbance, hypertension, hyperglycaemia
Risk of teratogenesis	Conflicting data but does not appear to increase overall risk of birth defects	Possible increased risk of oral clefts when used < 10 weeks gestation, but data are weak
Practice points	No sedation Expensive Available as tablets, wafers and oral dispersible formulations Ensure concurrent management of constipation – bowel obstruction has been reported Recommended as second-line agents	Consider withholding until after 10 weeks gestation if alternate therapy an option Restrict to refractory cases

Dosing: BD = twice a day; TDS = three times per day; QID = four times per day; max = maximum recommended total daily dose.
Source: Adapted from Society of Obstetric Medicine of Australia and New Zealand (SOMANZ) Guidelines for nausea and vomiting in pregnancy and hyperemesis gravidarum, 2019. Lowe SA, Bowyer L, Beech A, et al (Table 4, p26).

that are also reported in the literature are: dizziness, headaches, hypotension; effects on the gut such as pain, **constipation**, or diarrhoea; loss of appetite; and painful mouth and tongue.

Non-sedating histamine H1 antagonists are usually recommended rather than sedating antihistamines. Medications such as cyclizine, promethazine and cinnarizine are used.

Sedating antihistamines such as doxylamine may be used if the effect of sedation is not a concern.

Dopamine antagonists

D2 antagonists work directly on the chemical trigger zone (CTZ), situated within the medulla and connected to the vomiting centre, by blocking the action of dopamine. In addition to the antiemetic effects, dopamine antagonist medication also affects the gastrointestinal tract, causing increased gastric emptying and diarrhoea. Central nervous system effects include sedation, mood changes, and brainstem function changes (thermoregulation, respiratory effort and cough reflex may be depressed). Posture and movement disorders are also reported, with long-term and high doses because of the D2 antagonists on the basal ganglia in the brain. Reported disorders include acute dystonia, restlessness, and pseudoparkinsonism.

D2 antagonist medications include metoclopramide, domperidone and phenothiazines (prochlorperazine and chlorpromazine). Note that promethazine is a phenothiazine but acts as an antihistamine.

Serotonin antagonists

Serotonin receptor antagonists are the most effective antiemetic drugs available outside of pregnancy, but there remains controversy about their use in pregnancy. Multiple studies have shown that ondansetron is more effective than other drugs in reducing vomiting, with some effect on reducing nausea. Some concern has been highlighted regarding birth defects, in particular cleft palate, associated with ondansetron use. Huybrechts et al (2018) analysed data from more than 1.8 million pregnancies in America looking at the association between ondansetron use and overall congenital malformations, cardiac anomalies, or oral clefts. Of the 88,467 infants whose mothers had taken ondansetron, there was no increase in congenital malformations. There was, however, a slight increase in infants born with oral clefts – specifically cleft palate, not lip. However, the medication is still recommended if other medications are ineffective.

Corticosteroids

Corticosteroids act to reduce inflammation in the gut and therefore the messaging to the vomiting centre.

Gastro-oesophageal reflux

Gastro-oesophageal reflux – more commonly referred to as heartburn or reflux – is common in pregnancy, with reports of 30–80% of women experiencing symptoms (Le et al 2022). Symptoms are due to the hormonal effects of pregnancy: an increase in progesterone, a decrease in motilin, and an increase in enteroglucogon cause the lower oesophageal sphincter to relax, thereby decreasing gastric motility and gastric emptying. These hormonal effects lead to stomach acid entering the lower oesophageal tract. Symptoms often worsen towards the end of pregnancy, peaking at around 36 weeks as the pregnant uterus expands, putting physical pressure on the stomach and gastrointestinal tract. These physiological changes increase the risk of gastric aspiration if a pregnant woman loses consciousness or requires an emergency general anaesthesia.

Symptoms may include a burning sensation or pain to the throat, back and chest, reflux, nausea, and vomiting.

Management and treatment for gastro-oesophageal reflux

As for NVP, recommended first-line management is to make changes to diet and lifestyle, such as eating small meals, avoiding fatty foods, and sitting upright to eat.

Antacids

If symptoms persist, the Society of Obstetric Medicine of Australia and New Zealand (SOMANZ) recommends **antacids** containing magnesium, calcium, or aluminium. Antacids are considered safe in pregnancy; however, a long-term reduction in stomach acid can lead to disruption of the normal process of digestion. As heartburn and reflux is a condition that is usually experienced later in pregnancy, the concerns related to organogenesis are not relevant for most cases.

A variety of antacids are available as OTC medications in both liquid and tablet form. Antacids act quickly if taken on an empty stomach and can provide immediate relief of symptoms. Antacids are weak bases, aluminium, magnesium, sodium, calcium, and potassium. The bases combine with hydrochloric acid and decrease the acidity of the stomach by neutralising the acid content in the stomach. Of these compounds, the most common are aluminium hydroxide and magnesium carbonate, which are often combined.

Adverse effects: Aluminium hydroxide has a constipating effect and magnesium compounds can act as a laxative; therefore combining the two compounds cancels out the effects on the bowel. The use of antacids may increase gastric acid secretion, leading to worsening symptoms.

Magnesium antacids

Magnesium carbonate and magnesium hydroxide are found in most OTC preparations. They reduce symptoms of heartburn by neutralising hydrochloric acid by forming insoluble magnesium chloride.

Magnesium trisilicate is also found in some antacids. When neutralised with hydrochloric acid it forms a jelly-like silica which absorbs the enzyme pepsin, thereby making it inactive. Preparations containing magnesium trisilicate are longer acting, but when used alone it is not a very effective antacid.

Aluminium hydroxide neutralises hydrochloric acid and becomes insoluble aluminium chloride which absorbs pepsin. A side effect of aluminium hydroxide is constipation; therefore, it is not usually recommended in pregnancy.

Sodium bicarbonate neutralises hydrochloric acid; however, this reaction forms carbon dioxide which increases the production of gastric acid. Sodium bicarbonate is absorbed and secreted in the kidney. High doses can cause oedema, metabolic alkalosis, and kidney stones, and therefore it is not recommended during pregnancy or breastfeeding. Other side effects include stomach distention (bloating), belching, flatulence, and stomach pain.

Calcium salts

Some antacid preparations may contain calcium salts. Extended use may lead to kidney stones.

Alginates

Alginates are derived from seaweed and are present in many antacids. Alginates combine with gastric acid to form a viscous jelly which reduces gastric reflux. They form a protective raft that localises to the proximal stomach (Meteerattanapipat et al 2017).

Antacids should be taken 1–2 hours after meals and before bedtime. Antacids are available in both liquid and tablet preparations; liquids are reported as being more effective.

Adverse effects: Antacids should only be taken to treat symptoms and not used as a preventative medication. The use of antacids can worsen symptoms due to the overproduction of gastric acid, and this is more common with antacids containing calcium and sodium.

Caution should also be taken with the administration of other medications as antacids react with many drugs. Medications should not be taken within 1–3 hours of taking antacids. For women with a history of kidney stones, or where there is concern regarding renal function (e.g. preeclampsia), antacids should be avoided if possible.

Sucralfate

Sucralfate is a complex of sucrose and aluminium hydroxide. Sucralfate needs acid to react so will only be effective if the gastric contents are acidic. It forms a thick paste-like substance which sticks to the stomach lining, protecting it from the acid.

Adverse effects: As it is not absorbed, sucralfate has minimal side effects; however, it has been reported to cause constipation, dry mouth, nausea and vomiting, and headaches. Sucralfate should not be taken with other antacids and, like other antacids, it will interfere with absorption of medications. Therefore, medications should be administered 1–3 hours after taking sucralfate.

Acid suppressants: Histamine antagonists (H2)

Acid secretion in the gut is stimulated by the release of H2 receptors. H2 antagonists inhibit histamine from binding to histamine H2 receptors, thereby inhibiting gastric acid secretion, and pepsin and gastrin output. H2 antagonist drugs can be useful in controlling symptoms. H2 histamines are easily absorbed and take effect within one hour of administration. H2 antagonists can be taken orally or intravenously, and the effects can be long lasting (4–12 hours depending on the drug). Common drugs used are cimetidine, ranitidine, nizatidine and famotidine. Although ranitidine has been available for use for over 40 years, and has been shown to be effective in multiple studies of use in pregnancy without teratogenic or adverse outcomes, it is no longer the preferred option and is currently unavailable in Australia and New Zealand. The current preferred option for use in pregnancy is famotidine.

Multiple animal studies have demonstrated most of the H2 antagonist drugs to be safe for use during pregnancy (Thelin & Richter 2020) However, some caution is recommended with some of the newer drugs on the market, such as nizatidine. Although animal studies have been conducted, the results are mixed, and no adequate or well-controlled studies have been conducted on pregnant women's use of nizatidine (Thelin & Richter 2020).

Adverse effects: The most common side effects reported from the use of H2 antagonists are headaches, dizziness, nausea and vomiting, and constipation. In rare cases and in long-term use, there is a risk of anti-androgen effects but these symptoms resolve quickly if medication is ceased.

Acid suppressants: Proton pump inhibitors

Proton pump inhibitors inhibit acid formation in the cells in the lining of the stomach by inhibiting hydrogen ions from being produced in the stomach parietal cells. There are several proton pump inhibitors available, such as omeprazole; however, these medications should only be recommended if other treatments are unsuccessful, as the use of proton pump inhibitors has the potential to increase the risk of infection and to reduce vitamin B12 levels (Swarnakari et al 2022). Although these medications are the most effective drug treatment for gastric reflux, their use in pregnancy has not been extensively researched; therefore, data relating to their safety in pregnancy is limited. Some recent studies have also linked an increase in pregnant women's use of gastric acid suppression drugs in pregnancy and subsequent childhood allergies.

There are many PPI available on the market. The most common are omeprazole, lansoprazole, pantoprazole and rabeprazole, which are all considered relatively safe in pregnancy. However, as previously stated, minimal research has been conducted and to date, very little research has been undertaken with pregnant women. Omeprazole is the most prescribed proton pump inhibitor and can be administered orally 20 mg once or twice daily or IV 40 mg once daily.

Adverse effects: These drugs are generally well tolerated. Common reported side effects from proton pump inhibitors are headache, dizziness, nausea, vomiting, diarrhoea, abdominal pain, constipation, and flatulence. Rarer adverse effects include rash and itchiness, insomnia, dry mouth, oedema hypersensitivity reactions, hepatic and renal changes (Thelin & Richter 2020). (Table 7.6.)

Constipation

Constipation is defined as difficulty in defecating. Normal bowel movements vary between individuals; therefore, it is not the frequency of bowel movements but the associated discomfort that defines constipation.

TABLE 7.6 Acid suppression for symptoms of gastro-esophageal reflux

THERAPY	DOSE	RISK	COMMENT
First-line: Antacids containing magnesium, calcium, or aluminium	As required for mild symptoms	No increase in congenital malformations	Constipation or diarrhoea in high doses
Second-line: H2 antagonists	Ranitidine 150–300 mg BD Famotidine 20 mg OD or BD	No increase in congenital malformations	Well tolerated
Third-line: Proton pump inhibitors	Omeprazole 20 mg OD-BD Lansoprazole 15 mg OD-BD Rabeprazole 20 mg OD-BD Esomeprazole 40 mg OD-BD Pantoprazole 40 mg OD-BD	No increase in congenital malformations	Well tolerated

Source: Adapted from Nikfar S, Abdollahi M, Moretti ME, et al. Use of proton pump inhibitors during pregnancy and rates of major malformations: a meta-analysis. Diges Dis Sci. 2002;47(7):1526–1529; Mahadevan U, Kane S. American Gastroenterological Association Institute medical position statement on the use of gastrointestinal medications in pregnancy. Gastroenterol. 2006;131(1):278-282; Gill SK, O'Brien L, Koren G. The safety of histamine 2 (H2) blockers in pregnancy: a meta-analysis. Dig Dis Sci. 2009;54(9):1835-1838; Gill SK, O'Brien L, Einarson TR et al. The safety of proton pump inhibitors (PPIs) in pregnancy: a meta-analysis. Am J Gastroenterol. 2009;104(6):1541-1545.

Many pregnant women complain of difficulty passing faeces, making constipation a common complaint in pregnancy.

Constipation in pregnancy has multiple causes, including hormonal changes. Increased levels of progesterone and relaxin cause relaxation of the smooth muscle of the gut, decreased motilin and an increase in enteroglucogen. The effects of progesterone and oestrogen slow down the activity of the bowel and increase the absorption of salt and water absorption in the gut. The pressure of the growing uterus on the bowel affects the ability of the bowel to function optimally. Changes in diet and fluid intake and reduced activity can contribute to constipation. As with other common discomforts of pregnancy, lifestyle changes are recommended as first-line management.

Management and treatment for constipation

Dietary changes are recommended, such as increasing fibre and fluid in the diet by eating more whole foods, grains, fruits, and vegetables. Prunes and/or prune juice are also recommended to reduce constipation. Lifestyle changes, such as changing the sitting position on the toilet, leaning forward with feet on a low stool or similar so that the knees are higher than hips, can aid defecation. Going to the toilet as soon as the urge is felt and increasing daily exercise is also recommended.

Laxatives

Laxatives are used in managing constipation if dietary and lifestyle adaptations are unsuccessful. Laxatives are grouped into several different categories depending on their action. All laxatives have the potential to disrupt the normal function of the bowel, cause dehydration and electrolyte imbalances, and can cause a disruption to normal gut flora so should be taken with caution (Edwards et al 2017). The gut microbiome is a critical component of an individual's metabolism and overall health, and the removal of healthy gut flora can lead to recolonisation by other microorganisms, which has the potential to cause increased bacteria in the bowel, infections, and other associated problems. Abdominal pain and flatulence are also associated with laxative use.

Laxatives can be taken orally or administered directly into the rectum as suppositories or enemas. However, per rectum administration has the potential to irritate the uterus so is usually avoided unless other methods are unsuccessful. Per rectum administration can also cause irritation and pain to the rectum and anal area. Laxatives should be administered 1–2 hours post administration of other medicines to ensure the medications are absorbed completely.

Bulk-forming laxatives

Bulk-forming laxatives are the first choice for management of constipation in pregnancy if lifestyle and dietary changes are unsuccessful. Bulk laxatives are undigested polysaccharides that attract water by osmosis. This increases their volume and stimulates peristalsis. Bulk laxatives are considered safer than other laxatives in pregnancy as they do not act on the gut motion. Caution must be taken to ensure that adequate fluid is taken when taking bulk laxatives, as they have the potential to cause faecal impaction. Women should be advised to drink at least 500 ml of fluid with the laxative. They are not as quick to act as other laxatives and may take 1–3 days to be effective.

Common side effects include a feeling of fullness, decrease in appetite, bloating, flatulence, and abdominal cramping. Common types of bulk-forming laxative are bran supplements, methylcellulose, ispaghula husk (Fybogel), psyllium (Metamucil).

Faecal softeners

Faecal softeners, also referred to as stool softeners, include docusate, liquid paraffin and poloxamer. They are commonly used to treat acute constipation and to prevent straining. Compounds act as detergent to hold water molecules into the faeces. This makes the faeces softer and therefore easier to expel. The compounds do have a mild stimulant effect; however, the main property of these laxatives is to hold water, not stimulate the bowel. They therefore do not work quickly and may take several days to be effective. A common stool softener is docusate.

Liquid paraffin, a mixture of liquid hydrocarbons obtained from petroleum, is not digested and absorption is minimal. Liquid paraffin penetrates and coats the faecal mass and prevents excessive absorption of water. Liquid paraffin can impair the absorption of fat-soluble vitamins A, D, E and K. If liquid paraffin is taken with meals, gastric emptying time may be delayed. If used in large doses it has the potential to leak or seep from the rectum which can be uncomfortable and embarrassing to women. Poloxamer is a surfactant that increases penetration of fluid into faeces, thereby softening the faecal mass. It is a component of Coloxyl.

Osmotic laxatives

The osmotic laxatives include macrogols or polyethylene glycols (PEGs), glycerol, lactulose and sorbitol. These are not absorbed. By exerting an osmotic effect, they increase the volume of fluid in the lumen. This increased volume accelerates the transfer of the gut contents and leads to increased defecation. These types of laxatives act by a physical mechanism. Small molecules are not effectively absorbed in the intestines. This makes a stronger than normal solution in the colon. The contents are hypertonic, which means the water is retained. Osmotic pressure means that water can be pulled from the gut into the bowel. This increases volume and pressure in the bowel and rectum which, in turn, stimulates the defecation reflex.

Glycerol suppositories act as osmotic agents by absorbing water, but they also lubricate and increase stool bulk. Local irritation of the mucous membrane of the rectum may promote peristalsis, and evacuation occurs 5–30 minutes after insertion.

Saline laxatives retain and increase the water content of faeces by virtue of an osmotic effect and stimulate peristalsis. Saline laxatives are soluble salts (e.g. magnesium salts, sodium salts and PEG macrogol electrolyte solutions) that are only slightly absorbed from the alimentary canal. Because of their osmotic effect, they retain and increase the water content of faeces. The water in the intestinal lumen produces fluid accumulation and distension, leading to peristalsis and eventual evacuation of bowel contents. The result is a faecal mass of liquid or semi-liquid stools.

Magnesium sulphate (Epsom salts) is a common, quick-acting laxative which has an effect within 3 hours. These types of laxatives are generally not recommended in pregnancy as they are usually used to treat moderate to severe constipation and have the potential to cause dehydration and electrolyte imbalances.

Stimulants

Stimulant laxatives promote accumulation of water and increase peristalsis in the colon by irritating intramural sensory nerve plexi endings in the mucosa. The principal stimulant laxatives are bisacodyl, sodium picosulfate and preparations of senna. These agents promote accumulation of water and electrolytes in the lumen and stimulate nerve endings to increase intestinal motility. The stimulant laxatives usually act in 6–12 hours. Their primary effect is on the small and large intestines, which explains their tendency to produce griping and cramping pains. Stimulant laxatives are generally avoided in pregnancy unless other methods are unsuccessful and constipation is severe, as they can cause uterine irritation.

Bisacodyl is a relatively non-toxic laxative agent that stimulates peristalsis on contact with the mucosa of the colon. It is the chemical triphenylmethane, related to the pH indicator phenolphthalein. The enteric coating is formulated to dissolve in intestinal fluids and, when released, produces its stimulating effects on the colon. It should not be chewed, crushed, or taken with milk or antacids because it can irritate the stomach, causing severe abdominal cramps. Oral medication is effective in 6–12 hours, and suppositories and enemas act within 15–60 and 5–15 minutes, respectively. Suppositories may cause anal and rectal irritation.

Senna is derived from the dried leaves of the Cassia plant. Oral administration is effective within 6–12 hours; however, senna commonly causes abdominal pain and griping pain. It is found in proprietary remedies such as Laxettes and Senokot. Adverse effects of stimulant laxatives include abdominal cramping and fluid and electrolyte imbalance.

Candidiasis

A balanced and healthy vaginal microbiome is important for maintaining female reproductive health (Willems et al 2020). During pregnancy, most women will experience a normal increase in vaginal discharge. However, if the discharge is offensive or accompanied by pain or itching, further assessment may be warranted. Treatable infections include bacterial vaginosis, vaginal trichomoniasis (see Chapter 12) and vaginal candidiasis.

Candida albicans is usually part of the normal flora of the skin, mouth, intestines, and vagina. Candidiasis (thrush) is often referred to as an opportunistic infection, as in certain circumstances (e.g. antibiotic use) an overgrowth of this bacteria can occur, resulting in a systemic infection. Pregnancy increases the frequency of vaginal candida colonisation, and it is thought to be caused by increased levels of circulating estrogens and the deposition of glycogen and other substrates in the vagina during pregnancy.

Management and treatment for Candidiasis
Azole antifungals

The evidence on the use of medications to treat symptomatic vaginal discharge due to vaginal candidiasis is limited. Treatment is usually by administration of azole antifungals. A 2001 Cochrane review (Young & Jewell 2001) showed imidazole drugs were more effective than other drugs. A more recent review by National Guideline Alliance (2021) for the treatment of symptomatic vaginal discharge due to vaginal candidiasis in pregnant women, critiqued three RCTs. All the included studies used vaginal imidazole-based antifungal treatments and showed that the treatment was effective, with over 80% of women who received antifungal treatment having a negative culture following the treatment.

Azole antifungals that contain two nitrogens in the azole ring are called imidazoles, and those with three nitrogens are called triazoles. These agents are fungistatic and affect the biosynthesis of fungal ergosterols by interfering with the cytochrome P450 (CYP)-dependent enzyme lanosterol demethylase (also called 14α-sterol demethylase) that catalyses ergosterol formation. Ergosterol is a major component of the fungal cell membrane, and the azoles cause depletion of ergosterol and accumulation of 14α-methylated sterols. This results in inhibition of fungal growth, interference in nutrient transport and, ultimately, cell leakage and death. At therapeutic concentrations, the azoles have a greater affinity for the fungal 14α-sterol demethylase than for the human liver equivalent CYP 14α-sterol demethylase. This selective toxicity allows for the use of these drugs in humans.

Azole antifungals in pregnancy are usually administered topically to the vulva and/or with a vaginal pessary inserted into the vagina, although in some cases oral administration may be indicated. Low-dose oral fluconazole is often used in pregnancy for treatment of severe vulvovaginal candidiasis that is unsolved by topical treatment. However, caution is required due to recent studies that show an increased risk of spontaneous abortion, and the risk of fetal anomalies among users of high-dose (> 150 mg) fluconazole during the first trimester of pregnancy (Nørgaard et al 2008; Mølgaard-Nielsen et al 2013).

The first-line management for treatment of vaginal candidiasis in pregnancy is clotrimazole pessary and cream. These treatments are available over the counter. Other treatment options are miconazole and nystatin, but these are not as effective as clotrimazole.

Clotrimazole

Pessaries contain 100 mg, 200 mg or 500 mg.

The pessary dose to treat thrush is:

- 100 mg – use 1 pessary every night for 6 nights in a row or 2 pessaries for 3 nights in a row.
- 200 mg – use 1 pessary (or 2 × 100 mg pessaries) every night for 3 nights in a row
- 500 mg – use 1 pessary for 1 night only

Clotrimazole internal cream contains 500 mg of clotrimazole in every 5 g of cream. It comes as a single application that you use once.

Clotrimazole external cream is used 2 or 3 times a day for at least 2 weeks.

Adverse effects: Common side effects from the pessary or internal cream:

- discomfort or swelling in or around vagina
- pain or a burning or stinging feeling after putting the pessary in
- lower stomach pain or pain in the pelvic area
- bleeding from the vagina.

Side effects usually go away when pessaries or internal cream use are stopped.

Common side effects from the external cream:

- red, irritated skin
- pain, burning or stinging sensation.

Probiotics

Probiotics are live microorganisms that exert health benefits to the host upon consumption in sufficient amounts. Although probiotics have been used commonly for gut health, increasing evidence over the years has illustrated the benefits of probiotics beyond that of gut maintenance. Probiotics have been documented to maintain and modulate microbiota profiles in the gut and vagina, and they are able to inhibit pathogenic *Candida* spp.

Probiotic therapy has been suggested for the treatment or prevention of *Candida* vaginitis. Pericolini and colleagues (2017) found that vaginal administration of the probiotic *S. cerevisiae* reduced inflammation and symptoms in women. A randomised, double-blind and placebo-controlled study (SynForU-HerCare trial) involving 78 pregnant women with vaginal candidiasis showed that the oral administration of lactobacilli putative probiotics for 8 weeks reduced symptoms and recurrences of symptoms. Women who received the intervention also experienced improved social and emotional wellbeing compared to women receiving the placebo. The study's authors concluded that probiotics could be a potential strategy for the maintenance of vaginal health during pregnancy (Ang et al 2022).

Combined treatment

A recent follow-on RCT from the SynForU-HerCare study combined azole antifungal treatment with oral probiotics. This study demonstrated that for women who received vaginal clotrimazole alone, the current infection was treated but recurrences were not prevented. However, with the addition of probiotics, recurrent infections were reduced. The authors suggest that routine use of probiotics during pregnancy can inhibit and treat candida infections and prevent recurrences and reduction of vaginal inflammation.

Rh (D) immunoglobulin

Each individual carries unique antigens on the surface of their cells, thus the immune system will recognise cells of another individual. Blood groups are determined by the ABO system and rhesus factors. Maternal Rh D antibodies may develop during pregnancy when an Rh D negative pregnant woman carries an Rh D positive fetus. Development of antibodies occurs when fetal red blood cells (RBCs) enter the maternal circulation, and antibodies are produced towards the fetal Rh D antigen. The most common sources of fetal RBCs entering the maternal circulation are thought to be small feto-maternal haemorrhages (FMHs) at birth and silent transplacental haemorrhages in the antenatal period.

Rh positive individuals carry the D antigen on their red blood cells and have no rhesus antibodies in their blood plasma (Sarwar et al 2023). Rh negative individuals do not have the D antigen but on exposure to Rh positive cells can produce anti D antibodies (1gG) which can cross the placenta. The maternal response to the fetal RBCs is known as 'sensitisation' or alloimmunisation.

In the first pregnancy/birth, sensitisation is often of little consequence; however, the maternal immune system will create antibodies, and then in subsequent pregnancies maternal antibodies will recognise the fetal cells as foreign and attack them. Fetal cells are split open giving rise to haemolytic disease of the fetus and newborn (HDFN). As fetal cells are destroyed the fetus becomes anaemic. Severe cases cause hydrops fetalis (gross oedema or accumulation of fluid leading to fetal death). Fetal treatment is the administration of an in-utero exchange blood transfusion (McBain et al 2015).

After birth, the neonate can become ill due to a buildup of bilirubin, as the placenta is no longer removing the bilirubin from the fetal circulation. Bilirubin is the waste product of the destroyed RBCs and can accumulate to cause jaundice. If SBR levels rise above 120 micromoles/litre, the bilirubin can cross the blood–brain barrier into the cerebral tissue and cause permanent brain damage (kernicterus). In the absence of intervention, HDFN affects 1% of neonates, and is a significant cause of perinatal mortality and morbidity, and long-term disability (Zwiers et al 2018).

Before Rh D immunoprophylaxis became available in the late 1960s, approximately 16% of women who had given birth to an Rh D positive, ABO-compatible baby developed alloantibodies in their subsequent pregnancy.

Rh D immunoglobulin is manufactured from plasma of Rh D negative blood donors who are stimulated to produce elevated levels of anti-D antibodies. Through a process of plasmapheresis, anti-D is extracted from the plasma and pasteurised as an immunoglobulin for prophylactic administration It is given to Rh D negative women with no preformed anti-D antibodies (during pregnancy and immediately postpartum) to prevent Rh D alloimmunisation. In Australia, routine prophylactic anti-D for Rh negative women is recommended at 28 and 34 weeks. (Tables 7.7–7.9.)

7.5 Complementary and alternative medicines (CAMs)

Complementary and alternative medicines are becoming more widely used during pregnancy. There is a common misconception that natural therapies are always safe, so it is essential that midwives have a basic understanding of some of the CAM therapies a woman may use during her pregnancy to allow for an open and honest discussion about the risks and benefits of their use (Illamola et al 2020; Kam et al 2019). Common CAMS used during pregnancy are aromatherapy, herbal medicines, and homeopathy.

Aromatherapy

Concentrated essential oils that are extracted from plants contain chemical components which can cause physiological and psychological effects. Advising on the

TABLE 7.7 Summary of guidance on the use and timing of Rh D immunoglobulin for routine immunoprophylaxis

CLINICAL INDICATION	RH D IMMUNOGLOBULIN DOSE AND TIMING	TARGET GROUP
Routine antenatal immunoprophylaxis	625 IU At 28 and 34 weeks of pregnancy	Rh D negative pregnant women with no preformed anti-D antibodies (unless NIPT for fetal RHD has predicted that they are not carrying an Rh D positive fetus).
Routine postnatal immunoprophylaxis	625 IU After giving birth	All Rh D negative women with no preformed anti-D antibodies after giving birth to an Rh D positive baby (based on cord blood or neonatal Rh D typing a). If the baby is Rh D positive administer Rh D immunoglobulin even if the NIPT predicted an Rh D negative baby. If the baby is Rh D positive and is born preterm, give the postnatal dose even if the birth is within 72 hours of a dose given for routine antenatal immunoprophylaxis or for a sensitising event. A cord blood or neonatal testing should be performed regardless of NIPT results for fetal RHD.

FMH = fetomaternal haemorrhage; IM = intramuscular; IU = international units; NIPT = non-invasive prenatal testing
anti-D – refers to circulating antibodies; Rh D – refers to genotype; Rh D immunoglobulin – refers to the product; Rh D positive/negative – refers to blood type
Source: Adapted from Guideline for the prophylactic use of Rh D immunoglobulin in pregnancy care 2024. National Blood Authority (NBA). www.blood.gov.au/anti-d-0

TABLE 7.8 Summary of guidance on the use and timing of Rh D immunoglobulin for sensitising event immunoprophylaxis

CLINICAL INDICATION		RH D IMMUNOGLOBULIN DOSE AND TIMING	TARGET GROUP
Sensitising event immunoprophylaxis in the first 12 weeks of pregnancy	Miscarriage. Termination of pregnancy (medical after 10 weeks gestation or surgical) Ectopic pregnancy. Molar pregnancy. Chorionic villus sampling.	250 iu as soon as practical within 72 hours. If delayed beyond 72 hours, the dose should be given up to 10 days from the sensitising event, but may have lower efficacy. For ongoing uterine bleeding alone, a repeat dose of Rh D immunoglobulin (250 iu if before 12 weeks and 625 iu if after) may be appropriate after an interval of 6 weeks.	All Rh D negative women with no preformed anti-D antibodies
Sensitising event immunoprophylaxis after 12+6 weeks of pregnancy	Genetic studies (chorionic villus sampling, amniocenesis and cordocentesis). Abdominal trauma considered sufficient to cause fetomaternal haemorrhage, even if FMH testing is negative. Each occasion of revealed or concealed antepartum haemorrhage. (Where the woman suffers unexplained uterine pain the possibility of concealed antepartum haemorrhage [and the need for immunoprophylaxis] should be considered.) External cephalic version (successful or attempted). Miscarriage or termination of pregnancy.	625 iu as soon as practical within 72 hours. If delayed beyond 72 hours, the dose should be given up to 10 days from the sensitising event, but may have lower efficacy. For ongoing uterine bleeding alone, a repeat dose may be appropriate at 6-weekly intervals.	All Rh D negative women with no preformed anti-D antibodies (unless NIPT for fetal Rh D has predicted the fetus to be Rh D negative).
Large FMH ≥6 ml of fetal red cells (equivalent to 12 ml of whole blood)	Antepartum Postpartum	625 iu as soon as possible. Follow laboratory or specialist obstetric advice for additional doses of im Rh D immunoglobulin or iv Rh D immunoglobulin, and for follow-up testing.	All Rh D negative women with no preformed anti-D antibodies (unless NIPT for fetal Rh D has predicted the fetus to be Rh D negative).

FMH = fetomaternal haemorrhage; im = intramuscular; iu = international units; iv = intravenous; NIPT = non-invasive prenatal testing; anti-D – refers to circulating antibodies; Rh D – refers to genotype; Rh D immunoglobulin – refers to the product; Rh D positive/negative – refers to blood type
Source: Adapted from Guideline for the prophylactic use of Rh D immunoglobulin in pregnancy care 2024. National Blood Authority (NBA). www.blood.gov.au/anti-d-0

TABLE 7.9 Products available under the national blood arrangements

PRODUCT	PRESENTATION	DOSE	VOLUME	ADMINISTRATION
Rh(D) immunoglobulin-vf	Single vial	250 iu	Up to 2 mL	Slow deep intramuscular injection
Rh(D) immunoglobulin-vf	Single vial	625 iu	Up to 2 mL	Slow deep intramuscular injection

use of aromatherapy is outside the scope of practice of the midwife and women should be referred to a qualified aromatherapist. Women can self-administer essential oils by inhaling the scent of the oil or applying it to the skin. Some essentials oils can be toxic if applied neat to the skin, therefore it is recommended that oils be diluted with a carrier oil (e.g. olive, grape seed, calendula, or almond oil) before applying to the skin. Essential oils can also be added to an emulsifier such as full fat milk to aid distribution in bathwater.

Some essential oils can be teratogenic and therefore it is recommended that women avoid using essential oils during the first trimester. A few essential oils are emmenogogic, which means they can cause bleeding during pregnancy and have the potential to abort the pregnancy – these essential oils are sometimes used to stimulate labour (see Chapter 8).

Common essential oils used during pregnancy are:

- Chamomile: calming, reduces tension
- Frankincense: calming, mood stabilising
- Jasmine: evokes feeling of joy, happiness, peace, and self-confidence.
- Lavender: used to relax and calm. Can reduce blood pressure and eases muscular tension
- Lemon oil: can ease nausea
- Neroli: decreases anxious nerves. Depressant. Avoid in low mood

- Mandarin: has a balancing effect on the mind. Can help with nightmares, insomnia, fatigue and fluid retention
- Peppermint: can ease nausea
- Rose oil: relaxing
- Sweet orange: mood lifting, energy boost and a refreshing scent
- Teatree: antiseptic and antiviral
- Ylang ylang: contains a component called linalool, which helps with anxiety. It reduces pain, stress, blood pressure, and muscle tension.

Herbal medicines

Herbal medicine is the therapeutic use of plants, including essential oils and herbal teas. Herbal medicines are absorbed into the body, and should therefore be treated as a drug. Some common herbal treatments used in pregnancy are:

- Alfalfa (*Medicago sativa*) – one of the most nutritionally rich herbs, packed with vitamins and minerals, including vitamin K
- *Aloe vera* – when taken orally, can be used for asthma, dry skin and constipation. Topically, *Aloe vera* is used for acne and wound healing
- Astragalus (*Astragalus membranaceus*) – improves blood circulation to the liver and helps improve liver function
- Calendula (*Calendula officinalis*) – topically, antiseptic, soothes wound inflammation, useful for general wound healing
- Comfrey (*Symphytum officinale*) – topically, promotes new cell growth and controls bleeding. A great overall healer. Not to be taken internally. Do not use on broken skin
- Cranberry – commonly used for the prevention or treatment of urinary tract infections (UTIs)
- Dandelion leaf (*Taraxacum officinale*) – rich in vitamin A, calcium, and iron. A natural diuretic and antioxidant which relieves mild oedema and nourishes the liver
- Echinacea – commonly used to treat the common cold, sore throat and other upper respiratory tract infections
- Garlic – used to prevent and treat the common cold and respiratory tract infections
- Ginger – has been used to manage nausea and vomiting
- Globe artichoke (*Cynara scolymus*) – a hepatic and choleretic herb to support healthy digestion and liver function
- Horse chestnut (*Aesculus hippocastanum*) – topically, is an astringent, a circulatory tonic, with anti-inflammatory properties. Improves microvascular circulation and reduces swelling
- Hibiscus rosella (*Hibiscus sabdariffa*) – rich in antioxidants and vitamin C

- Mugwort (*Moxa*): Moxibustion (moxa therapy on the acupuncture point Bladder 67) has successfully been used to turn breech presentation
- Nettle (*Urtica dioica*) – depurative, rich in iron, calcium, magnesium and vitamin K. Nourishes the immune system. Combats anaemia. Relieves muscle spasm and leg cramps. Topically: strong astringent useful for cuts, sores and haemorrhoids
- Oat straw (*Avena sativa*) – nourishes the nervous system, rich in calcium and magnesium. Helps the body to lower blood sugar levels and blood pressure when needed. Helpful for insomnia
- Olive leaf extract – used for viral or bacterial infections including influenza and the common cold
- Plantain (*Plantago lanceolate*) – has a soothing, cooling effect and is considered an effective remedy for healing haemorrhoids
- Red raspberry leaf (*Rubus idaeus*) – used traditionally to prepare the body for labour and to relieve nausea. A uterine tonic, rich in many nutrients, which nourishes the female reproductive system. Supports, tightens and tones the muscles and ligaments of the uterus
- Rosehip (*Rosa canina*) – anti-inflammatory, astringent, also rich in antioxidants and vitamin C
- Spearmint (*Mentha spicata*) – calming for the nervous system and helps to settle the stomach and support digestion
- St. Mary's thistle (*Silybum marianum*) – a hepatic herbs which cleanses and strengthens the liver; supports protein synthesis in the liver and helps improve blood filtering systems
- Witch hazel (*Hamamelis virginiana*) – topically: an astringent, curbs bleeding and reduces inflammation, pain, itching and swelling.

Homeopathics in pregnancy

- *Calcarea phosphorica* – used to strengthen a woman who tends toward easy tiredness, poor digestion, cold hands and feet, and poor absorption of nutrients. Some women who need this remedy find only 'junk food' appealing during pregnancy, or have cravings for smoked and salty food
- *Carbo vegetabilis* – helpful to a woman who feels weak and faint during pregnancy
- *Ferrum phosphoricum* – helpful for nervous, sensitive women who often feel weak or tired, with easy flushing of the face and a tendency toward anaemia
- *Nux vomica* – may be useful for indigestion, heartburn, stomach pain, and constipation during pregnancy
- *Pulsatilla* – helpful at times of strong hormonal changes
- *Ferrum metallicum* – helpful in correcting anaemic tendencies

- *Sepia* – indicated for women who feel tired and irritable during pregnancy or with little enthusiasm for the pregnancy. Nausea, constipation, a feeling of weakness in the pelvic floor.

KEY POINTS

Complementary and alternative medicines

- Complementary and alternative medicines are becoming more widely used during pregnancy.
- Common CAMS used during pregnancy are aromatherapy, herbal medicines, and homeopathy.
- Caution is needed as some CAMS are contraindicated during pregnancy.

CONCLUSION

This chapter has provided an overview of the considerations that must be taken regarding the use of medicines during pregnancy. Common discomforts and conditions in pregnancy have been discussed and the recommended treatments. It is essential that the midwife has a good understanding of the implications of drug use in pregnancy, including the impact of medications on the fetus.

REVIEW QUESTIONS

Review the clinical scenario at the beginning of this chapter and consider the following questions.

1 What first- and second-line pharmaceutical or other options are available for the management of Bella's symptoms?

2 As Bella's primary midwife, which of the options discussed in the chapter would you discuss with her regarding management of her current symptoms to optimise pregnancy health status for herself and her baby?

3 What specific information do women want from their healthcare providers about medication use in pregnancy?

4 As midwives we talk to women about many aspects of their pregnancy. Reflect on how confident you feel about discussing the use of medicines in pregnancy. Do you feel confident discussing the risks and benefits of their use? Do you feel confident in recommending a particular treatment option?

5 How often are you asked about the use of aromatherapy or herbal treatments such as raspberry leaf tea?

6 How does the Australian categorisation of drugs and safety during pregnancy assist midwives in their decision making regarding safe use of medications for pregnant women?

7 What does the research say about the use of mugwort (moxibustion) in pregnancy?

REFERENCES

Ang XY, Chung FY, Lee BK, et al. Lactobacilli reduce recurrences of vaginal candidiasis in pregnant women: a randomized, double-blind, placebo-controlled study. J Appl Microbiol. 2022 Apr;132(4):3168-3180. doi.org/10.1111/jam.15158

Basirat Z, Moghadamnia AA, Kashifard M, et al. The effect of ginger biscuit on nausea and vomiting in early pregnancy. Acta Med Iran. 2009;47:51-56.

Bsat F, Bayer-Zwirello L, Seubert D, et al. Randomized study of three common outpatient treatments for nausea and vomiting of pregnancy [abstract]. Am J Obstet Gynecol. 2001;185(6 Suppl):S181.

Bsat FA, Hoffman DE, Seubert DE. Comparison of three outpatient regimens in the management of nausea and vomiting in pregnancy. J Perinatol. 2003 Oct;23(7):531-535. doi:10.1038/sj.jp.7210986

Chiossi G, Neri I, Cavazzuti M, et al. Hyperemesis gravidarum complicated by Wernicke encephalopathy: background, case report, and review of the literature. Obstet Gynecol Surv. 2006 Apr;61(4):255-268. doi.org/10.1097/01. ogx.0000206336.08794.65

Dante G, Pedrielli G, Annessi E, et al. Herb remedies during pregnancy: a systematic review of controlled clinical trials. J Matern Fetal Neonatal Med. 2013;26:306-312.

Ding M, Leach M, Bradley H. The effectiveness and safety of ginger for pregnancy-induced nausea and vomiting: a systematic review. Women Birth. 2013;26:e26-30. doi. org/10.1016/j.wombi.2012.08.001

Ebrahimi N, Maltepe C, Bournissen FG, et al. Nausea and vomiting of pregnancy: using the 24-hour Pregnancy-Unique Quantification of Emesis (PUQE-24) scale. J Obstet Gynaecol Can. 2009;31:803-807.

Edwards SM, Cunningham SA, Dunlop AL, et al. The maternal gut microbiome during pregnancy. MCN Am J Matern Child Nurs. 2017 Nov/Dec;42(6):310-317. doi:10.1097/ NMC.0000000000000372

Fejzo M, Rocha N, Cimino I, et al. GDF15 linked to maternal risk of nausea and vomiting during pregnancy. Nature. 2024;625:760–767. doi.org/10.1038/s41586-023-06921-9

Huybrechts KF, Hernández-Díaz S, Straub L, et al. Association of maternal first-trimester ondansetron use with cardiac malformations and oral clefts in offspring. JAMA. 2018 Dec;18(320):2429-2437. doi: 10.1001/jama.2018.18307

Huybrechts KF, Hernandez-Diaz S, Bateman BT. Contextualizing potential risks of medication in pregnancy for the newborn-the case of ondansetron. JAMA Pediatrics. 2020;174(8):747-748. doi: 10.1001/jamapediatrics.2020.1325

Kam PC, Barnett DW, Douglas ID. Herbal medicines and pregnancy: a narrative review and anaesthetic considerations. Anaesth Intensive Care. 2019 May;47(3):226-234. doi:10.1177/0310057X19845786

Kametas NA, Nelson-Piercy C. Hyperemesis gravidarum, gastrointestinal and liver disease in pregnancy. Obstetrics, Gynaecology and Reproductive Medicine. 2008 March;18(3) 69-70. doi:10.1016/j.ogrm.2008.01.003

Kennedy D. Classifying drugs in pregnancy. Aust Prescr. 2014;37:38-40. doi.org/10.18773/austprescr.2014.018

Le Y-LT, Luu MN, Mai LH, et al. Prevalence and characteristics of gastroesophageal reflux disease in pregnant women. Rev Gastroenterol Mex (Engl Ed). 2023 Oct-Dec;88(4):341-346. doi.org/10.1016/j.rgmx.2021.11.010

Lupattelli A, Spigset O, Twigg MJ, et al. Medication use in pregnancy: a cross-sectional, multinational web-based study. BMJ Open. 2014;4:e004365. doi.org/10.1136/bmjopen-2013-004365

Lynch MM, Squiers LB, Kosa KM, et al. Making decisions about medication use during pregnancy: implications for communication strategies. Matern Child Health. 2018 Jan;22(1):92-100. doi:10.1007/s10995-017-2358-0

Matthews A, Haas DM, O'Mathúna DP, et al. Interventions for nausea and vomiting in early pregnancy. Cochrane Database Syst Rev. 2015 Sep;(9):CD007575. doi.org//10.1002/14651858.CD007575.pub4

McBain RD, Crowther CA, Middleton P. Anti-D administration in pregnancy for preventing rhesus alloimmunisation. Cochrane Database Syst Rev. 2015 Sep;(9):CD000020 https://www.ncbi.nlm.nih.gov/pubmed/26334436

Meteerattanapipat P, Phupong V. Efficacy of alginate-based reflux suppressant and magnesium-aluminium antacid gel for treatment of heartburn in pregnancy: a randomized double-blind controlled trial. Sci Rep. 2017 Mar 20;7:44830. doi: 10.1038/srep44830.

Mølgaard-Nielsen D, Pasternak B, Hviid A. Use of oral fluconazole during pregnancy and the risk of birth defects. N Engl J Med. 2013 Aug 29;369(9):830-839. doi: 10.1056/NEJMoa1301066

Mousa A, Naqash A, Lim S. Macronutrient and micronutrient intake during pregnancy: an overview of recent evidence. Nutrients. 2019 Feb 20;11(2):443. doi: 10.3390/nu11020443

Nana M, Tydeman F, Bevan G, et al. Termination of wanted pregnancy and suicidal ideation in hyperemesis gravidarum: a mixed methods study. Obstet Med. 2022 Sep;15(3):180-184. doi.org/10.1177/1753495X211040926

National Guideline Alliance (UK). Management of symptomatic vaginal discharge in pregnancy: antenatal care: evidence review T. London: National Institute for Health and Care Excellence (NICE); 2021 Aug. (NICE Guideline, No. 201.) Available from: https://www.ncbi.nlm.nih.gov/books/NBK573944

Nørgaard M, Pedersen L, Gislum M, et al. Maternal use of fluconazole and risk of congenital malformations: a Danish population-based cohort study. J Antimicrob Chemother. 2008 Jul;62(1):172-176. doi.org/10.1093/jac/dkn157

Nuangchamnong N, Niebyl J. Doxylamine succinate-pyridoxine hydrochloride (Diclegis) for the management of nausea and vomiting in pregnancy: an overview. Int J Womens Health. 2014 Apr12;6:401-409. doi: 10.2147/IJWH.S46653

Pericolini E, Gabrielli E, Ballet N, et al. Therapeutic activity of a Saccharomyces cerevisiae-based probiotic and inactivated whole yeast on vaginal candidiasis. Virulence. 2017 Jan 2;8(1):74-90. doi: 10.1080/21505594.2016.1213937.

Rad MN, Lamyian M, Heshmat R, et al. A randomized clinical trial of the efficacy of KID21 point (Youmen) acupressure on nausea and vomiting of pregnancy. Iran Red Crescent Med J. 2012;14(11):697-701.

Sanders J, Blaylock R, Dean C, et al. Women's experiences of over-the-counter and prescription medication during pregnancy in the UK: findings from survey free-text responses and narrative interviews. BMJ Open. 2023;13:e067987. doi:10.1136/bmjopen-2022-067987

Sarman, I. Review shows that early foetal alcohol exposure may cause adverse effects even when the mother consumes low levels. Acta Paediatr. 2018 Jun;107(6);938–941. doi: 10.1111/apa.14221

Sarwar A, Citla Sridhar D. Rh hemolytic disease. [Updated 2023 Mar 6]. In: StatPearls [Internet]. Treasure Island (FL): StatPearls Publishing, 2023. Available from: https://www.ncbi.nlm.nih.gov/books/NBK560488/

Sharifzadeh F, Kashanian M, Koohpayehzadeh J, et al. A comparison between the effects of ginger, pyridoxine (vitamin B6) and placebo for the treatment of the first trimester nausea and vomiting of pregnancy (NVP). J Matern Fetal Neonatal Med. 2018 Oct;31(19):2509–2514. doi.org/10.1080/14767058.2017.1344965

Sheehan, P. Hyperemesis gravidarum: assessment and management. Aust Fam Physician. 2007 Sep;36(9):698-701.

Soma-Pillay P, Nelson-Piercy C, Tolppanen H, et al. Physiological changes in pregnancy. Cardiovasc J Afr. 2016 Mar-Apr;27(2):89-94. doi.org/10.5830/CVJA-2016-021

Swarnakari KM, Bai M, Manoharan MP, et al. The effects of proton pump inhibitors in acid hypersecretion-induced vitamin B12 deficiency: a systematic review (2022). Cureus. 2022 Nov 19;14(11):e31672. doi: 10.7759/cureus.31672

Tan M-Y, Shu S-H, Liu R-L, et al. The efficacy and safety of complementary and alternative medicine in the treatment of nausea and vomiting during pregnancy: a systematic review and meta-analysis. Front Public Health. 2023;11:1108756. doi: 10.3389/fpubh.2023.1108756

Thelin CS, Richter JE. Review article: the management of heartburn during pregnancy Aliment Pharmacol Ther. 2020 Feb;51(4):421-434. doi.org/10.1111/apt.15611

Thomson M, Corbin R, Leung L. Effects of ginger for nausea and vomiting in early pregnancy: a meta-analysis. J Am Board Fam Med 2014;27:115-122.

Willems HME, Ahmed SS, Liu J, et al. Vulvovaginal candidiasis: a current understanding and burning questions. J Fungi (Basel). 2020 Feb 25;6(1):27. doi: 10.3390/jof6010027

Zwiers C, Scheffer-Rath M, Lopriore E, et al. Immunoglobulin for alloimmune hemolytic disease in neonates. Cochrane Database Syst Rev. 2018 Mar;3(3):CD003313. doi: 10.1002/14651858.CD003313.pub2.

ONLINE RESOURCES

Australian Government Department of Health and Aged Care: Clinical Practice Guide Pregnancy Care (2020 edn): https://www.health.gov.au/resources/pregnancy-care-guidelines

Australian Government Department of Health and Aged Care: Therapeutic Goods Administration – Vitamin B6 Pyridoxone: https://www.tga.gov.au/news/safety-alerts/vitamin-b6-pyridoxine

https://amhonline-amh-net-au.eu1.proxy.openathens.net/chapters/gastrointestinal-drugs/drugs-dyspepsia-reflux-peptic-ulcers/proton-pump-inhibitors

Australian Medicines Handbook 2024: https://shop.amh.net.au/products/books/2024

National Blood Authority: Guideline for the Prophylactic use of Rh D immunoglobulin in pregnancy care (2021). National Blood Authority, Canberra: https://www.blood.gov.au/sites/default/files/Guideline%20for%20the%20prophylactic%20use%20of%20Rh%20D%20immunoglobulin%20in%20pregnancy%20care.pdf

The New York Times. (2013, September 24). The shadow of the thalidomide tragedy. YouTube: https://www.youtube.com/watch?v=41n3mDoVbvk

SOMANZ: Guideline for the management of nausea and vomiting in pregnancy and hyperemesis gravidarum (2019): https://www.somanz.org/content/uploads/2020/07/NVP-GUIDELINE-1.2.20-1.pdf

Prophylactic use of Rh (D) immunoglobulin in pregnancy care (2021): https://www.blood.gov.au/sites/default/files/Guideline%20for%20the%20prophylactic%20use%20of%20Rh%20D%20immunoglobulin%20in%20pregnancy%20care.pdf

Hyperemesis gravidarum: https://www.hyperemesis.org/research/

Pregnancy sickness support: https://pregnancysicknesssupport.org.uk/

World Health Organization. Nutritional interventions update: vitamin D supplements during pregnancy (2020, July 29): https://www.who.int/publications/i/item/9789240008120

World Health Organization. WHO recommendations on antenatal care for a positive pregnancy experience (2016, November 28): https://www.who.int/publications/i/item/9789241549912

Young GL, Jewell D. Topical treatment for vaginal candidiasis (thrush) in pregnancy. Cochrane Database System Rev. 2001: (4): CD000225. doi.org/10.1002/14651858.CD000225 (accessed 27 August 2023).

CHAPTER 8

LABOUR AND BIRTH

Clare Davison, Roslyn Donnellan-Fernandez

Key Abbreviations

ARM	artificial rupture of membranes
CAM	complementary and alternative medicines
CNS	central nervous system
IOL	induction of labour
GA	general anaesthetic
5-HT	hydroxytryptamine (serotonin)
IUGR	intrauterine growth restriction
LA	local anaesthetic
N_2O	nitrous oxide
OR	opiod receptor
OTC	over the counter
PCA	patient controlled analgesia
PCEA	patient controlled epidural analgesia
PCIA	patient controlled intravenous analgesia
PG	prostaglandin
PPH	postpartum haemorrhage
TXA	tranexamic acid
VE	vaginal examination

Key Terms

agonist 131
amides 153
amines 147
analgesics 128
anaphylaxis 153
anaesthetics 128
antiemetics 128
augmentation 128
benzodiazepines 144
caudal 152
cervix 127
contractions 127
dermatome 151
epidural 149
ergot alkaloids 128

ergot alkaloid hypersensitivity 131
esters 147
fundus 127
involution 131
oxytocics 128
paraesthesia 153
prostaglandins 128
sedatives 156
spinal 135
tocolytics 128
tranexamic acid 132
uterotonics 128

Chapter Focus

This chapter focuses on the use of pharmacology during labour and birth and the immediate post-birth period. Topics covered include the use of uterotonics and tocolytics, drugs used in induction and augmentation of labour, and pharmacological pain management during labour and birth. The chapter will also discuss the use of complementary and alternative medicines during labour and birth.

Key Drug Groups

Uterotonics:

- oxytocin, carbetocin, ergometrine, prostaglandins E2 and E1, F2α, carboprost, dinoprost, mifepristone

Inhalation anaesthetic:

- nitrous oxide
- methoxyflurane

Analgesics:

- NSAIDs, paracetamol, diclofenac

Opioids:

- morphine, fentanyl, pethidine

Local/regional anaesthetics:

- lignocaine, bupivacaine, ropivacaine

General anaesthetics:

- inhalational – desflurane, isoflurane, evoflurane
- IV – thiopental, propofol

Learning Outcomes

- Outline the indications and contraindications of pharmacological pain relief during labour and birth.
- Discuss the history of pharmacological use during labour and birth.
- Outline the different drugs commonly used during an induction and augmentation of labour.
- Describe the different uses of uterotonics.
- Describe the drugs used to actively manage the birth of the placenta, and treatment of a postpartum haemorrhage.
- Describe the different types of analgesia used during childbirth.
- Discuss the side effects and contraindications of drugs used during labour and birth.
- Demonstrate an understanding of CAM use during labour and birth and the immediate postnatal period.

CRITICAL THINKING SCENARIO

Olive is 32 years old and is 41 weeks pregnant with her first child. She is having an induction of labour (IOL) for intrauterine growth restriction (IUGR), and you have recommended active management of the birth of the placenta. As Olive's IOL progresses she requests analgesia, stating that she would prefer to have an injection rather than an epidural as she wants to move around. She has heard that moving and remaining upright can progress labour and is worried that an epidural will lead to a caesarean. Olive also wishes to establish early breastfeeding.

1 What information would you provide to Olive so she could make an informed decision in regard to her induction of labour options and the recommended active management of the birth of the placenta?

2 What information will you provide so she can make an informed decision regarding pain management during labour and birth?

3 When Olive questions you about the impact of any pharmacologic analgesia on her baby in the immediate period after birth, what would you advise?

Introduction

Over the last century birth has moved from the community to the hospital, and this move has resulted in increasing numbers of women experiencing induction of labour and medically managed birth. In Australia and New Zealand this translates into most women experiencing labour and birth in a hospital setting. In most developed countries, including Australia and New Zealand, intrapartum care is dominated by a medicalised and technocratic model. In both countries the number of women having their labour induced has continued an upward trend over the last 10 years including discussion of outcomes for women and newborns where IOL is made available as a 'choice' (Ananthram et al 2022). Recent statistics show that nearly half of Australian first-time mothers have their labour induced compared with about a quarter of women in 2010 (Australian Institute of Health and Welfare [AIHW] 2021). Many women who commence labour spontaneously will have medical intervention to speed their labour up (augmentation). Within this medicalised model, if birth is not completed within the expected time frame, the process is often deemed pathological, and intervention is recommended to meet the perceived appropriate timelines allowed for labour and birth.

While the use of herbal medicines for induction of labour is common globally, and is suggested to be effective, the effects are not well understood and there is inconclusive evidence of safety due to the absence of good quality data (Zamawe et al 2018). Another upward trend is that of women using pharmacological pain relief, including epidurals, to cope with the sensations experienced during childbirth. Increased use of pharmacological pain relief is associated with medical induction, where cervical ripening and uterine **contractions** are initiated pharmacologically and often in combination with mechanical stimuli, for example cervical balloon catheter dilation (Gill et al 2023).

8.1 Physiology of labour and birth

During pregnancy the uterus increases in weight by about 20-fold (50 g to 1000 g), and by 10-fold in length. Control of uterine activity is via sympathetic fibres: noradrenaline (acting at α2-adrenoceptors) causes excitation and muscle contraction; adrenaline causes inhibition (relaxation of uterine muscle).

During the last few weeks of a full-term pregnancy, painless uterine contractions become increasingly frequent, and the lower uterine segment and **cervix** become softer and thinner, preparing the uterus for labour. Basal levels of oxytocin increase 3–4-fold during pregnancy. The key event stimulating labour is still not determined. It involves complex interactions of several placental, fetal, and maternal hormones, including a rise in the estrogen:progesterone ratio (which increases the number of oxytocin receptors), increased sensitivity of the uterus to oxytocin released from the posterior pituitary gland, and prostaglandins (PGs) produced from amnion and chorion (Hundley et al 2020).

Oxytocin is commonly referred to as the hormone of love and has an essential function during labour and birth. In normal physiology, blood oxytocin levels gradually rise in pregnancy. During labour oxytocin continues to rise with pulses of oxytocin becoming progressively bigger and more frequent. After labour has been initiated, regular uterine contractions moving downwards from the **fundus** help expel the fetus. The process of birth usually takes several hours. The cervix must fully dilate to allow the fetus to move into the birth canal. Once the cervix is fully dilated the baby descends, and expulsive contractions and maternal effort lead to the birth of the baby. Following birth of the baby, the placenta must also be expelled to complete the birth process. In many textbooks, labour and birth has been divided into three stages, first stage (dilation of the cervix), second stage (expulsion of the baby), and third stage (birth of the placenta). However, contrary to popular belief, the birth process is a continuum and progress is often not linear (Dixon et al 2013).

Oxytocin is one of two hormones secreted by the posterior pituitary; the other is vasopressin. The effect of oxytocin causes the uterus to contract, promoting the progress of labour. Oxytocin also influences the brain and induces beneficial adaptive effects during labour and birth and postpartum. During labour, oxytocin is released into both the blood and brain, with high oxytocin levels in the cerebrospinal fluid (CSF). Oxytocin has many positive effects; it reduces anxiety, stress and pain in labour and switches on brain pleasure and reward centres. A large oxytocin pulse occurs with the birth, and pulses continue afterwards, which help the new mother to birth the placenta, prevent bleeding, and warm her chest for skin-to-skin contact with her baby (Buckley 2015; Uvnas-Moberg et al 2019).

Within a physiological birth, mother and baby work together. The fetal adrenal medulla responds by secreting high amounts of catecholamines, and the adrenal cortex secretes corticosteroids, which clear the infant's lungs, provide surfactant for breathing, mobilise nutrients and promote increased blood flow to brain and heart, all preparing the infant for independent existence. However, as discussed, most births are medicalised in Australia and New Zealand. A medicalised birth can be more stressful for both mother and baby and it is essential that midwives are aware of the common drugs used and their effects on both the mother and baby, during labour and birth and postnatally. This includes the impact on provision of evidence-based midwifery care during 'the golden hour' immediately following birth encompassing optimisation of human bonding and initiation of breastfeeding (Brimdyr et al 2015; Neczypor et al 2017).

8.2 Overview of drugs used during labour

The pharmacokinetics of drugs may be altered during labour and birth. During labour, gastric emptying is delayed and vomiting may result, which can alter drug absorption; therefore, parenteral routes are often recommended. Drug metabolism and excretion may be prolonged. Drugs commonly used during childbirth include those listed below.

1 For increasing or reducing uterine contractility (**uterotonics**):
   ○ **prostaglandins** – to induce labour
   ○ **oxytocics** – to increase uterine contractility and assist in induction of labour and reduction of postpartum haemorrhage (PPH)
   ○ **ergot alkaloids** – to manage the birth of the placenta, reduce and treat postpartum haemorrhage
   ○ **tocolytics** – to decrease uterine contractility (from the Greek stem 'tokos', meaning 'birth').
2 For pain relief:
   ○ **analgesics** – opioids (e.g. morphine, pethidine, and fentanyl) and over-the-counter medications (e.g. paracetamol)
   ○ *non-steroidal anti-inflammatories (NSAIDs)* – for post-perineal suturing/repair (e.g. slow-release diclofenac) are discussed in Chapter 9
   ○ **anaesthetics –** the most common is nitrous oxide ('gas'). Also epidural with local anaesthetics (e.g. lignocaine and bupivacaine) which are often administered via epidural injection or patient controlled epidural analgesia (PCEA). An opioid and local anaesthetic can be co-administered for effective obstetric analgesia, for caesarean section or vaginal birth. General anaesthetic may be used for caesarean section birth in an emergency or if unable to use spinal or epidural.
3 Other:
   ○ **antiemetics** – may be used during labour if women feel nauseous, particularly if using opioid analgesia or post caesarean section. These are discussed in Chapter 7.

8.3 Uterotonics

Oxytocics

As discussed, increased medicalisation of birth means that a large majority of women will have their labours induced or augmented by pharmacological means. Induction and **augmentation** may be medically indicated for mothers and babies experiencing complexity and co-morbidity during pregnancy, for example, preeclampsia, pre-gestational diabetes, preterm prelabour rupture of membranes, chorioamnionitis (woman) or fetal intrauterine growth restriction or intrauterine fetal death (baby) (Gill et al 2023). Agents that stimulate contraction of the smooth muscle of the uterus, resulting in contractions and labour, are called **oxytocics**. Synthetic oxytocin, alkaloids of the plant fungus ergot, and prostaglandins (PGs) of the E and F series cause uterine contractility and will now be discussed.

Synthetic oxytocin

In 1906, Sir Henry Dale found that a pituitary extract stimulated uterine contractility in cats, leading him to identify the hormone oxytocin. Nearly 50 years later, in 1954, the chemical structure of oxytocin was described by American biochemist Vincent du Vigneaud and was synthesised the following year.

Synthetic oxytocin is indicated to induce, augment, and manage labour, and to treat postpartum haemorrhage (PPH); it is administered IM or by IV infusion (Table 8.1).

TABLE 8.1 Uterotonics/medicines used to control bleeding and manage the birth of the placenta

MEDICINE	DOSE AND ROUTE	ADMINISTRATION ADVICE	SIDE EFFECTS	COMMENTS
Oxytocin (syntocinon)	IV infusion, 2 milliunits/minute, increased by 2 milliunits/minute at intervals of > 30 minutes to a maximum of 32 milliunits/minute. (1000 milliunits = 1 unit.) Monitor fetal heart rate and uterine activity so that dose can be adjusted according to response. Active management of the birth of the placenta: IM or slow IV injection, 10 units given with or after birth of the shoulder. After caesarean section. Slow IV injection, 5 units immediately after birth. Treatment of postpartum haemorrhage. IM, 10 units or slow IV injection 5–10 units. In severe cases may be followed by an IV infusion.	Induction after rupture of membranes and augmentation of labour. Give IV bolus injection slowly (avoid rapid injection due to risk of cardiovascular effects). Induction and augmentation of labour, a suggested dilution for IV infusion is 10 units oxytocin in 1 L Hartmann's solution or sodium chloride 0.9% to give a strength of 10 milliunits/mL. An infusion rate of 12 mL/hour is equivalent to 2 milliunits/minute of oxytocin. Post birth of the placenta for increased risk of bleeding: 40 iu in 1 L Hartmann's solution or sodium chloride 0.9% at rate of 250 mL/hour. Practice points when using an infusion, monitor fluid balance to prevent water intoxication. It is unclear whether induction or augmentation of labour using uterine stimulants increases the risk of amniotic fluid embolism.	Infrequent (0.1–1%) nausea, vomiting. Rare (< 0.1%) water intoxication, arrhythmias, anaphylactic/anaphylactoid reactions, severe (tetanic) uterine contraction leading to uterine rupture or fetal hypoxia and death; flushing, ECG changes (including prolonged QT interval), transient hypotension, reflex tachycardia (common with rapid IV injection). Water intoxication. Oxytocin has weak antidiuretic properties and may contribute to maternal and neonatal hyponatraemia if used in high doses.	
Carbetocin	After caesarean section: IV injection slowly over 1 minute. 100 micrograms as a single dose following birth. Active management of the birth of the placenta: IV/IM, 100 micrograms as a single dose following birth.	Oxytocin receptor agonist. Used for uterine atony and postpartum haemorrhage after caesarean section. Used as an alternative oxytocic if a single dose is ineffective. Has a longer duration of action than oxytocin although carbetocin has been available for many years, data regarding its efficacy and safety are limited compared to oxytocin, carbetocin may reduce the use of additional oxytocics after caesarean section (evidence is unclear for vaginal birth) but the risk of postpartum haemorrhage is similar; there are limited data for use under general anaesthesia.	Common (> 1%) nausea, vomiting, abdominal pain, itch, flushing, feeling of warmth, sweating, dizziness, hypotension.	
Ergometrine	Prevention of postpartum haemorrhage: IM, 200 micrograms following birth of the placenta. Treatment of postpartum haemorrhage: IV, 25–50 micrograms; repeat every 2–3 minutes, if needed, up to a usual total of 250 micrograms. IM, 250 micrograms.	If giving IV, consider diluting 250 micrograms (0.5 mL) to 5 mL (to give 50 micrograms/mL) with sodium chloride 0.9%.	Common (> 1%) nausea and vomiting. Infrequent (0.1–1%) hypertension, abdominal pain, headache. Rare (< 0.1%) MI, cerebral infarction, gangrene, pulmonary oedema. Contraindications: Hypertension Preeclampsia Fibroids Multiple pregnancy	
Syntometrine	Combined oxytocin and ergometrine: oxytocin 5 IU/mL, ergometrine 500 mcg/mL, in 1 mL.	1 mL IM repeat if necessary to a maximum of 3 mL total.	As above for oxytocin and ergometrine. Nausea, vomiting and hypertension.	As above for oxytocin and ergometrine. Alternative first-line management for the active management of the birth of the placenta and treatment of PPH.

Continued

TABLE 8.1 Uterotonics/medicines used to control bleeding and manage the birth of the placenta—cont'd

MEDICINE	DOSE AND ROUTE	ADMINISTRATION ADVICE	SIDE EFFECTS	COMMENTS
Carboprost (15-methyl prostaglandin F2α)	0.25 mg in 1 mL ampoule via IM injection. Total dose should not exceed 2 mg (8 doses).	Used for intractable PPH when other management is not successful.	Common (> 1%) nausea, vomiting, diarrhoea, pyrexia and bronchospasm.	Carboprost should only be used by medically trained personnel in a hospital with 24-hour medical cover. Carboprost is available via the Special Access Scheme (SAS). An SAS Category A form must be completed.
Dinoprost (prostaglandin F2α)	5 mg in 1 mL ampoule Intamyometrial injection.	Used for intractable PPH when other management is not successful. Intramyometrial injection. Maximum dose of 3 mg. Preparation Dilute (5 mg) 1 mL to 10 mL with sodium chloride 0.9% to give 0.5 mg Dinoprost per ml. Discard 4 mL from 10 mL to leave the maximum dose of 3 mg (6 mL).	Common (> 1%) bronchospasm, acute hypertension – usually transient, abdominal cramps, diarrhoea and vomiting. Rare (< 0.1%) convulsions, flushing, shivering, uterine rupture. Hypotension secondary to myocardial failure, cardiac arrhythmia including ventricular tachycardia, pulmonary oedema due to raised pulmonary artery pressures, hypoxia due to pulmonary shunting.	
Misoprostol	400 or 600 micrograms.	Oral/sublingual/buccal/rectal Oral 400–600 mcg (2 to 3 tablets) Rectal 600 mcg (3 tablets)	Incidence and severity of adverse effects depend on the dose and route of administration. Common (> 1%) nausea, vomiting, diarrhoea, back pain, transient hypertension or hypotension, bronchoconstriction, headache, epigastric pain, vasovagal symptoms (e.g. flushing, shivering), blurred vision, fever, altered fetal heart rate, uterine hypercontractility and hypertonus. Rare (< 0.1%) uterine hyperstimulation leading to uterine rupture or fetal hypoxia and death, serious cardiovascular events (e.g. coronary vasospasm, MI, stroke).	May be an alternative for prevention of postpartum haemorrhage when other agents are unavailable but should not be used routinely. Oral has a quicker administration and quicker onset with peak plasma concentration around 15–30 minutes after administration. Rectal administration has slower onset (45–120 minutes).
Tranexamic acid	1 g in 10 ml ampoule of tranexamic acid	IV controlled delivery via pump at rate of 1 mL per minute over 10 minutes. Or 1 g in 10 mL given over 10 minutes by slow IV push. A second dose can be given within 30 minutes if bleeding continues.	Common (> 1%) nausea, vomiting. Rare (< 0.1%) thrombosis, visual disturbances including transient disturbance of colour vision, hypotension and dizziness (particularly after rapid administration), nausea, vomiting, diarrhoea.	Second-line management of PPH when unresponsive to oxytocin and ergometrine. When bleeding is caused by trauma. If there is a likely delay for theatre or transfer to hospital as administration may reduce the overall blood loss.

Source: Australian Medicines Handbook 2024.

Carbetocin, an analogue, has longer duration of action and is administered as a single slow IV injection, 100 microgram dose. A recent advance in heat-stable carbetocin makes this a useful drug in low resource settings as it does not require cold chain transport and storage (see Online resources: FIGO/ICM 2023).

Ergot alkaloids

Ergot alkaloids are naturally occurring fungal compounds with varied actions on several types of receptors. Ergometrine produces prolonged, strong contractions of the uterus, especially postpartum, and has vasoconstrictor actions, so is useful in the treatment of PPH. However, in

> ## DRUG MONOGRAPH 8.1
> ## Ergometrine
>
> ### Actions and mechanism
>
> Ergometrine increases the force and frequency of uterine contractions by direct stimulation of the smooth muscle of the uterine wall. Increased contractions and muscle tone, and vasoconstriction of bleeding vessels at the placental site, arrest postpartum haemorrhage.
>
> ### Indications and contraindications
>
> Ergometrine is administered after the birth of the placenta to contract the uterus and uterine blood vessels, and promote **involution** of the uterus, to prevent PPH. Ergometrine is contraindicated to induce labour or during the labour and birth because contraction of the cervix would cause fetal distress and compression, and delay birth.
>
> ### Pharmacokinetics
>
> Ergometrine has unpredictable bioavailability, so is given parenterally. It is formulated for IM administration (or, in emergency, IV) and has rapid onset of action within 1–3 minutes. The duration of uterine contractions after IM injection is about 3 hours. The drug is metabolised in the liver and excreted mainly in faeces.
>
> ### Drug interactions
>
> Ergometrine has significant interactions with many drugs that also affect receptors for noradrenaline or 5-HT. Effects of other vasoconstrictors are enhanced, whereas those of antianginal vasodilators are antagonised. Drugs that reduce metabolism of ergometrine (e.g. erythromycin, clarithromycin, and some antivirals) may cause ergotism and ischaemia if given concurrently.
>
> ### Adverse reactions
>
> These include nausea, vomiting, hypertension, headache, allergic reactions and, rarely, infarction, pulmonary oedema and gangrene. A dose-related effect is abdominal cramping.
>
> ### Warnings and contraindications
>
> Use with caution in people with hypocalcaemia. Avoid use in women with **ergot alkaloid hypersensitivity**, cardiac or vascular disease, eclampsia or preeclampsia, sepsis, or liver or kidney impairment. It is contraindicated in pregnancy (Category C), during labour and birth of the fetus or to induce labour, or in multiple pregnancies.
>
> ### Dosage and administration
>
> To prevent PPH, a dose of 200 micrograms is administered IM; in emergencies or in those with excessive uterine bleeding 25–50 micrograms repeated up to total 250 micrograms by slow IV route is recommended. Ergometrine 0.5 mg/mL is also formulated in combination with oxytocin 5 IU/mL (Syntometrine) for active management of the birth of the placenta and prevention of PPH.

the active management of the birth of the placenta, oxytocin is generally preferred to the combination of ergometrine with oxytocin (Syntometrine) which is associated with a higher incidence of nausea, vomiting and hypertension with little advantage over oxytocin alone in terms of blood loss (small reduction in risk of blood loss > 500 mL; no difference in risk of blood loss > 1000 mL) (Drug Monograph 8.1).

Prostaglandins

Prostaglandins were discovered in the 1930s and named after the prostate as they were first isolated in semen and thought to be made by the prostate gland. It is now known that many tissues in the body make prostaglandins. Prostaglandin function depends on where it is found. Endogenous prostaglandins have a very short half-life and their action is usually confined to the tissues where they are made. Derived from the fatty acid arachidonic acid, prostaglandins are produced in the endometrium and myometrium with production increased towards the end of pregnancy, following induction of cyclooxygenase 2 by inflammatory cytokines at term. Prostaglandin Es and prostaglandin Fs contract uterine smooth muscle and are implicated in disorders of menstruation. Prostaglandin F_{2a} is a vasoconstrictor, while prostaglandin E_2 and prostacyclin are vasodilators. The uterus becomes increasingly sensitive to PGs during pregnancy, increasing 10-fold at term compared to earlier in pregnancy. Prostaglandins also upregulate oxytocin receptors.

Several synthetic prostaglandin **agonists** and analogue preparations can be used clinically.

Prostaglandins have been used to induce labour since the 1960s. The aim of their use is to soften, efface (often referred to as cervical ripening or cervical priming), and dilate the cervix and stimulate contractions (Pierce et al 2018). Prostaglandins can be given orally, intra-cervically, intravenously, or in the extra-amniotic space. The intra-cervical route is more invasive and has been shown to be less effective than vaginal administration (Boulvain 2008).

Effect of prostaglandins on smooth muscle cells according to receptor subtypes

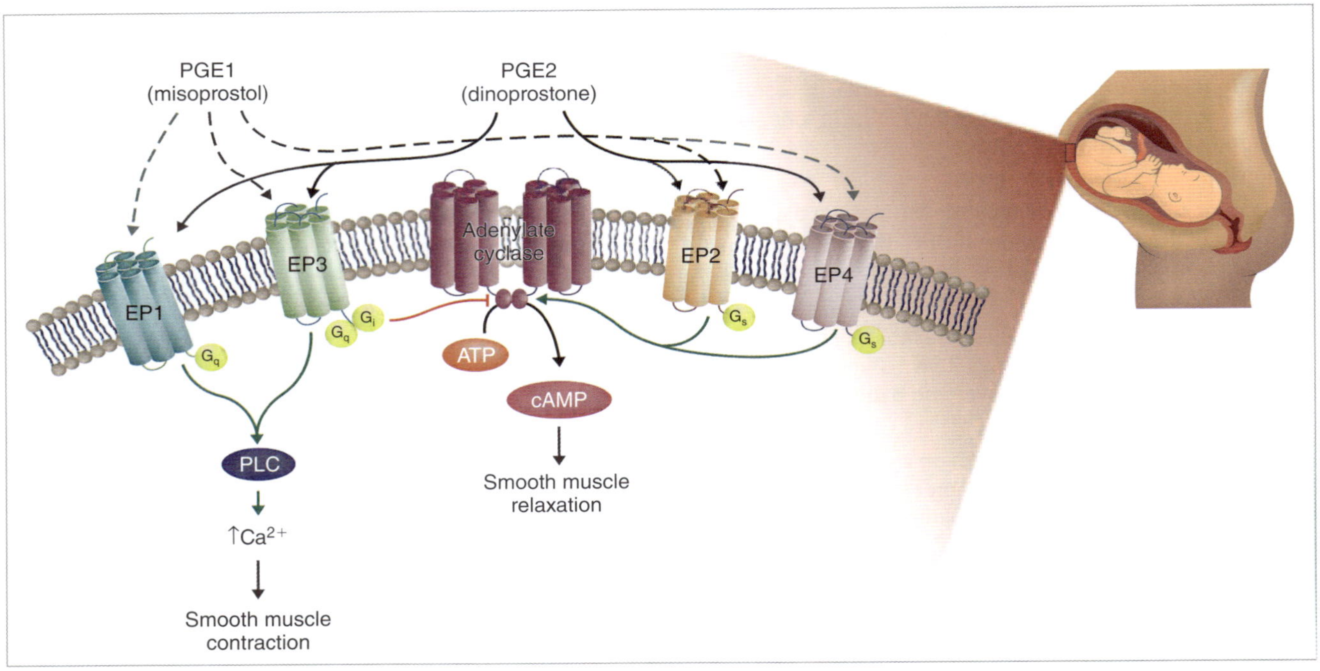

FIGURE 8.1 Abbreviations: ATP = adenosine triphosphate; cAMP = cyclic adenosine monophosphate; EP = E prostanoid; PGE = prostaglandin E; PLC = phospholipase C

Source: Pierce S, Bakker R, Myers DA, Edwards RK. Clinical insights for cervical ripening and labor induction using prostaglandins. AJP Rep. 2018 Oct;8(4):e307-e314. doi: 10.1055/s-0038-1675351. Epub 2018 Oct 29. PMID: 30377555; PMCID: PMC6205862.

Common prostaglandins

Prostaglandin E_2 – an analogue, dinoprostone, is usually the prostaglandin of choice for induction of labour at term. It is usually given vaginally as a gel, tablet, or pessary.

Prostaglandin $F_2\alpha$ – an analogue, dinoprost and carboprost, are used for intractable PPH when other management is not successful. They can also be used in termination of first- or second-trimester pregnancy, by intravaginal or intrauterine administration. Dinoprost is administered via intramyometrial injection. Carboprost is administered via intramuscular injection.

Prostaglandin E_1, misoprostol and gemeprost – misoprostol was discovered in 1973 and was initially licensed for the prevention and treatment of gastrointestinal ulcers. For this indication, the dose starts from 200 micrograms twice daily; therefore, it was manufactured in 200 microgram tablets. It can be taken orally with few side effects and remains stable at room temperature. Misoprostol is usually given orally, sublingual or buccally, or per rectum (PR) for prevention and treatment of PPH, and for management of miscarriage or termination of pregnancy. Gemeprost can also be used in medical termination during the first or second trimester of pregnancy or to ripen the cervix prior to a surgical termination and is administered via vaginal pessary. (See Table 8.2.)

Antifibrinolytic and haemostatic agents

Tranexamic acid

Tranexamic acid is a synthetic analogue of the amino acid lysine that binds to the lysine building site on plasminogen and inhibits breakdown of clots by blocking binding of plasminogen and plasmin to fibrin, which inhibits fibrinolysis. Fibrin breakdown starts when the glycoprotein pro-enzyme plasminogen, which is produced by the liver, is converted into the fibrinolytic enzyme plasmin by tissue plasminogen activator. A recent randomised controlled trial, the WOMAN trial, clearly demonstrated that tranexamic acid is a safe and effective treatment for PPH. The WHO recommends that women with PPH receive 1 g of tranexamic acid intravenously as soon as possible after giving birth, followed by a second dose if bleeding continues after 30 minutes or restarts within 24 hours since the first dose. Research shows that if given early, tranexamic acid reduces deaths due to bleeding by one-third (Brenner et al 2019; Mielke et al 2020).

TABLE 8.2 Dose, pharmacological effects, pharmacokinetics, adverse events re comparison of dinoprostone and misoprostol

CHARACTERISTIC	DINOPROSTONE	MISOPROSTOL
Description	PGE2	Synthetic PGE1 analogue
Formulation	• 10 mg vaginal insert placed in the posterior fornix	• Tablet, 100 or 200 mcg; administered vaginally or orally
Dose	• 0.3 mg/h released over 12 h	• 25–50 mcg vaginally, every 4–6 h • 25–100 mcg orally, every 2–4 h
Receptor binding	EP1, EP2, EP3, EP4	EP3 (potent); possibly EP2
Pharmacologic effects	• Induces cervical remodelling • Inconsistent effects on uterine contractions; may be related to cervical ripening vs direct myometrial effect • Mild stimulation of the GI tract	• Induces cervical remodelling • Generation of uterine contractions • Increased contractility vs PGE2 • Decreases total myometrial collagen and connective tissue vs PGE2 • Stimulates the GI tract and may stimulate the fetal gut, resulting in meconium-stained amniotic fluid
Pharmacokinetics	• Half-life: 2.5–5 min	• Half-life (oral): 20–40 min • Half-life (vaginal): 60 min
Adverse effects	• Tachysystole (vaginal insert: 2.0%; cervical gel: 6.6%) • Chills/fever (vaginal insert: <1%; cervical gel: 1.4%) • Diarrhoea/vomiting/nausea (vaginal insert: <1%; cervical gel: 5.7%)	• Tachysystole (vaginal: 16.6%; oral: 7.0%) • Chills/fever (≤5%) • Diarrhoea/abdominal pain/nausea (≤5%; increased with oral administration)
Cost	• Vaginal insert: approximately $215.00–250.00; cervical gel: approximately $315.00	• Approximately $2.00

Source: Pierce S, Bakker R, Myers DA, Edwards RK. Clinical insights for cervical ripening and labor induction using prostaglandins. AJP Rep. 2018 Oct;8(4):e307-e314. doi: 10.1055/s-0038-1675351. Epub 2018 Oct 29. PMID: 30377555; PMCID: PMC6205862.

Tocolytics

Drugs that relax the uterus are described as **tocolytics** and are discussed in more detail in Chapter 17. Tocolytics may be used to delay labour or inhibit threatened miscarriage, or during a complex labour to relax the uterus and stall contractions and allow for a management plan to be made for a compromised fetus. Preterm labour, occurring before the 37th week of pregnancy, is a complication in 10–15% of all pregnancies and preterm birth increases the possibility of neonatal morbidity and mortality. Delaying labour, if appropriate, may allow time for transport of the woman to a specialist centre for the birth of a significantly preterm infant or for administration of corticosteroids to the mother to facilitate fetal production of lung surfactant.

Tocolytics are not used when prolongation of pregnancy is hazardous for the fetus or mother. Most tocolytics effectively delay labour for 2–3 days, but they do not improve perinatal outcomes (mortality, respiratory distress syndrome) or decrease the rate of preterm birth. Responses of both fetus and mother (heart rate, glycaemia) must be carefully monitored (WHO 2022). Rarely, drugs such as terbutaline may be administered as acute tocolysis for management of hypertonus occurring during induction of labour or spontaneous labour.

KEY POINTS

Uterotonics

■ Synthetic oxytocin, alkaloids of the plant fungus ergot, and prostaglandins of the E and F series cause uterine contractility.

■ Synthetic oxytocin (syntocinon) can be used to induce, augment, and manage labour, and to treat postpartum haemorrhage.

■ In the active management of the birth of the placenta, oxytocin is preferred to the combination of ergometrine with oxytocin (syntometrine).

8.4 The pathophysiology of pain

There are many options for pain management during labour and birth. These include:

• non-pharmacological – such as breathing exercises, massage, acupuncture, and sterile water injections (Box 8.1 CAM considerations)

BOX 8.1   CAM considerations

Complementary and alternative medicines (CAMs) are becoming more widely used during labour and birth. There is a common misconception that natural therapies are always safe, so it is essential that midwives have a basic understanding of the CAM therapies a woman may use during her labour and birth to allow for an open and honest discussion about the risks and benefits of their use. Common CAMs used during labour and birth are aromatherapy, herbal medicines, and homeopathy (Tiran 2000; Turpin 2022).

Aromatherapy

Concentrated essential oils that are extracted from plants contain chemical components which can cause physiological and psychological effects. Aromatherapy can be administered by inhaling the scent of the oil; applying the essential oil to the skin during massage; or adding it to water in a bath. *Note: essential oils should not be added to a birth pool.*

Common essential oils used in labour and birth

Chamomile: calming, reduces tension

Clary sage: used as a uterotonic to increase contractions and induce labour, reduce pain perception and shorten labour. *Note: Clary sage should not be used before 37 weeks gestation. Midwives caring for pregnant women should be cautious in exposure to clary sage oil. It should not be used in a diffuser in hospital settings to limit exposure to pregnant women.*

Frankincense: calming, mood stabilising

Jasmine: evokes feeling of joy, happiness, peace and self-confidence

Lavender: to relax and calm. Can reduce blood pressure and ease muscular tension

Neroli: to reduce anxiety and nervous tension, decrease anxious nerves

Mandarin: to decrease fatigue and fluid retention

Peppermint: to ease nausea

Rose oil: for relaxation

Sweet orange: to lift mood and boost energy. Has a refreshing scent

Teatree: an antiseptic and antiviral

Ylang ylang: contains a component called linalool, which helps with anxiety. Reduces pain, stress, blood pressure, and muscle tension

Herbal medicines

Herbal medicine is the therapeutic use of plants, including essential oils and herbal teas. Note: Herbal medicines are absorbed into the body, and should therefore be treated as a drug.

Some common herbal treatments are:

Adhatoda (Adhatoda vasica): oxytocic action, has been used to treat PPH

Angelica archangelica: a uterine stimulant. Traditionally used to release the placenta. Believed to tone the uterus while relaxing the cervix

Black cohosh: a uterine tonic and spasmolytic herb, indicated to 'prepare for labour'. Traditionally used with blue cohosh to strengthen labour contractions and support labour progress

Blue cohosh: tones the uterus, with oxytocic actions, indicated to 'assist with labour'

Raspberry leaf: nourishes the uterus and increases uterine tone, indicated to prevent and treat PPH

Ginger root: for exhaustion and nausea. Ginger increases circulation so may increase risk of bleeding post birth

Lady's mantle (Alchemilla vulgaris): a blood coagulant, used to reduce bleeding post birth

Motherwort (Leonurus cardiac): promotes uterine tone and effective contractions. Also used to relieve anxiety

Mugwort (moxa): used to decrease postpartum bleeding and increase blood circulation to the pelvic area to treat pain. Moxibustion (moxa therapy on the acupuncture point Bladder 67) has been used successfully to turn breech presentation

Shepherd's purse (Capsella bursa-pastoris): a blood coagulant and vasoconstrictor. Used to reduce bleeding post birth. Traditionally used to treat PPH before synthetic oxytocins were available

Schisandra chinensis: used to enhance labour contractions during birth, particularly during a long, tiring or protracted labour.

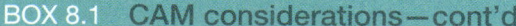

BOX 8.1   CAM considerations—cont'd

Homeopathy

Homeopathy is based on the theory of treating 'like with like'. Homeopathy claims to stimulate healing responses to diseases by administering minute doses of substances that mimic the symptoms of those diseases in healthy people. The most common homeopathics used during labour and birth are:

Arnica: for relief of soreness that comes from physical exertion and muscle strain. Relieves soft tissue damage (perineum or abdomen) following birth – reduces swelling, bruising, and risk of infection, and promotes healing

Caulophyllum: used either to induce labour or augment labour if contractions are short and irregular or stop

Cimicifuga: used to ease the fear of labour and birth in women who have a history of traumatic childbirth and/or miscarriage

Gelsemium: used to ease fear during labour and birth 'stage fright'

Pulsatilla: helpful at times of strong hormonal changes.

Bach Flower Remedies

Bach Flower Remedies are used to treat emotional symptoms associated with a disease or disorder. There are 38 Bach remedies but the most used Bach Flower Remedy during labour and birth is Rescue Remedy, a combination of five remedies, that is said to reduce stress, fear and nervous tension. The remedies are preserved in alcohol, although the amount is very small so is considered safe unless there is a known intolerance to alcohol.

- pharmacological – over-the-counter medicines (e.g. paracetamol), anaesthetic agents, and opioids.

Note that NSAIDs should be avoided because of increased risk of bleeding (especially after aspirin) and adverse effects on the fetal cardiovascular, respiratory, and renal systems.

Many women request the use of pharmaceutical pain relief options during labour and birth and many report mixed experiences of different pain relief methods (Thomson et al 2019) Currently, around four in five women who labour in Australia receive pain relief. In 2021 the most common types were nitrous oxide (inhaled) (52%), followed by epidural or caudal analgesic (42%) and systemic opioids (11%) (AIHW 2023; see Online resources). Midwives must be able to provide evidence-based information to enable women to make informed decisions in relation to the effects and side effects, on themselves and on their baby, of drugs taken at this time. Ideally this information should be provided to women during pregnancy.

The experience of pain

Pain is a subjective experience that involves both physiological and emotional responses. Nociception, or the perception of noxious stimuli, is only one component of pain. There is much ongoing research into the physiological mechanisms of pain. Pain is detected by nociceptors (pain receptors). Tissue injury in the periphery releases many mediators, such as bradykinin, PGs, adenosine triphosphate and histamine, which can enhance or initiate firing of the nociceptive fibres (Fig 8.2). These nociceptive fibres are A-delta fibres (mediating sharp, transient, fast pain) or C-fibres (mediating burning, aching, slow, visceral pain). Signals are transmitted to the **spinal** cord via these primary (first-order) afferent fibres terminating in the dorsal horn of the spinal cord (substantia gelatinosa). Several neuropeptides are released from neurons; substance P (a neurokinin) and calcitonin gene-related peptide are present, especially in nociceptive primary afferent neurons (Fig 8.2). Voltage-gated calcium channels are opened, and the transmitter glutamate is released and crosses the synaptic gap, activating AMPA (at the first synapse). Activation of NMDA receptors is a slower response and associated with activity-dependent plasticity, a progressive increase in the response of dorsal horn nociceptive neurons to repeated stimuli. (Known as 'windup', this greatly increased sensitivity is associated with hyperalgesia.) The ascending nerve axons (second-order neurons) continue upwards in the anterolateral spinothalamic tracts (left-hand side of Fig 8.2) to the ventral and medial parts of the thalamus where they synapse with third-order neurons connecting to specific areas of the limbic system and somatosensory cortex, where the messages are perceived as pain.

The gate control theory

Although there are further developments in the understanding of pain, the gate control theory of pain transmission put forward by Melzack and Wall in 1965 greatly enhanced the understanding of pain. It proposes that a physiologically analgesic spinal 'gate' mechanism in the dorsal horn of the spinal cord can modify the transmission of painful sensations from peripheral nerve

Physiology of pain

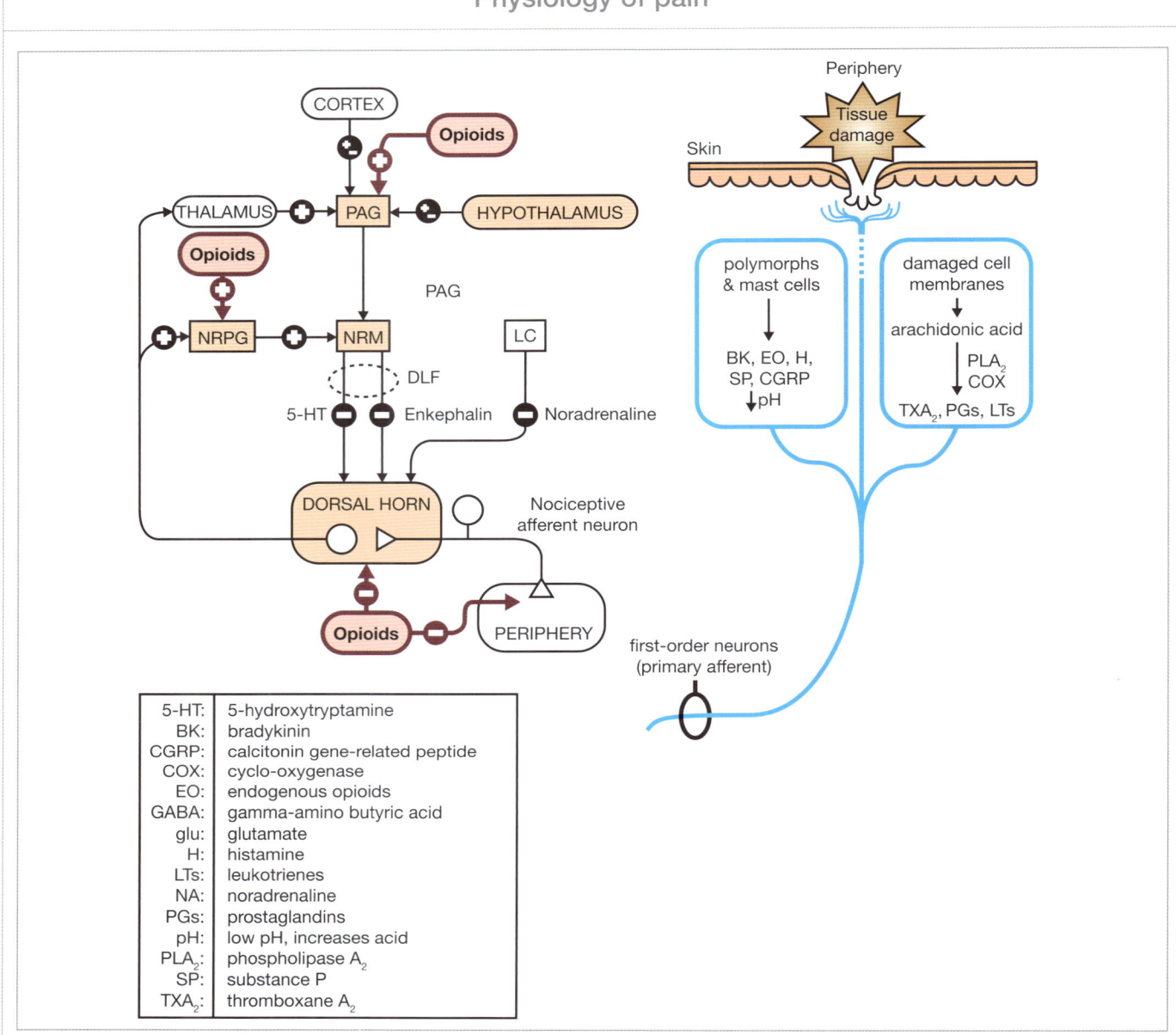

FIGURE 8.2 Right-hand side: periphery – some mediators, neurotransmitters and nerve pathways involved in pain sensation. Left-hand side: the descending control system, showing the main sites of action of opioids. 5-HT = 5-hydroxytryptamine; BK = bradykinin; COX = cyclooxygenase; DLF = dorsolateral funiculus of spinal cord; EO = endogenous opioids; H = histamine; LC = locus coeruleus; LTs = leukotrienes; NRM = nucleus raphe magnus; NRPG = nucleus reticularis paragigantocellularis; PAG = periaqueductal grey matter; PGs = prostaglandins; low pH = increasing acidity; PLA 2 = phospholipase A 2; SP = substance P; TXA 2 = thromboxane A 2

Sources: Adapted from Argoff 2011; Rang et al 2007; used with permission.

fibres to the thalamus and cortex of the brain. The gate is influenced by descending inhibition from the higher centres of the brain: efferent anti-nociceptive (analgesic) pathways from the cortex descend via the periaqueductal grey matter down the spinal cord. (These descending pathways are shown on the left-hand side of Figure 8.2, and the descending pain control system in Figure 8.3.) The important transmitters in this pathway are 5-HT, noradrenaline, enkephalins and GABA. In the dorsal horn areas, they act directly on or via the short interneurons modifying afferent impulses, thus reducing transmission of incoming pain sensation.

Sites of action of opioids to relieve pain

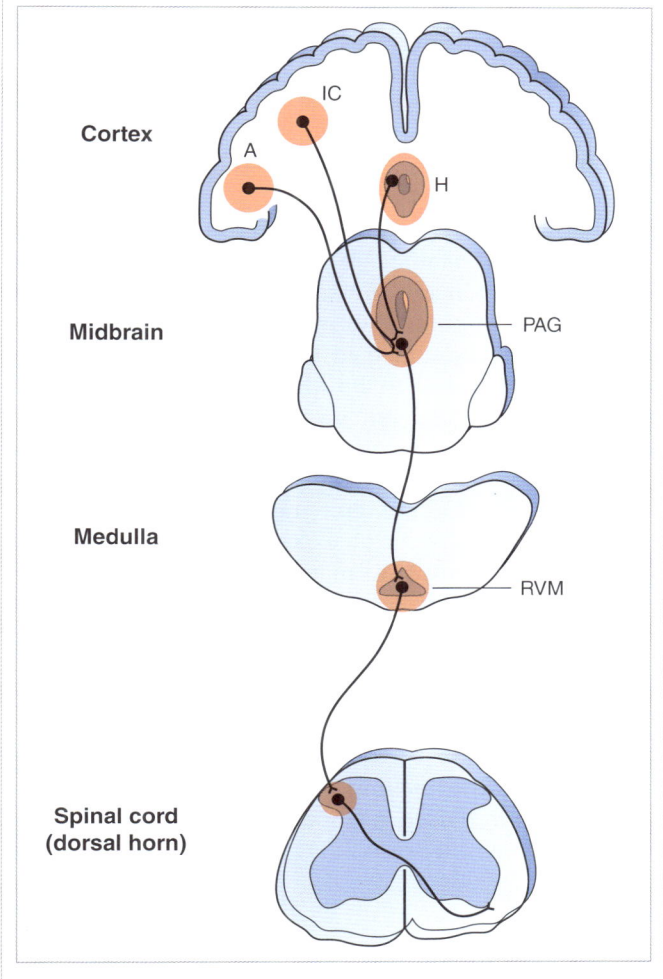

FIGURE 8.3 A = anterior cingulate cortex; IC = insular cortex; H = hypothalamus; PAG = periaqueductal grey; RVM = rostral ventromedial medulla

SWI injection points

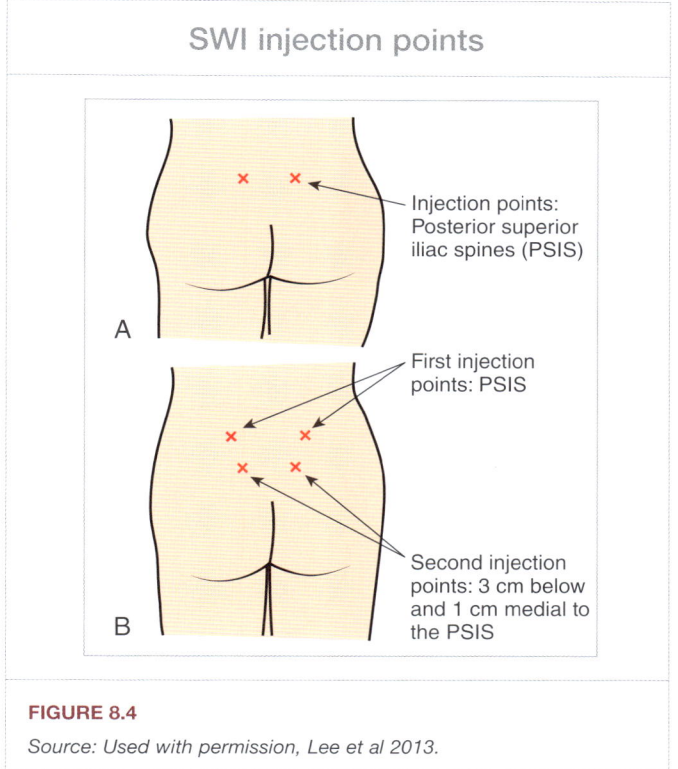

FIGURE 8.4

Source: Used with permission, Lee et al 2013.

Non-pharmacological pain management: Sterile water injections

About one in three labouring women experience low back pain in labour which persists during contractions. This may or may not relate to the position of the baby in the woman's pelvis. Many women request epidural analgesia to cope with the pain and lack of rest during contraction; however, sterile water injections (SWIs) offer a non-pharmacological option for relief. SWIs are a relatively simple and inexpensive method of providing relief for women with low back pain in labour (Lee et al 2013; Mårtensson et al 2008). Several systematic reviews and RCTs have demonstrated that sterile water injected into the skin of the lumbar-sacral area of labouring women can provide analgesic effects without detrimental side effects

(Fig 8.4). The SWI initiates relief from pain almost immediately after the injection and has been reported to last up to 2 hours 30 minutes after administration (Mårtensson et al 2008; Mårtensson et al 2017; Stulz et al 2021; Fouly et al 2018; Lee et al 2020; Lee et al 2013).

SWI administration

An injection of sterile water of 0.1–0.3 (intracutaneous) or 0.5 (subcutaneous) is administered into the skin of the woman's lumbar-sacral area, bordered by the rhombus of Michaelis (Fouly et al 2018; Lee et al 2013; Mårtensson et al 2018; Mårtensson et al 2022). SWI can be injected as a single injection, or two or four injections (Fig 8.5). There is a short-lived discomfort associated with the intervention because of somatic and mechanical irritation from the injections, causing a brief (15–30 s) burning and stinging sensation (Fouly et al 2018; Lee 2013; Lee et al 2020). The four technique injections provide the highest efficacy regarding low back pain relief among the two other techniques, despite the little discomfort of injection pains with the procedure (Almassinokiani et al 2020; Bahasadri et al 2006; Lee et al 2020; Lee et al 2013; Lee et al 2022). Repeated injections can be administered at the request of the woman.

The following sections discuss the different options for pharmacological relief of pain commencing with the least invasive and progressing to the most invasive.

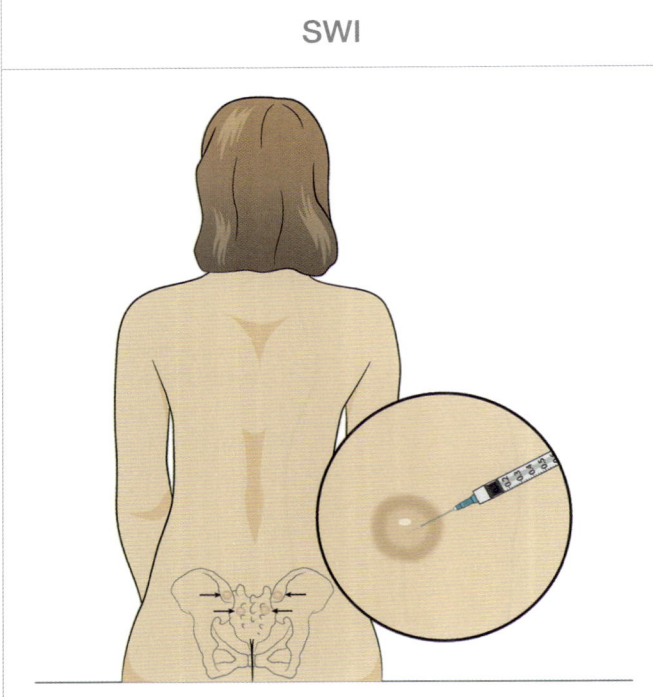

SWI

FIGURE 8.5

Source: With permission from Emily E. Sharpe MD (Assoc. Prof). Image taken from Sharpe EE, Rollins MD. Beyond the epidural: alternatives to neuraxial labor analgesia. Best Prac Res Clin Anaesthesiology. 2022;36(1):37-51.

8.5 Pharmacological relief of pain

Paracetamol

The exact mechanism of paracetamol (acetaminophen), a non-opioid analgesic, is unclear. It is assumed that it inhibits prostaglandin synthesis in the CNS and hence is an effective antipyretic analgesic. Although its anti-inflammatory effects are minimal, paracetamol does appear to inhibit COX in some tissues in some species. There is recent evidence that paracetamol also acts as a prodrug, with one of its metabolites, AM404, being active at cannabinoid receptors in the CNS, thus mimicking the analgesic actions of marijuana.

In recommended levels, paracetamol is generally believed to be a safe over-the-counter analgesic with:

- adverse effects and allergic reactions rare at therapeutic doses
- low risk of gastric upset, peptic ulceration or bleeding, tinnitus or renal impairment
- negligible plasma-protein binding; hence no risk of displacement causing drug interactions
- few serious adverse drug interactions.

However, in recent years some authors have questioned the safety of paracetamol use in pregnancy.

Studies have analysed large data sets, which demonstrate acute and chronic defects and impairments may occur in children who have been exposed to paracetamol during pregnancy (asthma, ADHD, child development, male fertility) (Brandlistuen 2013; Jensen 2010; Liew 2014; Snijder 2012). The quality of these studies is rightly criticised as they are considered low quality; however, caution is recommended in assessing the risk/benefit ratio of using this medication during pregnancy, labour, and birth (Brune et al 2015).

As noted in Drug Monograph 8.2, adverse effects are rare with paracetamol in recommended therapeutic doses, although in some instances nausea and rash have occurred. Ingestion of 20 or more tablets (10 g) can cause potentially fatal damage to the liver and kidneys and hypoglycaemia, due to buildup of a toxic metabolite (Brune et al 2015). Even normal doses (4 g/day) can cause hepatotoxicity, especially in people who are fasting, have regular excessive alcohol use or are taking drugs that induce the enzyme CYP2E1. Inadvertent overdose can also occur by exceeding the recommended daily dose in attempts to manage increasing pain or by additive effects of paracetamol present in more than one over-the-counter preparation.

In recent years caution has been advised with respect to regular paracetamol use during pregnancy. Analyses of databanks and case–control studies show that the use of paracetamol during pregnancy may increase the incidence of asthma in children of mothers having used paracetamol during pregnancy (for review, see McBride 2011; Jensen et al 2020; Brune et al 2015).

Opioids

History of opioids

Opium is the dried extract of seed capsules of the opium poppy *Papaver somniferum* (meaning 'the poppy bringing sleep'). Opium contains many pharmacologically active alkaloids (nitrogenous compounds), including morphine, codeine and papaverine. The term 'opiate' strictly refers only to opium derivatives, whereas 'opioid' means any opium-like compound and includes endogenous pain relieving substances as well as synthetic drugs mimicking opiates. Compounds directly derived from opium are called opiates and synthetically derived compounds are called opioids.

The medicinal effects of opium have been known in many cultures for over 6000 years. Opium (which contains 8–14% morphine) was almost literally 'the panacea for all ills', as it is effective against pain, diarrhoea, cough, and sleeplessness. A Latin synonym for opium preparations was 'laudanum', meaning 'praiseworthy'. Opium was widely advertised and available well into the 20th century for even mild conditions such as coughs and infants' teething pains.

Opioids are commonly used during labour and birth in Australia and New Zealand and may be administered

DRUG MONOGRAPH 8.2
Paracetamol

Paracetamol, having little anti-inflammatory action, is rather different from the other NSAIDs, but is safer than aspirin as an analgesic.

Mechanism of action

Paracetamol's analgesic and antipyretic (anti-fever) actions are thought to be due to inhibition of PG synthesis in CNS tissues via cyclo-oxygenase inhibition; it may also modulate inhibitory descending serotonin (5-HT) pathways, and a metabolite may activate cannabinoid receptors.

Indications

Paracetamol is indicated for relief of fever and mild-to-moderate pain associated with headaches, muscular aches, period pain, acute sinusitis, otitis media, arthritis, migraine and postoperative pain.

Pharmacokinetics

After oral administration, paracetamol is rapidly and completely absorbed from the GIT; peak plasma concentration is reached in 10–60 minutes, and pain relief begins after 30 minutes. Absorption is delayed by food in the GIT. Distribution via the bloodstream is uniform, with an apparent volume of distribution of 1–1.2 L/kg, implying some sequestration (binding) of paracetamol in tissues. There is negligible plasma-protein binding. Paracetamol does cross the placenta in small amounts and so can affect the fetus. It is excreted in only small amounts in the milk of lactating women; hence it is the analgesic of choice in breastfeeding mothers.

The metabolism of paracetamol occurs in the liver by hepatic microsomal enzymes. In adults the main metabolites (65–85%) are the glucuronide and sulfate conjugates, whereas in children it is the sulfate derivative. Excretion is via the urine as metabolites (95%) within 24 hours. The elimination half-life is 1–3 hours; hence, doses must be given regularly every 3–4 hours to maintain therapeutic blood levels.

Adverse drug reactions

In normal doses, paracetamol rarely causes adverse effects; dyspepsia (stomach upsets), allergy, raised aminotransferase levels and blood disorders may occur. Because of the high therapeutic index (safety margin), accidental overdose is rare. If taken in acute overdose, it is potentially fatal, with acute liver failure occurring 2–3 days later. As there may be few symptoms in the early stages (vomiting, abdominal pain, hypotension, sweating and CNS effects), treatment is instituted as soon as overdose is suspected, with attempts to remove the drug by gastric lavage or activated charcoal and administration of the specific antidote acetylcysteine.

Drug interactions

There are few clinically significant drug interactions. Paracetamol is a substrate for CYP1A2, so may interact with inducers of this enzyme (e.g. phenytoin, tobacco) or inhibitors (amitriptyline, warfarin). Thus paracetamol may prolong bleeding times in patients previously stabilised on warfarin.

Precautions and contraindications

Caution should be used before administering paracetamol to people with renal or hepatic dysfunction, as the drug or its metabolites may accumulate. Paracetamol is considered safe in pregnancy (Category A) and in breastfeeding. Products may contain appreciable amounts of sodium or aspartame.

Dosage and administration

Paracetamol is available in multiple formats: tablets, capsules, chewable tablets, elixirs, suppositories and as an injection. The recommended adult dose of paracetamol is 1 g (usually administered in two 500 mg tablets or capsules) 4–6-hourly. There are also controlled-release options available of 665 mg per tablet which lasts for 8 hours. The maximum daily dose of paracetamol is 4 g.

Paracetamol is available in a multitude of formulations (oral and IV infusion), and mixed with other active ingredients, so it is important to check the total paracetamol dose in people taking more than one formulation. The standard adult dose is 1–2 tablets, capsules or suppositories, each containing 500 mg paracetamol, administered every 3–4 hours, not exceeding a maximum of 4 g per day. Formulations suitable for children include infant drops, elixirs, suspensions and suppositories; dose recommendations on the basis of the child's age and weight should not be exceeded (children 1 month to 12 years, medically unsupervised: maximum 60 mg/kg daily for up to 48 hours, not to exceed 4 g daily). Small elderly patients should have doses lower than 1 g four times daily.

via intramuscular, intravenous, epidural, intrathecal, buccal, oral, or transdermal route, depending on the setting and desired effect.

Common opioids used during labour and birth are morphine and fentanyl. These are discussed in further detail later in this section.

Pharmacokinetics

Opioids act on the CNS and suppress the perception of pain. Centrally acting opioids are opioid agonists and stimulate opioid receptors within the CNS. The opioid receptors within the body means that we respond to painful stimuli and make naturally occurring analgesic compounds called 'endogenous compounds'. These neuromodulators suppress centrally controlled pain mechanisms within the CNS. The compounds are polypeptides (endorphins, enkephalins, dynorphins) and are distributed widely in the CNS in areas associated with pain transmission. There are many different opioid receptors in the body. At the cellular level, the opioid receptors are G-protein-coupled receptors that are linked to membrane-bound enzymes as well as calcium and potassium channels in the nerve membrane. Activation of the opioid receptors inhibits the enzyme production reducing the cyclic adenosine monophosphate (cAMP) levels which leads to a complex chain of effects on the body resulting in decreased neuronal excitability and reduced pain. Receptors in the limbic system of the brain produce the euphoric effect associated with opioid use. For many people, opioids do not take away the pain; however, the euphoric and sedative effect of the drug is sometimes more prominent and effective at achieving a beneficial effect.

Clinical considerations when using opiates during labour and birth

Effects on the central nervous system

Opioids may cause euphoria, restlessness, anxiety, and hallucinations. Vision can also be blurred, and speech slurred which can make it difficult for the woman to communicate with her caregivers. Drowsiness and sedation are very common side effects of opioid analgesia. If opiates are given close to the time of birth, the woman may have difficulty pushing and the instinctual 'mothering' behaviours may be affected. A study by Jonas et al (2008) found that opioid distribution of the oxytocin surge at birth affected the mothers' responses to her newborn infant at birth and for up to 6 months postpartum.

Respiratory distress

Opioids cause depression on the respiratory centres in the CNS, leading to respiratory depression; therefore, women should not be left alone if they have used opioids during their labour. Respiratory depression of a woman in labour can lead to retention of carbon dioxide and respiratory acidosis in both the woman and fetus. Hypoxia in the mother directly affects the fetus leading to fetal heart decelerations.

Hypotension/bradycardia

Opioids affect the cardiovascular centres in the medulla which decreases the activity of the sympathetic nervous system. This can cause bradycardia and hypotension in the woman, and a reduction in placental perfusion and corresponding changes in the fetal heart rate, such as reduced variability and depression of the fetal heart. Although this may only be transient, because of the opioids it can be interpreted as fetal distress and lead to medical intervention.

Effects on the gastrointestinal tract

The chemoreceptor trigger zone within the medulla is stimulated by many opioids which can lead to severe nausea and vomiting. Between 30–60% of women who receive opioids during their labour report nausea and vomiting. Because opioids also cause sedation the woman is at risk of aspiration, and therefore antiemetics are recommended to women who receive opioids. The gastrointestinal tract also has opioid receptors. Stimulation of these receptors reduces peristalsis and increases water absorption, leading to constipation.

Renal function

The use of opioids also affects the woman's renal system and can lead to decreased urine output and retention of urine. A reduction in renal perfusion can lead to a reduction in diuretic hormones and urine formation. Opioids inhibit smooth muscle and this will affect the bladder and the urge to urinate, leading to an increased chance of urinary retention which can be exacerbated by the effects of hormones and the physiology of labour and birth.

Effects of histamine

Histamine release is also triggered by opioids which can lead to vasodilatory responses such as sweating, skin flushing particularly of the face and chest, urticaria (hives) and pruritis (itchiness).

Neuroendocrine actions

Although the administration of opioids will affect the secretion of hypothalamic hormones, the short-term use of opioids should not be a problem unless the woman has preexisting conditions that affect adrenals or thyroid functions.

Effects on the fetus

Opioid analgesia is transferred rapidly via the placenta to the fetus. Opioid concentration is higher in the fetal circulation than in the maternal circulation. There are fewer plasma proteins in the fetal circulation which leads to a high concentration of unbound opioids in the fetal circulation. The fetus has a lower pH, which means some drugs are more likely to be ionised, and the liver is immature and therefore unable to excrete the opioids efficiently. Opioids can increase variations in fetal heart rate patterns during labour and depress breathing in the newborn.

Effects on the newborn infant

If a mother has opioids during her labour and birth the newborn may have depressed breathing, be drowsy, and thermoregulation and normal reflexes may be affected. The effect of the opiates in the infant is one of narcosis, including reduced muscle tone and depressed CNS, leading to a delay in the rooting and sucking responses which can impact breastfeeding. Pethidine, an opioid used to relieve labour pain, is metabolised to norpethidine. The half-lives of pethidine and norpethidine in neonates are extremely prolonged (20 and 60 hours respectively), therefore clearance time from the baby's body is extended (van den Anker 2021). It is therefore essential that the newborn baby is closely observed and monitored for signs of respiratory depression, CNS depression and narcosis.

Administration

Opioids are not usually given orally during labour and birth due to the delay in absorption and metabolism. The usual mode of administration is intramuscular or via an epidural or intrathecal catheter.

Morphine

Morphine gets its name from Morpheus, the Greek god of dreams and sleep, and is the most commonly used opioid during labour. Morphine is the prototype opioid analgesic; all new analgesics are compared with morphine for potency and for therapeutic effects or adverse reactions. Morphine is available in many dosage forms, including injection, oral mixture, modified-release capsules, and tablets (Drug Monograph 8.3); and slow-release epidural injection.

DRUG MONOGRAPH 8.3
Morphine

Morphine is a strong analgesic with central actions on pain perception; it mimics the actions of enkephalins and endorphins at ORs.

Mechanism of action of opioids
See text for specific mechanisms of action.

Indications
IM, IV, epidural/spinal for acute pain relief during labour and birth, sedation to enable and maintain intubation.

Pharmacokinetics
Morphine may be administered by many routes – PO (i.e. by mouth), IM, IV, SC, epidural, intrathecal and rectal. It is rapidly absorbed and is subject to extensive first-pass metabolism in the liver, leading to poor bioavailability (about 40% when taken orally), so the oral dose may need to be 2–6 times the parenteral dose (Table 8.3). The main metabolites are active M6G and morphine-3-glucuronide.

Morphine is distributed widely in most body tissues, but only a small fraction crosses the blood–brain barrier. Metabolites are excreted primarily via the kidneys, with 7–10% undergoing enterohepatic circulation, which extends the half-life. The mean elimination half-life is 2–3 hours, but this is increased with slow-release preparations (tablets, capsules, oral suspension), such that the peak morphine concentrations during chronic use occur 4–8 hours after dosing and therapeutic effects may extend for 16–24 hours.

Drug interactions
See Drug Interactions 8.1.

Adverse reactions
The most common adverse reactions reported are constipation, nausea and vomiting, itch, urinary retention, sedation, circulatory and respiratory depression and miosis (pin-point pupils); overdose with opioids can cause cessation of respiration. Tolerance occurs to analgesia as well as to depressant effects (but not to constipation), requiring higher dosages. Constipation should be pre-empted with prophylactic laxative or a diet high in fibre. Respiratory depression, dependence and withdrawal reactions are not usually problems when opioids are used clinically for relief of pain during labour and birth.

Warnings and contraindications
- Avoid the use of opioids in people with known opioid drug hypersensitivity, or a history of drug abuse.
- Use opioids with caution in women with acute respiratory depression, acute asthma, or other respiratory impairment, and in patients with elevated intracranial pressure (may be exacerbated).
- Use with caution in biliary colic or pancreatitis (may cause spasm of biliary tract muscle and sphincter), acute abdominal conditions or severe inflammatory bowel disease (risk of obscuring the diagnosis, or risk of toxic megacolon).
- Doses need to be reduced in women with renal or liver impairment.
- Administration during pregnancy may result in dependence in the infant; use during labour may cause respiratory depression in the infant, treated with naloxone.

Dosage and administration
Standard morphine doses are 10 mg IV/IM/SC. Epidural dosages are discussed below.

TABLE 8.3 Selected opioid dosage forms

DRUG/DOSE FORM	USUAL DOSE	FREQUENCY OF ADMINISTRATION (HOURLY OR PER DAY)	NOTES
Morphine			The 'gold standard'; analgesic for severe pain, acute and chronic pain; has an active metabolite M6G
Oral solution	5–20 mg	4-hourly	30 mg oral morphine is considered equivalent to 10 mg parenteral morphine
Tablets	5–20 mg	12-hourly	
CR tablets	5–200 mg	12-hourly	
IM/SC/IV	0.5–10 mg 5–20 mg (MIMS)	4–6-hourly	
Epidural, IT	100–200 micrograms 2–3 mg epidural	12–24-hourly	Slow-release form for anaesthetist-only use in hospital; patient requires close monitoring for 48 hours
Buprenorphine			For chronic pain or opioid dependence; slow onset; partial agonist, low dependence liability
IM, IV	0.3–0.6 mg	6–8-hourly	Also 8 mg and 16 mg oral fast-dissolving tablets
Sublingual film	0.4, 2 and 8 mg	6–8-hourly	
Transdermal patch	5, 10, 15, 20, 25, 30 and 40 micrograms/h	Every 7 days	For moderate-to-severe pain
Codeine			Weak opioid, metabolised to morphine; for mild-to-moderate pain; cough suppression; diarrhoea
Oral Linctus	30–100 mg 5 mg/mL	4–6-hourly maximum 240 mg in 24 hours	Combination formulations contain sub-therapeutic doses
Fentanyl			Highly potent (dosed in microgram); for moderate-to-severe pain, during anaesthesia, chronic pain, breakthrough pain. Note: various preparations are not equivalent.
Orally disintegrating	100, 200, 300, 400, 600 and 800 micrograms		
Sublingual tablets	100, 200, 300, 400, 600 and 800 micrograms		Sublingual tablets: Initial dose may be repeated after 30 minutes if necessary (but 2 hours should elapse before retreatment of breakthrough pain)
SC/IV, epidural (obstetric analgesic slow IV), IT	50–100 micrograms	1–2-hourly	
Transdermal patch	12–100 micrograms/h	Every 3 days	Patches release 12–100 micrograms/h; not for opioid-naive
Lozenge ('lollipop')	200–1600 micrograms	6–8-hourly. Max. 4 doses per day	Absorbed via buccal mucosa; for breakthrough pain and children
Intranasal	Child 1.5 mcg/kg to max. 100 mcg		If needed second dose of 0.75–1.5 mcg/kg to max of 100 mcg may be given after 5–10 minutes
Hydromorphone			Less sedative
Oral:			Morphine 10 mg IM/SC is equivalent to hydromorphone 1.5–2 mg IM/SC
Solution	1 mg/mL dose 2–4 mg	4-hourly	Morphine 30 mg oral is equivalent to 6 mg hydromorphone
Tablets	2, 4 and 8 mg	4-hourly	
CR tablets	4, 8, 16, 32 and 64 mg	Every 24 hours	
IM/SC/IV	1–2 mg	4–6-hourly	

TABLE 8.3   Selected opioid dosage forms—cont'd

DRUG/DOSE FORM	USUAL DOSE	FREQUENCY OF ADMINISTRATION (HOURLY OR PER DAY)	NOTES
Methadone			Severe postoperative or chronic pain; maintenance of dependence; long half-life, so risk of accumulation
Oral:			
Tablets	10 mg	6–8-hourly, short term Chronic: max. 12-hourly	
Syrup	5 mg/mL dose 10–20 mg (max. 80 mg) per day	6–8-hourly, short term Chronic: max. 12-hourly	
IM/IV/SC	5–10 mg	6–8-hourly	
Oxycodone			Oral bioavailability variable, 50–90%
Oral:			
Tablets	5 mg only	6-hourly	
CR tablets	5, 10, 15, 20, 40 and 80 mg	12-hourly	CR formulations have longer duration of action (12–24 h)
Capsules	5, 10 and 20 mg	4–6-hourly	
Liquid	5 mg/5 mL Dose 5 mg	4–6-hourly	
SC	2.5–10 mg	4–6-hourly	1 mg parenteral = 2 mg oral
Slow IV	Dose 1–5 mg (max. 10 mg)	4-hourly	
Rectal	30 mg	6–8-hourly	Rectal bioavailability also variable
Pethidine			Risk of excitement, poor oral efficacy; useful in labour, renal and biliary colic pain; interactions with drugs affecting 5-HT levels
IM/SC	25–100 mg	3–4-hourly	
Slow IV	25–50 mg	3–4-hourly	
Epidural	25–50 mg	Single dose duration of action 2–5 hours	Obstetric analgesia
Tramadol			Weak opioid; moderate-to-severe pain; monoamine uptake inhibitor, useful for neuropathic pain; low misuse potential
Oral:			
Capsules	50–100 mg	4–6-hourly	
CR formulation	100, 150 and 200 mg	12–24 hours	
IM, IV	50–100 mg	Every 12 hours	

CR = controlled-release; IM = intramuscular; IT = intrathecal; IV = intravenous; SC = subcutaneous
Note: Doses need to be titrated depending on age, level of pain, tolerance, and renal or hepatic impairment; doses for high-potency opioids buprenorphine and fentanyl are in micrograms or fractions of a mg.
Source: Adapted from information in MIMS Online and Australian Medicines Handbook 2021.

Fentanyl

Fentanyl is a lipid soluble opioid often used in epidural analgesia. Fentanyl is a potent opioid and much stronger than morphine. The rapid action of fentanyl, the increased duration of the action and the smaller volumes needed give it an advantage over other opioids like morphine (see Drug Monograph 8.4).

8.6 Inhalation agents

Inhalation analgesia has been used by women during childbirth for over 100 years. Queen Victoria is said to have used chloroform for her births. The chemistry of anaesthetic agents is diverse. They share the properties of lipid solubility and the ability to bind to cell membranes

---

DRUG MONOGRAPH 8.4
Fentanyl

Fentanyl is a strong opioid analgesic with a mechanism and actions like morphine. Its clinical potency ranges from 50–100 times that of morphine, and it mimics the actions of endogenous enkephalins and endorphins at opioid receptors (ORs).

Indications

During labour and birth fentanyl is used in epidural anaesthesia in combination with bupivacaine or ropivacaine and as an adjunctive analgesic during general anaesthesia.

Pharmacokinetics

The plasma-protein binding of fentanyl is about 84%. Fentanyl is rapidly and extensively metabolised primarily by CYP3A4 in the liver to several pharmacologically inactive metabolites. The minimum effective analgesic serum concentration of fentanyl ranges from 0.3–1.2 ng/mL, while surgical anaesthesia and profound respiratory depression occur at serum levels of 10–20 ng/mL. Within 72 hours of IV fentanyl administration, approximately 75% of fentanyl is excreted in the urine, and about 9% in the faeces, mostly as inactive metabolites.

Drug interactions

See Drug Interactions 8.1. In addition, as fentanyl can contribute to serotonin toxicity, it is contraindicated with monoamine oxidase inhibitors (MAOIs) or other drugs implicated in serotonin syndrome. Azole antifungals can impair the metabolism of fentanyl, leading to prolonged half-lives and risk of adverse effects.

Severe and unpredictable potentiation by MAOIs has been reported with opioid analgesics, and the use of fentanyl in patients who have received MAOIs within 14 days is not recommended. Due to additive pharmacological effect, the concomitant use of **benzodiazepines** or other CNS depressants increases the risk of respiratory depression, profound sedation, coma, and death.

Adverse reactions

The most common adverse reactions are bradycardia, rash and itch at the site of administration, constipation, nausea, somnolescence (drowsiness), and headache. The most serious potential adverse reactions associated with opioid use are respiratory depression, hypotension, and shock.

Warnings and contraindications

- Fentanyl should only be used by experienced doctors and in patients who are under constant supervision.
- Respiratory depression is the most marked and dangerous side effect, and fentanyl should be used with caution in patients with severe impairment of pulmonary function. The respiratory depressant effect of fentanyl persists longer than the measured analgesic effect. Respiratory depression can be reversed by opioid antagonists; however, appropriate surveillance should be maintained.
- Fentanyl should be used with caution in impaired hepatic or renal function or in patients susceptible to respiratory depression.
- Fentanyl may induce hypotension, particularly in hypovolaemic patients, and may produce bradycardia and possibly asystole.
- Contraindications include known hypersensitivity or intolerance to fentanyl, other opioid analgesics or to any of the excipients, bronchial asthma, head injuries and increased intracranial pressure.
- Fentanyl may cause muscle rigidity, particularly involving the muscles of respiration. This effect is related to the dose and speed of injection and may be reduced by slow intravenous injection.
- Profound sedation, respiratory depression, coma, and death may result from the concomitant use of fentanyl with benzodiazepines or other CNS depressants.
- Fentanyl can produce drug dependence and therefore has the potential for being abused.

Dosage and administration

Doses may vary widely depending on the indication for which it is given, the route of administration, tolerance developed, level of pain, and opioid familiarity/naivety of the patient.

Sources: Based on information from Australian Medicines Handbook 2024; Medsafe NZ database – see Online resources.

DRUG INTERACTIONS 8.1

Opioids

DRUG	POSSIBLE EFFECTS AND MANAGEMENT
Alcohol or other CNS depressants (other opioids, anaesthetics, sedatives, psychotropics)	May result in enhanced CNS depression, respiratory depression and hypotension. Reduce dosage and monitor closely.
Buprenorphine (partial agonist)	May result in additive effect of respiratory depression if given concurrently with low doses of μ- or κ-receptor agonists; avoid concurrent usage. Partial agonists given with an opioid agonist may reduce the analgesic effects of the full agonist or precipitate withdrawal symptoms.
Monoamine oxidase inhibitors (MAOIs) (phenelzine, tranylcypromine, moclobemide and selegiline)	Intensify the effects of opioids (especially pethidine, tramadol and fentanyl) and may cause serotonin syndrome.[3] Caution should be exercised and dosages of opioids reduced.
Opioid antagonists (naltrexone, naloxone)	Will produce withdrawal symptoms in patients dependent on opioid medications. Avoid concurrent administration.
Diltiazem, erythromycin and fluconazole	May inhibit metabolism and increase concentration of alfentanil, thus exacerbating respiratory depression. Dose may need to be decreased.
Rifampicin	May enhance metabolism and decrease concentration of morphine, codeine and alfentanil, thus reducing their effects. Effects should be monitored, and dose may need to be increased or another analgesic substituted.
Many drugs (including anticonvulsants, antivirals, antifungals, rifampicin and St John's wort)	May enhance metabolism and decrease concentration of methadone, thus reducing its effects. Effects should be monitored, and dose may need to be increased.

at certain sites. Nowadays, inhaled analgesia during labour involves the self-administered inhalation of sub-anaesthetic concentrations of agents while the woman remains awake, and her protective laryngeal reflexes remain intact. Most of the agents are easy to administer, can be started in less than a minute and become effective within a minute. Inhaled anaesthetics used during a general anaesthetic will be discussed later in this chapter.

Nitrous oxide

Nitrous oxide (N_2O) is the most used inhaled analgesia during childbirth. The first device to administer inhaled N_2O to labouring women was developed in 1881; however, the apparatus was large and the gas was expensive, so it was not used widely. Fifty years later this changed when in 1933 the Minnitt apparatus, which delivered a fixed 50% N_2O mixed with air, was developed. The UK Royal College of Obstetricians and Gynaecologists certified the Minnitt apparatus, and in 1936, endorsed its administration by midwives. Following the development of the Entonox system, which mixed 50% N_2O with 50% oxygen (O_2) by Turnstall in 1965, the use of N_2O became widespread. The use of N_2O continues today, with over two-thirds of women in Australia and New Zealand using it during labour and birth. It is ideal for use in labour as it is short acting. Women remain in control by self-administering the gas using a mask or mouthpiece. Nitrous oxide use in labour and birth does not stop a woman from being mobile or upright.

Pharmacokinetics

Nitrous oxide is a colourless, non-flammable, slightly sweet tasting and smelling gas which has low anaesthetic potency and low blood solubility; therefore, it is not metabolised to any significant effect (Baysinger 2019). The low solubility is what allows for the rapid onset and offset of the drug with peak brain concentration within 20 to 60 seconds of inhalation and rapid elimination from the body. As the gas is lipid soluble it will cross the placenta into the fetus. The concentration of N_2O in the fetus reaches 80% of maternal values within 3 minutes of administration; however, it is rapidly eliminated (Klomp et al 2012; Likis et al 2014). The mechanism of action is complex. Central nervous system potassium channel inhibition leads to the release of endogenous opioids with k-receptor activation, and anxiolysis of GABA receptor activations. The precise mechanism of action of anaesthetics remains uncertain; however, the inhibition of NMDA receptor activity is thought to mediate the primary analgesic effect.

As with any anaesthetic, N_2O has the potential to cause CNS depression and hypoxia, so the woman

---

[3]Serotonin syndrome is an adverse effect due to excessive stimulation of $5-HT_{2A}$ receptors caused by drugs such as antidepressants; it is characterised by mental state changes (confusion, delirium and hypomania), gastrointestinal tract effects (diarrhoea), neuromuscular hyperactivity (hyperreflexia, incoordination and tremor), autonomic instability, sweating, fever and shivering (see Chapter 22 for more detail).

should not be left alone when using N_2O. Women with preexisting respiratory disease are at increased risk of hypoxia, and the use of N_2O has the potential to increase fetal hypoxia, so caution should be taken if there are any signs of fetal compromise.

Interestingly, despite common use, there is a dearth of up-to-date research available. The most cited research is Klomp et al's (2012) Cochrane review which included 26 RCTs, with a total of 2959 women. Komp et al (2012) investigated the effectiveness and safety of inhaled analgesia as pain relief for women in labour. The authors concluded that inhaled analgesia may help relieve labour pain without adversely increasing assisted birth rates (forceps or vacuum extraction) or caesarean section, or affecting neonatal wellbeing (Klomp et al 2012). Within the review a comparison was made with another less common inhaled gas, methoxyflurane, commonly referred to as flurane (see below). Flurane derivatives were found to be slightly more effective than N_2O for the reduction of pain and for pain relief although N_2O also helped to relieve pain

when compared with no treatment. Women who used N_2O were more likely to experience nausea compared with flurane derivatives. When compared with no treatment or placebo, N_2O resulted in side effects such as nausea, vomiting, dizziness and drowsiness. The review concluded that women should be informed that inhaled analgesia may help relieve pain during labour but warned that they may experience side effects, such as nausea, vomiting, dizziness and drowsiness. (Drug Monograph 8.5.)

Methoxyflurane

Methoxyflurane is a halogenated ether. Renal toxicity limits its regular use as an anaesthetic; however, it is a powerful analgesic administered to stable, conscious patients by paramedics in pre-hospital settings. It is administered via a hand-held 'puffer' in which 3 mL of the solution is vaporised and then inhaled. Onset of analgesia occurs after a few breaths, and intermittent use provides effective pain relief for 20–30 minutes. Drowsiness and amnesia may occur, but there are few cardiovascular

---

DRUG MONOGRAPH 8.5
Nitrous oxide

Nitrous oxide is a simple inorganic molecule with the chemical formula N_2O. It should not be confused with nitric oxide, now recognised as a gas generated in many body cells involved in vasodilation and immune responses, and as a chemical mediator in the CNS in neurotransmission and neurodegeneration.

Mechanism of action

Its analgesic action may be mediated via opioid receptors, while the hypnotic/anxiolytic action is mainly due to enhancement of GABA-mediated CNS depression and the anaesthetic action due to NMDA receptor inhibition.

Indications

Nitrous oxide is commonly used for dental surgery, minor surgery and obstetric analgesia. It is indicated for induction and maintenance of GA. It is a powerful analgesic, a useful anxiolytic but a weak anaesthetic, so is often combined with other (volatile) anaesthetics to enhance its effects. It is presented as a compressed gas – for example, in a 50:50 mixture with oxygen (Entonox).

Pharmacokinetics

Nitrous oxide is inhaled and absorbed via the lungs; it has low solubility in blood and tissues, so has a rapid onset of action and recovery time. It is excreted 100% unchanged through the lungs.

Adverse effects and drug interactions

It is non-irritant and virtually without odour. Its few adverse effects are hypoxia, mild cardiac depression, and nausea, vomiting or delirium. It has no known significant drug interactions. Prolonged inhalation (> 6 hours) can cause adverse haematological and neurological effects. It may be abused; escaped gas should be scavenged to avoid occupational exposure and contribution to the greenhouse effect. It is considered safe in pregnancy and is widely used as an inhaled analgesic during labour and birth, as it can be administered by the mother (and/or midwife) during contractions and does not accumulate or cause respiratory depression in the neonate.

Warnings and contraindications

There is risk of hypoxia if inadequate oxygen is provided. Precaution is advised in instances of heart failure, and there is a risk of increased volume in air-containing cavities in conditions such as abdominal distension and pneumothorax, At the termination of N_2O anaesthesia, the rapid movement of large amounts of N_2O from the circulation into the lungs may dilute the oxygen in the lungs (diffusion hypoxia). To prevent this, the anaesthetist usually administers supplementary oxygen for 3–5 minutes to clear the N_2O from the lungs.

Dosage and administration

Women self-administer a 50:50 mixture of $N_2O:O_2$.

adverse effects. Due to renal toxicity, it should not be used on consecutive days or in renal impairment.

8.7 Local anaesthetic

Local anaesthetic (LA) drugs were developed following the introduction of the natural compound cocaine into medicine and ophthalmic surgery in the 1870s and 1880s. The main problems with cocaine were its CNS actions, acute toxicity, and addictive properties, so other benzoic acid **esters** were studied. The amide compound lidocaine (lignocaine), developed in 1943, rapidly became widely used and is still considered the prototype LA. A long-acting drug from the bupivacaine-type group is used when longer duration of activity is required, and more recently a combination of lidocaine (lignocaine) and prilocaine (EMLA: eutectic mixture for local anaesthesia) has been formulated as a cream and a patch for topical application. An ideal LA would produce nerve blockade only in sensory nerves when administered topically or parenterally (by injection) and would be rapidly reversible, non-toxic to both local tissue and major organs, with rapid, painless onset of action for a reasonable operating time. While no LA is perfect, two that are commonly used during childbirth are lidocaine (see Drug Monograph 8.6) and the longer acting bupivacaine.

Chemistry and dissociation of local anaesthetic drugs

Chemically, LA drugs have similar structures: they generally have at one end an aromatic (phenyl) group, joined through an intermediate chain of carbons to an amine (nitrogen-containing) group. The aromatic group helps make that end of the molecule lipid-soluble (lipophilic) and the amine group makes the other end water-soluble (hydrophilic). This allows the LA molecules to align and act within nerve cell membranes, which can be considered as phospholipid bilayers.

Esters and amides

The intermediate carbon chains contain either an ester link (O_C–O-) or an amide link (O_C–N-). The ester-type LAs (cocaine, procaine, tetracaine [amethocaine] and benzocaine) are metabolised rapidly by plasma esterase enzymes to p-aminobenzoic acid (PABA) metabolites, which can cause allergic reactions in some patients; ester LAs are not often used now. Amide anaesthetics (e.g. lidocaine [lignocaine], prilocaine, bupivacaine and ropivacaine) are not metabolised to PABA derivatives, and rarely induce allergic reactions.

Amines can be charged or uncharged

Because the LAs are all **amines** (except benzocaine), they can exist in solution as the uncharged tertiary amine form NR_3 (analogous to ammonia, NH_3) or as the charged quaternary amine form NR_3H (like the ammonium ion, NH_4). The forms are in equilibrium, as shown in the dissociation reaction at the top of Figure 8.6. The proportion of each form depends on the chemistry of the individual LA molecule and the pH of the solution or tissue it is in.

Mechanism of action

LAs reversibly prevent the generation and conduction of impulses in excitable membranes and thus decrease sensitivity to pain. The basic mechanism of action of these drugs is as follows: the nonionised form enters the cell by diffusion through membranes where it readily becomes ionised and binds to a modulatory site in the voltage-dependent sodium channel, blocking the channel and interfering with their transient opening, thus preventing the transient inrush of sodium. Hence, threshold potential is not reached, the cell membrane is not depolarised, the development of the action potential and its propagation are prevented, and the nerve is blocked. The LA drugs are said to be ion channel modulators or membrane stabilisers. Other drug groups with similar actions are the antidysrhythmic agents and anticonvulsants. (Lidocaine [lignocaine] is in fact used for these effects.)

Autonomic and sensory nerves are blocked preferentially

All potentially excitable membranes are affected, so LAs have actions not only on sensory nerve cells but also on autonomic and motor nerves, muscle cells (cardiac, smooth, skeletal), secretory cells and neurons in the CNS. The susceptibility of a nerve to LA action depends on the fibre diameter, myelination, tissue pH and length of nerve fibre exposed to LA solution. Autonomic and sensory fibres are blocked preferentially because they are thinner, unmyelinated, and more easily penetrated by drugs. Loss of pain is followed in sequence by loss of responses to temperature, proprioception (position of body parts), touch and pressure. Motor fibres may also be

---

DRUG MONOGRAPH 8.6
Lidocaine (lignocaine)

Mechanism of action
Lidocaine (lignocaine) is an amide-type LA that prevents the initiation and propagation of nerve impulses. It also has antidysrhythmic properties because it stabilises all potentially excitable membranes, including the conduction system of the heart.

Indications
Lidocaine (lignocaine) is used commonly for production of local anaesthesia by topical, infiltration, nerve block, epidural and intrathecal, spinal, ophthalmic, dermal (patches, cream, ointment) and IV regional anaesthesia routes. It is also used to treat or prevent ventricular dysrhythmias.

Pharmacokinetics
Onset of action is rapid (5–10 minutes) and duration of nerve blockade is 1–1.5 hours. After absorption into the general circulation or after IV injection, the drug is redistributed rapidly to tissues, especially the heart.
Metabolism occurs in the liver and excretion is via the kidneys; less than 10% is excreted unchanged. The elimination half-life is 90–120 minutes.

Adverse effects
Excessive dosage, rapid absorption or delayed elimination can lead to toxic depressant effects in the central, autonomic and peripheral nervous systems and the cardiovascular and respiratory systems. Allergic reactions are rare.

Drug interactions
Other antidysrhythmics, phenytoin and alcohol may potentiate the cardiovascular effects of lidocaine (lignocaine). The clearance of lidocaine (lignocaine) may be reduced by drugs including beta-blockers, cimetidine, erythromycin and itraconazole.

Warnings and contraindications
Reduced doses should be given to children, elderly patients and those with cardiac, neurological, liver or kidney disease; cardiovascular function should be monitored during IV administration. Lidocaine (lignocaine) is contraindicated in patients with hypersensitivity to amide LAs, inflammation or sepsis at the site of injection, severe shock or hypotension, diseases of the CNS or supraventricular dysrhythmias.

Dosage and administration
Lidocaine (lignocaine) is formulated as an oral liquid (2%), oral paint (2.5%), topical liquid (4%), injection (0.5–2%), gel (2%), ointment (5%), cream (4%), spray (5%) and in various combination products. For local anaesthesia, the lowest effective dosage should be used, depending on the area to be anaesthetised, technique to be used, vascularity of the tissues and patient factors. The typical maximum safe dose is 3 mg/kg (solution without adrenaline) or 7 mg/kg with adrenaline; the specific dose depends on the route and usage. The most commonly used preparation in direct midwifery clinical practice is 5–10 mL of lidocaine 1% (50 mg) for infiltration prior to episiotomy followed by 10–15 mL of lidocaine 1% (150 mg) for the subsequent repair.

---

anaesthetised if adequate concentration of the drug is present over sufficient time.

Pharmacokinetics

An LA is administered for local analgesic action in the tissue or nerve pathway into which it is injected. It is only later that the drug is absorbed from the tissues into the bloodstream and distributed around the body, where it affects other systems and is metabolised and excreted.

Local disposition and action

An injected LA will first undergo local disposition (i.e. moving around) in the tissue. Onset of action is determined by the speed with which it diffuses into nerve cells, depending on its lipid solubility, which, as noted above, depends in turn on the pH of the tissue and the degree of ionisation of the LA molecules (a function of the p K a [negative logarithm of the ionisation constant] of the drug). Binding of the LA to tissue proteins and the presence of a vasoconstrictor in the solution help retain the drug in the tissues for longer action. Other potential factors include the volume and concentration of solution injected, speed of injection and local blood flow.

Diffusion, distribution, and metabolism

Local action is terminated by diffusion away, dilution and uptake into the vasculature (i.e. systemic absorption from the tissue) and distribution around the body. Lipid solubility is again the major determining factor, and a vasoconstrictor will decrease the rate of absorption into the general circulation. Metabolism of amide LAs occurs on first pass through the liver; this explains why LAs are inactive if

Mechanism of action of local anaesthetics

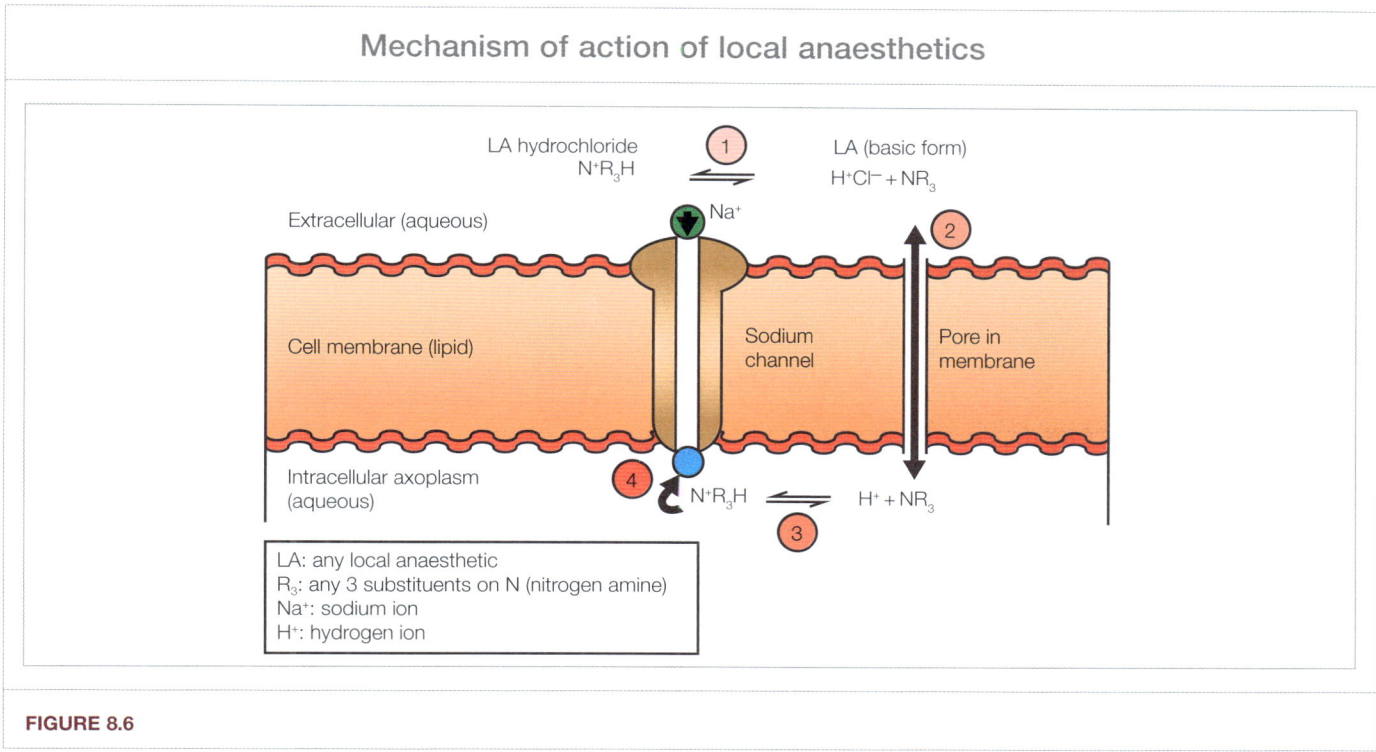

FIGURE 8.6

taken orally. (Oral administration would not allow for localised actions except in the upper gastrointestinal tract.) Inactive metabolites are excreted via the kidneys.

Duration of action

Overall, the onset and duration of action of an injected LA depend on pharmacokinetic factors. The half-lives of LAs are generally short (1–2 hours); however, the bupivacaine-type LAs have longer durations of action. The choice of LA for a particular procedure depends largely on the duration of drug action desired. These drugs may be used for assisted births such as forceps births, when a pudendal nerve block may be used rather than an **epidural**.

Long-acting local anaesthetics

Bupivacaine was the first long-acting LA developed, soon followed by others with high lipid solubility and high protein binding, giving them longer durations of action – up to 14 hours for major nerve blocks. Bupivacaine and ropivacaine differentiate well between sensory and motor blockade; however, bupivacaine is more cardiotoxic. Most are indicated for infiltration, nerve block, epidural and intrathecal anaesthesia; bupivacaine and ropivacaine are each also formulated combined with fentanyl for epidural anaesthesia/analgesia, and bupivacaine with adrenaline (epinephrine) for more prolonged action.

Use of a vasoconstrictor

Most LAs produce vasodilation by direct action on blood vessels and by anaesthetising sympathetic fibres to vasculature. This can cause rapid absorption of the drug into the systemic circulation; when the rate of absorption exceeds the rate of elimination, toxic effects can occur. Vasoconstrictors such as adrenaline (epinephrine) or felypressin may be formulated in the LA solution to decrease systemic absorption and detain the drug in local tissue, prolonging the duration of action of the anaesthetic and reducing the risk of systemic toxicity.

Parenterals

For injection by infiltration and nerve block techniques, the LA must be formulated as a parenteral solution that is sterile, particle-free, stable and preferably isotonic and buffered to the pH of body solutions. Particular cases are those of LA solutions with added vasoconstrictor (e.g. adrenaline [epinephrine], 1 in 200,000); and heavy solutions (for spinal anaesthesia) such as Marcain Spinal 0.5% Heavy Injection, a hyperbaric bupivacaine solution containing glucose at 80 mg/mL. Parenteral solutions of LA may also be formulated with an opioid analgesic such as fentanyl or morphine.

Techniques for local anaesthesia

There are several techniques by which local anaesthestics (LAs) are administered (Table 8.4). They may be:

- applied to an area (topical) e.g. cream applied to the skin before inserting an intravenous cannula, or
- injected into tissues (infiltration) e.g. for perineal repair.

TABLE 8.4 Local anaesthetic techniques

METHOD	TISSUE AFFECTED	DOSE FORM USED	EXAMPLES OF DRUGS USED	THERAPEUTIC INDICATIONS
Topical	Sensory nerve endings in mucous membranes and dermis	Solution, ointment, cream, eyedrops, spray, etc.	Cocaine, benzocaine, lidocaine (lignocaine), tetracaine (amethocaine), prilocaine	Relief of pain or itching; examination of conjunctiva; minor surgery; instrumentation
Infiltration	Sensory nerve endings in subcutaneous tissues or dermis	Injection	Prilocaine, lidocaine (lignocaine)	Minor surgery; skin lesions
Nerve block	Nerve trunk	Injection	Articaine, prilocaine, lidocaine (lignocaine), bupivacaine	Dental, eye and limb surgery; sympathetic block; obstetrics; postoperative pain relief
Epidural block	Spinal roots	Injection	Lidocaine (lignocaine), bupivacaine, levobupivacaine, ropivacaine	Thoracic and abdominal surgery; labour pain; caesarean section; postoperative pain relief
Spinal (subarachnoid) block	Spinal roots	Injection	Bupivacaine, levobupivacaine, ropivacaine	Abdominal surgery; surgery of the lower extremities; muscle relaxation
Intravenous regional anaesthesia	Upper limb	Injection	Prilocaine	Surgery on upper limb

LAs produce their effect in the immediate area only, hence the term 'local anaesthesia'. LAs can be injected around a nerve or nerve trunk (e.g. perineal nerve block, spinal or epidural techniques) to anaesthetise a large region of the body (regional anaesthesia). The LA should be injected slowly, with frequent aspirations (gentle 'sucking back' on the syringe) to ensure the needle tip is not in a blood vessel; pauses between bolus injections allow monitoring for systemic effects (Fig 8.7).

Infiltration anaesthesia is the use of LAs in a small area that circles the operative field; it is produced by injecting dilute solutions of the agent, usually with adrenaline, into the skin and then subcutaneously into the region to be anaesthetised. Repeated injection extends the anaesthesia as long as needed. Sensory nerve endings are anaesthetised, but not motor nerves. This method is used for perineal repair following birth (Fig 8.8).

In **nerve (conduction) block anaesthesia**, LA injected in the vicinity of a nerve trunk inhibits conduction of impulses to and from the area supplied by that nerve, the region of the operative site. A single nerve may be blocked, or LA may be injected where several nerve trunks emerge from the spinal cord (paravertebral block). During peripheral nerve block, motor nerves are usually blocked as well as sensory pathways. A concentrated solution is required because of the thickness of nerve trunk fibres; overall, less LA is needed than for the infiltration technique. This method of anaesthesia is often used for obstetric procedures (pudendal block) and for postoperative pain relief.

Central nerve block: Epidural anaesthesia

Epidural analgesia is widely used by women during labour and birth in Australia and New Zealand (42%; 40% respectively) and is associated with increased medical intervention (AIHW 2023; NZ Health 2023). Epidural analgesia is achieved by the administration of medications; usually an opioid analgesia combined with a local anaesthetic into the epidural space in the woman's spine. The epidural space is in the lumbar region of the spine (Fig 8.9). This space is approximately 4 mm wide and contains blood vessels and fatty tissue. It is situated around the dura mater, with the spinal nerves passing through it. The engorgement of blood vessels during pregnancy decrease this space and it is also affected by the increased blood flow from uterine contractions during labour.

The epidural catheter is inserted by an anaesthetist through a spinal needle. The needle is removed, and the catheter is left in place to enable medications to be given either as a bolus, a continual infusion or a pump (PCEA) controlled by the woman. The aim of an epidural is to reduce sensation and pain during contractions by blocking transmission of the pain signals to the spinal nerves. Historically, medications given via epidurals were usually given in large dosages, rendering the woman numb from the waist down and unable to move her lower limbs. However, recent advances in the administration of the medications mean that 'low dose' epidurals are available which enable the woman to move and even stand.

Epidural and spinal blocks are specialised central nerve blocks in which spinal roots are blocked where they emerge from the spinal canal. Autonomic nerves may also be blocked, so there is a risk of autonomic adverse effects. To enhance analgesia, an opioid such as morphine or fentanyl is often co-administered by these

The routes of administration of local anaesthetic drugs

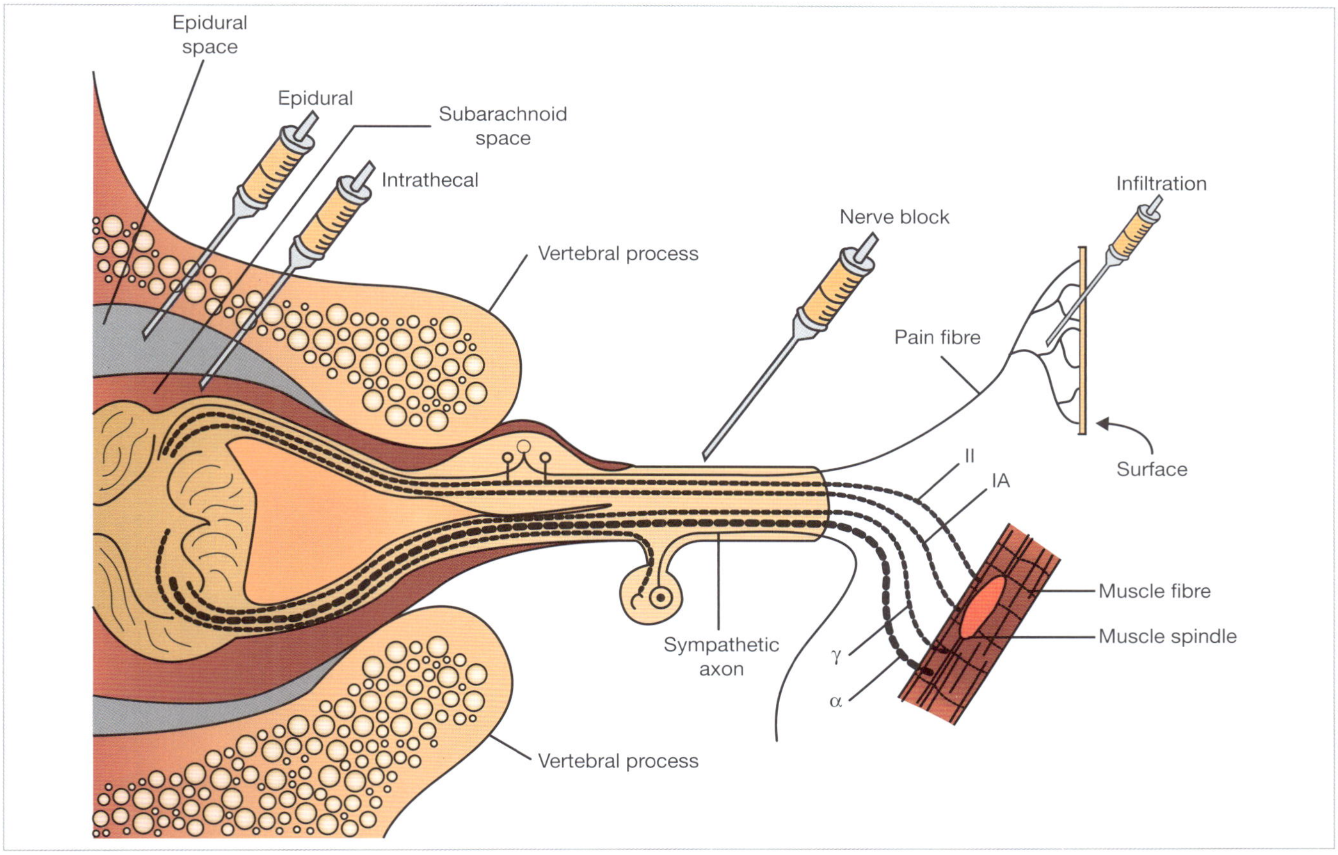

Epidural space

Epidural

Subarachnoid space

Intrathecal

Vertebral process

Nerve block

Infiltration

Pain fibre

II

IA

Surface

Muscle fibre

Muscle spindle

Sympathetic axon

γ

α

Vertebral process

FIGURE 8.7

Infiltration of perineum

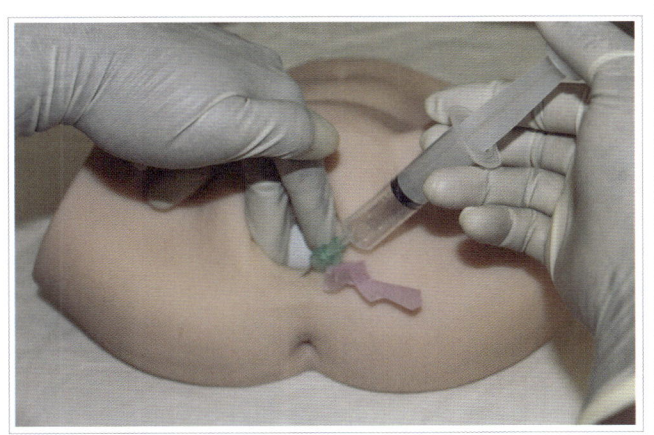

FIGURE 8.8

Source: With permission from Peri Health London.

techniques. Central nerve block is contraindicated if there is systemic anticoagulation, coagulation abnormality or raised intracranial pressure (e.g. low platelets from preeclampsia).

Midwives caring for women with epidural analgesia in labour should be experienced and competent and provide care in accordance with the facility's policy and guidelines. Women should be closely monitored.

Dermatome assessment

Dermatome assessment is used to monitor the level and extent of analgesia, using a standard dermatome chart (showing the areas of skin supplied with afferent nerve fibres by a single posterior root). Sensory block is assessed to ensure that the spinal/epidural/caudal LA is covering the patient's pain, and that the block is not so extensive as to cause complications. Since pain and temperature nerves are blocked similarly, reaction to temperature stimulation indicates that pain is still felt. Cold stimulation can be done with an ice-block on the skin,

Epidural and spinal anaesthesia

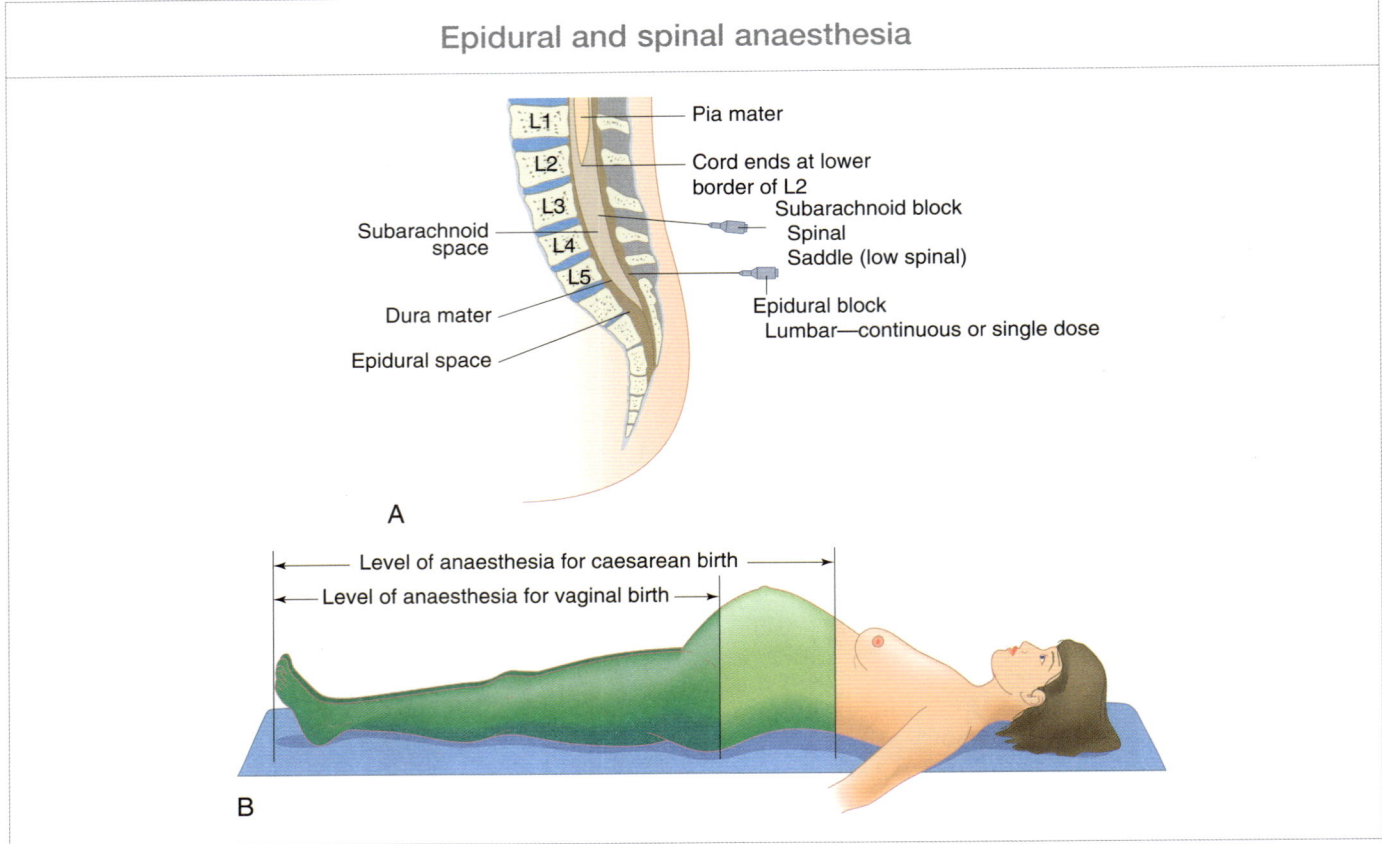

FIGURE 8.9 **A** The insertion sites for the needle in epidural, subarachnoid, and spinal blocks. **B** Levels of anaesthesia for vaginal birth compared with minimum level required for caesarean birth.

Source: Matteson PS. Women's health during the childbearing years: a community-based approach. Mosby; 2001.

starting with an area away from the area likely to be affected (e.g. face or forearm), then testing areas likely to be blocked, plus areas above and below, to establish the level of block on both sides of the body. Anaesthetised areas are indicated on a dermatome chart – for example, R: T8–L1; L: T10–L2.

Epidural (extradural) anaesthesia

An epidural is an injection of LA into the space between the dura mater and the ligamentum flavum, at spinal cord levels C7–T10. The 'space' is filled with loose adipose tissue, lymphatics, and blood vessels; LA solution tends to remain localised at the level where it is injected. The solution does not contact the spinal cord or CSF, so there is less risk of CNS infection than with spinal injection. The dose is determined by the number of spinal segments to be blocked. Postoperative urinary retention is common, due to blockade of parasympathetic nerves. To provide additional analgesia with epidural anaesthesia, ropivacaine 2 mg/mL is formulated with the opioid analgesic fentanyl (2 or 4 micrograms/mL). **Caudal** anaesthesia is an epidural procedure in which the anaesthetic solution is injected into the caudal canal,

the sacral part of the vertebral canal containing the cauda equina or the bundle of spinal nerves that innervate the pelvic viscera. It is used in obstetrics.

Patient controlled epidural analgesia

Patient controlled epidural analgesia (PCEA) is a method that enables the woman to control the administration of medication into the epidural catheter. The PCEA can be self-administered as a bolus and can be combined with a background infusion.

Central nerve block: Spinal (subarachnoid) anaesthesia

In spinal anaesthesia (also called subarachnoid, intradural or intrathecal block), the LA is injected into the CSF in the subarachnoid space, below the level of termination of the spinal cord (i.e. at L3–4 or L4–5) and affects the lower part of the spinal cord and nerve roots. As the needle and solution meet the CSF, sterility and aseptic procedures are essential to prevent infections such as meningitis. The effects of a spinal anaesthetics are more rapid than an epidural so can be used where fast-acting analgesia/anaesthesia is needed, such as for an emergency caesarean section. The onset of anaesthesia usually occurs within 1–2 minutes of injection; duration is 1–3 hours, depending on the anaesthetic used.

The specific gravity of the LA solution and the patient's position determine the level of anaesthesia: a solution with a specific gravity greater than that of CSF will tend to diffuse downward. The success and safety of spinal anaesthesia depend primarily on the anaesthetist's skill and knowledge.

Disadvantages of this method include marked hypotension, decreased cardiac output and respiratory depression due to depression of medullary centres and sympathetic pathways. Hypotension may be treated with sympathomimetic agents such as ephedrine or metaraminol. Postoperatively, headache is the most common complaint; it may be accompanied by difficulty in hearing or seeing or may be postural and occur only in certain positions. Headache may be due to the opening in the dura made by the large spinal needle; the opening may persist for days or weeks, permitting loss of CSF and risk of infection (meningitis). **Paraesthesias** such as numbness and tingling may occur, usually limited to the lumbar or sacral areas and disappearing within a relatively short time.

Combined spinal/epidural analgesia

A combined spinal epidural combines the rapid onset of analgesia/anaesthesia with the longer-term option of an epidural.

Adverse drug reactions

Because LAs are potentially toxic drugs, dosage must be determined carefully. Adverse reactions can occur quickly, so patients must never be left alone; equipment for resuscitation and airways management should be available. Most reactions to LAs result from overdosage, inadvertent IV administration, and rapid absorption into systemic circulation or individual hypersensitivity or allergic response.

Adverse reactions can be classified as:

- local complications at the site of injection – inflammation, haematoma, nerve injury, abscess formation, necrosis
- psychogenic reactions – hyperventilation or vasovagal syncope (fainting) secondary to the injection stress (these may occur even before injection)
- adverse drug reactions specific to the individual LA
- systemic effects of the vasoconstrictor – sympathetic or central stimulation
- local effects of the vasoconstrictor – ischaemia, necrosis, gangrene
- reactions specific to epidural and spinal LAs – headache, hypotension, infections, neuropathies, paraesthesias and autonomic dysfunction

- allergies and hypersensitivity reactions – rash, bronchospasm, **anaphylaxis** (more common with esters than **amides**; can also occur in response to preservatives in the solution)
- systemic effects of the LA after absorption – numbness of tongue, CNS stimulation (tremor, visual disturbances, irritability, convulsions, due to blockade of inhibitory pathways) then CNS depression, relaxation of smooth and skeletal muscle, cardiovascular and respiratory depression; hypotension and inhibition of sympathetic pathways contribute to the risk of fainting.

Adverse reactions may require treatment. For minor reactions, conservative resuscitation and first-aid efforts are effective. For major reactions, oxygen, assisted ventilation and IV infusion of fluids and drugs to counteract convulsions, cardiovascular and respiratory depression may be necessary. Accidental overdose with an LA may prove fatal due to cardiotoxicity leading to cardiac arrest resistant to the usual resuscitation measures. IV administration of a lipid emulsion (e.g. Intralipid, normally used to provide parenteral nutrition) is an effective antidote, acting as a 'lipid sink' absorbing excess LA and counteracting toxic effects on the myocardium.

Significant drug interactions

Significant drug interactions and unexpected responses can occur (Drug Interactions 8.2), so close observation is needed. Anaesthetics containing a vasoconstrictor are used with caution in patients receiving antihypertensives, monoamine oxidase inhibitors and tricyclic antidepressants, as the combination may produce hypertension.

8.8 General anaesthetic

For most instances during labour and birth an epidural or epidural/spinal is used if surgery is required; however, in rare circumstances (e.g. emergency caesarean birth, manual removal of a retained placenta or repair of extensive perineal trauma) a general anaesthetic may be indicated.

General anaesthetics are divided into two groups: (1) inhalation anaesthetics, which include gases and volatile liquids; and (2) intravenous (IV) general anaesthetics, such as thiopental and propofol. Early inhaled anaesthetics included ether and chloroform as volatile liquids, and cyclopropane and nitrous oxide as gases.

Inhalation anaesthetics

Inhalation anaesthetics are gases or volatile liquids that can be administered by inhalation when mixed with oxygen. These rapidly reach a concentration in the blood and brain sufficient to depress the CNS and cause anaesthesia,

DRUG INTERACTIONS 8.2
Local anaesthetics

DRUG OR DRUG GROUP	LIKELY EFFECTS AND MANAGEMENT
Drugs that depress the cardiovascular system, including phenytoin	Additive cardiovascular depressant effects if LA is significantly absorbed; use LA cautiously and monitor effects
Antihypertensive agents	Enhanced hypotension with epidural or spinal LA
Drugs that predispose to methaemoglobinaemia (sulfonamides, primaquine, sodium nitroprusside)	Exacerbate methaemoglobinaemia from prilocaine; use cautiously
Drugs that cause dysrhythmias or prolong QT interval	Effects exacerbated by LA; avoid combination
Ciprofloxacin, fluvoxamine	Increase concentration, duration of action and toxicity of ropivacaine; avoid prolonged administration of the LA
Cimetidine, erythromycin, fluvoxamine, itraconazole, metoprolol, propranolol	May inhibit metabolism of lidocaine (lignocaine) and/or increase its concentration (depends on route of LA administration); monitor for effects and toxicity and decrease LA dose if necessary
Suxamethonium	Lidocaine (lignocaine) IV may decrease plasma cholinesterase activity and prolong muscle relaxation; monitor respiratory function
Anticholinesterase drugs	May inhibit the metabolism of ester-type LAs (procaine, cocaine)

expressed as the minimum alveolar concentration (MAC) for anaesthesia, which is inversely related to potency and lipid solubility. MAC provides a correlation between anaesthetic dose and immobility. It is the MAC of inhaled anaesthetic at sea level required to suppress movement to a surgical incision in 50% of the patients. Inhalation anaesthetics have the following characteristics:

- They provide controllable anaesthesia, as depth of anaesthesia is readily varied by changing the inhaled concentration.
- As the route of administration (and most excretion) is via the airways, lung function is critical to effective use of inhaled agents.
- The agents are good anaesthetics and thus can abolish superficial and deep reflexes. However, they may not have useful analgesic actions, so they are used in combination with an adjunct analgesic such as an opioid.
- Rapid recovery can occur as soon as administration ceases because the anaesthetic is excreted in expired air.
- Allergic reactions to these agents are uncommon.

Volatile liquid anaesthetics

Volatile liquid anaesthetics now in use include safer analogues of the halogenated hydrocarbon series: desflurane, isoflurane and sevoflurane. Sevoflurane has become the drug of choice for most procedures owing to its fast action and low toxicity. Historically drugs such as ether or chloroform were originally administered by placing a pad soaked in the liquid over the patient's

mouth and nose, so that the fumes were inhaled. This unpleasant procedure caused struggling, skin reactions, uncertain levels of dosage and absorption and a slow progression through the stages of anaesthesia. The more civilised technique used now involves controlled vaporisation of the volatile liquid into a flow of gas (oxygen with or without nitrous oxide), so a known concentration of volatile agent in oxygen is administered via a mask or endotracheal tube. All volatile agents require the use of a vaporiser. Desflurane has a boiling point close to room temperature. This may result in a large variation in concentrations. A heated, temperature-controlled vaporiser is therefore required.

IV anaesthetic agents

IV anaesthetic agents are used for induction or maintenance of GA, for conscious sedation, to induce amnesia and as adjuncts to inhalation-type anaesthetics. The major groups are ultrashort-acting barbiturates (thiopental) and non-barbiturates (propofol) (Drug Monograph 8.7).

Advantages and disadvantages

Advantages of IV anaesthetics are that they:

- rapidly induce unconsciousness and suppress reflexes, allowing external control of airways
- are readily controllable
- have amnesic effects
- reduce the amount of inhalational agent required
- allow prompt recovery with minimal doses

DRUG MONOGRAPH 8.7
Propofol

This white emulsion is fondly referred to as 'milk of amnesia' by anaesthetists.

Propofol is a rapidly acting, non-barbiturate hypnotic with no analgesic effects. It is formulated in an emulsion for IV injection or infusion and can be used for TIVA.

Mechanism of action

Its CNS depression is probably mediated through GABA receptors. It may also shorten channel opening times at nicotinic receptors and sodium channels in the CNS.

Indications

Propofol is used for the induction and maintenance of GA.

Pharmacokinetics

Propofol has a rapid onset of action within 30 seconds and duration of effect of only 3–5 minutes, owing to rapid redistribution from the brain to other tissues; hence, there is a short recovery period and few hangover effects. It is almost completely metabolised to the glucuronide, with a long terminal elimination half-life of 3–8 hours.

Adverse effects

Propofol is a respiratory and cardiac depressant and can produce apnoea, bradycardia and hypotension, depending on dose, rate of administration and drugs concurrently administered. Pain on injection, nausea, vomiting and involuntary muscle movement are commonly reported.

Drug interactions

Sedative and bradycardic effects of other drugs are increased. Bradycardia and cardiac arrest may occur after treatment with suxamethonium and neostigmine; the emulsion is physically incompatible with atracurium or mivacurium.

Warnings and contraindications

Raised intracranial pressure can occur; there is potential for abuse. Respiratory depression is prolonged in those with muscular disorders, and may affect the fetus or neonate if used on pregnant women (Category C).

Propofol infusion syndrome is a rare syndrome affecting patients receiving high doses over a long period. One or more of rhabdomyolysis, metabolic acidosis and cardiac and kidney failure may occur.

IV induction dose for propofol is by slow bolus injection or infusion is usually 2–2.5 mg/kg. Dosage regimen for adults is 4–12 mg/kg/hour as required.

- are simple to administer and provide pleasant induction (most patients prefer an IV line to a mask)
- do not pose a hazard of fire or explosion. Disadvantages of IV anaesthetics are that they:
- have high lipid solubility such that they can cross the placenta and affect the fetus
- have minimal muscle relaxation and analgesic effects
- are subject to elimination by hepatic metabolism and renal excretion
- commonly cause hypersensitivity reactions (to drug or vehicle)
- cause tissue irritation if drug or vehicle infiltrates tissue or if arterial injection occurs
- cause hypotension, laryngospasm and respiratory failure after overdosage or prolonged administration.

Pharmacokinetics

IV anaesthetics are rapidly taken up by brain tissue because of their high lipid solubility. Equilibrium between brain and blood levels occurs within one arm–brain circulation time (patients asked to count backwards from 10 as the agent is injected rarely reach 4 or 3). Short action results from the drug being quickly redistributed into the fat depots of the body; due to two-compartment distribution of the drug, the greater the amount of body fat, the briefer the effect of a single IV dose. With prolonged administration or large doses, however, saturation of fat depots leads to prolonged drug action and delayed recovery as drug is slowly released back into the circulation to be eliminated (10–15% per hour).

Pharmaceutics

IV anaesthetic agents present an interesting pharmaceutical formulation problem: an IV anaesthetic agent must be highly lipid soluble (to cross the blood–brain barrier and act) yet sufficiently water-soluble to be formulated as a solution that can be safely injected IV. This problem has been solved for some drugs with very low water solubilities by formulating them as oil-in-water emulsions (like milk) – for example, diazepam or propofol in a soya oil/egg lecithin/glycerol emulsion.

Ultrashort-acting barbiturates

The prototype ultrashort-acting barbiturate-type agent is thiopental (also known as thiopentone), a CNS depressant that potentiates the inhibitory transmitter GABA and thus produces hypnosis and anaesthesia without analgesia. GA with ultrashort-acting barbiturates is believed to result from suppression of the RAS, with respiratory and cardiovascular depression. Thiopental is often combined with a muscle relaxant and analgesic in balanced anaesthesia. Being very lipid soluble, it has a rapid action, then short duration due to redistribution mainly to muscle tissues. Thiopental also has anticonvulsant effects and reduces intracranial pressure; it is particularly useful in emergency anaesthesia.

The most common adverse effects post anaesthetic are shivering and trembling, and other CNS depressants effects such as nausea, vomiting, drowsiness and headache. Serious adverse reactions include emergence delirium (increased excitability, confusion and hallucinations), cardiac dysrhythmias or depression, allergic responses, bronchospasm and respiratory depression.

Because CNS-active drugs are lipid soluble, they are likely to cross the placenta and reach significant levels in the fetal bloodstream or be secreted in the milk of lactating mothers; expected drug benefits should be considered against the possible risk to the fetus. General anaesthetics, LAs, analgesics and **sedatives** must be dosed and monitored carefully if used during pregnancy, and fetal wellbeing must be closely monitored post-surgery.

KEY POINTS

Clinical aspects of general anaesthetic use

- Most patients will be administered a maintenance anaesthetic by inhalation, so the first rule of anaesthesiology is to keep a clear airway.

- To maintain a reliable airway, most patients will be intubated. A dose of a skeletal muscle relaxant is normally administered to facilitate intubation.

- Supraglottic airway devices, including the laryngeal mask airway, are used to keep the upper airway open to provide unobstructed ventilation.

- Balanced anaesthesia is the use of a combination of agents to achieve unconsciousness, analgesia, muscle relaxation and amnesia.

- Premedication may include an antianxiety agent (e.g. midazolam) and atropine to suppress secretions. Adjuncts to anaesthesia include depolarising and non-depolarising NM blockers. Antiemetics and opioids are used for postoperative nausea and pain.

- Common adverse effects and drug interactions are the potentiation of CNS depression and the risk of malignant hyperthermia from suxamethonium plus a general anaesthetic.

- As many disease states and risk factors can alter a person's response to anaesthesia, preoperative assessment of the patient's health status should be undertaken. Factors such as age, concurrent disease states, medications, lifestyle factors and possibility of pregnancy should be taken into consideration.

- Postoperative care includes the administration of antiemetics for nausea and vomiting, opioid analgesics and NSAIDs for pain, and aspirin to prevent postoperative thrombosis.

CONCLUSION

This chapter provides an overview of the drugs a midwife may encounter when providing care for a woman during labour and birth, including the immediate post-birth period. Essential knowledge of key drug groups involved in induction and augmentation of labour, and active management of placental birth and postpartum haemorrhage, including a range of pharmacological pain options available for labour and birth have been covered. Aspects of CAM have been included. It is important midwives have a sound understanding of the indications, contraindications, and potential interactions for the use of the drugs and CAMs covered in this chapter. This knowledge must encompass an understanding of the effects and side effects of drugs and CAM on the woman and baby, and includes responsibility for midwifery practice and care provision for both, in accordance with relevant evidence-based clinical guidelines.

REVIEW EXERCISES

1 What drugs are used in an induction of labour? When are they contraindicated?

2 What drugs are available to aid the birth of the placenta?

3 What are the dosages and route of administration for each drug in Q1 and Q2?

4 Describe the side effects and potential for other drug interactions.

5 What are the benefits and disadvantages for use of each drug in Q1 and Q2?

6 What are the differences between an epidural and combined spinal/epidural? What circumstances would one be more beneficial than the other?

7 Describe how dinoprostone works to induce labour.

8 Nitrous oxide is commonly used during labour and birth. What type of drug is it, how is it used, and what are the common side effects of using nitrous oxide during labour and birth?

REFERENCES

Almassinokiani F, Ahani N, Akbari P, et al. Comparative analgesic effects of intradermal and subdermal injection of sterile water on active labor pain. Anesth Pain Med. 2020 Apr 25;10(2):e99867. doi: 10.5812/aapm.99867

Ananthram H, Rane A. Head in the sand: contemporary Australian attitudes towards induction of labour. Aust N Z J Obstet Gynaecol. 2022;62:483–486. doi: 10.1111/ajo.13512

Australian Institute of Health and Welfare. Australia's mothers and babies report 2021. https://www.aihw.gov.au/reports/mothers-babies/australias-mothers-babies/contents/summary (accessed 21 August 2023)

Bahasadri S, Ahmadi-Abhari S, Dehghani-Nik M, et al. Subcutaneous sterile water injection for labour pain: a randomised controlled trial. Aust N Z J Obstet Gynaecol. 2006;46(2):102–106.

Baysinger CL. Inhaled nitrous oxide analgesia for labor. Curr Anesthesiol Rep. 2019;9:69–75. https://doi.org/10.1007/s40140-019-00313-4

Brandlistuen RE, Ystrom E, Nulman I. Prenatal paracetamol exposure and child neurodevelopment: a sibling-controlled cohort study. Int J Epidemiol. 2013;42:1702–1713.

Brenner A, Ker K, Shakur-Still H, et al. Tranexamic acid for post-partum haemorrhage: what, who and when. Best Pract Res Clin Obstet Gynaecol. 2019 Nov;61:66-74. doi: 10.1016/j.bpobgyn.2019.04.005. Epub 2019 Apr 30. PMID: 31128974; PMCID: PMC6891248.

Brimdyr K, Cadwell K, Widstrom A-M, et al. The association between common labor drugs and suckling when skin-to-skin during the first hour after birth. Birth (Berkeley, Calif). 2015;42(4):319–328.

Brune K, Renner B, Tiegs G. Acetaminophen/paracetamol: a history of errors, failures and false decisions. Eur J Pain. 2015 Aug;19(7):953-965. doi: 10.1002/ejp.621. Epub 2014 Nov 27. PMID: 25429980.

Buckley S. Hormonal physiology of childbearing: evidence and implications for women, babies, and maternity care. Washington DC: Childbirth Connection Programs; National Partnership for Women and Families; 2015. http://refhub.elsevier.com/S1521-6934(20)30033-X/sref19 (accessed 21 August 2023)

Dixon L, Skinner V, Foureur M. Women's perspectives of the stages of labour. Midwifery. 2013;29:10-17. http://refhub.elsevier.com/S1521-6934(20)30033-X/sref35 (accessed 21 August 2023)

Fouly H, Herdan R, Habib D, et al. Effectiveness of injecting lower dose subcutaneous sterile water versus saline to relief labor back pain: randomized controlled trial. Eur J Midwifery. 2018 Mar 14;2:3. doi: 10.18332/ejm/85793. PMID: 33537564; PMCID: PMC7848597.

Gill P, Lende MN, Van Hook JW. Induction of labor. [Updated 2023 Feb 20]. In: StatPearls [Internet]. Treasure Island (FL): StatPearls Publishing; 2024 Jan-. Available from: https://www.ncbi.nlm.nih.gov/books/NBK459264/ (accessed 13 March 2024)

Hundley V, Downe S, Buckley S. The initiation of labour at term gestation: physiology and practice implications. Best Pract Res Clin Obst Gynaecol. 2020;67:4-18. https://doi.org/10.1016/j.bpobgyn.2020.02.006 (accessed 21 August 2023)

Jonas et al (2008). Effects of opioids on mothers during and post birth. In, Conaboy C, (2022) Mother brain: separating myth from biology – the science of the parental brain. London: Blackwell 2022.

Jensen MS, Rebordosa C, Thulstrup AM, et al. Maternal use of acetaminophen, ibuprofen, and acetylsalicylic acid during pregnancy and risk of cryptorchidism. Epidemiol. 2020; 21(6):779–785. doi: 10.1097/EDE.0b013e3181f20bed

Klomp T, van Poppel M, Jones L, et al. Inhaled analgesia for pain management in labour. Cochrane Database Syst Rev. 2012;(9):CD009351 (accessed 14 March 2024)

Lee N, Webster J, Beckmann M, et al. Comparison of a single vs a four intradermal sterile water injection for relief of lower back pain for women in labour: a randomised controlled trial. Midwifery. 2013;29:585-591. doi: 10.1016/j.midw.2012.05.001. Epub 2012 Jul 7.

Lee N, Gao Y, Collins SL, et al. Caesarean delivery rates and analgesia effectiveness following injections of sterile water for back pain in labour: a multicentre, randomised placebo controlled trial. EClinicalMedicine. 2020;25:100447. doi: 10.1016/j.eclinm.2020.100447

Lee N, Leiser B, Halter-Wehrli MS, et al. Two versus four sterile water injections for managing back pain in labour. Women and Birth. 2022;35:8. doi:10.1016/j.wombi.2022.07.023

Liew Z, Ritz B, Rebordosa C, et al. Acetaminophen use during pregnancy, behavioral problems, and hyperkinetic disorders. JAMA Pediatr. 2014;168:313-320. doi: 10.1001/jamapediatrics.2013.4914

Likis FE, Andrews JC, Collins MR, et al. Nitrous oxide for the management of labor pain: a systematic review. Anesth Analg. 2014;118(1):153-167. doi: 10.1213/ANE.0b013e3182a7f73c

Mårtensson LB, Gunnarsson BM, Karlsson S, et al. Effect of topical local anaesthesia on injection pain associated with administration of sterile water injections – a randomized controlled trial. BMC Anesthesiol. 2022;22(35). doi.org/10.1186/s12871-022-01573-0

Mårtensson LB, Wallin G. Sterile water injections as treatment for low-back pain during labour: a review. Aust N Z J Obstet Gynaecol. 2008;48:369-374. doi:10.1111/j.1479-828X.2008.00856.x

Mårtensson LB, Hutton EK, Lee N, et al. Sterile water injections for childbirth pain: an evidenced based guide to practice. Women and Birth. 2017;31(5):380-385. doi: 10.1016/j.wombi.2017.12.001

Mielke RT, Obermeyer S. The use of tranexamic acid to prevent postpartum hemorrhage. J Midwifery Women's Health. 2020 May;65(3):410-416. doi: 10.1111/jmwh.13101.

Neczypor JL, Holley SL. Providing evidence-based care during the golden hour. Nurs Womens Health. 2017;21(6):462–472.

New Zealand Ministry of Health (2023). Maternity and newborn data and stats. https://www.health.govt.nz/nz-health-statistics/health-statistics-and-data-sets/maternity-and-newborn-data-and-stats

Smith P, Papadopoulou WR, Thomas A, et al. Uterotonic agents for first-line treatment of postpartum haemorrhage: a network meta-analysis. Cochrane Database Syst Rev. 2020 Nov 24;11(11):CD012754. doi.org//10.1002/14651858.CD012754.pub2

Pierce S, Bakker R, Myers DA, et al. Clinical insights for cervical ripening and labor induction using prostaglandins. AJP Rep. 2018 Oct;8(4):e307-e314. doi: 10.1055/s-0038-1675351. Epub 2018 Oct 29. PMID: 30377555; PMCID: PMC6205862. (accessed 14 March 2024)

Snijder CA, Kortenkamp A, Steegers EA, et al. Intrauterine exposure to mild analgesics during pregnancy and the occurrence of cryptorchidism and hypospadias in the offspring: the generation R study. Hum Reprod. 2012;27:1191–1201. doi: 10.1093/humrep/der474. Epub 2012 Feb 2.

Thomson G, Feeley C, Moran VH, et al. Women's experiences of pharmacological and non-pharmacological pain relief methods for labour and childbirth: a qualitative systematic review. Reprod Health. 2019;16:71. https://doi.org/10.1186/s12978-019-0735-4

Tiran D. Complementary therapies for pregnancy and childbirth, 2nd edn, Elsevier, 2000.

Turpin G, Ritmejerytė E, Jamie J, et al. Aboriginal medicinal plants of Queensland: ethnopharmacological uses, species diversity, and biodiscovery pathways. J Ethnobiol Ethnomed. 2022 Aug 10;18(1):54. doi: 10.1186/s13002-022-00552-6. PMID: 35948982; PMCID: PMC9364609.

Uvnas-Moberg K, Ekstrom-Bergstrom A, Berg M, et al. Maternal plasma levels of oxytocin during physiological childbirth – a systematic review with implications for uterine contractions and central actions of oxytocin. BMC Pregnancy Childbirth. 2019 Aug 9;19(1):285. http://refhub.elsevier.com/S1521-6934(20)30033-X/sref23

Van den Anker J. Neonatal effects of drugs administered during pregnancy, chapter 4.7. In, Jacqz-Aigrain E, Choonara I (eds), Paediatric clinical pharmacology. Boca Raton: CRC Press, 2021. https://doi.org/10.1201/9780367800666

WHO recommendation on tocolytic therapy for improving preterm birth outcomes. Geneva: WHO, 2022. Licence: CC BY-NC-SA 3.0 IGO. https://www.ncbi.nlm.nih.gov/books/NBK585023/pdf/Bookshelf_NBK585023.pdf (accessed 21 August 2023)

Zamawe C, King C, Jennings HM, et al. Effectiveness and safety of herbal medicines for induction of labour: a systematic review and meta-analysis. BMJ Open. 2018;8:e022499. doi: 10.1136/bmjopen-2018-022499

ONLINE RESOURCES

Australian Institute of Health and Welfare. Australia's mothers and babies report 2021 – Analgesia: https://www.aihw.gov.au/reports/mothers-babies/australias-mothers-babies/contents/labour-and-birth/analgesia

Australian Medicines Handbook 2024: https://amhonline.amh.net.au/auth (accessed 11 March 2024)

Australian Indigenous Health InfoNet, Bush medicines: https://healthinfonet.ecu.edu.au/key-resources/resources/32414/?title=Noongar+bush+medicine++medicinal+plants+of+the+south+west+of+Western+Australia&contentid=32414_1

International Federation of Gynecology and Obstetrics, International Confederation of Midwives. Guidance on the use of heat-stable carbetocin as an alternative to oxytocin in the prevention of postpartum haemorrhage. 2023: https://www.figo.org/sites/default/files/2023-03/FIGO-ICM%20Statement_Heat-stable%20carbetocin_EN.pdf (accessed 14 March 2024)

RANZCOG. Clinical Guidelines for Abortion Care 2024: https://ranzcog.edu.au/resources/abortion-guideline/ (accessed 14 March 2024)

SA Health Analgesia for Labour and Birth (Pharmacological) 2020: https://www.sahealth.sa.gov.au/wps/wcm/connect/052c4527-f3dd-4a18-809d-9d948302cdc9/Analgesia+for+Labour+and+Birth+%28Pharmacological%29_PPG_v1_1.pdf?MOD=AJPERES&CACHEID=ROOTWORKSPACE-052c4527-f3dd-4a18-809d-9d948302cdc9-obo-O6v

CHAPTER 9

THE POSTNATAL PERIOD

Clare Davison, Roslyn Donnellan-Fernandez

Key Abbreviations

BMD	bone mass density
CAM	complementary and alternative medicine
COC	combined oral contraceptive
COX	cyclo-oxygenase
EMA	early medical abortion
LARC	long-acting reversible contraceptive
NSAID	non-steroidal anti-inflammatory drug
OTC	over the counter
PG	prostaglandin
POP	progesterone-only oral contraceptive
STI	sexually transmitted infection
IUD	intrauterine device
VTE	venous thromboembolism

Key Terms

analgesia 160
barrier method 176
contraception 164
contraceptive 164
emergency
contraception 173
natural family
planning 176
perineal trauma 160
postnatal 160
postpartum 160
rhythm method 176
termination 173
vasectomy 176
vasovasostomy 176

Chapter Focus

This chapter focuses on the postnatal period (also referred to as the puerperium or postpartum period) and care of the new mother within the first few weeks following birth. The postnatal period refers to the 6–8 weeks following the birth of the baby. This is the time for many changes, physical and psychological, as the woman's body adapts following the birth. While postpartum recovery is a normal and generally healthy phase of the continuum of childbearing for a woman, some may also experience the onset of other health challenges or chronic illness, physical and/or psychological, for the first time.

This chapter is divided into sections related to the most common reasons for the woman to require pharmaceutical support, including contraception. Many of the medications have been discussed in previous chapters, so these are cross-referenced to the relevant chapters.

Key Drug Groups

Analgesics:

- over-the-counter medications; paracetamol, NSAIDs (ibuprofen, naproxen, diclofenac, celecoxib)
- opioids; morphine, tramadol. (Opioids are discussed in detail in Chapter 8.)

Antibiotics:

- amoxicillin with clavulanic acid, cefalexin and metronidazole. (Antibiotics are discussed in detail in Chapter 12.)

Contraceptives:

- hormonal contraceptives; estrogen (EE), mestranol or estradiol
- synthetic progestogens; norethisterone, levonorgestrel, ulipristal acetate, medroxyprogesterone acetate

Learning Outcomes

- Identify the different medications commonly used during the postnatal period, including indications for their use.
- Outline your approach and rationale for conducting a comprehensive medication history and review with a woman postnatally, following hospital discharge.
- Describe the action and effects of hormonal contraceptives.
- Discuss the most suitable type of contraceptives for the postnatal woman's individual circumstances, including breastfeeding women.
- Identify some of the CAM products commonly used by women in the postnatal period and discuss potential interactions with other prescription drugs the woman may be taking, including the implications of these interactions and possible side effects.

CRITICAL THINKING SCENARIO

Jasmine gave birth via caesarean section to her first baby, Poppy, 4 weeks ago. Jasmine is exclusively breastfeeding and coping well with Poppy and the transition to parenting. During your postnatal visit Jasmine states she does not want to take the pill as she has heard it is not suitable for use during breastfeeding, but she does not want to have another baby for at least 3 years. Jasmine confides there have been challenging conversations with her partner in the past in relation to mode of contraception preferences, and it is important for her to get this issue sorted out as early as possible with assistance from supportive health professionals.

1   What advice and information can you provide Jasmine in relation to contraceptives that are suitable for use while breastfeeding? What other health information and history might you also want to collect from Jasmine at this point regarding her consideration of suitable contraceptive options?

2   What choice does Jasmine have in relation to contraception?

3   What specific educational components or other considerations might be relevant to Jasmine's situation and options that her midwife should cover during this consultation?

Introduction

In the early **postnatal** period, the first 10–14 days, there are many hormonal changes taking place as the body's systems revert to the pre-pregnancy state and make the physiological adaptions to support lactation. The postnatal period is a time for the reproductive organs to heal and regain their shape and structure, and for the body's other systems to transition to their pre-pregnancy state. Recovery and care required will depend on many factors such as the woman's health pre-pregnancy, during pregnancy, the type of birth, and whether she has any preexisting medical conditions or **postpartum** risks or complications, including psycho-social aspects that need to be considered. This care should encompass a comprehensive medication review, as many relevant studies indicate that up to 50% of postnatal women are taking at least one medicine during this period (Saha et al 2015). The midwife should always ensure that a full case history is taken and all aspects of postnatal care are discussed with the woman, including mental health, as this is a particularly vulnerable time for many women and the care received during this time can impact the person's long-term health.

9.1 Analgesia

The management of postpartum pain is extremely important. There are multiple reasons for **analgesia** in the postnatal period. Women recovering from caesarean section will require analgesia due to the impact of surgery. For some women, the contractions caused by the involution of the uterus result in pain, often referred to as 'afterpains'. These sensations are usually felt after the birth of the placenta, at their most intense between 12–24 hours postpartum, and usually resolve by the end of the first week. The afterpains are generally more intense during breastfeeding and can be experienced as severe pain, complicated by nausea and vomiting in multi-gravid women. Non-pharmacological pain relief such as heat packs can help, but for some women the afterpains are as painful and intense as labour pain and pharmacological pain relief may be needed. Some women may also choose to incorporate CAM therapies including herbal tinctures for management of afterbirth pains, for example, *Arnica montana* (arnica), *Bellis perennis* or *Viburnum opulus* (aptly known as 'cramp bark'). **Perineal trauma** and bruising are another indication for pain relief. Perineal pain can make sitting very uncomfortable, and this can impact breastfeeding in the early days following birth. Movement can also be difficult due to pain, and everyday activities such as going to the toilet, standing, walking and caring for the baby and herself can be challenging, leading to a detrimental effect on the woman's postnatal recovery and experience. The woman is now able to take pharmacological pain medication without worrying about harming the fetus. However, if the woman is breastfeeding caution will be needed. Some medications, especially opioids, are contraindicated and unsuitable for use when breastfeeding due to their transfer in breast milk; the transferred effects include sedation and central nervous system depression in the breastfeeding infant (see Chapter 10).

There are several types of analgesic medications that can be used in the postnatal period, including drugs that are safe during breastfeeding. Analgesic medications are discussed in more detail in Chapter 8. The following section will briefly highlight different types of analgesia use in the postnatal period, from over-the-counter preparations to prescription-only medications.

Women are often directed to use 'simple' analgesia for postnatal pain. The most used are paracetamol and non-steroidal anti-inflammatory drugs (NSAIDs).

Paracetamol

As discussed in Chapter 8, paracetamol is generally believed to be a safe over-the-counter (OTC) analgesic. Adverse drug interactions, adverse effects and allergic reactions are rare with therapeutic doses. Oral paracetamol is rapidly absorbed, with bioavailability approximately 90%, reaching peak serum levels in 15–60 minutes and its elimination half-life is 1–3 hours.

Paracetamol is available in multiple formats: tablets, capsules, chewable tablets, elixirs, suppositories and as an injection. The recommended adult dose of paracetamol is 1 g (usually administered in two 500 mg tablets or capsules) 4–6-hourly. There are also controlled-release options available of 665 mg per tablet which lasts for 8 hours. The maximum daily dose of paracetamol is 4 g. (See Chapter 8.)

Non-steroidal anti-inflammatory drugs (NSAIDs)

Non-steroidal anti-inflammatory drugs are one of the most used groups of drugs worldwide. Generally, NSAIDs are either prescribed or purchased over the counter for their analgesic, anti-inflammatory and antipyretic properties. NSAIDs are used for treatment of mild-to-moderate pain and inflammation. All the NSAIDs possess the same therapeutic properties – analgesic, antipyretic and anti-inflammatory effects. Unfortunately, they share to varying degrees the same adverse reactions. This is because inhibition of prostaglandin (PG) synthesis, which accounts for all the therapeutic effects (e.g. antipyretic/anti-inflammatory), also accounts for the adverse renal and gastrointestinal effects.

A recent Cochrane review found that NSAIDs appear to be the most effective analgesia for treating women experiencing pain postpartum from uterine cramping and involution after vaginal birth. Paracetamol may be a possible alternative where the use of NSAIDs is not appropriate, but it can also be used in addition to NSAIDs. Opioids may be more effective than placebo, but with more adverse effects. Unfortunately, 11 out of the 28 studies that were included in this review excluded breastfeeding mothers, making the evidence less generalisable to a broader group of women (Deussen et al 2020). Opioids are unsuitable for breastfeeding mothers as they can cause infant drowsiness which may progress to severe central nervous system depression (see Online resources: LactMed 2024 and Chapter 10).

Cyclo-oxygenase enzymes and prostaglandin synthesis

Cyclo-oxygenase (COX) catalyses the oxygenation of arachidonic acid, which is a 20-carbon fatty acid esterified to phospholipids of cell membranes. Arachidonic acid is released from the cell membrane by a variety of physical, chemical and hormonal stimuli through the action of acylhydrolases, principally phospholipase A2. Once released, arachidonic acid is metabolised principally to prostaglandins (PGs) and LTs. At the time, this single enzyme was thought to be responsible for the synthesis of all PGs, which fall into several main classes, designated by letters and distinguished by substitutions on the cyclopentane ring (e.g. PGE 1, PGE2, PGI2).

PGs are synthesised by most cells in the body and bind to several PG receptors. PGE2 is the main PG that contributes to inflammatory erythema and pain. It does not cause pain directly but appears to potentiate the pain induced by mediators such as bradykininase or histamine by sensitising nociceptors on sensory nerve terminals to painful stimulation. This property of hyperalgesia is also shared by PGI2. PGE2 also causes fever. Following its release by inflammatory mediators from endothelial cells in blood vessels of the hypothalamus, PGE2 binds to EP3 receptors in a specialised region of the hypothalamus, interfering with temperature control and thus producing a pyretic effect. In the kidney, PGE2 and PGI2 play an important role in maintaining glomerular filtration, acting as vasodilators increasing renal blood flow, inhibiting sodium reabsorption and stimulating renin release. Within the GI tract, PGE2 (acting on EP3 receptors) and PGI2 (acting on prostacyclin receptors) reduce the secretion of gastric acid and, through a vasodilator action, increase gastric mucosal blood flow. In addition, PGE2 stimulates production of a viscous mucus that plays a major role in protecting the gastric mucosa against gastric acid-induced damage. By 1990, a second COX enzyme (COX-2) had been identified. It was soon established that COX-1 (the original enzyme identified) is expressed in most tissues and catalyses the synthesis of protective mucosal PGs in the GI tract and vasodilatory PGs in the kidneys. COX-2 is constitutively expressed in many tissues – for example, brain, kidney, placenta and GI tract (often at low levels) – and is upregulated in cancer tissues and by inflammatory cytokines, laminar shear stress and various growth factors.

NSAIDs have significant anti-inflammatory actions which lead to an analgesic effect. NSAIDs inhibit the synthesis of prostaglandin by blocking the activity of the COX enzyme. COX inhibitors also lower body temperatures as they block prostaglandin synthesis in the hypothalamus, the temperature-regulating centre of the body. Many NSAIDs, therefore, can be used as an anti-inflammatory, analgesic and antipyretic, making them a very useful medication in the postnatal period. NSAIDs are effective for mild-to-moderate pain. They have useful opioid-sparing effects, allowing reduction of opioid dosage when combined with opioid analgesics in people with moderate pain.

Mechanism of action

Aspirin and the older NSAIDs (e.g. the -profens) inhibit both COX-1 and COX-2 and it was thought at the time that inhibition of COX-2 accounted for the anti-inflammatory actions of NSAIDs, whereas inhibition of COX-1 explained the GI and renal toxicity. This led to the search for drugs that would inhibit COX-2 selectively (the -coxibs).

NSAIDs in current clinical use non-selectively inhibit both COX-1 and COX-2. In addition to inhibition of COX, the non-selective NSAIDs also reduce synthesis of superoxide radicals, inhibit expression of adhesion molecules, reduce the activity of nitric oxide synthase, induce apoptosis, modify lymphocyte activity and cell membrane function, and decrease activity of proinflammatory cytokines. All these actions may contribute variously to the anti-inflammatory action of NSAIDs, but this remains to be established. In general, by interfering with PG synthesis, NSAIDs tend to reduce the inflammatory process and ultimately provide pain relief. Some NSAIDs are available OTC, and the differences between the prescription and OTC NSAIDs are usually in the strengths of the products and the indications for which they are recommended.

Pharmacokinetics

Oral absorption of these drugs is very good. Although eating prior to taking this medication may delay absorption, due to the adverse effects on the GI tract it is usually recommended that NSAIDs are taken with food. Plasma protein binding is high and most of these drugs are metabolised to varying degrees by the liver and the metabolites excreted by the kidneys.

The main NSAIDs used in the postnatal period are ibuprofen, naproxen and diclofenac. More recently the COX-2 inhibitor celecoxib (Celebrex) has been used with good effect.

NSAID dosage and administration

- Ibuprofen:
  ○ oral 200–400 mg 3–4 times a day (6-hourly). Up to 2400 mg daily may be used short term
- Diclofenac:
  ○ oral 75–150 mg daily in two or three doses. Maximum 200 mg
  ○ per rectum 75–150 mg suppositories in two or three doses. Maximum of 200 mg a day
- Naproxen:
  ○ oral conventional tablet: 250–500 mg twice daily
  ○ controlled-release tablet: oral 750–1000 mg once daily
  ○ maximum 1250 mg daily
- Celecoxib:
  ○ oral 400 mg as a single dose on the first day, then 200 mg once or twice daily if needed. Maximum 5 days treatment.

Common side effects

The most common adverse reaction for NSAID use is gastrointestinal irritation; therefore, these medications should never be taken on an empty stomach.

- Common (> 1%):
  ○ nausea, dyspepsia, GI ulceration or bleeding, raised liver enzymes (especially diclofenac), diarrhoea, headache, dizziness, salt and fluid retention, hypertension
- Infrequent (0.1–1%):
  ○ oesophageal ulceration, rectal irritation (with suppositories), heart failure, hyperkalaemia, renal impairment, confusion, bronchospasm, rash
- Rare (< 0.1%):
  ○ blood dyscrasias, interstitial nephritis, cystitis, nephrotic syndrome, acute renal failure, papillary necrosis, MI (infrequent with diclofenac), stroke, hepatitis, aseptic meningitis, tinnitus, photosensitivity, severe skin reactions (e.g. Stevens-Johnson syndrome, toxic epidermal necrolysis), hypersensitivity (e.g. anaphylaxis, asthma, angioedema, urticaria)

(Australian Medicines Handbook 2024)

Opioids

Opioids are recognised as the strongest analgesic available for acute severe pain. The use of opioids is limited to the lowest dose for the shortest duration of use. Opioids are covered in extensive detail in Chapter 8.

Codeine

Prior to early 2018, many women were advised to take medicines containing codeine in the postnatal period. Codeine is often combined with a non-opioid analgesic such as aspirin, paracetamol, or ibuprofen in compound analgesic tablets to provide stronger relief than the NSAID alone can achieve; however, misuse of combination products can lead to toxicity. Codeine, the 3-methyl ether of morphine, is a prodrug, being rapidly metabolised in most people to morphine (by CYP2D6). Inter-individual variation in pharmacokinetics leads to variable effectiveness, so codeine is not generally recommended. Constipation is a frequent adverse effect and may limit clinical usefulness. Therefore, it is no longer recommended in the postnatal period.

KEY POINTS

Analgesia

- The control of pain in the postnatal period is an important and essential part of midwifery care. There are multiple reasons that women may require analgesia in the postnatal period, from involution pain to postoperative pain.

- The main types of pharmacological analgesia used in the postnatal period are simple analgesics such as paracetamol, NSAIDs, and opioids.

- Opioids are recognised as the strongest analgesic available for acute severe pain. The use of opioids is limited to the lowest dose for the shortest duration of use.

- The choice of analgesia will depend on the woman's history, clinical picture and severity of pain, and should be made in consultation with the woman.

9.2 Infection, bladder and bowel care

Perineal trauma and repair

If perineal trauma occurs during the birth, it should be inspected thoroughly by the midwife and the extent of the trauma should be explained to the woman. The decision to repair the trauma or not is beyond the scope of this text. However, if the woman decides she would like her perineum repaired, adequate analgesia will be required. If the woman already has an epidural in place this should provide adequate cover. For women without epidurals local anaesthetic will be required prior to repair. The most common anaesthetic used for infiltration of the perineum is lignocaine (0.5% or 1% with or without adrenaline). Adrenaline will constrict the blood vessels, reduce bleeding, and allow greater visibility of the wound. The maximum dose is 200 mg (20 mL). For most repairs 70–100 mg of 1% lignocaine is adequate (7–10 mL). However, the longer acting bupivacaine may be used for more extensive repairs. Local anaesthetics are discussed in more detail in Chapter 8.

Prophylactic antibiotics

Prophylactic antibiotic therapy is generally recommended following severe perineal trauma repair (third- or fourth-degree tear) due to the increased risk of infection. Recommended antibiotics include amoxicillin with clavulanic acid:

- oral, 500–875 mg every 12 hours for 5 days, or
- IV, 1 g every 8 hours. Maximum dose 2 g.

If the woman is allergic to penicillins, use cefalexin 500 mg orally, 6-hourly for 5 days and metronidazole 400 mg orally, 12-hourly for 5 days.
Antibiotics are discussed in Chapter 12.

Wound infection

The woman is at risk of developing an infection in the postnatal period. Trauma to her perineum and damage to nipples from breastfeeding are potential sites for infection. The woman who has given birth by caesarean section also has the potential for infection from her surgical wound site. Another potential source of infection is endometritis caused by retained products following the birth. Retained products can be placenta membranes or blood clots. Symptoms include persistent heavy lochia, pain, tachycardia, and pyrexia. Treatment for infection caused by retained products is ampicillin (amoxicillin) 2 g IV initial dose then 1 g IV every 4 hours and gentamicin 5 mg/kg IV daily and metronidazole 500 mg every 12 hours.

Group A β-Haemolytic Streptococcus (GAS) is the most common bacteria linked to sepsis in the postnatal period. In recent years GAS has become the most common cause of maternal mortality. Due to the non-specific symptoms, diagnosis can be difficult, causing a delay in treatment and adverse outcomes. If any wound infection is suspected, treatment should be offered, as delay in treatment may lead to increased maternal morbidity and mortality. Treatment of sepsis and antibiotics are discussed in Chapter 12. The treatment of mastitis is discussed in Chapter 10.

Bladder and bowel care

Women need to be provided with information in relation to supporting healthy bladder and bowel function post birth.

Bladder care

Women should be informed that there are multiple risk factors for bladder injury during labour and birth, for example delays in progress during labour and birth, assisted births (forceps or vacuum), perineal trauma, epidural, analgesics, caesarean section birth, bruising to vagina and perineum, and haemorrhoids. Additionally, hormonal changes in the postnatal period can impact bladder function. Some women may find the use of a urinary alkaliniser useful in the early postnatal period. Urinary alkalisers are medications that reduce the acidity of urine, therefore, can reduce 'stinging' during micturition. Urinary alkaliniser can be bought over the counter from most chemists. Cranberry juice has traditionally been used to prevent urinary tract symptoms. Methenamine hippurate (also known as Hexamine hippurate) is a urinary antiseptic that fights bacteria in the urine and may also be useful in supporting a healthy bladder. Women may be at increased risk of urinary tract infection in the postnatal period and if this is suspected early diagnosis and treatment is recommended. Please see Chapter 12 for more information on the treatment of infections during the childbirth continuum.

Bowel care

Constipation following the birth is common. As discussed in Chapter 7, hormonal changes impact the function of the bowel. The same dietary changes recommended during pregnancy are recommended in the postnatal period, such as increasing fibre and fluid in diet by eating more whole foods, grains, fruits, and vegetables. Prune juice is a natural alternative to pharmacological laxatives or bulking agents. The idea of keeping bowel movements soft and easier to pass is beneficial, particularly if the woman has perineal trauma, bruising or haemorrhoids. Some women may be advised to take laxatives to support bowel function, and these are discussed in detail in Chapter 7.

KEY POINTS

Infection, bladder and bowel care

- Postnatally, the woman is at risk of developing an infection. Potential sites for infection are the perineum, uterus, bladder, and breasts.

- Swift treatment with antibiotics for any suspected infection is recommended as delays can lead to increased maternal morbidity and mortality.

- Bladder and bowel care are essential in the postnatal period. Constipation can be common following birth and may require pharmaceutical interventions such as laxatives or bulking agents.

9.3 Postnatal contraception

The midwife has an extremely important role in reproductive health in the postnatal period and conversations around pregnancy planning can be initiated during the antenatal period, where planning for postnatal **contraception** can be commenced. The provision of timely advice and supported access to contraception aims to enable women to plan subsequent pregnancies and reduce unintended pregnancies and short interpregnancy intervals. Even if women would prefer to wait before committing to a contraception method, this important discussion should be initiated and recorded to ensure women get the information they need regarding their options and easy access to contraception they prefer.

Women who become pregnant a short time after a previous pregnancy can have increased complications in their pregnancies, births, and neonatal outcomes, regardless of whether the pregnancy is planned or unplanned (Ni et al 2023). Research demonstrates that an interpregnancy interval of less than 12 months increases the risk of preterm birth, low birth weight, stillbirth, and neonatal death (Sedgh et al 2014; Islam et al 2022; Klebanoff 2019; Ni et al 2023).

An ideal contraceptive technique should be safe, 100% effective, immediately functional, easy to use, rapidly reversible after discontinuation, and should not interfere with sex life. Although no technique totally fulfils these criteria, many methods have remarkably low failure rates when used correctly by a highly motivated couple. Most contraceptive techniques, while protecting against pregnancy, do not protect against

transmission of sexually transmitted infections (STIs) (only condoms do the latter). Readiness of availability, requirement for prescription or fitting by a health professional, and cost may be significant factors in decision making and choice of method. In Australia, preparations subsidised on the Pharmaceutical Benefits Scheme (PBS) are usually significantly cheaper than others.

Contraception for women

The availability of effective and acceptable contraception is critical to women's sexual health. **Contraceptive** methods in women include oral tablets (usually provided in monthly calendar packs), IUDs, intravaginal rings and diaphragms, intramuscular implants and female condoms. Some typical products are shown in Figure 9.1. Estimates for 'who uses what' in Australian couples suggest that about 30% use combined oral contraceptives (COC), 23% a barrier method, 16% sterilisation (male or female), 5% a long-acting method, and the rest another or no method.

Since the 1960s, millions of women have used combined oral contraceptives (COCs; an estrogen–progestogen combination in various doses in a 28-day cyclical regimen), or an oral progestogen-only formulation, for decades during their reproductive lives (CFB 9.1).

CLINICAL FOCUS BOX 9.1

A short history of the oral contraceptive pill

The rationale for thinking that estrogens and progestogens might act as reversible contraceptive agents was the fact that ovulation does not occur during pregnancy, when levels of estrogens and progestogens are high. Important stages in the development of oral contraceptives (OCs) are as follows:

- In the 1930s, advances in steroid chemistry facilitated the chemical synthesis of steroid hormones; research into methods of chemically modifying plant hormones to mass-produce steroids led to the development of some inexpensive orally active preparations.

- In the 1950s, combinations of mestranol (metabolised to EE) and norethynodrel as OCs were tested in large-scale clinical trials in Puerto Rico and Haiti and provided successful reversible contraception with acceptable levels of adverse reactions.

- In 1960, the first OC preparation was marketed in the United States; it was a combination containing mestranol 150 micrograms and ethynodiol diacetate 10 mg. In 1961, OCs were available in Australia.

- Early OC formulations were indeed pills (small spherical masses containing active drugs, prepared by rolling techniques), but now the hormones are formulated into small tablets; the term 'pill' has remained in the OC context.

- Typical early preparations contained EE 100–150 micrograms per tablet plus 1–4 mg norethisterone, now rec-

Different types of female contraceptive products

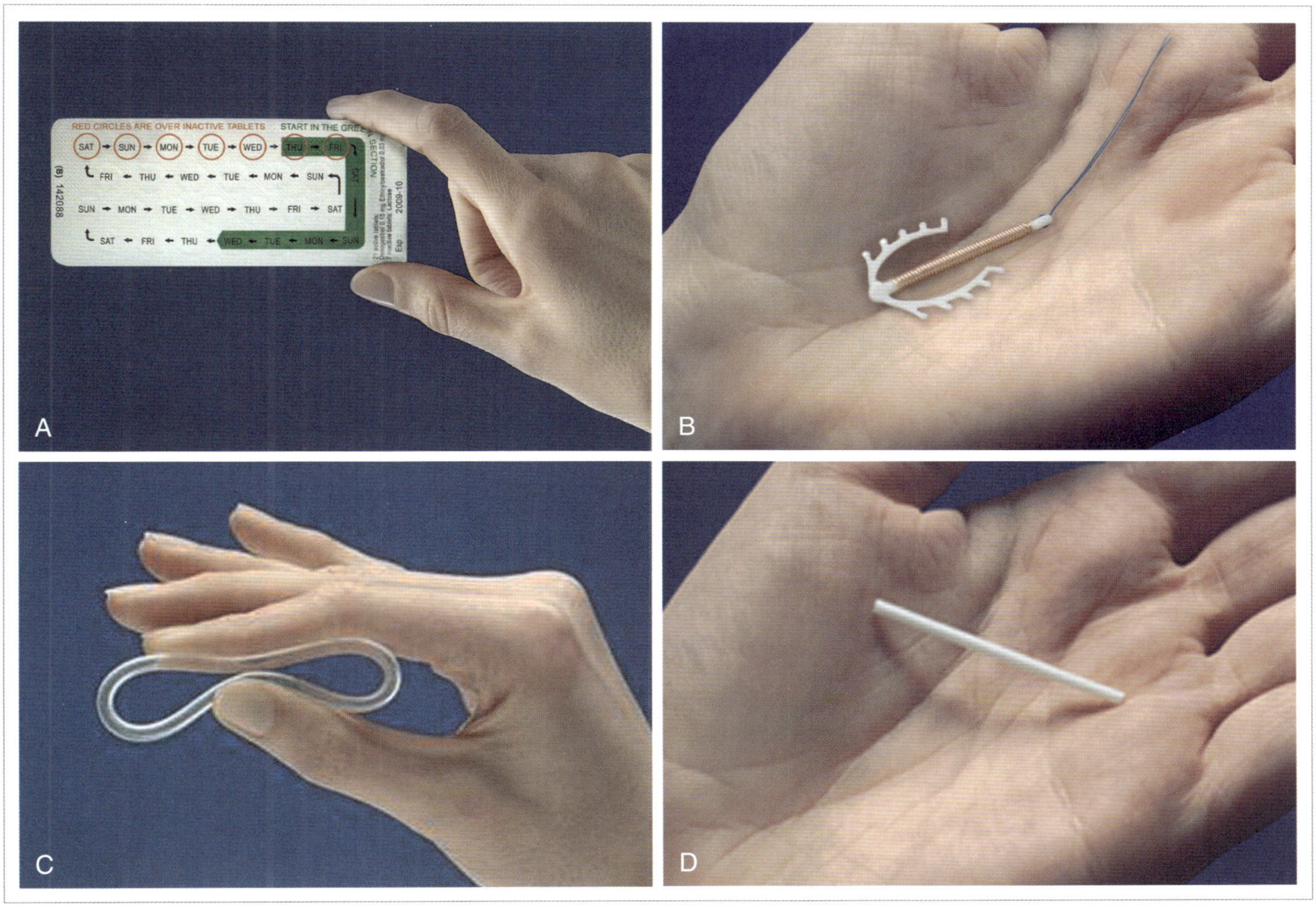

FIGURE 9.1 A 28-day pack of COC. **B** Copper IUD. **C** Intravaginal ring. **D** Intramuscular implant.

Source: Merck Sharp & Dohme (Australia) Pty Ltd; reproduced with permission.

ognised as unnecessarily large amounts of estrogen. Current formulations include only 20–50 micrograms EE plus 0.5–1 mg norethisterone or equivalent.

- The importance of taking a 'pill' every day was recognised, so tablets were soon packaged in calendar packs (Fig 9.1A) with the days marked, and with seven placebo (sugar) tablets included in most packs to avoid a break in tablet-taking.

Today there are many formulations of the pill. Monophasic and multiphasic options are available. All COCs contain an estrogen and a progestogen.

Availability of an OC pill heralded not only a pharmacological revolution but also sexual and social revolutions: for the first time, women had a reliable, safe, and reversible method of controlling their fertility, which allowed them to be sexually active without fear of pregnancy, to separate career choices from family planning, and to compete more equally with men in the workforce.

Many factors determine what form of contraception suits a particular woman: age; postpartum, breastfeeding or perimenopause status; whether family is complete; concurrent medical conditions (e.g. cancer, cardiovascular disease, liver function, diabetes, pre- or post-surgery, epilepsy); predisposition to thromboembolism, acne, or hirsutism; concurrent drugs; adverse reactions to previous pharmacological contraceptives; smoking status; and individual preferences.

Oral contraceptives are indicated in regular and emergency contraception, menstrual disorders and to treat endometriosis and acne. Precautions are needed in women with migraine; unexplained vaginal bleeding; obesity or malabsorption syndromes; early postpartum mothers; women over 40; those on drugs that induce CYP3A4 enzymes; and smokers. COCs are contraindicated in women with a history of hypertension, breast cancer, cardiovascular disease or liver disease, at risk of venous thromboembolism (VTE), or having major surgery.

It is extremely important that women who are breastfeeding and choosing the contraceptive pill are counselled appropriately and prescribed the most appropriate oral contraceptive pill as some formulas are contradicted in breastfeeding women.

Hormone components of COC formulations

The aim of most COC formulations is to mimic closely the sequence and levels of hormones in the menstrual cycle, in which estrogen levels are low early in the cycle, high in mid-cycle, and medium late in the cycle; progestogen levels are very low or absent until the mid-cycle surge of gonadotrophins, then rise late in the cycle (Fig 9.2). The typical 21/7 COC regimen for 1 month contains 21 days of active hormone tablets, then 7 days with placebo or no tablets, which precipitates the withdrawal bleed – that is, the next menstrual cycle. Note that menstruation can be effectively suppressed by 'tricycling' – that is, taking only the active tablets from 3-monthly packs of COCs for 9 weeks in a row, then placebo (or no) tablets for 7 days. This decreases the frequency of withdrawal bleeds and heavy or painful periods, which is useful when menstruation would be inconvenient. A commercially available 3-month pack (84 tablets with 150 micrograms levonorgestrel plus 30 micrograms EE, followed by seven tablets with 10 micrograms EE) achieves the same results.

Beneficial effects

More than 50 years of worldwide clinical experience have shown the OC pill to be safe and effective. Beneficial effects include: avoidance of unwanted pregnancy and pregnancy-related morbidity and mortality; lower rates of ectopic pregnancies, atheroma, thyroid disease, menstrual problems, anaemia, premenstrual dysphoric disorder, benign cysts, pelvic inflammatory disease, ovarian cancer and endometrial cancer, STIs, acne and hirsutism; and protection against endometriosis and fibroids.

Provided that risk factors are minimised, COCs are safe for most women for most of their reproductive lives. However, there are some adverse effects that need to be considered when women are choosing the right contraception for them and their individual circumstances.

Adverse effects

Possible adverse effects or disadvantages:

- weight gain and fluid retention (anabolic effects)
- breast tenderness, impaired glucose tolerance and skin changes (estrogenic effects)
- general symptoms (nausea, depression, chloasma, acne)
- short-term amenorrhoea after cessation
- increased risk of thrombosis and myocardial infarction, especially in smokers, obese women and those aged over 35 (CFB 9.2)
- breakthrough bleeding
- possible association with breast cancer, cervical cancer, liver cancer, gall bladder disease, inflammatory bowel disease and rheumatoid arthritis.

Adverse effects usually diminish over time, with continued use of the same method.

CLINICAL FOCUS BOX 9.2

Combined oral contraceptives and venous thromboembolism risk

A venous thromboembolism (VTE) is a rare but serious side effect of COCs. That is, the blockage of leg and pulmonary vessels by a venous thrombosis (blood clot). A thrombosis in the lower leg, thigh or pelvis vessels is known as a deep vein thrombosis, while a blockage in the pulmonary vasculature is known as a pulmonary embolism. A pulmonary embolism can be life-threatening and can cause sudden death.

Different COCs have different thromboembolism risk. Higher estrogen doses are correlated with higher VTE risk, as increased levels of plasma estrogen increase the hepatic synthesis of procoagulant proteins and decrease the synthesis of fibrinolytic and anticoagulant factors, leading to hypercoagulability.

COCs that contain third- and fourth-generation progestogens (desogestrel, dienogest, gestodene, or drospirenone) have a higher relative risk of VTE when compared with second-generation progestogens (norethisterone, levonorgestrel). For every 10,000 women taking third- or fourth-generation progestogens, 9–12 women will develop a VTE in a year. This is reduced to 5–7 women taking second-generation progestogens (Butcher et al 2016).

It is important for health professionals to educate their patients who are prescribed the COC to recognise the signs and symptoms of VTE. The most common signs and symptoms of deep vein thrombosis include pain, swelling, heaviness, redness and cramping in the legs. The most common clinical symptoms of pulmonary embolism include shortness of breath, rapid breathing, cough, sharp chest pain that worsens during breathing (pleuritic chest pain), and syncope (fainting).

Other factors that increase VTE risk include cigarette smoking, obesity, increasing age, migraines and a family history of VTE.

Source: Butcher B, Donovan C, Farrell L, et al. Risk of venous thromboembolism in women taking the combined oral contraceptive: a systematic review and meta-analysis. AJGP. 2016;45(1):58-67.

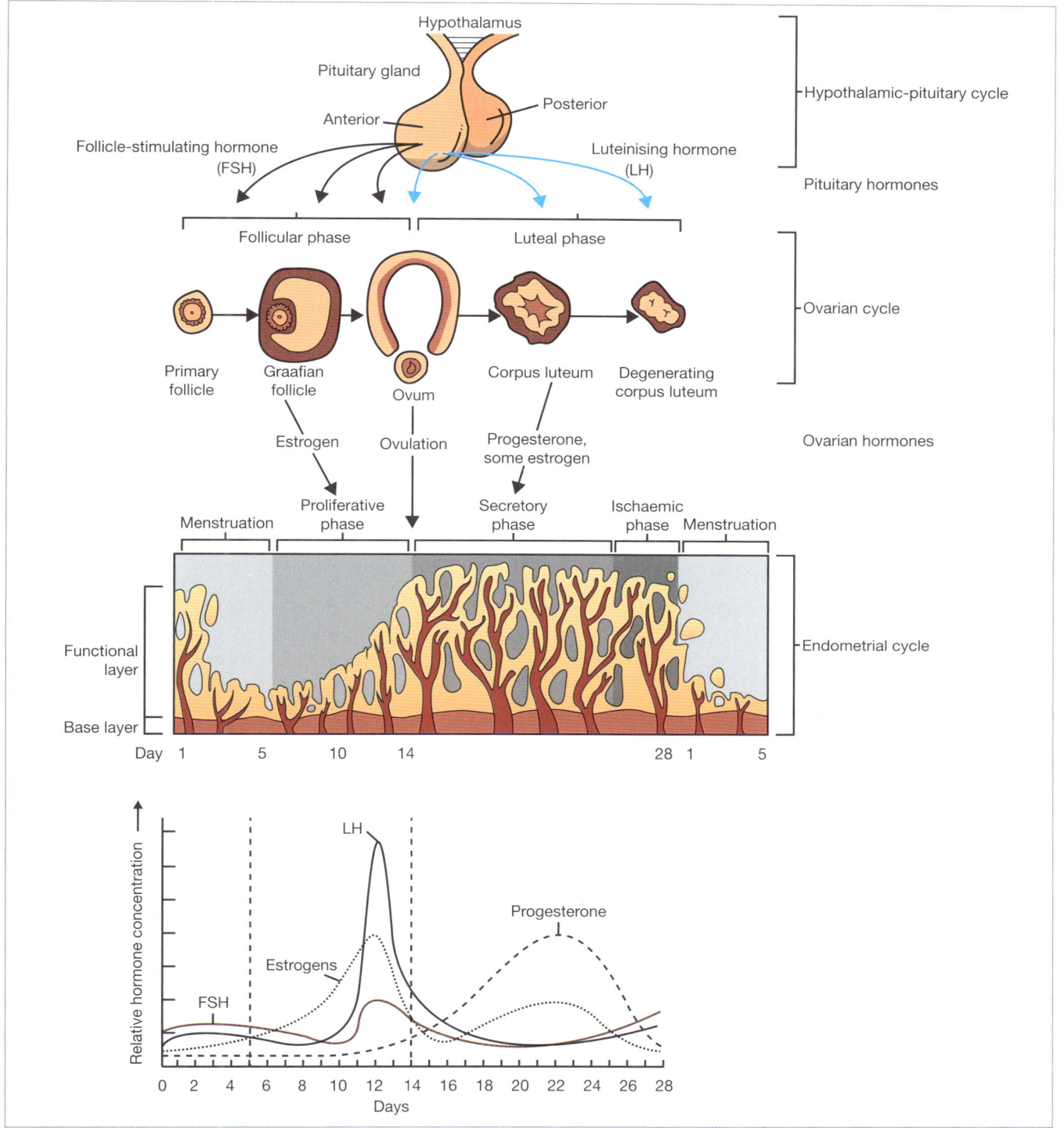

FIGURE 9.2

Source: Adapted from Salerno 1999; used with permission.

Contraindications and interactions

Because OC preparations are taken by millions of women for most of their reproductive lives, it is crucial that long-term safety, risks and benefits be identified and compared with risks associated with pregnancy and childbirth, particularly in countries where maternity care is inadequate and access to a safe abortion may be difficult. Major long-term studies have demonstrated that the low-dose OCs incur fewer risks than does pregnancy.

Absolute contraindications for OCs are: thromboembolic disease, coronary artery disease, stroke, active liver disease, estrogen-dependent cancers, focal migraine, porphyrias and pregnancy. As discussed earlier, OC use is relatively contraindicated in hypertension, diabetes, previous cholestasis, undiagnosed vaginal bleeding, elective surgery within 4 weeks, sickle cell disease and severe depression, and in women aged over 35 years with risks for coronary artery disease.

There are many potential drug interactions with COCs, especially with drugs that induce CYP3A4 enzymes, enhancing clearance of sex hormones (estrogen and progesterone) and leading to contraception failure; barbiturates, many anticonvulsants, some antivirals and rifamycin antibiotics are particularly implicated. It is essential that the midwife take a full medical history, including any medications the woman may be taking, prior to prescribing the oral contraceptive pill. The Australian Medicines Handbook 'Drug Interactions' is available online and is a valuable resource.

Note: Those with EE dose under 30 micrograms or estradiol dose under 1.5 mg are considered low-dose; an EE dose of 30–35 micrograms is standard; and EE 50 micrograms is high-dose. Women taking these drugs are recommended to use IUDs with levonorgestrel or copper, or medroxyprogesterone depot for contraception, discussed later in this chapter.

Actions and mechanisms

For detailed information on the physiological actions, mechanisms, pharmacokinetics, adverse effects, drug interactions and contraindications of the component drugs, for typical estrogens see Drug Monograph 9.1

DRUG MONOGRAPH 9.1
Estradiol valerate

Indications

Estradiol valerate is used for its estrogenic actions on ovary and uterus in HRT to prevent and treat estrogen-deficiency symptoms after ovariectomy or menopause, and in the COC 'pill' for contraception.

Actions and mechanisms

Estradiol valerate is an ester derivative of the natural hormone. See text.

Pharmacokinetics

Estradiol valerate is a prodrug of estradiol-17β. It is rapidly and completely absorbed (peak plasma concentration within 6 hours), and quickly metabolised in the liver to estradiol, then to various metabolites, of which estriol and estrone have estrogenic activity. Estradiol is highly protein-bound and has a half-life of 18–24 hours. Metabolites are excreted in bile, and undergo enterohepatic recycling.

Drug interactions

See Drug Interactions 9.1.

Side effects and adverse reactions

Typical estrogenic effects are breast pain and enlargement, changes in menstrual bleeding, headaches, nausea, vomiting, a change in libido, oedema of lower extremities, chloasma (darkened patches of skin on the face) and increased risk of thromboembolism. Administration by skin patch can cause irritation and dermatitis.

Warnings and contraindications

Estrogens should be used with caution in smokers and in women with endometriosis, diabetes, migraine or epilepsy. Avoid use in pregnancy and in women with estrogen hypersensitivity, thromboembolic disorders or severe cardiovascular or liver disease, breast cancer and other estrogen-dependent tumours, or hypercalcaemia (see also later discussion of risks with COC or HRT). Estrogens reduce lactation and are excreted in breast milk, so administration to breastfeeding mothers is not recommended.

Dosage and administration

In HRT: a cyclical dosing schedule of 3 weeks estradiol administration (1–2 mg daily by mouth) and 1 week off, possibly with addition of a progestogen for the last 10–14 days of the cycle, most closely approximates the natural menstrual cycle. The progestogen must be added to HRT in postmenopausal women with an intact uterus to avoid endometrial hyperplasia or carcinoma. The prescriber should re-evaluate the patient at least annually.

Transdermal estradiol is also used for women with estrogen deficiency, particularly as HRT in menopause (used with a progestogen in women with an intact uterus). Applied topically to intact skin, the patch releases 25–100 micrograms (0.025–0.1 mg) daily. It is usually worn continuously and should be replaced twice weekly. Sensitivity reactions at the application site often occur. Estradiol is also formulated in many COC tablet types (Table 9.1) and as a vaginal pessary and transdermal gel.

TABLE 9.1 Examples of hormonal contraceptives

BRAND NAME	ESTROGEN (micrograms)	PROGESTOGEN (mg)
Monophasic COC		
Femme-tab ED, Lenest 20 ED, Loette, Microgynon 20 ED, Microlevlen ED, Micronelle 20 ED	EE 20	Levonorgestrel 0.1
Petibelle, Yasmin, Yaz, Yaz Flex	EE 20 or 30	Drospirenone 3.0
Madeline, Marvelon 28	EE 30	Desogestrel 0.15
Valette	EE 30	Dienogest 2.0
Eleanor 150/30 ED, Evelyn 150/30 ED, Femme-Tab 30/150 ED, Lenest 30 ED, Levlen ED, Microgynon 30 ED, Micronelle 30 ED, Monofeme, Nordette	EE 30	Levonorgestrel 0.15
Minulet	EE 30	Gestodene 0.075
Brenda-35 ED, Carolyn-35 ED, Chelsea-35 ED, Diane-35 ED, Estelle-35 ED, Jene-35 ED, Juliet-35 ED, Laila-35 ED	EE 35	Cyproterone acetate 2.0
Brevinor, Brevinor-1; Norimin, Norimin-1	EE 35	Norethisterone 0.5 or 1.0
Norinyl-1	Mestranol 50	Norethisterone 1.0
Microgynon 50 ED	EE 50	Levonorgestrel 0.125
Zoely	Estradiol 1.5 mg	Nomegestrol 2.5
Multiphasic COC		
Triphasil, Logynon ED, Trifeme, Triquilar ED (6/5/10/7 tabs)	EE 30/40/30/0	Levonorgestrel 0.05/0.075/0.125/0
Qlaira (2/5/17/2/2 tabs)	Estradiol 3/2/2/1/0	Dienogest 0/2/3/0/0
Combined, depot		
NuvaRing (vaginal ring, for 3 weeks)	EE 2.7 mg	Etonogestrel 11.7 mg
Progestogen-only (oral)		
Noriday 28	None	Norethisterone 0.35
Microlut	None	Levonorgestrel 0.03
Levonelle-1, NorLevo-1, Postella-1, Postinor-1	None	Levonorgestrel 1.5 (for emergency contraception)
Progestogen-only (depot/IUD)		
Depo-Provera, Depo-Ralovera	None	Medroxyprogesterone acetate 150 mg IM every 3 months
Implanon NXT	None	Etonogestrel 68 mg subdermal every 3 years
Mirena IUD	None	Levonorgestrel 52 mg; replaced every 5 years

Note: Those with EE dose under 30 micrograms or estradiol dose under 1.5 mg are considered low-dose; an EE dose of 30–35 micrograms is standard; and EE 50 micrograms is high-dose.
ED = extended dose
Source: Australian Medicines Handbook 2021.

(estradiol valerate) and for progestogens see Drug Monograph 9.2 (levonorgestrel). Relevant to contraceptive effects is that the estrogen component decreases FSH release and thus impairs selection and development of a follicle; this decreases the likelihood of ovulation and implantation. The progestogen component thickens uterine mucus, decreases LH release, and impairs ovulation and tubal motility, decreasing the likelihood of fertilisation. Over a few cycles, estrogen–progestogen combinations inhibit secretion of hypothalamic GnRH, pituitary gonadotrophins FSH and LH and endogenous ovarian steroids. Overall, pregnancy does not occur.

The mechanisms of action of female contraceptive methods are compared diagrammatically in Figure 9.3.

Counselling points

All women prescribed the contraceptive pill should be appropriately counselled by a health professional and the information below should be given:

- When to start taking a pack of tablets. (Most should be taken within the first 5 days of the cycle, i.e. days of menstrual bleeding)
- What to do if one or more active tablets are missed or in the case of vomiting or diarrhoea. (Generally, if more than 24 hours late or a tablet may not have been absorbed, or if pack was started on other than days 1–5 of the cycle, additional contraception methods should be used for 7 days)
- Adverse effects to watch for and report (severe chest pain or headache, vision changes, leg pain or swelling, acne, weight gain) (Fig 9.3)
- The greater risks of adverse effects for smokers
- There are many effective methods of contraception and many formulations of COCs
- How to change formulations if prescribed. (Skip the inert tablets for the first cycle and keep taking the active tablets; another contraceptive method may be needed)
- The pill does not protect against STIs
- If taking the progestogen-only pill (POP or minipill), it must be taken at the same time each day
- Many antiepileptic medicines and rifamycin antibiotics may reduce the effectiveness of some COCs due to increased metabolism of EE; a COC with higher EE doses and/or other contraceptive method may be necessary
- It is possible to delay menstruation temporarily by tricycling.

Oral COC formulations

*(Note: these are **not** suitable for use by women who are breastfeeding)*

Many different types of COC formulations are available, with different combinations and sequences of semisynthetic hormones selected to optimise activity and minimise adverse effects. Combined oral contraceptive pills are contraindicated in women who are breastfeeding, especially during the first 6 weeks post birth. Ethinyl estradiol in doses greater than 30 micrograms daily can suppress lactation, resulting in more supplementation and earlier discontinuation of breastfeeding than non-hormonal or progestin-only contraception. Introduction of an estrogen before 3 weeks postpartum may also increase the risk of thromboembolism in postpartum women, while rare cases of reversible breast enlargement in breastfed infants have also been reported (See Online resources: LactMed 2024).

Most formulations of the COC in Australia and New Zealand contain an estrogen (EE); other estrogens used are mestranol or estradiol (DM 9.1). Several synthetic progestogens are used in COCs: norethisterone, levonorgestrel (DM 9.2), desogestrel, gestodene or drospirenone (the latter three are less likely to have androgenic effects), or cyproterone, dienogest or nomegestrol (with anti-androgen activity). Drospirenone also has useful anti-mineralocorticoid actions, and may help reduce blood pressure and body weight; however, it carries increased risk of VTE (CFB 9.2). Formulations containing EE 35 micrograms or less plus norethisterone or levonorgestrel are considered first-line (Stewart et al 2015).

Monophasic OCs containing a fixed ratio of estrogen and progestogen are taken for 21 (or 24) days of the normal menstrual cycle, then inactive tablets may be taken for the next 7 (or 4) days. Tri- or multi-phasic COCs most closely mimic the normal estrogen and progesterone levels during the menstrual cycle. The dose of estrogen is kept at a low level during the 21-day dosing period, or may increase (mid-cycle surge) in the middle of the cycle, while the progestogen is progressively phased up (increased twice) to mimic the natural release of hormones; inactive tablets are taken for the last 7 days. Because of the lower doses, adverse reactions reported are lower than with the monophasic formulations; however, controlled trials show little difference in cycle control.

Table 9.2 lists the compositions, doses and brand names of some typical OCs used in these methods; a typical calendar pack is shown in Figure 9.1A. (However, formulations change frequently, so current references should be consulted.)

'The minipill' *suitable for use by women who are breastfeeding

Low-dosage progesterone-only OCs (the minipill) were developed for women unable to take estrogens, for example women who are breastfeeding, or those with a history of thromboembolic disorders or who smoke. Progesterone-only OCs are less effective than COCs and have a higher incidence of breakthrough bleeding and menstrual irregularity.

The progestogen-only pills (POP) do not contain estrogen; therefore they are suitable for women who are breastfeeding. Most postpartum women will not ovulate for at least 6 weeks; however, in approximately one-third of women, the first cycle is preceded by ovulation and so they are potentially fertile. Therefore, midwives should be discussing contraception in the early postnatal period to ensure that women who wish to consider contraceptives are counselled and informed of their choices. The POP can be commenced in the immediate postnatal period.

POP contain lower doses of hormones; therefore, the timing of taking the tablet each day is critical. It is recommended that, if administration is delayed by more than 3 hours, an additional method of contraception be used for 48 hours. The minipill may be unreliable in women who are overweight (see Online resources: CDC 2023).

Sites of action of various contraceptive methods in the female reproductive tract

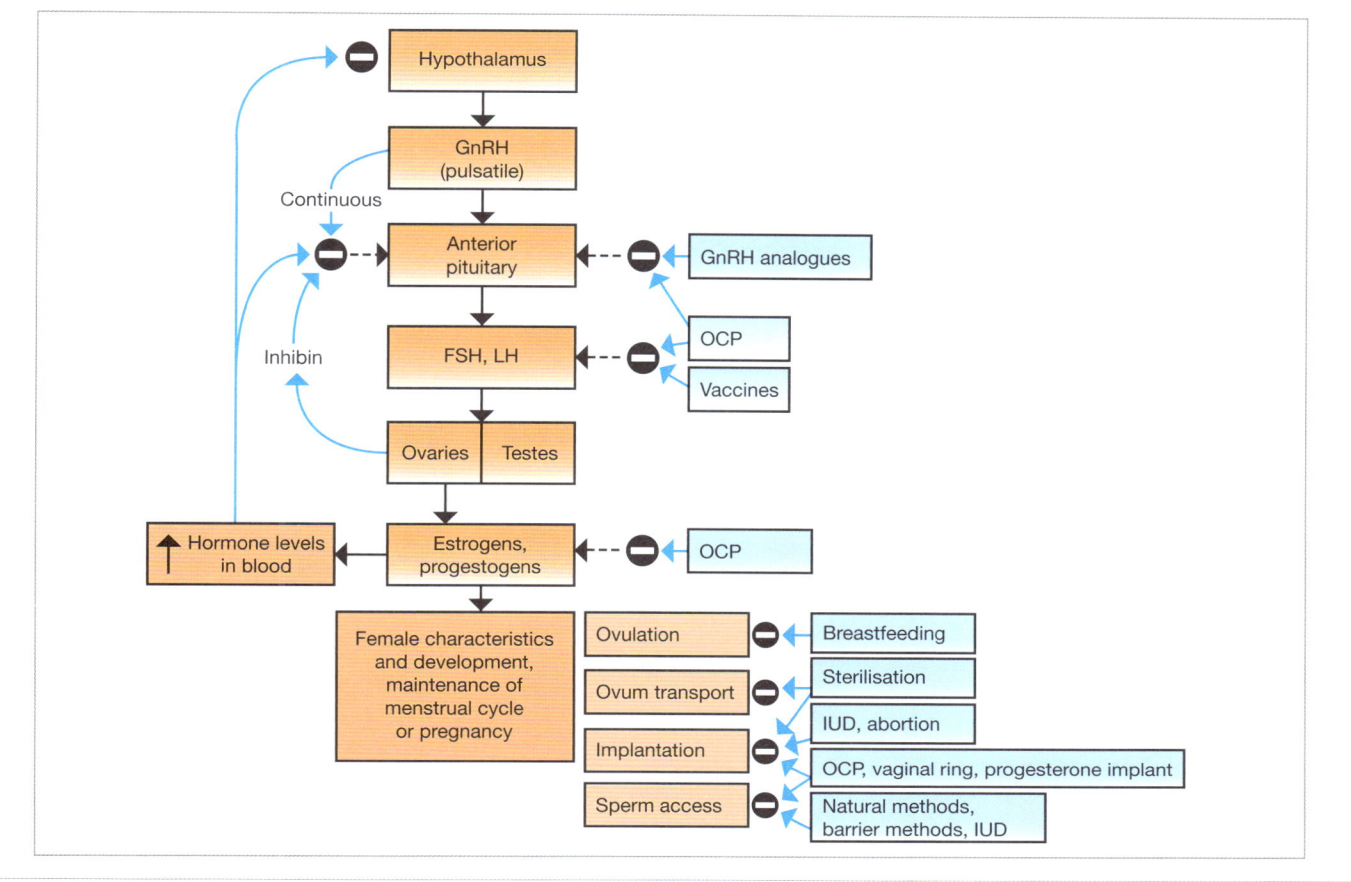

FIGURE 9.3 [–] = effect decreased or inhibited; GnRH = gonadotrophin-releasing hormone; IUD = intrauterine device; OCP = oral contraceptive pill

DRUG INTERACTIONS 9.1

Some potentially significant interactions with estrogens

DRUG	POSSIBLE EFFECTS AND MANAGEMENT
Enzyme inducers (barbiturates, some antiepileptics, aprepitant, bosentan, modafinil, some antivirals, rifamycins, St John's wort)	May accelerate metabolism of estrogens and reduce their activity; additional contraception such as condoms should be used if required; effects in HRT may be reduced
Atazanavir, etoricoxib	Increase concentrations of EE and risk of adverse effects; low-dose EE (30 micrograms) OC formulations should be used or a different interacting drug selected
Antibiotics (e.g. ampicillin)	May reduce potency of estradiol because of metabolism by altered gut flora
Tobacco (smoking)	Tobacco smoking increases risk of serious cardiovascular adverse reactions and venous thromboembolism; risk is higher in women over 35 who smoke; OCs not recommended
Orlistat	Orlistat-induced diarrhoea may reduce estrogen levels; additional contraception may be necessary
Selegiline	COCs may increase selegiline concentration, enhancing its effects and adverse effects; reduce selegiline dose or avoid combination
Drugs affecting blood glucose	Estrogens can increase blood glucose levels, thus affecting diabetes control
Thyroid hormones	Estrogens may alter concentrations of thyroid hormones, requiring increased thyroxine dose; thyroid function should be monitored

Notes: (1) See Australian Medicines Handbook 2024, Drug interactions, under 'Combined Oral Contraceptives' and 'Hormone Replacement Therapy'. (2) Doses of estrogens in HRT formulations are considerably lower than in COC, so fewer drug interactions are expected.

TABLE 9.2 Comparison of contraceptive methods

FAILURE RATE[1]	ADVANTAGES	DISADVANTAGES
COCs		
0.3–9%[2]	• regular, lighter, less painful periods • can choose when periods occur • improve acne and menstrual disorders • reduce risk of PID, anaemia, ovarian and endometrial cancer	• efficacy affected by some drugs, vomiting and severe diarrhoea • need to be taken each day • may cause spotting, nausea, vomiting, breast enlargement and tenderness, headache, fluid retention, increase in BP, mood changes, VTE (rare) • increase risk of MI and stroke in smokers > 35 years or those with hypertension
Combined hormonal vaginal ring		
0.3–9%[2]	• no daily tablets • regular periods (and can choose when they occur) • woman inserts and removes	• requires monthly insertion and removal • may cause vaginal irritation, infection or discharge • ring may be expelled
Progestogen-only contraceptives		
Drospirenone tablets		
0.3–9%[2]	• useful when COC is contraindicated/less appropriate (e.g. breastfeeding, migraine) or not tolerated	• need to be taken every day • efficacy affected by some drugs, vomiting and severe diarrhoea • may cause amenorrhoea, irregular bleeding, breast tenderness, acne
Levonorgestrel or norethisterone tablets		
0.3–9%[2]	• useful when COC is contraindicated/less appropriate (e.g. breastfeeding, migraine, history of VTE, smokers > 35 years) or not tolerated	• need to be taken at the same time every day (within 3 hours) • efficacy affected by some drugs, vomiting and severe diarrhoea • may cause amenorrhoea, irregular bleeding, breast tenderness, acne
Medroxyprogesterone IM depot		
0.2–6%	• no daily tablets • prolonged contraception (12 weeks) • efficacy unaffected by drug interactions	• injection every 12 weeks • cannot be removed • return to fertility may be delayed after stopping (rarely > 12 months) • may cause amenorrhoea, irregular bleeding, breast tenderness, acne, weight gain, decreased BMD
Etonogestrel implant		
0.05%	• no daily tablets • long-term contraception (3 years)	• doctor inserts and removes • efficacy affected by some drugs • may cause amenorrhoea, irregular bleeding, acne, breast tenderness
Levonorgestrel IUD		
0.2%	• lighter, less painful periods • efficacy unaffected by drug interactions • no daily tablets • long-term contraception (5 years)	• doctor inserts and removes • may cause amenorrhoea, irregular bleeding, acne • increases risk of pelvic infection for 3 weeks after insertion, device may be expelled (especially in first year)
Copper IUD[3]		
0.6–0.8%	• efficacy unaffected by drug interactions • long-term contraception (5 or 10 years)	• doctor inserts and removes • may cause heavy periods, period pain • increases risk of pelvic infection for three weeks after insertion, device may be expelled (especially in first year)
Barrier methods		
2–18% (male condom) 5–21% (female condom) 6–12% (diaphragm)	• condoms are easy to use, readily available • condoms reduce risk of most STIs including HIV • polyurethane male or female condoms suitable in latex allergy or with oil-based products	• *condoms* may break or slip off • *diaphragm* initially fitted by nurse or doctor; woman needs to be taught how to use it; needs refitting if weight change > 3 kg or after pregnancy, miscarriage or abortion; effectiveness may be increased by use with a spermicide (not available in Australia) • oil-based products (e.g. petroleum jelly, baby oil) can damage latex • latex may rarely cause allergy

[1] estimated percentage of women with an unintended pregnancy within first year of use; the lower number is for perfect use, the higher number is for typical use
[2] based on combined data for COCs and progestogen-only pills (POPs); efficacy of POPs likely to be lower than COCs as less likely to be taken perfectly; no data for vaginal ring (failure rate assumed to be similar to COC)
[3] replace Copper TT380 Short® and Load 375® every 5 years or Copper TT380 Standard® every 10 years
Source: Australian Medicines Handbook 2024.

DRUG MONOGRAPH 9.2
Levonorgestrel

Levonorgestrel is a prototype synthetic progestogen. Levonorgestrel's contraceptive effects are by preventing ovulation and fertilisation if intercourse has taken place in the pre-ovulatory phase when the likelihood of fertilisation is the highest. *(For actions and mechanisms, see text.)*

Indications

Levonorgestrel is indicated for oral contraception (alone or combined with an estrogen), emergency contraception, in long-term contraception (as an IUD), in postmenopausal HRT, in treatment of hormonal imbalances in dysmenorrhoea and in specific carcinomas (breast, endometrial, renal cell – specialist oncologist uses only).

Pharmacokinetics

Levonorgestrel is rapidly absorbed after oral administration, reaching maximum plasma concentration after 2 hours, with a mean elimination half-life of about 26 hours. It is highly protein-bound to sex-hormone-binding globulin. It is metabolised in the liver, with inactive metabolites excreted in urine and faeces.

Drug interactions

Effectiveness of oral progestogens, and possibly of the IUD, may be reduced by CYP3A4 enzyme-inducing drugs, particularly rifamycins, many anticonvulsants and some antivirals; contraceptive failure may result, so alternative contraception is necessary. (For details see reference texts such as the Australian Medicines Handbook, Appendix B, under 'Combined Oral Contraceptives' and 'Progestogens'.)

Adverse reactions

High doses for emergency contraception may cause breast pain, nausea and vomiting, vaginal bleeding, and headache; lower long-term doses may cause reversible ovarian cysts. IUD insertion may cause pain or cramps and irregular bleeding.

Warnings and contraindications

Should be used with caution in women with uterine, genital, or urinary tract bleeding (undiagnosed) or malabsorption syndromes. Avoid use in women with progestogen hypersensitivity, breast, or genital tract cancer (contraceptive use), severe liver or thromboembolic disease and in pregnancy.

Dosage and administration

Low physiological dosages are used for progestational effects in replacement therapy, and higher doses to suppress ovulation, menstruation and gonadotrophin production. Examples of dosing regimens are:
- in IUD, for contraception or HRT: 52 mg (replaced every 5 years)
- as component of COC: 50–150 micrograms
- as emergency contraceptive: 1.5 mg single dose, taken within 72 hours of unprotected intercourse.

Emergency contraception

The emergency contraceptive pill, sometimes misnamed the 'morning-after pill', is indicated for use within 72 hours of unprotected sexual intercourse or in possible failure of contraceptive method in women not wanting to conceive. Small amounts of the hormonal preparations will pass into the breast milk; however, breastfeeding is still recommended (Shaaban et al 2019; Bateson 2021; Sääv et al 2010). The available methods are:

- ulipristal acetate, 30 mg, an SPRM; most effective oral emergency contraceptive pill, effective in 99% of cases up to 5 days after unprotected intercourse.
- levonorgestrel, 1.5 mg, within 72 hours of unprotected intercourse; 85% effective; less effective in obese women. Ulipristal and levonorgestrel as an emergency contraceptive pill are Pharmacist-Only Medicines (Schedule 3) in Australia. **Emergency contraception** has been shown in societies in which it is readily available to reduce the rate of abortion. The main contraindication to these regimens is known pregnancy.

The use of antiprogestogens such as mifepristone, RU486, at a single dose of 200 mg, followed by a PG analogue, to terminate pregnancy is classified as medical **termination** rather than as emergency contraception.

An alternative, non-oral, non-hormonal method of emergency contraception is insertion of a copper-impregnated intrauterine device (IUD), which is 99% effective if inserted for up to 5 days after unprotected intercourse (discussed in more detail later in this chapter).

Oral contraception

- Oral contraception with combinations of an estrogen and a progestogen is the most widely and frequently used method of female contraception.

- Progesterone-only contraceptives are suitable for women who are breastfeeding.

- Types of contraceptive formulations include combined continuous and phased preparations, progestogen-only tablets and implants, and emergency contraception regimens.

- Risk–benefit analysis shows that, for most women, use of oral contraception is safe, effective, reversible, and inexpensive, and protects against many gynaecological problems. Adverse reactions are mild with low- or no-estrogen formulations.

- Because OCs are primarily for self-administration, education is important for accurate and safe administration and for early recognition of adverse reactions, particularly thromboembolism.

- Women should also be aware of potential interactions with other prescription drugs such as antibiotics which may render their oral contraceptive less effective and/or CAM therapies, for example St John's wort. St John's wort interacts with hormonal contraceptives resulting in increased metabolism of norethindrone and ethinyl estradiol. Women consuming St John's wort should be counselled to expect breakthrough bleeding and advised to add a barrier method of contraception as it can increase their risk of an unplanned pregnancy (see Online resources: BMJ 2020).

Non-oral hormonal contraception

The non-oral hormonal methods of contraception – depot injection, vaginal ring, depot intramuscular (IM) implantation, and hormonal IUD – have many advantages over oral formulations, including:

- they avoid problems with impaired gastrointestinal tract (GIT) absorption (e.g. from vomiting or diarrhoea)
- they avoid hepatic first-pass metabolism, so lower estrogen doses are effective
- controlled-release formulations readily achieve steady plasma concentrations
- long durations of action (3–10 years)
- improved compliance and effectiveness, as no daily action (or memory) or regular maintenance is required
- scant or no menstrual bleeding or pain (excluding copper IUD)
- they are more effective than OCs at preventing unintended pregnancies (in the first year of use, the failure rates of long-acting reversible contraceptives [LARCs] are 0.05–0.8%, compared with 9% with the OC)
- a good safety profile with few contraindications.

Long-acting reversible contraceptives

There is robust evidence that the provision of immediate LARC postnatally is safe and effective in preventing rapid repeat pregnancy (Stark et al 2022). There are multiple LARC options available, but they all have one thing in common: the plan for a longer term contraception. In Australia and New Zealand, LARC use is increasing. Approximately, 11% of Australian women use a LARC (6.1% for IUDs and 4.9% for implants) (see Online resources: MSI Australia 2024).

Progestogen-only depot preparations *suitable for women who are breastfeeding

Depot injections of progestogen (e.g. depot medroxyprogesterone acetate [DMPA]) have the lowest failure rate of all reversible contraceptive methods. Progestogen contraceptives thicken cervical mucus to stop the passage of sperm and change the endometrium, reducing the potential for implantation. They act on the hypothalamus and suppress pituitary LH surge. The depot injection reliably suppresses ovulation. This method is suitable for women who do not want to take a daily tablet or who cannot take estrogens. DMPA 150 mg is administered via deep intramuscular injection into the gluteus maximus or deltoid muscles. Doses are repeated every 12 weeks; however, DMPA provide contraceptive cover for up to 14 weeks allowing for a 2-week leeway.

Adverse effects

- Common (> 1%)
  - IM: 50% become amenorrhoeic within 12 months, delayed return of menstrual periods after stopping (may take > 6 months), weight gain
  - loss of bone mass density. IM depot use is associated with a small decrease in BMD that is greatest in the first few years of use. At least partial recovery of bone loss occurs after stopping use. The effect on osteoporosis or risk of fractures is not yet known. Ensure adequate calcium and vitamin D intake, and encourage weight-bearing exercise and smoking cessation.
- Rare (< 0.1%)
  - injection site reactions (e.g. nodules, atrophy, lipodystrophy).

Additionally, there may be a period of infertility for some months after completing the course. For some women this may be up to a year.

Implant *suitable for women who are breastfeeding

A subdermal depot implant containing a progestogen is also available and works in the same way as the depot injection to inhibit sperm and stop ovulation. The implant consists of a polymer rod impregnated with the progesterone (Fig 9.1D). It is implanted using aseptic procedures under the skin of the inner aspect of the upper arm and is left in place for 3–5 years, during which there is a gradually reducing rate of release of active drug. Women using a subdermal implant can experience varying bleeding patterns from no bleeding at all to irregular and frequent bleeding. Like other progesterones, headaches, weight gain, acne and changes in mood are reported side effects. The progesterone in the implant is metabolised by the CYP3A4 system in the liver. Caution is advised for women who are taking some antiepileptic medications, HIV medications and over-the-counter products, including herbal (particularly St John's wort), as the effectiveness of the contraceptive may be reduced (see Online resources: AMH 2024).

There are two types of implants available:

- Implanon NXT:
  - single rod implant, 68 mg etonogestrel. 40 mm long, 2 mm diameter. Releases 60 g per day and lasts 3 years (available in NZ and Australia)
- Jadelle:
  - double rod implant, 75 mg levonorgestrel. 43 mm long, 2.55 mm diameter. Releases 100 g in the first month, reducing to 30 per day by 2 years and beyond. Lasts for 5 years; however, has been reported to have an increased failure rate in the final year (only available in NZ).

Fertility will return very quickly after removal of the implant, within a few days. Return to normal menstrual periods is usually very quick.

Combined vaginal ring *Not suitable for women who are breastfeeding

The vaginal ring provides controlled release of a progestogen/estrogen combination (Fig 9.1C). It is a flexible polymer ring that slowly releases EE (15 micrograms/24 hours) and etonogestrel (120 micrograms/24 hours). It is inserted by the woman into her vagina and left for 3 weeks, then removed; her next menstrual period usually starts within 2–3 days. Absorption of the steroid hormones through vaginal epithelium is rapid, and first-pass metabolism is avoided. The ring has similar contraceptive efficacy, possible adverse effects, precautions and contraindications as combined estrogen–progestogen products taken orally in the COC pill.

Intrauterine devices (IUDs) *Suitable for women who are breastfeeding

An intrauterine device is a small device in the shape of a 'T' which is placed inside the uterus (Fig 9.1B). IUDs alter the intrauterine environment to decrease sperm motility and viability, inhibit or decrease ovulation and follicular development and inhibit nidation (attachment of the fertilised ovum in the endometrium). They can cause dysmenorrhoea, pelvic inflammatory disease or uterine perforation, and the IUD can be expelled from the uterus. There are two types of IUDs, copper and hormone infused. IUDs are used for long-term (5–8 years) reversible contraception. The IUD should only be fitted by trained practitioners (Johnson 2005). Insertion of an IUD is usually a relatively short sterile procedure, usually completed within 10 minutes. Insertion may be uncomfortable rather than painful; however, for some women it can be painful. Analgesia such as a NSAID can be taken an hour prior to the procedure and a local anaesthetic may also be applied prior to the insertion. The device is fitted via the vagina. The practitioner inserts a speculum to enable the cervix to be visualised then the IUD is inserted into the uterus via the cervix with an insertion tube. Once the IUD is in place the insertion tube is removed, the IUD remains in the uterus with the threads hanging through the cervical os into the vagina. Threads are trimmed to approximately 3 cm and this should be recorded in the woman's notes (Johnson 2005). The woman should also be advised to check she is able to feel the strings monthly.

Copper IUD

In addition to the IUD effects, a copper IUD is impregnated with copper which is toxic to sperm. Copper IUDs do not have any hormonal component so are suitable for use with breastfeeding women. In Australia and New Zealand there are three main options available:

- TT-380 (licensed for up to 10 years)
- TT-380s (licensed for up to 5 years)
- LOAD Cu-375 (licensed for up to 5 years).

Some women experience increased bleeding with the copper IUD and this is the main reason cited for its removal (see Online resources).

Hormone-releasing IUD

A plastic IUD impregnated with levonorgestrel, a slow-release progestogen, is also available. It is useful for long-term contraception (5 years). The IUD releases a small amount of levonorgestrel per day into the uterine cavity which thickens the cervical mucus plug and alters the endometrial environment, making it hostile to sperm. Efficacy, safety, and satisfaction have been demonstrated in a broad population, including parous, nulliparous, and young women (Jensen et al 2022).

In Australia two hormonal IUDs are available, the Mirena® and the Kyleena®. They are both available on the PBS which makes a hormonal IUD a cost-effective option for most women. In New Zealand women have the option of two hormonal IUDs: the Mirena® and the slightly smaller Jaydess; however, the woman must cover the full cost of the device (see Online resources).

The Mirena® IUD contains 52 mg levonorgestrel and releases 20 micrograms of levonorgestrel per day over 5 years. The Kyleena contains 19.5 mg levonorgestrel. More information and comparison of the two IUDs is available from Sexual Health Victoria (see Online resources).

The Jaydess IUD contains 13.5 mg levonorgestrel. The hormonal release rate is approximately 14 micrograms/ 24 hours after 24 days and is reduced to approximately 10 micrograms /24 hours after 60 days. It then declines progressively to 6 micrograms/24 hours after one year and 5 micrograms/24 hours after 3 years. The average levonorgestrel in vivo release rate is approximately 8 micrograms/24 hours over the first year of use and 6 micrograms/24 hours over the period of 3 years.

Non-drug contraceptive methods

Non-drug methods (except for condoms) generally have much lower success rates in preventing pregnancies, but as there are no hormonal elements they are suitable for women who are breastfeeding.

Barrier methods

Barrier methods of contraception impose a physical barrier between sperm ejaculated during sexual intercourse and an oocyte in the woman's uterine tube. Some offer protection against STIs and cervical cancer; male condoms are especially effective. The female condom, a thin rubber pouch inserted in the vaginal canal, also protects against STIs.

'Diaphragms' or 'caps' inserted in the vagina prevent access of sperm to the cervical canal. They are inserted before intercourse and left in place for at least 6 hours afterwards. Complications include irritation or pain and allergic reactions. They do not prevent STIs.

'Natural' methods

The 'natural' methods of family planning or contraception include total abstinence from sexual activity, periodic abstinence planned to avoid the most fertile days of a woman's cycle (**rhythm method**), withdrawal of the penis before ejaculation (coitus interruptus) and reliance on the anti-ovulation effects of prolactin during breastfeeding.

Rhythm method

Natural family planning methods are commonly used by people who prefer not to use devices or drugs to prevent conception. They rely on attempts to predict the day of ovulation and avoidance of intercourse for several days before and after ovulation (as the ovum is viable for about 2 days and sperm for up to 7 days after intercourse). The method works only if the woman has regular periods and can predict the time of ovulation (usually 14 days before her next period). The methods require abstinence from sexual intercourse for at least half the cycle (days 8–20 in a 28-day cycle). Accuracy in predicting the day of ovulation can be improved by measuring the small rise in basal body temperature occurring in response to the mid-cycle rise in progesterone, or by identifying changes in mucus secretions, abdominal pain, breast tenderness or cervix or mood changes before, during and after ovulation. The unreliability of such methods contributes to the high birthrates and/or high abortion rates in societies or couples relying on these methods.

Sterilisation

Sterilisation is virtually 100% effective as a contraceptive method and is the most widely used form of contraception worldwide. The techniques in women involve ligation or clipping of the fallopian tubes (tubal ligation) and in men, **vasectomy** – that is, surgical interruption of the vas deferens to prevent transport of sperm. New Zealand has the highest rate of male vasectomy globally, followed by Australia, with approximately one in four men over the age of 40 having had a vasectomy. Although considered a permanent form of sterilisation, vasectomy can be reversed (**vasovasostomy**) in most men. Severe complications are rare.

KEY POINTS

Non-oral hormonal and non-drug methods

- The non-oral hormonal methods of contraception are depot injection, vaginal ring, depot intramuscular (IM) implantation and hormonal IUD.

- Longer term contraception such as IUD and implants are very effective and are being increasingly used by women in Australia and New Zealand.

- Depot injections of progestogen (e.g. depot medroxyprogesterone acetate [DMPA]) have the lowest failure rate of all reversible contraceptive methods.

- Depot implants containing a progestogen are also available and work in the same way as the depot injection to inhibit sperm and stop ovulation. The subdermal implant consists of a polymer rod impregnated with the progesterone which is implanted.

- Intrauterine devices (IUDs) are small, T-shaped devices that are inserted into the uterus to prevent pregnancy. They offer long-term contraception (between 5–10 years) but can be removed at any time by a health professional. IUDs alter the intrauterine environment to decrease sperm motility and viability, inhibit or decrease ovulation and follicular development, and inhibit nidation.

- There are two types of IUDs available, including the hormonal IUD (Mirena/Kyleena) and the non-hormonal IUD (copper).

- The hormonal IUD works by slowly releasing a very low dose of the hormone levonorgestrel.

- The copper IUD is made from copper. It does not contain hormones and works by constantly releasing a small amount of copper which is toxic to sperm.

- Barrier methods of contraception impose a physical barrier between sperm ejaculated during sexual intercourse and an oocyte in the woman's uterine tube.

- Condoms are the only form of contraception that protect against most STIs as well as preventing pregnancy.

Failure of contraception

Unintended pregnancy despite contraception can be considered an adverse event of failed therapy. More than 50% of women with an unplanned pregnancy report that they had been using some contraceptive method, obviously unsuccessfully. Of women in many countries using the COC pill, 50% admit to having missed at least one pill in the previous 3 months. Common reasons for stopping contraception, leading to 'accidental' pregnancies, include concerns about long-term effects and adverse media stories.

A common way of expressing the ineffectiveness (likely failure rate) of a contraceptive method is the Pearl Index, which gives a statistical estimate of the number of unintended pregnancies in 100 women over one year of use.

It is calculated as follows:

number of pregnancies × 12 divided by total number of women months of usage × 100

Reported failure rates of methods are shown in Table 9.3.

TABLE 9.3 Failure rates for contraceptive methods

CONTRACEPTIVE METHOD	CONTRACEPTIVE FAILURE RATE (%)
No method	85
Periodic abstinence ('rhythm method')	1–25
Withdrawal ('coitus interruptus')	4–22
Female condom	5–21
Male condom	2–18
Diaphragm	6–12
OC pill: combination	0.3–9
OC pill: progestogen-only	0.3–9
Combined hormone vaginal ring	0.3–9
Depot MPA	0.2–6
IUD + copper	0.6–0.8
Sterilisation (female)	0.2–0.5
IUD + levonorgestrel	0.2
Vasectomy (male)	0.1–0.15
Implant etonogestrel	0.05

Failure rates are expressed as % women with pregnancy during 1 year of use.
Ranges are lowest expected rate (perfect use) to typical rate in use.
IUD = intrauterine device; MPA = medroxyprogesterone acetate; OC = oral contraceptive
Sources: Australian Medicines Handbook 2024.

Medical termination

In some instances a woman may choose to terminate her pregnancy. Women should be counselled as to their options if they choose not to continue with the pregnancy. One of the options available to women in Australia and New Zealand is a medical termination, often referred to as early medical abortion (EMA). To confirm the pregnancy, serum HCG concentration levels are taken; this also provides a baseline for comparison post termination. An ultrasound is also needed to confirm an intrauterine pregnancy. There are few contradictions to medical termination and women can self-administer the medications, enabling privacy.

Mifepristone is a progestational and glucocorticoid hormone antagonist. Its inhibition of progesterone induces bleeding during the luteal phase and in early pregnancy by releasing endogenous prostaglandins from the endometrium or decidua. For early medical termination (at less than 63 days gestational age), oral mifepristone 200 mg (RU486, an antiprogestogen) followed 36–48 hours later by misoprostol self-administered at home has been shown to be a safe and effective treatment option (Bateson et al 2021; Mazza et al 2020; RANZCOG 2024 – see Online resources). (DM 9.3, DM 9.4.)

Women should be advised that follow-up is recommended to confirm there is no ongoing viable pregnancy and for any extra support that may be required. Serum HCG concentration can be measured 7 days post termination, and should be 80% lower than the baseline test taken prior to the termination. Alternatively, women may choose to take a low-sensitivity urine pregnancy test 16–21 days after the mifepristone has been taken. Low-sensitivity tests only detect HCG concentrations over 1000 IU/L, whereas standard pregnancy tests measure HCG concentrations above 25 IU/L. Women should also be provided with resources for emotional and mental health support, should it be needed, and ongoing contraception advice.

A post procedure information sheet should also be provided (see Table 9.4).

KEY POINTS

Failure of contraception

- More than 50% of women with an unplanned pregnancy report that they had been using some form of contraception.

- Women should be counselled as to their options if they choose not to continue with the pregnancy. One of the options available to women in Australia and New Zealand is a medical termination, often referred to as early medical abortion.

- There are few contraindications to medical termination and women can self-administer the medications. An essential component of offering women a medical termination is ensuring there is a follow-up plan. Women should be advised that follow-up is recommended to confirm there is no ongoing viable pregnancy and for any extra support that may be required.

DRUG MONOGRAPH 9.3
Mifepristone

Mode of action
Progesterone receptor antagonist that dilates the cervix and sensitises the myometrium to the effects of prostaglandins. It also has dose-dependent antiglucocorticoid effects (whether this occurs after a single dose of 200 mg is unclear).

Indications
Termination of first or second trimester intrauterine pregnancy, with misoprostol or gemeprost.

Adverse effects
Some of the following adverse effects may be caused by the prostaglandin given after mifepristone.
- Common (> 1%): nausea, vomiting, diarrhoea, abdominal pain, headache, dizziness, fatigue, fever, breast tenderness
- Infrequent (0.1–1%): hot flush, rash, itch, vaginal haemorrhage
- Rare (< 0.1%): uterine rupture

Dosage
According to local protocol or seek specialist advice. The following dose has been used.
- Oral: 200 mg as a single dose, followed 36–48 hours later by misoprostol or gemeprost.

Practice points
- Women must be followed up 14–21 days after taking mifepristone to ensure termination of pregnancy is complete and vaginal bleeding has stopped.
- Vaginal bleeding usually starts 1–2 days after taking mifepristone, may be heavy for 2–3 days, and lasts for 10–16 days on average.
- Medical practitioners and pharmacists must be registered and certified with MS Health before prescribing or dispensing mifepristone.
- For further information see the statement on the use of mifepristone for medical abortion at ranzcog.edu.au.

Source: Australian Medicines Handbook 2024.

DRUG MONOGRAPH 9.4
Misoprostol

Prostaglandin E1 analogue

Mode of action
Softens and dilates the cervix and induces uterine contractions via action on smooth muscle (may also have other effects, e.g. on blood vessels, bronchi, GIT).

Indications
Termination of intrauterine pregnancy up to 63 days gestation, with mifepristone.

Contraindicated
Previous caesarean section or major uterine surgery—contraindicated due to increased risk of uterine rupture.

Breastfeeding
Appears safe; theoretical possibility of diarrhoea in child.

Dosage
According to local protocol or seek specialist advice. The following doses have been used.
- Termination up to 63 days gestation:
  - Give 36–48 hours after mifepristone.
  - Oral, buccal: 800 micrograms as a single dose (or in two doses of 400 micrograms 2 hours apart). A repeat dose may be appropriate.
  - Buccal route: put tablets in the mouth between the cheeks and gums. Let them dissolve over 30 minutes before swallowing what is left of the tablets.
  - Do not use oral route after 49 days gestation as it is less effective than buccal route.
  - Surgical termination, vaginal: 400 micrograms (2 tablets) inserted into the vagina 3 hours before surgery.
- First trimester miscarriage:
  - Initial course, sublingual: 400 micrograms every 3 hours to maximum of four doses.
  - If no progress within 3 hours of last dose of misoprostol, after a 12-hour break from treatment, insert 800 micrograms (4 tablets) into the vagina, then insert 400 micrograms (2 tablets) into the vagina every 3 hours to maximum of three doses. (Total dose 2000 micrograms.)

DRUG MONOGRAPH 9.4
Misoprostol—cont'd

- Second trimester miscarriage:
  - Sublingual: 400 micrograms every 3 hours to maximum of four doses. Course may be repeated if no progress after 24 hours.
  - Vaginal: 400 micrograms (2 tablets) inserted into the vagina every 6 hours to maximum of four doses. Course may be repeated if no progress after 24 hours.
- Intrauterine fetal death:
  - < 34 weeks gestation: 200 micrograms (1 tablet) sublingually or vaginally every 3–6 hours until birth. If response is inadequate after giving 1200 micrograms over 24 hours, consider alternative treatments or repeat the regimen after 24 hours.
  - > 34 weeks gestation: 100 micrograms (half a tablet) sublingually or vaginally every 3–6 hours until birth. If response is inadequate after five doses, consider alternative treatments or repeat the regimen after 24 hours.

Counselling

- Buccal, put tablets in the mouth between the cheeks and gums. Let them dissolve over 30 minutes before swallowing what is left of the tablets.

Source: Australian Medicines Handbook 2024.

TABLE 9.4 Advice after a medical abortion

GENERAL ADVICE AFTER A MEDICAL ABORTION

A follow-up blood test is very important to check that the abortion has been successful. The test needs to be taken 7 days after you took the first tablet (mifepristone). Other forms of testing may be appropriate for some people, but your clinic will discuss these with you if they are an option. For 7 days after taking the second tablet (misoprostol), to reduce the risk of infection, avoid:
- sexual intercourse
- use of tampons or menstrual cups
- swimming
- taking a bath or using a spa.

WHEN TO GO TO AN EMERGENCY DEPARTMENT

Go to an emergency department if at any time you have:
- very heavy bleeding, such as any of the following:
  - your bleeding fills more than two large pads in an hour for more than 2 hours in a row
  - you are passing clots the size of a small lemon or larger
  - you feel faint and think the bleeding is heavy even if you are not sure about how much you are bleeding
- any of the following symptoms (which could mean an ectopic pregnancy in the Fallopian tube):
  - severe abdominal (tummy) pain
  - pain in your pelvis on one side
  - pain in the tips of your shoulders
- other concerns and you don't have access to medical advice (e.g. from the prescribing clinic).

WHEN TO CONTACT THE CLINIC THAT PRESCRIBED THE ABORTION DRUGS

If you have any of the symptoms below, you might still be pregnant. Contact the clinic if:
- at 24 hours after taking misoprostol, you either:
  - have had no or little bleeding (less than a normal period), or
  - have not passed any pregnancy tissue, or any clots larger than a small grape
- at 48 hours after taking misoprostol, you still have nausea
- you had some initial bleeding, but it stopped within 4 days of taking misoprostol
- at 14 days after taking misoprostol, you still have breast tenderness.

If you have any of the symptoms below, there might still be some pregnancy tissue (e.g. placenta) in the uterus (womb). Contact the clinic if:
- at 7 days after taking misoprostol:
  - you are still passing clots
  - you still have cramping pain
  - you still have bleeding that is heavier than a period
  - you have bleeding that stopped and restarted and has been as heavy as a period for the last 24 hours or more
- at 14 days after taking misoprostol you have bleeding that is not much less than when it started
- at 4 to 5 weeks after taking misoprostol you still have bleeding that is different to your usual menstrual cycle.

Continued

TABLE 9.4 Advice after a medical abortion—cont'd

Contact the clinic if you have any of the symptoms below, as they can indicate that you have an infection of the uterus: • pelvic pain • pain during sex • unusual vaginal discharge • fever (over 38°C) • tenderness on touching the abdomen (tummy) or pelvis • nausea or vomiting • feel unwell.
Contact the clinic that prescribed the abortion drugs if you have any concerns about the medical abortion.

Source: Published in eTG complete, December 2020. ©Therapeutic Guidelines Ltd https://ccmsfiles.tg.org.au/s3/PDFs/pdf_SRG2_Table20.21_MedicalAbortion_v1.pdf

9.4 Postnatal mental health

The postnatal period can be a challenging time for women's mental health as they negotiate the transition to motherhood. Perinatal and postnatal mental health disorders, including posttraumatic stress disorder (PTSD), are increasing globally. Australia and New Zealand have seen an increase in women dying by suicide in recent years. The risk of suicide is increased in women with preexisting mental health illness. Early assessment and identification of potential risk factors and referral for appropriate support is essential. Preexisting mental health conditions should be monitored as these can be exacerbated in the postnatal period due to lack of sleep and changes in hormones. Women are often reluctant to take medications in the postnatal period if they are breastfeeding; however, some medications are suitable for use in lactating women. Mental health is discussed in detail in Chapter 19, including medications that may be prescribed for women during pregnancy and postpartum for acute and chronic mental health issues. Medication suitable for lactating and breastfeeding women is discussed in Chapter 10.

9.5 Complementary and alternative medicine

Complementary and alternative medicines (CAMs) are becoming more widely used throughout the childbirth continuum and this includes the postnatal period. In the postnatal period CAM may be used to prevent infection, as analgesia to relieve sore muscles, to promote wound healing, relieve perineal bruising and soreness, and to treat haemorrhoids (Weed 1986).

Herbs

Alfalfa (Medicago sativa) – contains vitamins A, D, E and K as well as chlorophyll and carotene; and minerals such as potassium, calcium, magnesium. Helps remedy anaemia and balances hormones

Black cohosh (Cimicifuga racemosa) – a uterine tonic and spasmolytic, helps treat afterpains

Celtic sea salt – helpful in soothing, cleansing and healing of wounds

Chamomile (Matricaria recutita) – analgesic, anti-inflammatory, antibiotic, and has anti-inflammatory properties

Cinnamon (Cinnamomum cassia) – a warming herb which improves circulation and reduces uterine cramps

Comfrey (Symphytum officinale) – promotes new cell growth and controls bleeding. A great overall healer. Not to be taken internally. Do not use on broken skin

Crampbark (Viburnum opulus) – muscle relaxant and anti-spasmodic, this herb also nourishes and soothes the nervous system with its nervine and sedative effects

Corydalis (Corydalis ambigua) – a mild sedative and analgesic herb

Fennel (Foeniculum vulgare) – a spasmolytic herb, can be used for postnatal afterpains and balances hormones. Also has galactogogue actions

Ginger (Zingiber officinale) – relaxes spasms and soothes stressed nerves

Horse chestnut (Aesculus hippocastanum) – an astringent, and a circulatory tonic with anti-inflammatory properties. Improves microvascular circulation and reduces swelling

Lady's mantle (Alchemilla vulgaris) – an astringent herb which has a strengthening effect on the endometrium and uterine wall and helps protect healing elastin fibres

Lavender (Lavandula officinalis) – antiseptic, analgesic and antibacterial properties

Lemon balm (Melissa officinalis) – a balancing, calming herb

Marigold (Calendula officinalis) – antiseptic, soothing wound inflammation, general wound healing

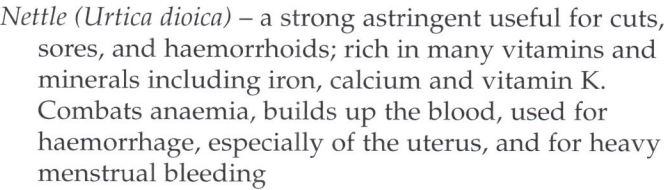

Nettle (Urtica dioica) – a strong astringent useful for cuts, sores, and haemorrhoids; rich in many vitamins and minerals including iron, calcium and vitamin K. Combats anaemia, builds up the blood, used for haemorrhage, especially of the uterus, and for heavy menstrual bleeding

Plantain (Plantago lanceolate) – has a soothing, cooling effect and considered an effective remedy for healing haemorrhoids

Raw honey – has natural antibacterial properties which have proven health benefits when taken internally or applied to the skin and wounds

Red clover (Trifolium pratense) – a blood-building tonic rich in iron and copper salts, improves platelets and haemoglobin counts

Red raspberry leaf (Rubus idaeus) – a uterine tonic, rich in many nutrients including calcium, iron, magnesium, and vitamins, which nourish the female reproductive system. Supports and tones the muscles and ligaments of the uterus

Rosemary (Rosmarinus officinalis) – astringent, antibacterial and anti-inflammatory properties

Sage (Salvia officinalis) – astringent, antiseptic and anti-inflammatory properties

Shepherd's purse (Capsella bursa-pastoris) – astringent, antiseptic and useful to reduce bleeding and bruising

St John's wort – along with comfrey, relieves pain and reduces inflammation and swelling

Wild yam (Dioscorea villosa) – has anti-spasmodic and hormone-modulating actions, reduces the intensity of postnatal afterpains

Witch hazel (Hamamelis virginiana) – an astringent, curbs bleeding and reduces inflammation, pain, itching and swelling. Useful for relief of haemorrhoids and perineal trauma

Withania (Withania somnifera) – used for recovery and convalescence

Yarrow (Achillea millefolium) – astringent and antibacterial properties; the anti-spasmodic effects reduce inflammation. A superior remedy for wounds and cuts.

Homeopathy

Arnica – commonly used for bruising and can aid in healing the perineum and other tissues after birth. It can also be used for afterpains

Aconite – for insomnia, feelings of anxiety, restlessness and worry

Bellis perennis – for bruising and trauma related to birth, as well as afterpains

Calms forte – gentle sleep aid, helpful for women who are exhausted but having trouble sleeping and adjusting to their drastically altered sleeping rhythms

Calcarea carbonica – can help women with feelings of being overwhelmed in the postpartum

Cimicifuga – for emotionally and hormonally based depression

Mag phos – for spasmodic cramping pain

Sepia – for supporting and balancing postnatal hormonal changes, the baby blues and postpartum depression

Pulsatilla – for supporting emotionally sensitive women who are prone to tears in the postpartum

Phosphorus – for anxiety and fear in the postnatal period.

Essential oils/aromatherapy

Soothing – a blend of rosemary, hypericum, lavender and arnica oils in the bath or as a massage is soothing

Exhaustion – oils such as lavender, geranium, neroli and orange can be used in an oil burner or added to the bath or a massage blend.

KEY POINTS

CAMs

- Complementary and alternative medicines (CAMs) are becoming more widely used throughout the childbirth continuum and this includes during the postnatal period.

- It is essential that midwives have a basic understanding of the CAM therapies a woman may use to allow for an open and honest discussion about the risks and benefits of their use.

- Common CAMs used are aromatherapy, herbal medicines and homeopathy.

CONCLUSION

The postnatal period is a time of major transition for women, both physically and psychologically. The midwife is ideally placed to be able to provide information and support the woman to treat any postnatal challenges she may have that require medicines. Use of prescription drugs, over-the-counter preparations, limited CAM therapies, and contraceptives are common features of care for the majority of women in the postnatal period. A comprehensive approach to the care of the woman and her infant at this time encompasses a thorough history of medication use, past and present. It also includes regular review and education to ensure the health status of both the woman and her baby are optimised.

REVIEW QUESTIONS

1 What is the most appropriate analgesia for the postpartum woman following a vaginal birth with perineal trauma? Describe your rationale and reasoning.

2 What is the most appropriate analgesia for the postpartum woman following a caesarean section? Describe some specific aspects of the woman's history and plan for ongoing care that may be relevant to the selection of analgesic in this context.

3 What advice would you give to a postnatal woman with extensive perineal trauma in relation to prophylactic antibiotics? Include any additional advice and education, including comfort measures and evidence for use of CAM therapies that may be appropriate.

4 What are the different types of hormonal contraceptives, and which are most suitable for women who are breastfeeding? Are there other factors (additional to breastfeeding status) that should be considered with respect to selection of a post-birth hormonal contraceptive?

REFERENCES

Bateson D, McNamee K, Harvey C. Medical abortion in primary care. Aust Prescr. 2021;44:187-192. doi.org/10.18773/austprescr.2021.050 (accessed 21 August 2023)

Butcher B, Donovan C, Farrell L, et al. Risk of venous thromboembolism in women taking the combined oral contraceptive: a systematic review and meta-analysis. AJGP. 2016;45(1):58-67.

Deussen AR, Ashwood P, Martis R, et al. Relief of pain due to uterine cramping/involution after birth. Cochrane Database Syst Rev. 2020, Issue 10. CD004908. doi:10.1002/14651858.CD004908.pub3

Islam MZ, Billah A, Islam MM, et al. Negative effects of short birth interval on child mortality in low- and middle-income countries: a systematic review and meta-analysis. J Glob Health. 2022;12:04070.

Jensen JT, Lukkari-Lax E, Schulze A, et al. Contraceptive efficacy and safety of the 52-mg levonorgestrel intrauterine system for up to 8 years: findings from the Mirena Extension Trial. Am J Obstet Gynecol. 2022;227:873.e1-12. doi.org/10.1016/j.ajog.2022.09.007 (accessed 1 April 2024)

Johnson BA. Insertion and removal of intrauterine devices. Am Fam Physician. 2005 Jan;71(1):95-102. PMID: 15663031. (accessed 1 April 2024)

Klebanoff MA. Interpregnancy interval after stillbirth: modifiable, but does it matter? Lancet. 2019;393:1482–1483.

Mazza D, Burton G, Wilson S, et al. Medical abortion. AJGP. 2020 Jun;49(6). doi: 10.31128/AJGP-02-20-5223 (accessed 21 August 2023)

Ni W, Gao X, Su X, et al. Birth spacing and risk of adverse pregnancy and birth outcomes: a systematic review and dose-response meta-analysis. Acta Obstet Gynecol Scand. 2023 Dec;102(12):1618-1633. doi: 10.1111/aogs.14648. Epub 2023 Sep 7. PMID: 37675816; PMCID: PMC10619614.

Sääv I, Fiala C, Hämäläinen JM, et al. Medical abortion in lactating women—low levels of mifepristone in breast milk. Acta Obstet Gynecol Scand. 2010 May;89(5):618-622. doi: 10.3109/00016341003721037. PMID: 20367522.

Saha MR, Ryan K, Amir LH. Postpartum women's use of medicines and breastfeeding practices: a systematic review. Int Breastfeed J. 2015;10(28). doi.org/10.1186/s13006-015-0053-6

Sedgh G, Singh S, Hussain R. Intended and unintended pregnancies worldwide in 2012 and recent trends. Stud Fam Plann. 2014;45:301-314. doi: 10.1111/j.1728-4465.2014.00393.x.

Shaaban OM et al. 2019. Levonorgestrel emergency contraceptive pills use during breastfeeding; effect on infants' health and development. J Matern Fetal Neonatal Med. 32:2524–2528. doi:10.1080/14767058.2018.1439470.

Stark EL, Gariepy AM, Son M. What is long-acting reversible contraception? JAMA. 2022;328(13):1362. doi:10.1001/jama.2022.14239 (accessed 1 April 2024)

Stewart M, Black K, Choosing a combined oral contraceptive pill. Aust Prescr. 2015;38(1):6–11. In, Tiran D, Complementary therapies for pregnancy and childbirth, 2nd edn. Elsevier 2000. ISBN: 9780702023286

Weed, SS. Wise woman herbal for the childbearing year, volume 1. Woodstock NY: Ash Tree Publishing 1986.

ONLINE RESOURCES

Australian Medicines Handbook 2024: https://amhonline.amh.net.au/auth (accessed 11 March 2024)

Centre for Disease Control (2023). Progestin: https://www.cdc.gov/reproductivehealth/contraception/mmwr/spr/progestin.html (accessed 1 April 2024)

Drugs and Lactation Database (LactMed®). Bethesda (MD): National Institute of Child Health and Human Development (2006). Oxycodone: https://www.ncbi.nlm.nih.gov/books/NBK501245/ (accessed 1 April 2024)

RANZCOG. Clinical Guidelines for Abortion Care (2024): https://ranzcog.edu.au/resources/abortion-guideline/ (accessed 14 March 2024)

Sexual Health Victoria (2022). Hormonal IUDs available in Australia. A comparison chart tool for clinicians to use with patients to assist in decision making: https://shvic.org.au/assets/resources/SHV_Hormonal_IUDS_Clinician_with_Patient.pdf (accessed 1 April 2024)

Therapeutic Guidelines. Advice after a medical abortion (2020): https://ccmsfiles.tg.org.au/s3/PDFs/pdf_SRG2_Table20.21_MedicalAbortion_v1.pdf

Online resources (various) – Contraception:

https://www.bmj.com/company/newsroom/antibiotics-may-lessen-effectiveness-of-hormonal-contraception/

https://www.getthefacts.health.wa.gov.au/condoms-contraception/types-of-contraception

https://medsafe.govt.nz/profs/datasheet/j/jaydessIVD.pdf

https://www.mims.co.uk/drugs/contraception/contraceptive-devices/copper-t-380-a

https://www.thewomens.org.au/health-information/contraception/intra-uterine-device-iud

https://www.thewomens.org.au/health-information/contraception/your-contraception-choices/

https://www.msiaustralia.org.au/

CHAPTER 10

THE NEWBORN AND LACTATION

Roslyn Donnellan-Fernandez, Clare Davison

Key Abbreviations

ADH	anti-diuretic hormone
AED	anti-epileptic drug
G6PD	glucose-6-phosphate dehydrogenase deficiency
GH	growth hormone
GIT	gastrointestinal
HcG	human chorionic gonadotrophin
M/P	milk plasma
MW	molecular weight
NSAID	non-steroidal anti-inflammatory drug
OC	oral contraceptive
PB	protein binding
pKa	measure of the relative strength (degree of ionisation) of a weak acid or base
PRIF	prolactin release inhibiting factor (dopamine)
RID	relative infant dose
SSRI	selective serotonin reuptake inhibitor
T½	half-life – the time required for plasma concentration of a drug to decrease by 50%
TCA	tricyclic antidepressant
THC	tetrahydrocannabinol
Tmax	the time a drug takes to reach maximum concentration
TRH	thyrotropin-releasing hormone
Vd	volume distribution – a drug's propensity to remain in plasma or redistribute to other tissue compartments

Chapter Focus

This chapter focuses on pharmacology and medication use during lactation and breastfeeding. The basic principles of medication management in well newborns are covered, including common medications administered or prescribed by midwives. It provides the midwife with an understanding of the principles that regulate the passage of drugs into breast milk, and includes an overview of some common medications/CAMs used to support lactation. Classification systems for the safety of medications during lactation are described. Adverse effects and drug interactions between prescribed medications and breast milk reported in lactating women are covered, including potential developmental outcomes for infant health and recommendations for follow-up. Research on medications used by breastfeeding women and related ethical issues are discussed. The critical thinking scenario, case study and review questions covered in the chapter will equip the midwife to confidently describe principles of medication use, identify drug interactions and adverse effects in breast milk – including potential impact on infants – and apply enhanced clinical decision making in partnership with lactating and breastfeeding women.

Key Drug Groups

Dopamine antagonists:
- domperidone, metoclopramide

Dopamine agonists:
- cabergoline, bromocriptine

Analgesics:
- NSAIDs, acetaminophen/paracetamol

Anxiolytics and antidepressants:
- AEDs, SSRIs, TCAs

Anti-infectives

Contraceptives

Social drugs

Other:
- asthmatic, cardiovascular, antihistamines

Key Terms

agonist 188
antagonist 187
autocrine 186
daltons 190
dopamine 187
estrogen 186
endocrine 186
galactogogue 197
human placental
    lactogen 186

ionisation 190
lactation 187
mammary glands 186
off-label use 193
oral bioavailability 190
oxytocin 187
pituitary gland 187
plasma protein
    binding 188
prolactin 186

Learning Outcomes

- Understand the relationships between pharmacology, lactation and breastfeeding related to the woman and her newborn.
- Identify the principles that regulate the passage of drugs into breast milk.
- Describe classification systems for the safety of medications in lactation, and recommendations for follow-up where there are concerns regarding developmental outcomes for infant health.
- Outline the adverse effects and drug interactions between prescribed medications and breast milk, providing examples reported in lactating women.
- Understand the common medications/CAMs used to support lactation.
- Describe the principles of medication use and clinical decision making with breastfeeding women.
- Outline some of the ethical issues in therapeutic use and research of new medications with breastfeeding women.
- Understand the basic principles of medication management in well newborns.

CRITICAL THINKING SCENARIO

Fiona gave birth spontaneously to her twins, Bianca and Duncan, at 35 weeks gestation. After a 2-week stay in the newborn nursery, Fiona and the twins are discharged home, well and breastfeeding. Follow-up postnatal care has been arranged with the community midwife.

Fiona is a single parent who works from home as an established journalist and writer, and has the assistance of a live-in nanny to help care for the twins. Fiona is committed to breastfeeding but also has a hectic social schedule and increased work commitments a month after the twins' birth. Between the launch of her new book, *Super Mamas*, and other engagements she says she feels 'under pressure'. Fiona is worried that her breast milk supply will not be adequate for the twins, needs so has searched the internet for strategies and products that can increase her milk supply. You are the community midwife providing postnatal care to Fiona and the twins. During your first visit, Fiona tells you about her internet research on products to help increase her milk supply. She tells you she has found prescription and non-prescription items that may help.

1   What are some of the products and/or medications Fiona may have found? As her midwife, what information, advice and strategies do you discuss with her?

Fiona has been eagerly anticipating her interstate book launch when she will reconnect with Randall, the twins' father. She says she is looking forward to indulging her passion for champagne, alcohol, cigarettes, and some recreational drugs, all of which she was careful to avoid during her pregnancy. Fiona informs you that her nanny and the twins are travelling with her to the book launch and breastfeeding will be uninterrupted.

2   In view of Fiona's disclosures, what information may be essential for her decision making regarding the upcoming trip in relation to lactation, breastfeeding, and care of herself and the twins?

On her return from interstate, Fiona requests an urgent home visit. She is upset and angry. This morning her treating medical specialist advised that the recent onset of labile mood swings indicates that Fiona should resume pre-pregnancy medication to stabilise her mood. Fiona insists this is 'overkill' as she has been 'on top of the world' with many successes. She asks for your opinion about suitable complementary and alternative treatments she can use to manage her mood that will not interfere with breastfeeding, breast milk expression, or pharmaceutical contraception. She advises she has been taking St John's wort for the past 2 weeks, prior to travelling. As a last resort, Fiona asks about the 'best' prescription medication if she is 'compelled' to resume pharmacologic treatment for her mood swings as advised by her treating psychiatrist.

3   How will you advise Fiona?

Introduction

Abundant evidence reveals the benefits of breastfeeding for newborn infants and their mothers (see Online resources; AIHW 2023; COAG 2019). Breast milk provides complete nourishment to the infant, promotes healthy growth and development, and reduces the risk of diabetes, obesity, infection, leukaemia, and asthma development (Australian Breastfeeding Association 2024; Binns et al 2016). In addition, breastfeeding mothers have reduced risk of developing type 2 diabetes, breast cancer, and ovarian cancer (Kirkegaard et al 2018; Stordal 2023; Victora et al 2016). In Australia, the National Health and Medical Research Council (NHMRC) publishes infant feeding guidelines recommending that infants be exclusively breastfed until around 6 months of age, when solid food can be introduced. The guidelines also recommend that breastfeeding be continued until 12 months of age and beyond, 'for as long as the mother and child desire' (NHMRC 2013).

10.1 Use of medicines while breastfeeding

Use of medicines, including non-prescription items and CAM products, during breastfeeding is common and many mothers require medications while breastfeeding. A systematic review undertaken in 2015 indicated that more than 50% of postpartum women (breastfeeding or not) are required to take at least one medicine, and when vitamins and mineral supplements are included, this increases to almost 100% (Saha et al 2015). Maternal need for medication should not become a barrier to breastfeeding (Lynch et al 2018; McClatchey et al 2018). Drug therapy may be required to maintain the health of the woman experiencing acute or chronic illness and be essential for the ongoing welfare of the mother and baby. Breastfeeding women should therefore be provided with reliable sources of medication information. Women should also be informed of the importance of consultation with their primary health providers and prescribers prior to the initiation or modification of medication therapy during lactation and breastfeeding (Byerley et al 2022). Ethical issues may also arise in relation to the use of medications during lactation, especially where safety data may be inconclusive due to limited research on drugs in breastfeeding (Amir et al 2020; Illamola et al 2018; Mauvais-Jarvis et al 2021; Weld et al 2022). Typically, while most women demonstrate caution in relation to taking prescription medication while breastfeeding, this caution may not be observed in relation to CAMs or other herbal supplements (Barnes et al 2019). Some cautious considerations for the midwife caring for a breastfeeding woman and her infant if using CAM preparations are also provided in this chapter (McGuire 2018).

Safe drug therapy during lactation

Nearly all drugs, with few exceptions, transfer into breast milk and while most drugs can be considered 'safe' during breastfeeding, there are some exceptions that pose additional, significant risk to a breastfed infant, including drug–drug interactions. Medications that are compatible with breastfeeding and those that are contraindicated are discussed later in this chapter, including reference to useful quality sources of information and helplines for both health professionals and parents (see Online resources and Box 10.1). Some drugs taken by a breastfeeding mother may affect lactation and can be absorbed by the infant in sufficient amounts to cause pharmacological or toxic effects (Ahmadzai et al 2022). Factors that may influence this include the dose received through the breast milk and pharmacokinetics; therefore the effect of the drug in the breastfeeding infant should also be considered when prescribing medications for lactating women, including the potential for drug–drug interactions where the woman is taking multiple medications (Anderson & Momper 2020; Byrne & Spong 2019; Jones 2023). However, it is essential for the welfare of both mother and baby that the mother's health be maintained, and therefore drug therapy may be required. Women may hesitate to combine medicine use with breastfeeding, or may not initiate breastfeeding, or may stop taking medicines while breastfeeding (Scime et al 2023). They may also cease breastfeeding or choose formula feeding while taking medicines due to concern for their infant (Saha et al 2015).

Some healthcare practitioners mistakenly equate artificial feeding with breastfeeding as the infant's age increases (Biggs et al 2020; Quinn & Tanis 2020). Concerns over the risks of medication use in breastfeeding, and lack of knowledge on how to access information on the safety of medications in breastfeeding, have been found to be factors influencing health practitioners' decisions to recommend the cessation of breastfeeding in order to commence medications (McClatchey et al 2018). Stephens et al (2018) also point out that some healthcare practitioners believe that pregnancy contraindications for medications also apply to breastfeeding, highlighting that product information leaflets are designed to minimise the risk of litigation.

The above combined influences demonstrate why the recommendation to cease breastfeeding is common. It is therefore important that the advice and knowledge provided by midwives ensure optimal health outcomes for mothers and their babies as they make decisions about safe medication use during lactation. This encompasses awareness of which medications are appropriate for breastfeeding women and which are not. It is essential that the midwife obtains a full history, including the drugs they may be taking

BOX 10.1   Examples of drugs that should be avoided during breastfeeding

Alcohol (delay drinking until after a feed)	Iodine
Amiodarone	Lamotrigine
Anthracyclines (e.g. doxorubicin)	Lithium
Antineoplastic agents	Marijuana
Aspirin (high dose)	Methadone
Atenolol	Methotrexate
Chloramphenicol	Estrogens
Ciclosporin	Phenindione
Cocaine	Phenobarbital (phenobarbitone)
Combined oral contraceptives	Propylthiouracil
Cyclophosphamide	Radiopharmaceuticals
Diazepam	Retinoids
Dopamine agonists	Smoking (nicotine replacement is preferable)
Doxorubicin	Sotalol
Ephedrine hydrochloride	Tetracyclines
Ergotamine	Theophylline
Gold salts (e.g. auranofin, aurothiomalate)	Vigabatrin
Heroin	

Sources: Australian Medicines Handbook 2021; Hotham & Hotham 2015. Consult specialist pregnancy drug information centres for comprehensive advice.

independently for other illness or for chronic health conditions. The effects, side effects and interactions with other substances and medications may differ substantively for each mother/baby dyad (Datta et al 2019; McGuire 2019). Providing adequate and up-to-date information on medications prescribed, and the clear reasons for prescribing them, is essential so that women can make informed choices about the treatment they receive and the likely effect on themselves and their infants.

10.2 Pharmacology and breastfeeding

Anatomical overview and physiology – mammary glands

The **mammary gland** is a specialised organ, highly evolved, developing on each side of the anterior chest wall (Fig 10.1). The organ's primary function is to secrete milk. Although the gland is present in both sexes it is well developed in females, but rudimentary in males (Khan et al 2024).

Hormones and lactation

During pregnancy, the hormone levels of **estrogen**, progesterone, and prolactin rise, initiating the first stage of lactation by causing glandular tissue in the breasts to develop during the pregnancy period. It is important to be aware that non-gestational parents (adoptive or transgender) can induce lactation by stimulating breast milk production with hormone therapy. Following birth and during the transition from **endocrine** to **autocrine** control of lactation there are two principal hormones that directly affect breastfeeding: prolactin and oxytocin. These hormones are necessary for milk synthesis and secretion (let-down).

Prolactin – an anterior pituitary hormone – is the lactogenic hormone involved in proliferation and secretion of the mammary glands of mammals. Human prolactin is a protein hormone (198 amino acids in a single peptide chain), closely related chemically to GH and the placental hormone human chorionic gonadotrophin (**human placental lactogen**). Females have about 1.5 times the male concentration of prolactin. The physiological action of prolactin in females causes an increase in the amount of breast tissue during pregnancy (via actions of estrogens), and in milk

Anatomy of a lactating breast

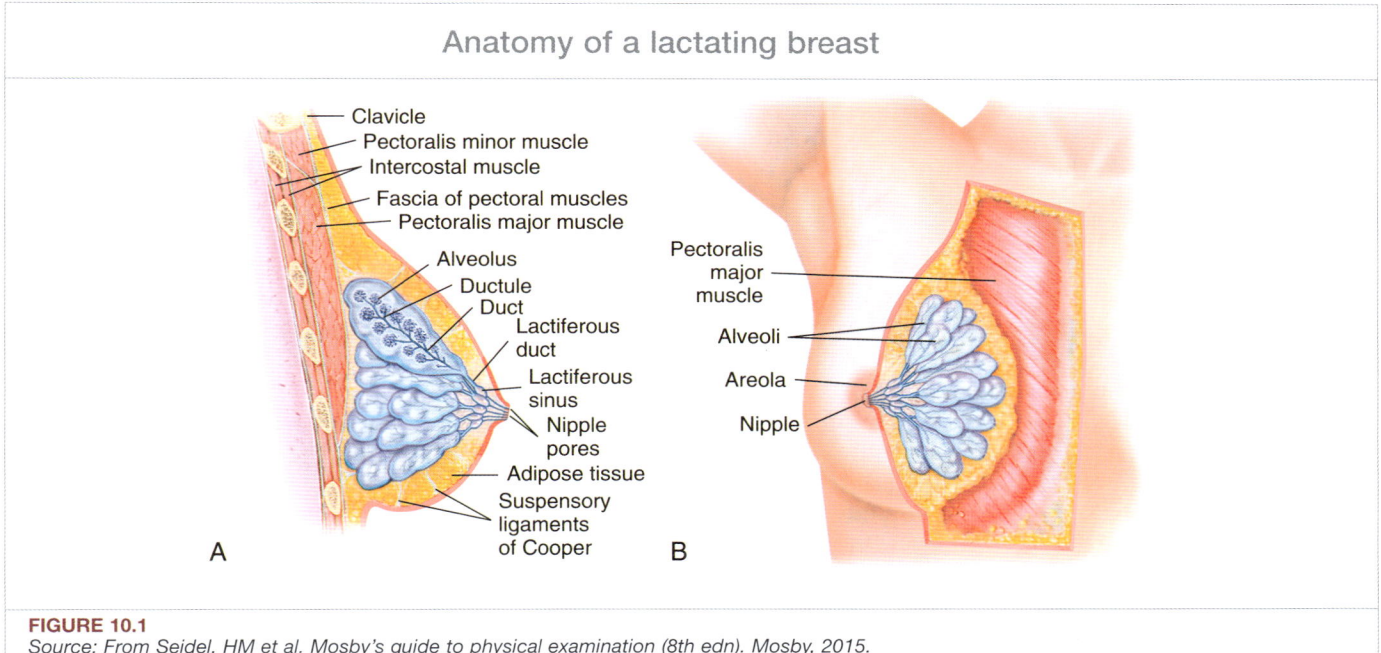

FIGURE 10.1
Source: From Seidel, HM et al. Mosby's guide to physical examination (8th edn). Mosby, 2015.

production, and possibly 'nest-building behaviour'. Gonadotrophin release and ovulation are suppressed which tends to have natural contraceptive effects in breastfeeding women. Prolactin is also secreted and has autocrine roles in other tissues, and signalling may be involved in other reproductive cancers (breast and prostate). The main hypothalamic control over prolactin release is inhibitory, via PRIF, which appears to be the central nervous system neurotransmitter, **dopamine**. Stimuli for release of prolactin include estrogens, suckling by a baby, dopamine antagonists (notably the neuroleptic agents used in schizophrenia) and TRH. Prolactin inhibits its own secretion by stimulating dopamine production in the brain, a short feedback loop (Grattan 2015). Prolactin enhances functions of the mammary glands; its release is inhibited by dopamine.

Oxytocin – a posterior pituitary hormone – stimulates the mammary glands to increase milk secretion (let-down); release during suckling by the infant helps reduce the uterus to pre-pregnancy size (involution). Oxytocin also has weak anti-diuretic hormone (ADH)-like actions but may have transient vasodilator action. It has been called the 'love hormone' and 'moral molecule' as it appears to be involved in personal relationships, trust, altruism, generosity, parenting, postnatal depression, autism, and the immune system (Zik & Roberts 2015). Mammals deprived of social contact when young have reduced levels of oxytocin and get less pleasure from rewarding stimuli.

Lactation promoters and inhibitors

Lactation – that is, production of milk from the mammary glands (breasts) – is initiated and maintained by the anterior pituitary hormone prolactin. Lactation begins when levels of progesterone and estradiol drop rapidly after birth. Suckling at the breast by the infant increases secretion of prolactin by neural reflexes, which act via the hypothalamus and **pituitary gland**, and triggers the milk let-down reflex, with oxytocin as a mediator. Prolactin release is inhibited by the hypothalamic prolactin release-inhibitory factor, the neurotransmitter dopamine. Suckling or mechanical stimulation of the nipple are the best stimulators of prolactin secretion.

Drugs can affect milk secretion or composition including mammary gland development, milk secretion and hormonal regulation of lactation (CFB 10.1). The dopamine **antagonists** domperidone and metoclopramide, normally prescribed as antiemetics or to stimulate motility of the upper GIT, have been used (off-label) to stimulate lactation by inhibiting prolactin release-inhibitory factor; however, there are safety concerns (Hale & Krutsch 2023; McGuire 2018). Dopamine antagonists, such as the phenothiazine psychotropic agents, may cause gynaecomastia and galactorrhoea. As domperidone use for lactation stimulation is 'off-label', recommendations/guidelines for use cautiously advise 10 mg of domperidone (1 tablet) three times a day until breast milk supply is well established. This may take several weeks. Occasionally, the prescriber may increase the dose to 20 mg (2 tablets) three times a day. The dose may vary depending on the woman's milk supply, but no more than 60 mg (6 tablets) should be taken in 1 day. Once milk supply is well established, the dose should be decreased gradually, for example 10 mg (1 tablet) two times a day for 1 week, before stopping the medicine altogether (see Online resources: Mothersafe). Drug side effects include headache (most common), abdominal pain, dry mouth, rash, and trouble sleeping. Other side effects such as restlessness and muscle spasm may occur, but they are rare. Women can be reassured that side effects such as tardive dyskinesia are associated with long-term use of dopamine antagonist medication only. However, domperidone should not be taken if women are taking other drugs such as antibiotics, antifungals, heart medication and some antidepressant/antipsychotic medication due to drug–drug interactions (AMH 2024).

It may be necessary, for clearly defined medical reasons, to inhibit lactation – for example, if the mother must take essential drugs that would be harmful to the infant when ingested in breast milk, or if the infant has died. Dopamine **agonists** cabergoline and bromocriptine inhibit release of prolactin from the anterior pituitary gland, resulting in suppression of lactation. Bromocriptine is no longer considered a suitable drug for lactation suppression due to case reports of associated maternal deaths from myocardial infarction (McGuire 2018), and cabergoline should only be used with caution.

Estrogens in combination contraceptive pill formulations also inhibit lactation; hence, estrogens are not used in oral contraceptive (OC) formulations in breastfeeding women. They are no longer indicated to treat postpartum breast engorgement. Conservative measures such as firm breast support (e.g. a supportive bra that is not restrictive, such as a sports bra) and ice packs are effective, with analgesics.

CLINICAL FOCUS BOX 10.1

Dopamine and lactation

When stimulation of lactation is required in a breastfeeding mother, a dopamine antagonist (e.g. domperidone) can be administered. However, natural methods facilitating breastfeeding are preferred (e.g. increased direct infant suckling and pumping to stimulate breast milk supply). When cessation of lactation is required (e.g. in cases of fetal or infant loss), drugs such as bromocriptine and cabergoline may be used to inhibit lactation.

Because dopamine is a neurotransmitter in many pathways in both the peripheral and central nervous systems, there are many adverse reactions and adverse drug interactions whenever dopamine agonists or antagonists are used; therefore ongoing monitoring and review of therapeutic aim, dosage, and pharmacologic effect, including side effects and potential for other drug interactions, is important. Adverse effects can occur particularly in the central nervous system, motor nervous system, cardiovascular system, endocrine glands, and gastrointestinal tract.

Passage of drugs into breast milk

There are complex interrelationships within the mother–baby dyad that govern how medications move from one to the other during breastfeeding. Understanding the basic principles enables the midwife to apply these concepts to most medications, even where there is limited research and evidence base for how the medication will affect a breastfed baby. Medications may pass from maternal plasma into breast milk by either passive diffusion, or less commonly, by active transport. The factors that influence the rate and amount of transfer vary depending on which pathway applies to the individual drug.

Almost all drugs in maternal circulation can be readily transferred to the colostrum (milk produced in the first week after birth) and breast milk; exceptions are large molecules such as heparin. Previously, insulin molecules were also thought to be too large, although research demonstrating the presence of both exogenous and endogenous insulin in breast milk now suggests there may be an 'active transport' mechanism involved. In general, the proven benefits of continuing breastfeeding must be weighed on an individual basis against the risks of exposure of the infant to maternal medications, and risks to the mother from ceasing essential drugs.

The mammary alveolar epithelium is more permeable to drugs during the colostrum stage of milk production; transfer of a drug or its metabolites into milk occurs predominantly by passive diffusion. Drug factors that enhance drug excretion into milk include dose and frequency, high maternal plasma drug concentration, low maternal **plasma protein binding**, low molecular weight (< 200) and greater lipid solubility. Central nervous system (CNS)-active drugs, being lipid-soluble, are likely to partition into breast milk, and hence the need for caution in prescribing (e.g. drugs used for management of epilepsy and seizures such as carbamazepine and phenytoin are highly lipid-soluble). So too is the recreational drug cannabis. Being 99% protein-bound, liposoluble, and of low molecular weight, THC can pass easily into breast milk to impact a newborn, including effects such as delayed motor development (Navarrete et al 2020).

CNS depressants may sedate the baby and depress suckling. Codeine, an opiate drug and respiratory depressant, is inappropriate to prescribe for a breastfeeding woman. Codeine is a prodrug and is metabolised hepatically by cytochrome P450 2D6 (CYP 2D6) into the active analgesic morphine. Codeine and morphine are excreted in breast milk. Genetic polymorphisms of CYP 2D6 are associated with varying responses to codeine. In one reported case study, the mother had a CYP 2D6 variation and was an ultra-rapid metaboliser of codeine. The breastfeeding baby had accumulated toxic levels of codeine and died (Gibson et al 2016). Other cases describing toxicity in breastfed infants have been reported. A systematic review published in 2008 identified 34 additional cases of non-fatal neonatal toxicities, including apnoea, drowsiness, and bradycardia (Gibson et al 2016; Online resources: LactMED 2006).

Some women will require ongoing drug therapy while lactating to support their mental health or to treat other preexisting chronic conditions, for example hypertension, asthma, diabetes, or thyroid conditions. Where antidepressants may be needed to treat postpartum depression, the selective serotonin reuptake inhibitors (SSRIs) appear to be safe with respect to transfer into breast milk, except for fluoxetine. Fluoxetine has a longer half-life than other SSRIs and achieves higher breast milk concentrations, therefore increasing the risk of adverse impacts in the breastfed infant (Molenaar et al 2018). Since development of the SSRIs, tricyclic antidepressants (TCIs) are now rarely used in lactating women. Sertraline and paroxetine appear to be the safest SSRI medications while breastfeeding.

All antidepressants have the potential to lead to neonatal adjustment syndrome (Cornet et al 2023). Neonatal adjustment syndrome, or poor neonatal adaptation syndrome (PNAS), also described as SSRI neonatal behaviour syndrome, comprises of central nervous system, respiratory, and gastrointestinal symptoms. If observed, changing or adjusting the mother's medication is indicated, including review of infant feeding. Use of lithium carbonate provides effective treatment in women with bi-polar (mood) disorder but is problematic in relation to breastfeeding. Lithium can permeate milk and is absorbed by the breastfed infant. This drug has a safety classification of L4 (Limited Data/Possibly Hazardous); however, some studies suggest that lithium administration is not an absolute contraindication to breastfeeding, provided the infant is closely medically monitored. Where the woman wishes to continue to breastfeed, the infant should be monitored for serum lithium levels, BUN/creatinine after 6 weeks or so, and cardiac defects such as Ebstein's anomaly. Thyroid function monitoring should also be considered (Hale & Krutsch 2023).

As these examples illustrate, the decision to breastfeed depends on case-by-case evaluation of the mother's illness course, risk factors, and personal preference, as well as the health of and potential risk to the infant. Alternative medications to lithium may be carbamazepine or lamotrigine (see Chapter 19 and Online resources: Hale & Krutsch 2023). Carbamazepine has drug–drug interactions with anticoagulants, antibiotics and antifungal drugs, including clarithromycin, erythromycin and fluconazole, hence the importance of a thorough medication history and review where women and their babies may be exposed to multiple prescription medications during breastfeeding.

Although breastfeeding is not usually contraindicated in mothers taking antiepileptic drugs (AEDs), CNS-depressant drugs may pass into breast milk; therefore breastfed infants should be monitored for drowsiness and feeding difficulties. These medications include gabapentin and lamotrigine. Minimal level one evidence is available on the comparative efficacy and safety of the newer AEDs in pregnancy and lactation, including the following medications: vigabatrin, tiagabine, topiramate, and levetiracetam.

The factors influencing drug transfer into breast milk and some further detailed examples, including consideration of drug–drug interactions in breastfeeding, are considered below and in the accompanying boxes.

Passive diffusion

Passive diffusion is the predominant pathway for drug transfer. Some factors are determined by the drug itself, and others by maternal or infant physiology.

Maternal medication level is the strongest determinant of breast milk medication concentration level. As most drugs and other substances pass into and out of breast milk via passive (or simple) diffusion, there is a direct relationship between the mother's plasma level and the breast milk medication concentration. Any factors that alter the maternal plasma concentration will also alter the breast milk concentration of the medication or substance. An example is maternal blood alcohol level. As the maternal blood alcohol level rises, the breast milk alcohol levels also rise. As the woman's body metabolises the alcohol and her blood levels fall, the alcohol moves out of the breast milk and back into the maternal circulation.

In the case of a choice between two NSAIDs, ibuprofen and naproxen, which are similar in many ways, there are important differences. Whereas ibuprofen has a half-life ($T\frac{1}{2}$) of approximately 2 hours, naproxen has a half-life of around 14 hours. To reduce infant exposure to a NSAID, ibuprofen is therefore the better choice as it is cleared in approximately 10 hours, with naproxen taking almost 3 days to clear.

Degree of protein binding in the maternal plasma will also influence the amount of drug transfer into breast milk. A drug that is highly protein-bound is held tightly in the maternal serum. The large molecule of protein bound to the drug is unable to cross into breast milk; only the free portion of the drug can pass through the lactocyte. High protein binding is considered as levels > 90%. In the example above, ibuprofen for example, is over 99% bound and therefore poorly transferred into breast milk.

Stage of lactation will also influence passive medication transfer into breast milk. Medication passes from the maternal plasma compartment through the capillary wall, then through both cell membranes of the lactocyte (alveolar cell) before it can pass into the breast milk. In general, medication transfer into breast milk in the first days postpartum is greater than later in lactation. The tight junctions between the lactocytes in the initial postpartum period allow the drug to pass between the cells easily. As the lactocytes swell at the onset of lactogenesis II, the tight junctions close. Following this closure the drug must pass from the plasma compartment through the capillary wall, through the wall of the lactocyte into the lactocyte and then out of the lactocyte into the alveolar lumen into the milk compartment.

Molecular weight of a medication affects the ability of a drug to passively diffuse into milk. The smaller the molecule the easier it is to transfer across cell membranes. Molecular size is measured in **daltons** (Da). In the absence of an active transport mechanism, large molecules (over 500 Da) are excluded from breast milk. For example, heparin has a molecular weight of 12,000 –15,000 Da and is not able to pass into breast milk. In contrast, alcohol has a molecular weight of 46 Da and is therefore readily transferred.

Lipophilic drugs refer to those medications which can easily dissolve in lipids/fats. Breast milk has variable concentration of lipids, with mean concentration about 4%. Cell membranes are mostly made from lipids. Drugs that have high lipid solubility transfer across the lactocyte cell membrane and dissolve in milk lipids readily. The concentration of lipids in maternal plasma is less than in milk so the capacity for lipid-soluble drugs to be accommodated in breast milk is higher than in serum. This means that milk levels of highly lipophilic drugs can be several times higher than those in serum. Drugs specifically targeted to affect the central nervous system (e.g. antiepileptic/seizure drugs) must be lipophilic to traverse the blood-brain barrier. This characteristic therefore means they can pass into breast milk easily.

Ionisation (the positive or negative electrical charge) of a molecule also affects the transfer of a drug into breast milk. Drugs that carry no electrical charge (non-ionised) pass more readily across cell membranes. Maternal serum sits at pH of 7.4, whereas breast milk is more acidic at pH of 7.2. Drugs that are slightly alkaline will be non-ionised in the slightly alkaline maternal serum, but once in milk will become ionised in the more acidic environment (e.g. lithium), and then cannot passively diffuse back through the cell membrane into serum. The process of ionisation of weakly alkaline drugs, trapping them in breast milk, is known as ion trapping. Once a drug has entered breast milk, it does not always mean the drug will also enter the infant in sufficient dose to produce an effect. For a drug to affect the infant it must absorbed from the gut, survive the passage through the infant's liver without substantial metabolism, and then be distributed to the site of action.

Oral bioavailability is a reliable predictor of the effect a medication will have in a breastfed baby. If a non-oral route of administration is used in the mother, it is generally because the medication has low oral bioavailability. Naloxone, a drug that may be administered to a woman to reverse the effect of narcotics administered during labour is given parenterally as it has low oral bioavailability. Any naloxone that enters breast milk will be broken down within the infant's gut and not absorbed. There will be no effect in the infant.

Active transport

For a small number of medications, there are active transport systems that transport medications selectively into breast milk. While the exact details of the type of pump systems are still yet unknown, it is understood that there are proteins that sit within the lactocyte cell membrane that bind to specific molecules, and using energy, move the molecule either into or out of the milk duct. For example, iodine, acyclovir, cimetidine, nitrofurantoin, and ranitidine appear to be actively transported into milk, and metformin appears to be transported out. Active transport mechanisms are now also proposed to explain the presence of insulin in breast milk. Povidone-iodine (Betadine) used on vaginal surfaces may concentrate in breast milk, potentially disrupting normal neonatal thyroid function if sufficient doses are used.

KEY POINTS

Factors influencing drug transfer into breast milk

- Maternal medication levels
- Maternal plasma protein binding
- Stage of lactation
- Molecular weight of the medication
- Lipid solubility
- Milk pH and medication pKa
- Medication oral bioavailability
- Age and physiological maturity of the baby
- Volume of milk intake

10.3 Pharmacokinetics in infants

Data on pharmacokinetics in infants are scant and conflicting. The age and maturity of an infant's physiology is different to adults and variable. It is believed that absorptive processes in the infant's GIT and drug distribution are like those in the adult, and that lipid-soluble drugs are well absorbed. A single measurement of a drug in human milk will not accurately reflect the total dose an infant receives. The infant's actual dose depends largely on the volume of milk consumed, which is on average 0.15 L/kg/day. The dose received via milk is generally much less than known safe doses given to an infant.

Immaturity of the gastrointestinal system, liver, and kidneys of all newborn infants will influence how the infant absorbs, metabolises, and excretes a medication. Gastric emptying times are longer in neonates and intestinal absorption rates are variable. Depending on the site of absorption of a drug from the intestinal tract, this can result in either increased or decreased medication absorption. The bioavailability of a medication in an infant is therefore not necessarily the same as the bioavailability of the same medication in an adult. In addition to affecting the medication dose absorbed, the altered physiology of the infant (particularly during the early neonatal period) may result in altered metabolism and excretion of medications, so that some medications may have extended half-lives in the infant, when compared to adults, prolonging the opportunity for adverse effects to occur. For example, in a 6-month-old infant caffeine has T½ of 2.6 hours, at 3–5 months it is 14 hours and in the neonatal period it is 97.5 hours. The adult T½ of caffeine is 4.9 hours for comparison. In a premature baby whose systems are compromised by illness, great care needs to be taken, as it can be very difficult to predict the pharmacokinetics of maternally administered medications in the breastfed baby.

Transfer of medications into breast milk prior to lactogenesis II is quite high. However, the volume of breast milk (or colostrum) being taken by the neonate is very small; therefore the total amount of medication ingested will also be very small. During weaning, as a child takes fewer breastfeeds the volume of medication ingested will also reduce (see Online resources; Hale 2015; Infant Risk Centre 2023).

The following factors are also relevant:

- If the drug is fat-soluble, it may be more highly concentrated in breast milk at the end of feeding (hindmilk), which contains more fat than at commencement of feeding.
- Because the infant's plasma protein concentration is lower compared with an adult's, a greater amount of free drug may be available to act.
- Metabolic reactions in the infant's liver are slower than in an older child's; hence, drug metabolism may be delayed.
- Drug excretion via the kidneys is delayed in the neonate since glomerular filtration and tubular functioning remain immature for months.
- Following assessment of risks and benefits for taking a drug while breastfeeding, the baby should be monitored for adverse effects such as irritability, sedation and/or weight faltering – less than expected weight gain/growth. While it is difficult to identify adverse reactions in neonates, feeding immediately prior to taking a dose may minimise

exposure as concentrations are usually lowest towards the end of the dosing interval. However, for some drugs, the milk concentration will lag behind the plasma concentration (Gardiner & Begg 2001).

Drug risk in breastfed infants

Drug risk in a breastfed infant depends on the concentration in the infant's blood and the effects of the drug in the infant. For drugs considered 'safe' in breastfeeding the arbitrary cut-off for an infant dose has been considered as 10% of the weight-adjusted maternal dose; however, the age of the infant and their likely ability to eliminate the drug (clearance) must also be considered. For example, in a premature infant, lower clearance may mean the infant concentrations are above those expected. A calculation of infant exposure to drugs can, to some extent, assist and guide safe use. As per Gardiner and Begg (2001):

The infant's dose (D_{infant}) received via milk can be calculated using the maternal plasma concentration ($C_{maternal}$), M/P_{AUC} ratio and the volume of milk ingested by the infant (V_{infant}) as follows:

$$D_{infant} \text{ (mg/kg/day)} = C_{maternal} \text{ (mg/L)} \times M/P_{AUC} \times V_{infant} \text{ (L/kg/day)}$$

Potential drug interactions and adverse effects between prescribed medications and breast milk

Medication in breast milk poses the greatest risk to premature babies, newborns, and babies who are medically unstable, especially those who have problems with kidney function. The risk is lowest for healthy babies 6 months and older, when drugs metabolise through infants' bodies efficiently. A useful method to assess the safety of medicines is the relative infant dose (RID), which is calculated by dividing the absolute infant dose (mg/kg/day) by the maternal dose (mg/kg/day) x 100.

Values less than 10% are considered compatible with breastfeeding (Hale & Krutsch 2023). For most medications the RID is less than 1%. Drugs that are contraindicated during breastfeeding include antineoplastic agents, ergotamine, methotrexate, cyclosporine, and radiopharmaceuticals. Examples of drugs to be avoided while breastfeeding are listed in Box 10.1.

Codeine should not be prescribed for breastfeeding women as metabolism varies between individuals and some breastfeeding mothers are ultra-rapid metabolisers of morphine and may concentrate the drug into milk. The underlying maternal pharmaco-genotype can alter metabolic or elimination pathways and lead to increased drug exposure in a breastfed infant. For example, a high degree of variability exists for CYP2D6-mediated conversion of codeine to morphine because of underlying genetic differences in CYP2D6 activity. People with certain CYP2D6 genotypes (i.e. ultra-rapid metabolisers) may convert codeine to morphine more extensively. This can result in neonatal death from morphine poisoning as confirmed by published report of a fatality in a breastfeeding neonate who was exposed to high levels of morphine in breast milk because his mother was a CYP2D6 ultra-rapid metaboliser (Wang et al 2017).

Drug interactions with prescription medication

Most, though not all, known drug interactions occur after absorption when medicines are administered concurrently, and result from either pharmacokinetic or pharmacodynamic mechanism of drug interaction (see Chapter 6). Many result from changes in enzyme activity which can lead to an accumulation of other drugs in the body and in breast milk (especially where the drug is highly lipid-soluble or ion-trapped), resulting in toxicity through delivery of concentrated infant dose in breast milk. Inducing or inhibiting CYP activity impacts metabolism of other drugs with the consequence that therapeutic effect can be much higher or lower than expected or desired. Because there are many possible drug–drug combinations, an awareness of those that affect liver enzymes is important. Caution should be exercised in prescribing drugs together where both drugs affect liver enzymes. Some examples of clinically significant CYP inhibitors and CYP inducers that may be relevant in prescription drugs being taken simultaneously are provided below (Table 10.1). This is followed by Table 10.2 for prescription medications and potentially harmful medication interactions and adverse events in breastfeeding.

Adverse effects of recreational drugs while breastfeeding

Alcohol

Alcohol passes into breast milk and is therefore not recommended for breastfeeding mothers. Any alcohol consumed will pass into breast milk in concentrations

TABLE 10.1 Examples of clinically significant inhibitors and inducers of CYP enzymes

CYP ENZYME	INHIBITORS	INDUCERS	DRUG GROUP
CYP3A	Azole antifungals Fluconazole SSRIs (fluoxetine, sertraline, paroxetine) Cimetidine	Phenytoin	Calcium channel blockers Protease inhibitors Carbamazepine Dexamethasone
CYP1A2	Ciprofloxacin, fluvoxamine Can increase plasma concentrations of other medication	Carbamazepine Smoking	SSRIs Anticonvulsant/AEDs
CYP2C8	Gemfibrozil, trimethoprim		Fibrates/lipid regulation Anti-folate antibiotic
CYP2C9	Azole antifungals Fluconazole	Rifampicin	NSAIDs Phenytoin Warfarin
CYP2C19	Azole antifungals Fluconazole Fluvoxamine, moclobemide Ticlopidine	Carbamazepine phenytoin Rifampin	SSRIs MAOI inhibitor
CYP2D6	SSRIs (fluoxetine, sertraline, paroxetine, fluvoxamine) Cimetidine Cinacalcet Doxepin Perhexiline Quinine	Dexamethasone Corticosterone Prednisolone Cortisol	Many antipsychotics Many β-blockers Codeine
CYP3A4	Clarithromycin Diltiazem Erythromycin Indinavir Itraconazole Ritonavir Saquinavir Verapamil	Phenytoin Ritonavir Rifampin	Macrolide antibiotics Protease inhibitors Calcium channel blockers

Source: Bryant & Knights, (5th edn) p.172; Bullock & Manias, (8th edn) p.150.

TABLE 10.2 Potentially harmful medication interactions/adverse events in breastfeeding

DRUG CLASS	MEDICATIONS/ SUBSTANCE	POTENTIAL ADVERSE EFFECT	RECOMMENDATION/POTENTIAL DRUG INTERACTIONS
ACE inhibitors	Enalapril is ACE drug of choice	Impaired kidney function	Milk levels low. ACE combined with other antihypertensives increases side effects: hyperkalaemia, hypotension, renal failure. Precaution with potassium-sparing diuretic, NSAIDs, cyclosporine, anticoagulants
Acetylsalicylic acid, salicylates, combined with other drugs; e.g. antacids, pain relievers, cough and cold medications	Aspirin	Risk of bleeding and Reye's Syndrome	Low dose only. Infant monitoring recommended. Drug interactions: mifepristone, acetazolamide, anticoagulants (warfarin, heparin), corticosteroids (prednisone), dichlorphenamide, valproic acid
AEDs	Carbamazepine: preferred Valproic acid: preferred	No consensus for safety of breastfeeding	Milk levels low with single AED. Interacts with MAOIs and other AEDs
Anabolic steroids	Testosterone **AVOID**	Masculinises infant; impairs lactation	*Avoid*
Analgesic/antipyretic	Acetaminophen	Safe in recommended dose	Milk levels < dose for infants
Anti-arrhythmic – class III – benzofuran derivative/ iodine containing compound	Amiodarone **AVOID**	Bradycardia; hypotension; arrhythmias; heart failure; peripheral neuropathy; hypothyroidism. Serum levels unpredictable; high active metabolite(14–74%) maternal levels	*Avoid* High infant exposure. Significant toxicity
Antiemetics/prokinetics: dopamine antagonists	Domperidone, metoclopramide	**Off-label use** to stimulate breast-milk production	No record of infant harm. Drug interactions: significant drug–drug interactions with antibiotics, antifungals, antidepressants and antipsychotics. **Contraindicated** with QT prolonging heart drugs
Antifungals	Fluconazole	Considered safe	Low excretion in breast milk < fluconazole neonatal dose. Drug interactions: quetiapine, lithium, escitalopram, erythromycin, clarithromycin
Antihistamines	Cetirizine: preferred Loratadine: preferred	Non-sedating antihistamines Sedation	Low levels in milk; safe. Can decrease milk supply. Drug interactions: MAOIs, antidepressants, sedatives, narcotic analgesia, cimetidine
Antimanic	Lithium **AVOID**	GI upset; risk of damage to CNS and kidneys	*Avoid where possible.* Infant monitoring. Drug interactions: ACE inhibitors, angiotensin II receptor antagonists, diuretics, NSAIDs
Antimicrobials/Antibiotics	Penicillins, cephalosporins, macrolides: preferred Nitromidazoles Tetracycline **AVOID** Quinolones and fluroquinolones **AVOID**	Affect infant gut flora; diarrhoea; possible allergy; hypersensitivity Infant teeth discolouration	Safe during breastfeeding. *Avoid* *Avoid*
Antipsychotics	Olanzapine: preferred Quesiapine: preferred	Sedation; CNS damage in animal studies	Limited safety data. Low milk excretion levels. Infant monitoring
Beta-blockers	Propranolol, labetalol, and metoprolol: preferred Atenolol, acebutolol, nadolol: **AVOID**	Bradycardia; hypoglycaemia; hypothermia	Infant monitoring. Drug interactions: antihypertensives, inotropic agents, anti-arrhythmics, NSAIDs, psychotropics, anti-ulcer drugs, anaesthetics, warfarin, oral hypoglycaemics, rifampicin

Continued

TABLE 10.2 Potentially harmful medication interactions/adverse events in breastfeeding—cont'd

DRUG CLASS	MEDICATIONS/SUBSTANCE	POTENTIAL ADVERSE EFFECT	RECOMMENDATION/POTENTIAL DRUG INTERACTIONS
Bronchodilators	Albuterol, levalbuterol, budesonide	Potential restlessness; tachycardia	Low bioavailability and maternal serum levels. Drug interactions: TCAs, MAOIs, diuretics
Caffeine	Theophylline	Jitteriness; inattention; poor feeding; poor sleeping	Restrict to < 300 mg/day
Combined oral contraceptives	Estrogen/progestogen **AVOID**	Can diminish milk supply in early weeks	General recommendation: avoid combined oral contraceptive, vaginal contraceptive ring, contraceptive patch
Corticosteroids	Prednisolone	Doses above 40 mg daily may suppress infant's adrenals	Monitoring of infant required
Cytotoxic drugs	**AVOID**	Damage to bone marrow, white blood cells; infection	*Avoid*
Delta-9-tetrahydrocannabinol	Cannabis **AVOID**	Delayed motor development	*Avoid*
Diuretics	Spironolactone	Can impair milk production	Poorly excreted into milk
Ethanol – depressant drug	Alcohol **AVOID**	Sedation, impaired suckling, feeding issues. Increases drug absorption by increasing GI solubility and GIT blood flow	Avoid breastfeeding within 2 hours of drinking. Drug interactions: opioids, antidepressants, antipsychotic medicines, benzodiazepines, sleeping tablets, antihistamines, cold and flu medicines, some antibiotics (metronidazole, azithromycin and nitrofurantoin)
Ergot-alkaloid derivatives	Bromocriptine: maternal deaths from myocardial infarction **AVOID** Cabergoline **AVOID** Ergotamine **AVOID** Ergometrine **AVOID**	Dopamine receptor agonists, block prolactin release	*Avoid* Suppresses lactation *Avoid* Suppresses lactation *Avoid* *Avoid*
H2 blockers – histamine H2-receptor antagonist	Cimetidine: may affect male infants – enlarged breasts. Famotidine: preferred	Potential hepatic enzyme inhibition	Slows clearance of some benzodiazepines. Drug interactions: interaction with the cytochrome P(CYP)450 enzyme which can affect drug metabolism and clearance
Halogen/trace element	Iodine **AVOID**	Hypothyroidism in neonate	RDA for iodine in breastfeeding is 290 mcg daily. *Avoid* Topical preparations can be absorbed
Immunomodulatory drugs	Calcineurin inhibitors and thiopurines: safe Azathioprine, sulfasalazine, mesalazine	Use with caution if baby is premature and has jaundice	Drug interactions: anti-infective agents directly inhibiting cytochrome P450 3A4
Monoclonal antibodies			Limited safety data available
NSAIDs	Ibuprofen: preferred Indomethacin: acceptable Naproxen: **AVOID**	Coagulation effect Seizures reported	Considered safe. Drug interactions: anticoagulants, ACE inhibitors, diuretics. Naproxen is for short-term use only under medical advice

TABLE 10.2 Potentially harmful medication interactions/adverse events in breastfeeding—cont'd

DRUG CLASS	MEDICATIONS/ SUBSTANCE	POTENTIAL ADVERSE EFFECT	RECOMMENDATION/POTENTIAL DRUG INTERACTIONS
Opioids	Codeine **AVOID** Buprenorphine **AVOID** Methadone **AVOID** (opioid use disorder)	Toxic accumulation; sedation; respiratory depression	*Avoid all* (exception: medical monitoring for treatment of substance use, withdrawal and/or opioid dependence disorders). Potential for physical dependence. Infant monitoring where woman being treated for opioid use
Retinoids	Isotretinoin **AVOID**	Can cause damage to sight, hearing, bones, liver; increased risk of convulsions	*Avoid* (including topical preparations)
Sedatives	Benzodiazepines Antipsychotics Prochlorperazine TCAs **AVOID**	Sedation; weak muscle tone; feeding difficulty	*Avoid*
Selective serotonin receptor agonist	Sumatriptan	Vasoconstriction risk	Milk levels low. Withhold breastfeeding 12 or 24 hours after administration if pre-term baby
SSRIs	Sertraline: preferred Paroxetine: preferred Citalopram: **AVOID** Escitalopram: **AVOID** Fluoxetine: **AVOID**	Limited long-term data; potential for neonatal adjustment syndrome	Drug interactions: serious drug–drug interactions with MAOIs and TCAs. Increased bleeding risk with NSAIDs, aspirin, warfarin
Stimulant laxatives Stool softeners Osmotic laxatives	Senna Docusate: preferred Lactulose, glycerol or macrogol: preferred	Diarrhoea in infant	Safe – all when used at recommended doses during breastfeeding
Stimulants	Ephedrine (cold cures) **AVOID**	Neonatal irritability; disruption to sleep. May reduce milk supply	*Avoid*
Sulphonylureas	Glipizide Glyburide	Small risk of hypoglycaemia in infant. Second-generation sulfonylureas likely safe during lactation	Drug interactions: fluoroquinolones, ciprofloxacin, levofloxacin, moxifloxacin. Majority due to induction or inhibition of cytochrome P450 enzymes in liver. Associated with both hyper and hypoglycaemia

like those of the mother's own bloodstream. Alcohol is not stored in breast milk; however, levels of alcohol in breast milk have proven adverse effects for the baby. Alcohol is associated with impaired motor development in the infant as well as altered sleep patterns and risk of hypoglycaemia. Alcohol may inhibit the let-down reflex; alter odour and taste of breast milk, and has been associated with decreased breast milk intake by the baby. Excessive alcohol consumption may impair a mother's ability to care for her baby. If the mother decides to consume alcohol on a limited basis, she can ensure baby is not exposed to any alcohol by carefully planning the breastfeeding schedule: breastfeed first, drink after; store expressed breast milk (EBM) uncontaminated by alcohol before drinking; and wait for complete alcohol elimination, a minimum of 2 hours post consumption.

Tobacco

Smoking is not recommended in breastfeeding mothers; however, breastfeeding remains the recommended method of infant feeding, even if the mother smokes. Nicotine rapidly concentrates in breast milk immediately after smoking. Nicotine and major metabolites are found in the breast milk of mothers who are exposed to secondhand smoke. The half-life of nicotine in breast milk is between 60–90 minutes.

Caffeine

Caffeine passes into breast milk and reaches peak levels within 60–120 minutes of maternal consumption. Excessive caffeine in breast milk can cause overstimulation in babies, and is manifested in hyper-alertness, sleeping difficulty, and feeding fussiness. Caffeine is in many foods and drugs in addition to beverages, for example chocolate, some analgesics, cold remedies, coffee, tea, cola soft drinks, and energy drinks. Limit caffeine intake to 300 mg per day from all sources. On average (where one cup is equal to 250 ml), 300 mg of caffeine would be contained in less than two cups of filter drip coffee; in three cups of instant coffee; or in six cups of tea. Advise the consumption of caffeinated beverages immediately after breastfeeding when the baby is sleeping for longer periods (Toronto Public Health 2017).

Medication for which there is limited evidence of long-term effects

Recently there has been an increased focus on the need for breastfeeding to be included alongside medicine use and neurodevelopmental outcomes in whole-population database investigations of the harms and benefits of medicines during pregnancy, the puerperium and postnatal period (Jordan et al 2022). These considerations are critical in avoiding long-term harm in newborn infants and as part of the ongoing evaluation of the safety and impact of maternal medicines on children, including their cognition, neurodevelopmental disorders, educational performance, and childhood ill-health.

There are many examples of health conditions where women undertake pharmacologic treatment, including while breastfeeding, where limited long-term data exists for the safety and impact of the drug on their developing infant. One example of a common area of treatment for women involving newer classes of drugs includes mental health issues, specifically, use of SSRIs as a treatment for depression postnatally. As highlighted by Jordan et al (2022), SSRI exposure in trimester 3 has direct effects on lactogenesis, as well as affecting monoamine metabolism and serotonin availability in infants, associated with a dose–response increase in restlessness, tremor, and incoordination. This is an example where longer-term evaluation of the impact of medications taken by women while pregnant and breastfeeding on neurodevelopmental and behavioural outcomes for children is essential, as is consideration of both the potential confounding and/or mediating effects of breastfeeding and breast milk on these outcomes, as compared to infants who are not breastfed.

While a comprehensive consideration of these issues is well beyond the scope of this text it is critical to highlight the importance and need for regular health assessment and ongoing follow-up of the developmental and behavioural outcomes for children. This includes assessment of cognitive and educational performance where there has been significant exposure to either new drugs and/or those for which safety data remains limited and studies confined to animal models only.

Drugs and breastfeeding guidelines

Midwives must know how a drug affects lactation and whether it is safe for a breastfeeding mother and child.

Guidelines have been drawn up based on clinical experience (see Online resources: Hotham & Hotham 2015 and *Pregnancy and Breastfeeding Medicines Guide*, The Royal Women's Hospital, Melbourne, 2023), with advice on specific drugs. In general, the following points are suggested:

- The benefits of breastfeeding to both infant and mother are important.
- Optimising the mother's health is in the best interests of mother and infant.
- Only essential drugs should be taken by breastfeeding women.
- Most prescription drugs are relatively safe for breastfed babies.
- Older drugs that appear safe should be prescribed in preference to new drugs for which there is little clinical experience.
- Many oral drugs reach maximum plasma concentrations within 2–3 hours, and babies tend to feed at 4–6-hour intervals, so the mother taking a dose of drug immediately after a feed and before the infant's longest sleep period usually minimises intake by the baby.
- If possible, surgery should be postponed; breastfeeding mothers requiring surgery can, generally, continue to breastfeed provided adequate hydration is maintained and the first quantity of milk after surgery is discarded.
- Local administration minimises both the dose and systemic absorption of a drug; hence, it minimises transfer into milk.
- Feeding can be withheld (or expressed milk given) if a one-off drug is needed – for example, a diagnostic agent.
- The milk-to-plasma ratio has been determined for some drugs; if this is high – for example, with antidepressants, some β-blockers and some NSAIDs – the drug may not be recommended or recommended only with caution and monitoring of the infant.

Breastfeeding is contraindicated:

- if any diagnostic radioisotope testing is scheduled (breastfeeding is interrupted until all the radioactive substance is absent from milk samples)
- when the drug is so toxic that minute amounts may profoundly affect the infant
- when the drug has high allergenic potential
- when the mother's renal function deteriorates (which augments drug excretion into breast milk)
- when serious pathological conditions require prolonged administration of high doses of drugs (e.g. cancer chemotherapy; antithyroid drugs).

See the Key Points box for principles to follow when administering drugs during breastfeeding.

Principles for drugs administered during breastfeeding

Drugs used by breastfeeding women must:

- be compatible with breastfeeding
- be taken at the minimum dose that is effective and for the shortest duration
- be used in paediatric drug therapy
- have the least toxic effect on the baby
- have the shortest half-life
- have the least concentration in breast milk, e.g. low breast-milk-to-plasma ratio
- have the poorest oral bioavailability to limit oral absorption
- be supported by published controlled studies.

If the woman is prescribed a drug contraindicated with breastfeeding, and there is no alternative drug compatible with breastfeeding the following guidelines apply:

- Discontinue breastfeeding until it is safe to resume.
- Express both breasts on a regular basis to maintain breast milk supply. Generally, this should be at least eight times a day; minimum of one expression overnight to simulate normal feeding pattern. May need to express more frequently if breasts are uncomfortable or full. Discard EBM.
- Feed the baby with a supplement using an alternative method (e.g. cup, spoon, syringe, finger feeding). Expressed breast milk collected prior to use of drug can be used as a supplement. If previously collected EBM is not available, an appropriate supplement should be offered.

10.4 Online clinical protocols and classification systems

Up-to-date, online clinical protocols related to breastfeeding and the use of drugs and supplements for specific indications (e.g. mastitis, **galactogogues**, substance use and abuse) and for diverse populations (e.g. LGBTQI+) can be located at the Academy of Breastfeeding Medicine (see Online resources; ABM, and Box 10.2).

Classification systems for the safety of drugs in lactation

Midwives who prescribe or recommend medications for breastfeeding mothers require access to up-to-date, well-referenced, quality sources that are specific to prescribing information during lactation. Several classification systems and reliable resources providing information on the safety of drugs in lactation are available. One of the best known is Thomas Hale's Lactation Risk Categories

---

BOX 10.2   Academy Breastfeeding Medicine: Useful evidence-based clinical protocols

ABM Clinical Protocol #36: The Mastitis Spectrum, Revised 2022

ABM Clinical Protocol #15: Analgesia and Anaesthesia for the Breastfeeding Mother, Revised 2017

ABM Clinical Protocol #28: Peripartum Analgesia and Anesthesia for the Breastfeeding Mother (2018)

ABM Clinical Protocol #18: Use of Antidepressants in Breastfeeding Mothers (2015)

ABM Clinical Protocol #13: Contraception During Breastfeeding, Revised 2015

ABM Clinical Protocol #21: Breastfeeding in the Setting of Substance Use and Substance Use Disorder (Revised 2023)

ABM Clinical Protocol #29: Iron, Zinc, and Vitamin D Supplementation During Breastfeeding (2018)

ABM Clinical Protocol #9: Use of Galactogogues in Initiating or Augmenting Maternal Milk Production, Second Revision 2018

ABM Clinical Protocol #33: Lactation Care for Lesbian, Gay, Bisexual, Transgender, Queer, Questioning, Plus Patients (2020)

See Online resources list: ABM (https://www.bfmed.org/protocols)

(Hale & Krutsch 2023). Hale has performed extensive research on the effects of medications in mothers' milk. Each medication is provided a rating from safest (L1) to hazardous (L5) (Table 10.3). While it is an extremely valuable, high-quality resource, the middle classification (Probably Safe: No studies, but expert opinion suggesting safety [L3]), is indicative of some of the limitations and ongoing ethical challenges associated with the absence of research and evidence-based safety data related to many medications and their use during lactation and breastfeeding. Therefore, while Hale's categories are useful, they represent an over-simplification of the complexity of decision making regarding drug use for a lactating woman. It is essential that advice is individualised to meet the needs and the unique situation of each person and their baby. Importantly, Mauvais-Jarvis et al (2021) provide additional evidence:

'Mauvais-Jarvis et al (2021) provide evidence that biologic sex differences result in genetic modification of the pharmacological response to drugs, including the PK and PD of multiple drugs. Effects include combinations of genetic, epigenetic and hormonal influences which produce different effects in male and female biologic systems at a cellular level. Additionally, co-morbidities and comedications can further modify drug response, as can polymorphisms, the menstrual cycle, pregnancy, and menopause (Mauvais-Jarvis et al., 2021).'

An example of a drug monograph from Hale's Medications and Mothers' Milk is reproduced below (DM 10.1).

TABLE 10.3 Thomas Hale's Lactation Risk Categories

LACTATION RISK CATEGORY	EXPLANATION
L1 Compatible	Drug which has been taken by many breastfeeding mothers without any observed increase in adverse effects in the infant. Controlled studies in breastfeeding women fail to demonstrate a risk to the infant and the possibility of harm to the breastfeeding infant is remote; or the product is not orally bioavailable in an infant.
L2 Probably Compatible	Drug which has been studied in a limited number of breastfeeding women without an increase in adverse effects in the infant. And/or the evidence of a demonstrated risk which is likely to follow use of this medication in a breastfeeding woman is remote.
L3 Probably Compatible	There are no controlled studies in breastfeeding women; however, the risk of untoward effects to a breastfed infant is possible, or controlled studies show only minimal non-threatening adverse effects. Drugs should be given only if the potential benefit justifies the potential risk to the infant. (New medications that have no published data are automatically categorised in this category, regardless of how safe they may be.)
L4 Potentially Hazardous	There is positive evidence of risk to a breastfed infant or to breast milk production, but the benefits from use in breastfeeding mothers may be acceptable despite the risk to the infant (e.g. if the drug is needed in a life-threatening situation or for a serious disease for which safer drugs cannot be used or are ineffective).
L5 Hazardous	Studies in breastfeeding mothers have demonstrated that there is significant and documented risk to the infant based on human experience, or it is a medication that has a high risk of causing significant damage to an infant. The risk of using the drug in breastfeeding women clearly outweighs any possible benefit from breastfeeding. The drug is contraindicated in women who are breastfeeding an infant.
Adult Concerns	This section lists the most prevalent undesired or bothersome side effects listed for adults. As with most medications, the occurrence of these is often quite rare, generally less than 1% to 10%. Side effects vary from one patient to another, with most patients not experiencing untoward effects.
Paediatric Concerns	This section lists the side effects noted in the published literature as associated with medications transferred via human milk. Paediatric concerns are those effects that were noted by investigators as being associated with drug transfer via milk. In some sections, I have added comments that may not have been reported in the literature but are well-known attributes of this medication.
Infant Monitoring	This section provides advice to the clinician regarding potential side effects that may occur in the infant from exposure to a medication in breast milk. The infant monitoring parameters can be used by the clinician to educate the mother about potential side effects that could occur in the infant.
Relative Infant Dose	The relative infant dose (RID) is calculated by dividing the infant's dose via milk in 'mg/kg/day' by the maternal dose in 'mg/kg/day'. This weight-normalising method indicates approximately how much of the 'maternal dose' the infant is receiving. Many authors now use this calculation because it gives a better indication of the relative dose transferred to the infant. I report RID ranges, as this gives the reader an estimate of all the RIDs published by the various authors. Note: Many authors use different methods for calculating RID. Some are not weight normalised. In these cases, their estimates may differ. Many researchers now suggest that anything less than 10% of the maternal dose is probably safe. This is usually correct. However, some drugs (metronidazole, acetaminophen) have much higher RIDs, but because they are quite non-toxic, they do not often bother an infant. When maternal weights are not published, most of the RIDs are calculated assuming a maternal average weight of 70 kg and a daily milk intake of 150 mL/kg/day in the infant.

Source: Adapted from Hale TW, Krutsch K. Hale's Medications & Mothers' Milk, 20th edn. Springer Publishing, 2023.

DRUG MONOGRAPH 10.1
Flucloxacillin

Trade: Flopen, Floxapen, Flu-Amp, Flu-Clomix, Flucil, Fluclox, Flucloxacillin, Magnapen, Staphylex
Category: Antibiotic, penicillin
L1 – Limited data-compatible
Drug last updated: 01/26/2022
Flucloxacillin is a penicillinase-resistant penicillin frequently used for resistant staphylococcal infections. Only trace amounts are secreted in human milk.[1] Its congener, cloxacillin, is commonly used to treat mastitis in breastfeeding mothers and has been used in thousands of breastfeeding patients without problem. Changes in gut flora are possible but unlikely.

DRUG MONOGRAPH 10.1
Flucloxacillin—cont'd

T½	1.5 h
M/P	
Tmax	1 h
PB	94%
MW	454
Oral	50%
Vd	0.11
pKa	2.7
RID	

Adult concerns

Nausea, vomiting, diarrhoea, constipation, skin rashes; hemolytic anaemia and interstitial nephritis have been reported rarely.

Adult dose

250–500 mg four times daily.

Paediatric concerns

None reported via milk.

Infant monitoring

Vomiting, diarrhoea, changes in gastrointestinal flora, and rash.

Alternatives

Cloxacillin, dicloxacillin.

[1]*Pharmaceutical manufacturer's prescribing information.*
Source: Example of a Drug Monograph provided in resource Hales Medications and Mother's Milk online would need to be sought from: Springer Publishing, HalesMeds.com (2022) https://www-halesmeds-com.libraryproxy.griffith.edu.au/monographs/61105?q=flucloxacillin

Helplines – safety of medicines in breastfeeding

Helplines also are available for direct contact by health professionals and women in Australia and New Zealand who are seeking information on the safety of medicines in breastfeeding and pregnancy (Table 10.4). In most of these services, information is provided by a qualified senior pharmacist. A list of quality online resource sites is also provided at the end of this chapter. Additionally, summary tables for a safety assessment of frequently used drugs and drug classification groups are provided by the following authors: Gardiner and Begg (2001); Amir (2011); McGuire (2018; 2019). For updated drug summary and breastfeeding recommendations see Table 10.5.

Management and treatment: Inflammatory mastitis and bacterial mastitis

Mastitis is inflammation and/or infection in a deep organ space (breast). Distinguishing inflammatory mastitis and bacterial mastitis in the breastfeeding mother is important, as effective pharmacologic management differs. Current evidence shows that antibiotics should be reserved for treatment of bacterial mastitis (see Online resources; ABM 2022, and Chapter 12). Recommended treatment for inflammatory mastitis includes continuing to breastfeed the infant on demand, and supportive comfort measures for symptomatic relief, such as the therapeutic use of ultrasound and ice packs as well as drugs that decrease inflammation and pain. Non-steroidal anti-inflammatory drugs (NSAIDs) can reduce oedema and inflammation, and acetaminophen/paracetamol can provide analgesia. Ibuprofen can be dosed 800 mg every 8 hours and acetaminophen/paracetamol 1000 mg every 8 hours.

Systematic review has shown that prophylactic antibiotics are not effective in the prevention of mastitis (Crepinsek et al 2020). The breast microbiome is significantly disrupted by the use of antibiotics to treat inflammatory mastitis, and there is a risk of progression to bacterial mastitis. Because many antibiotics and antifungal medications have anti-inflammatory properties, some women may experience relief when taking these drugs. However, non-selective antibiotic use promotes development of resistant pathogens and should be avoided for inflammatory mastitis.

TABLE 10.4 Services for information about medication safety for breastfeeding or pregnant women

NATIONAL SERVICES		
1300 MEDICINE	9 am to 5 pm AET	1300 633 424
Poisons Information	After hours and public holidays	13 11 26
STATE SERVICES (AVAILABLE DURING LOCAL BUSINESS HOURS)		
NSW	MotherSafe, Royal Hospital for Women, Randwick	(02) 9382 6539 (Sydney metro) 1800 647 848 (NSW non-metro)
SA	Medicines Information Centre Women's and Children's Hospital	(08) 8161 7555
VIC	Medicines Information Centre Royal Women's Hospital	(03) 8345 3190
	Medicines Information Centre Monash Medical Centre	(03) 9594 2361
WA	Obstetrics Medicine Information Service, King Edward Memorial Hospital	(08) 6458 2723
Resources for Families		

- Appropriate information for families can be found on the Australian Breastfeeding Association (ABA) webpage, Breastfeeding and medicines. Further information about common conditions and medications and their safety during breastfeeding are available to download from The Royal Women's Hospital, HealthyWA and MotherSafe.
- Mothers may require additional support with breastfeeding during periods of acute illness or when diagnosed with a chronic medical condition. ABA breastfeeding counsellors do not provide medical advice. However, a call to the National Breastfeeding Helpline on 1800 686 268 may provide reassurance and support for the mother at this potentially challenging time.
- Mothers with more complex health issues may benefit from ongoing breastfeeding support from an International Board Certified Lactation Consultant (IBCLC) or a Breastfeeding Medicine practitioner (see Online resources).

Online Resources
LactMed Database www.ncbi.nlm.nih.gov/books/NBK501922/   • A free, regularly updated online database with information on drugs and lactation aimed at health professionals and the breastfeeding mother.
Perinatology website www.perinatology.com/exposures/druglist.htm   • Features several links about drugs in pregnancy and breastfeeding.
Infant Risk Centre website www.infantrisk.com   • A US research centre focusing on medication safety during pregnancy and lactation. Includes digital resources for mothers and health professionals, and a web forum for questions from health professionals.
Lactation Consultants Australia New Zealand (LCANZ) www.lcanz.org   • A professional organisation for IBCLCs, health professionals and members of the public who have an interest in lactation and breastfeeding. Mothers can use the online database to find an IBCLC in their local area.
Breastfeeding Medicine Network Australia/New Zealand www.breastfeedingmed.com.au   • A non-profit organisation of medical doctors who specialise in breastfeeding medicine and support of breastfeeding. Mothers can use the member directory to find a Breastfeeding Medicine doctor in their local area.

* All services are available during local business hours, unless otherwise stated.
Source: Australian Breastfeeding Association – Medicines and breastfeeding. Breastfeeding Management Fact Sheet for Health Professionals 2024. Retrieved from https://abaprofessional.asn.au/fact-sheets/.

In contrast, bacterial mastitis progresses from ductal narrowing and inflammatory mastitis to a condition necessitating antibiotics or probiotics to resolve. Common organisms in lactational mastitis include Staphylococcus (e.g. *S. aureus, S. epidermidis, S. lugdunensis,* and *S. hominis*) and Streptococcus (e.g. *S. mitis, S. salivarius, S. pyogenes,* and *S. agalactiae*). Bacterial mastitis is not contagious and does not require interruption to breastfeeding (Mitchell et al 2022). In addition to principles of treatment applied for inflammatory mastitis, see recommended first- and second-line antibiotic treatment in Box 10.3.

Complementary medicines and breastfeeding recommendations

The increasing use of complementary and alternative medicines (CAMs) can add extra challenges to midwives providing care and support to the breastfeeding woman. Some CAMs may have adverse effects and are therefore contraindicated during lactation and breastfeeding. Others may interact with prescription medications and cause adverse events, side effects and interference with the intended therapeutic action, (e.g. contraception).

TABLE 10.5 Compatibility of commonly used medicines with breastfeeding

CONDITION	TREATMENT	BREASTFEEDING RECOMMENDATION	ADDITIONAL INFORMATION
Infection	**Antibiotics**		
	β-lactams (e.g. amoxicillin)	Compatible	Gastrointestinal flora changes possible; monitor infant for diarrhoea, vomiting, thrush
	Macrolides (e.g. erythromycin)	Compatible	Single dose of azithromycin considered safe
	Cephalosporins (e.g. cephalexin)	Compatible	May also affect infant gut flora (third generation more likely)
	Fluoroquinolones (e.g. ciprofloxacin)	Avoid if possible	Potential risk of arthropathies
	Trimethoprim	Compatible	
	Nitrofurantoin	Compatible	Avoid nitrofurantoin if infant less than 1 month old or premature
	Metronidazole	Avoid if possible	If single 2 g metronidazole dose given, discontinue breastfeeding for 12 hours
	Antifungals		
	Azoles (e.g. fluconazole)	Compatible	If applying miconazole oral gel to nipples, apply after breastfeeding
	Nystatin	Compatible	
	Antivirals		
	Aciclovir	Compatible	
Depressive disorders	**Antidepressants**		
	SSRIs (e.g. paroxetine)	Compatible	Paroxetine and sertraline preferred due to shorter half-lives
	TCAs (e.g. amitriptyline)	Less preferred due to potential toxicity	Amitriptyline compatible in doses up to 150 mg/day
	Anxiolytics		
	Benzodiazepines (e.g. temazepam)	Compatible in a single dose; avoid repeated doses	Short-acting benzodiazepines preferred as accumulation may occur. Monitor infant for drowsiness
Pain	**Analgesics**		
	Paracetamol	Compatible	Paracetamol analgesic of choice
	NSAIDs (e.g. ibuprofen)	Compatible	Avoid breastfeeding with long-term acetylsalicylic acid treatment
	Opiates (e.g. codeine)	Compatible in occasional doses	Monitor infant for drowsiness, apnoea, bradycardia and cyanosis. Use codeine with caution in rapid metabolisers
	Tramadol	Compatible	
Contraception	**Hormonal methods**		
	Progesterone	Compatible	See data sheet
	Oestrogen	Avoid if possible	May inhibit lactation

Continued

TABLE 10.5 Compatibility of commonly used medicines with breastfeeding—cont'd

Allergies and hay fever	Antihistamines		
	Sedating (e.g. promethazine)	Probably compatible	Occasional use probably safe. Monitor for sedation in mother and infant
	Non-sedating (e.g. loratadine)	Compatible	
	Topical		
	Corticosteroids (e.g. hydrocortisone)	Compatible	If applying to breasts, apply after feeding
Asthma	β2-adrenergics (e.g. salbutamol)	Compatible	
	Corticosteroids (e.g. budesonide)	Compatible	
Other	Warfarin	Compatible	
	Metformin	Compatible	

Source: MEDSAFE – New Zealand Medicines and Medical Devices Safety Authority https://www.medsafe.govt.nz/profs/puarticles/June2015/June2015Lactation.htm

---

BOX 10.3 Recommended antibiotic treatment for mastitis with systemic symptoms

In women with systemic symptoms of mastitis that have not resolved after 24–48 hours of increased breastfeeding and expressing of breast milk, antibiotic therapy is indicated to prevent breast abscess formation. Increased breastfeeding and expression of breast milk should continue alongside antibiotic therapy. The antibiotic regime summarised below is currently recommended in clinical guidelines in many Australian and New Zealand health facilities, as supported by the Therapeutic Guidelines (2023).

Oral
Flucloxacillin 500 mg every 6 hours for 5 days. If signs and symptoms are not resolved, then treatment should be continued for 10 days.

Alternatively

Dicloxacillin 500 mg every 6 hours for 5 days. If signs and symptoms are not resolved, then treatment should be continued for 10 days.

In women with non-severe or delayed hypersensitivity to penicillins

Cephalexin 500 mg every 6 hours for 5 days is suitable (unless the reaction involved amoxicillin or ampicillin). If signs and symptoms are not resolved, then treatment should be continued for 10 days.

In women with immediate hypersensitivity to penicillins

Clindamycin 450 mg orally, 8-hourly for 5 days is suitable. If signs and symptoms are not resolved, then treatment should be continued for 10 days.

IV
Flucloxacillin (or dicloxacillin) 2 g 6-hourly

In women with non-severe or delayed hypersensitivity to penicillins

Cefazolin (cephazolin) 2 g 8-hourly

In women with immediate hypersensitivity to penicillins

Clindamycin 600 mg 8-hourly, or

Vancomycin 1.5 g 12-hourly (only use if pathogen is resistant to first-line antibiotic therapy).

Source: Adapted from information in Therapeutic Guidelines. (2023). Lactational Mastitis. Therapeutic Guidelines online. Retrieved, 21 June 2024; and Infant Feeding – Mastitis and Breast Abscess. (2020). The Royal Women's Hospital, Victoria, Australia. https://thewomens.r.worldssl.net/images/uploads/downloadable-records/clinical-guidelines/infant-feeding-mastitis-and-breast-abscess_280720.pdf

While complementary medicines are often perceived as 'natural' and therefore safer than pharmaceutical medicine, this is not always the case (Barnes et al 2019).

Information on the use of herbal products while lactating and breastfeeding is limited (Budzynska et al 2012). While herbal galactagogues have been used for centuries in folk medicine, the plants contain lipophilic, pharmacologically active constituents. If taken in sufficient quantity, these can pass into the breast milk. Products sold in stores and online are not always evaluated for safety and effectiveness. Many are also not well studied regarding their safety to work as advertised and may lack specific standards for ingredients and strength. McGuire (2018) reviewed potential adverse effects of herbs used as galactogogues, and Amir (2011) the breastfeeding recommendations around some commonly used CAMs (Tables 10.6; 10.7).

Principles of safe prescribing to neonates

Prescribing drugs and supervising the use of medications for young infants is a complex and challenging professional

TABLE 10.6 Adverse effects of herbs used as galactogogues

HERB	ADVERSE EFFECTS
Alfalfa *Medicago sativa*	Dose-related bleeding
Blessed thistle *Cnicus benedictus*	Gastric irritation and potential allergies as it is part of the ragweed family
Chaste tree *Vitex agnus castus*	Nausea, vomiting, irritation, pruritis, rash, headache, increased menstruation
Dill *Anethum graveolens*	Alterations in sodium balance
Fennel *Foeniculum vulgare*	Allergic reactions and dermatitis (photo and contact)
Fenugreek seed *Trigonella foenum-graecum*	Hypoglycaemia, hypertension, diarrhoea and maple syrup body odour in mother. Allergy potential as part of the peanut family
Goat's rue *Galega officinalis*	Hypoglycaemia, hypotension, coughing, dose-related toxicity
Milk thistle (silymarin) *Silybum marianum*	Allergic reactions, diarrhoea
Malunggay *Moringa oleifera*	Hypoglycaemia, sedation
Raspberry leaf *Rubus idaeus*	Hypersensitivity reactions, changes in blood glucose
Shatavari *Asparagus racemosus*	Possible teratogenicity – avoid in pregnancy
Damiana *Turnera diffusa*	Hepatotoxicity, confusion, and hallucinations with high-dose *Turnera*

Source: McGuire 2018; Amir 2011.

Challenges in neonatal medication prescribing and administration

1 Consent

As the guardians of their baby, parents are the decision makers. If there are differences of opinion about management between parents, skilled communication to reach agreement may be required.

2 Safety

Aspects of medication safety in relation to neonates are heightened due to their vulnerability; therefore a systematic approach to medication review, assessment, drug calculation (including independent checking/verification), identification, prescribing and documentation is critical.

3 Drug calculations

In contrast to standard medication doses administered to adults, neonatal doses are usually calculated based on body weight. The risk for under- or over-dosing is heightened in this population, as is the risk for miscalculation. Because neonatal weight change can occur rapidly in the early weeks, drug dosages must be recalculated on a regular basis. Loss of birth weight can be common in the first few days (up to 10%), whereas full-term infants usually gain on average 30 grams a day over the first months of life after regaining birth weight.

4 Routes of drug administration

Few medications are reliably administered orally to a neonate unless these are directly given via a naso/orogastric feeding tube which is invasive and poses other iatrogenic risks. Incomplete dosing may therefore be delivered, even where oral liquid or drops are used, and these may be regurgitated.

Intramuscular

The IM route avoids the challenges associated with the oral route and ensures accurate and complete dosing on administration. Because muscle mass in a baby is small there are additional risks of neurological injury; therefore care must be taken in choosing the site of injection with reference to recognised landmarks. This is most usually the antero-lateral thigh. Absorption rates can also vary and the amount of medication that can be administered is also limited.

Topical

Apart from antifungal creams, this route is not often used. Because the skin of a neonate is thin and permeable, and highly influenced by the presence of radiant or skin-to-skin heat from the mother's body, absorption rates can vary and cause unpredictable response to drug dosing.

Intravenous

While reliable dosing is available from this route it also carries iatrogenic risk and is invasive, in addition to a requirement for trained staff and suitable equipment.

TABLE 10.7 Commonly used CAMs and supplements: Adverse effects and breastfeeding recommendations

COMPLEMENTARY MEDICINE (CAM) OR HERB	BREASTFEEDING RECOMMENDATION	POTENTIAL ADVERSE EFFECT
Aloe *Aloe vera*	Cautious use recommended. Topical use unlikely to cause adverse effects in infant	Reports of diarrhoea in infants whose mothers took extract of *Aloe vera* orally
Alfalfa *Medicago sativa*	Caution	Dose-related bleeding
Black cohosh *Cimicifuga racemose*	Not recommended	Selective estrogen receptor modulator activity; can lower breast milk production
Blessed thistle *Cnicus benedictus*	Caution	Gastric irritation and potential allergies
Chaste tree *Vitex agnus castus*	Compatible	Nausea, vomiting, irritation, pruritis, rash, headache, increased menstruation
Chamomile, German *Matricaria recutita*	Compatible	Safe at recommended doses
Cranberry *Vaccinium macrocarpon*	Compatible	
Dill *Anethum graveolens*	Caution	Alterations in sodium balance
Echinacea *Echinacea angustifolia; Echinacea purpura*	Use with caution	Possible diarrhoea, constipation, poor feeding, and skin rashes in infant
Evening primrose oil *Oenothera biennis*	Use with caution	Active constituents present in breast milk
Fenugreek *Trigonella foenum-graecum*	Use with caution at recommended doses	Hypoglycaemia, hypertension, diarrhoea, and maple syrup body odour in mother. Allergy potential as part of the peanut family
Feverfew	Not recommended for breastfeeding women	As an antiplatelet agent should not be used in people on anticoagulant therapy
Folic acid	Folic acid naturally found in breast milk. While breastfeeding, it is recommended to get 500 mcg (0.5 mg) of folic acid every day.	
Garlic *Allium sativum*	Safe in amounts usually used in food preparation. No information on safety of garlic supplements	May change smell of breast milk and affect baby's feeding
Ginger *Zingiber officinale*	Cooking with and eating ginger in natural form is compatible with BF	Not enough information known in relation to ginger supplements
Ginseng oriental *Panax ginseng*	Compatible	
Glucosamine	Compatible	
Goat's rue *Galega officinalis*	Caution	Hypoglycaemia, hypotension, coughing, dose-related toxicity
Iodine	Naturally occurring element. Recommended Dietary Allowance (RDA) for iodine during breastfeeding is 290 mcg daily	Too much iodine ($>$ 500 mcg to 1100 mcg) in the breast milk can cause problems with infant thyroid gland
Liquorice *Glycyrrhiza glabra*	Limited information	Use in medicinal amounts not recommended
Lysine	Compatible	
Malunggay *Moringa oleifera*	Caution	Hypoglycaemia, sedation

TABLE 10.7 Commonly used CAMs and supplements: Adverse effects and breastfeeding recommendations—cont'd

COMPLEMENTARY MEDICINE (CAM) OR HERB	BREASTFEEDING RECOMMENDATION	POTENTIAL ADVERSE EFFECT
Melatonin	Helps with circadian rhythm (sleep-wake-cycle). Melatonin made by human body is present in breast milk in higher amounts at night	Taking melatonin supplements while BF has not been well studied
Milk thistle/St Mary's thistle *Silybum marianum*	Traditional remedy to stimulate breast milk production	Scant evidence for safety and efficacy
Raspberry leaf *Rubus idaeus*	Generally safe in moderate amounts while BF	Hypersensitivity reactions, changes in blood glucose
Sage *Salvia officinalis*	Leaves in small amounts are safe	Decreases breast milk supply
St John's wort *Hypericum perforatum*	Limited information. Can interact with many medications, including contraceptives; TCAs, SSRIs, MAOIs and benzodiazepines	Reported side effects in BF infants are colic, drowsiness, lethargy
Vitamin C	Normal component of breast milk. RDI = 120 mg per day	

BOX 10.4   Principles of safe prescribing to neonates

- Work with a limited number of medications which have a long history of use that you know well.
- When prescribing decisions that are outside your knowledge and scope must be made, utilise a multi-disciplinary approach, including consultation and referral as indicated by midwifery professional practice guidelines and decision making framework.
- When writing prescriptions for drug dose determined by body weight, record the body weight, the dose in mg/kg, the strength of the formulation you are prescribing in mg/mL, and the final dose in mL.
- Always have another person check your calculations prior to administration.
- Provide parents with information and education regarding drug safety so they are enabled to safely calculate and administer common OTC medications themselves. Parents can also monitor the prescribing and administration practices of healthcare providers on behalf of the baby.
- Ensure access to quality drug reference sources when you are prescribing or administering medications.

---

activity (Box 10.4). A comprehensive understanding of the normal and pathological physiological changes in neonatal physiology over the first weeks of life is needed to inform both medication use and prescribing decision making. While the range of medications prescribed by midwives for well neonates is relatively limited, the range of medications administered for treatment of an unwell neonate is variable and dependent on the age and health status of the infant. It requires specialised knowledge and safety considerations (Krzyzaniak et al 2016) and is beyond the scope of this text. Nevertheless, as a midwife, it is important to have access to neonatal appropriate prescribing resources. The *Australian Medicines Handbook* publishes the AMH Children's Dosing Companion, a quality resource (see Online resources; AMH).

Neonatal vaccination

The *Australian National Immunisation Handbook* is a quality resource that will support your discussion with women regarding neonatal vaccination (see Online resources and Chapter 11). According to ACIPs General Best Practice Guidelines for Immunisation in Special Situations, except for smallpox and yellow fever vaccines, neither inactivated nor live virus vaccines administered to a lactating woman affect the safety of breastfeeding for women or their infants.

Drug Monograph 10.2 provides information about the administration and use of vitamin K as prophylaxis for newborn babies against haemorrhagic disease of the newborn, also referred to as vitamin K deficiency bleeding (VKDB).

DRUG MONOGRAPH 10.2
Vitamin K for newborn babies

Vitamin K (named from the German 'Koagulation Vitamin') is a composite name for methylnaphthoquinones – lipid-soluble vitamins critical in the blood-coagulation cascade. **Phytomenadione**, vitamin K1, is found in plants, especially green leafy vegetables; its name in the US is phylloquinone. The vitamin K2 form can be synthesised in the gut by bacteria.

Mechanism of action

Vitamin K is a necessary co-factor in the liver synthesis of clotting factors II (prothrombin), VII, IX and X; it is a coenzyme for vitamin K-dependent carboxylase, and possibly also involved in bone metabolism. Its actions are competitively antagonised by coumarin-type anticoagulants such as warfarin.

Indications

Vitamin K is administered routinely to all newborn babies to prevent haemorrhagic disease of the newborn and vitamin K deficiency bleeding (VKDB), which can cause catastrophic intracranial haemorrhages. Neonates have low prothrombin levels, as vitamin K does not readily cross the placenta, their gut flora is not yet established, and they are not eating a mixed diet. (In adults, vitamin K is given to treat deficiency caused by inadequate intake, severe liver disease, or prolonged use of antibiotics; and as an antidote to overdose with coumarin anticoagulants.)

Pharmacokinetics

Vitamin K is usually administered parenterally. Approximately 80% of an oral dose of the vitamin is absorbed, less when from the diet. The lipid-soluble vitamin is taken into mixed micelles via bile and pancreatic enzymes, thence to the liver where it is re-packaged into very low density lipoproteins and distributed throughout the body. It is rapidly metabolised, and excreted about 20% in urine and 40–50% in faeces; blood levels and body stores are low. Little is excreted in the breast milk.

Drug interactions (in adults)

- The most significant interaction is antagonism by warfarin-type anticoagulants which deplete the body of vitamin K-dependent clotting factors; people taking these drugs need to maintain a consistent intake of vitamin K in their diet.
- Bile acid sequestrants and orlistat reduce gut absorption of vitamin K, and antibiotics can reduce gut production of K2.
- Hepatic enzyme-inducers given to a pregnant woman may exacerbate the risk of VKDB in her newborn.

Adverse reactions

Common adverse reactions to IM injection in newborns include short-term pain, tenderness and erythema (reddening).

Precautions and contraindications

Parental consent is needed before vitamin K is administered to a newborn; verbal consent is usually adequate. Parents fearing adverse effects for their babies are encouraged to allow IM injection, as this is more effective and simpler than the oral dosing schedule. The single IM dose is given (usually by a midwife) before the baby is transferred to a ward from the birthing suite. It is particularly necessary for babies delivered via instrumental or caesarean section births, who are more prone to bleeding.

Dosage and administration

Vitamin K is supplied in a paediatric formulation, 10 mg/mL. The IM dose is 1 mg (0.1 mL), given into the thigh muscle. In very small babies ($<$ 1.5 kg), the dose may be reduced to 0.5 mg (0.05 mL). The dosage regimen for oral administration is three doses of 2 mg (0.2 mL): at birth, on day 3–5, and at 4 weeks. It is important to stress to parents the need for the three doses, as they will have to obtain a prescription for and administer the second and third doses.
(Doses in adults for severe hypoprothrombinaemia are complicated, depending on blood clotting test results; reference texts should be consulted.)

Acknowledgments: Prepared with the assistance of Midwife Denise Jenkins and Dr Alison Bryant-Smith, MRCOG, Melbourne.

CRITICAL THINKING EXERCISE

· ·

Siobhan and her baby Kyla were discharged home on day 3 by their treating private obstetrician following birth by emergency caesarean section after an induction of labour. As an endorsed midwife and authorised prescriber of the private midwifery practice providing postnatal follow-up care for Siobhan and Kyla, your home visit on day 4 at 24 hours following hospital discharge is your first meeting and interaction with this mother/baby dyad. Siobhan has a written hospital discharge summary for you, is teary and appears in significant pain. She states that this birth and initiating breastfeeding with Kyla is considerably more challenging than with Carlos, her active 2-year-old son, born vaginally, who still has the occasional breastfeed. Significant discomfort associated with ongoing nipple thrush that became exacerbated during pregnancy has also resulted in ongoing treatment with fluconazole, which was included with Siobhan's supply of discharge medication and which she advises she has taken, alongside the prescribed analgesia and laxative. Kyla has received one breastfeed only since discharge from hospital. Siobhan states the baby is constantly sleeping and 'not interested' in feeding. On the discharge summary you note that Siobhan has been issued with a one-week supply of oxycodone. Siobhan states that the discharge analgesia supplied is barely covering her pain and that she has exceeded the recommended daily allowance in addition to 'topping up' with some other OTC analgesia purchased by her husband last evening. Baby Kyla is difficult to rouse, and her breathing appears intermittent and irregular after unwrapping.

Questions

1. What is your immediate assessment and management for Kyla and Siobhan?

2. What concerns, if any, do you have in relation to Siobhan's discharge prescription medication, including review, potential medication interaction/adverse events, and ongoing care plan?

3. Explain your decision making, assessment and review, providing rationale for your approach to medication management.

4. What process of consultation, referral, and documentation – including with whom – is required in this scenario, and why?

5. What specific education/information must be discussed with Siobhan?

KEY POINTS

Summary of neonatal physiology influencing medication pharmacology

- Lung fluid that has been retained decreases the rate of passage of inhaled substances into the bloodstream.

- Circulating blood volume is low, relative to adult body weight, altering the volume of drug distribution, with higher circulating concentrations than would occur if a similar intravenous dose/kg body weight were given to an adult. Neonatal blood volume varies between infants depending on length of time elapsed prior to cord clamping.

- Glomerular filtration rate is reduced, reducing the rate of excretion of drugs via the kidney.

- Gastrointestinal mucosa is thin and permeable, increasing absorption of orally administered medications. Gastric emptying times change rapidly over the first days after birth, varying according to the feeds provided. Variable responses to the same dose of an oral medication may occur.

- Regurgitation is common, resulting in variable doses of orally administered medications entering the gut.

- Hepatic functions are immature, so drug metabolism is slow. This can reduce the effect of drugs that must be metabolised to be active and increase the effect of drugs that are metabolised to inactive metabolites.

CONCLUSION

Breastfeeding is recognised as the best way to provide complete nutrition to the infant, and women who require medication yet want to breastfeed need to be supported to do so. Many medications are unsuitable for use during lactation, so to enable women to make informed decisions regarding medications during breastfeeding, midwives must understand the pathophysiology of lactation and how medications are metabolised by the body and into breast milk. This chapter provided an overview of pharmacology and medication use during lactation and breastfeeding, including the basic principles of medication management in well newborns. A complete understanding of the use of medication during breastfeeding, and of common medications used in the neonatal periods, is an essential part of midwifery practice.

REVIEW EXERCISES

1. How can you, as a midwife, ensure you are providing evidence-based information about the safety of CAMs to women you are providing care for? What sources of information would you recommend they access?

2 What are the preferred analgesic options for women in the postpartum period while breastfeeding? Why are they preferred?

3 Describe and differentiate the pathophysiology of inflammatory mastitis, as contrasted with bacterial mastitis, including the pharmacological and other management strategies to resolve each condition. What principles guide the use of selected pharmacotherapy for each condition? Why are these principles important?

4 Identify three prescription drug–drug interactions in breastfeeding women that may result in adverse events and describe the pharmacokinetic or pharmacodynamic mechanism responsible.

ADDITIONAL CRITICAL THINKING EXERCISES

1 During a routine postnatal visit to a woman's home at 21 days, you note her baby to be very drowsy and difficult to rouse. The woman advises she is very happy that her baby is 'more settled' as for the past week she has been topping up her discharge analgesia for post-caesarean pain management with some 'spare' oxycodone left over from a knee operation last year and this is working well for everybody.

   i. What is your immediate midwifery assessment and management for mother and baby, including any education required?

2 Prior to becoming pregnant and giving birth to baby Norman, Geraldine received chemotherapy for bone cancer and has been in remission for 18 months. Norman is now 2 months old and fully breastfed when Geraldine receives the devastating news that there are signs the cancer has metastasised and that she will soon require further treatment with chemotherapy.

   i. What issues will need to be discussed in relation to breastfeeding in this situation?

   ii. Who should be involved and what is your role given you were Geraldine's primary midwife during her pregnancy and birth of Norman?

REFERENCES

Ahmadzai H, Tee LBG, Crowe A. Adverse drug reactions in breastfed infants: A cross-sectional study of lactating mothers. Breastfeed Med. 2022;17:1011-17 (accessed 6 February 2024)

Amir LH, Grzeskowiak LE, Kam RL. Ethical issues in use of medications during lactation. J Hum Lact. 2020;36(1):34-39. doi:10.1177/0890334419888156 (accessed 6 February 2024).

Amir LH, Pirotta MNV, Raval M. Breastfeeding – Evidence based guidelines for the use of medicines. Aust Fam Physician. 2011 Sep;40(9):684-690. https://www.racgp.org.au/getattachment/28bd8ca1-0e31-4428-ab55-ca5ad8095325/Breastfeeding.aspx (accessed 6 February 2024)

Anderson PO, Momper JD. Clinical lactation studies and the role of pharmacokinetic modeling and simulation in predicting drug exposures in breastfed infants. J Pharmacokinet Pharmacodyn. 2020 Aug;47(4);295–304. doi.org/10.1007/s10928-020-09676-2 (accessed 6 February 2024)

Australian Medicines Handbook. Australian Medicines Handbook Pty Ltd; Adelaide, 2004.

Barnes LAJ, Barclay L, McCaffery K, et al. Factors influencing women's decision making regarding complementary medicine product use in pregnancy and lactation. BMC Pregnancy Childbirth. 2019 Aug;19(1):280. doi.org/10.1186/s12884-019-2396-2

Binns C, Lee M, Low WY. The long-term public health benefits of breastfeeding. Asia Pacific J Public Health. 2016;28(1):7-14, doi: 10.1177/1010539515624964 (accessed 6 February 2024)

Budzynska K, Gardner ZE, Dugoua JJ, et al. Systematic review of breastfeeding and herbs. Breastfeed Med. 2012 Dec;7(6):489-503. doi: 10.1089/bfm.2011.0122. Epub 2012 Jun 11. PMID: 22686865; PMCID: PMC3523241.

Byerley EM, Perryman DC, Dykhuizen SN, et al. Breastfeeding and the pharmacist's role in maternal medication management: identifying barriers and the need for continuing education. J Pediatr Pharmacol Ther. 2022;27(2):102-108. doi: 10.5863/1551-6776-27.2.108. Epub 2022 Feb 9. PMID: 35241980; PMCID: PMC8837210 (accessed 6 February 2024)

Byrne JJ, Spong CY. 'Is it safe?' – The many unanswered questions about medications and breast-feeding. N Engl J Med. 2019 Apr 4;380(14):1296-1297. doi: 10.1056/NEJMp1817420. PMID: 30943334 (accessed 6 February 2024)

COAG (2019) Australian National Breastfeeding Strategy: 2019 and beyond. https://www.health.gov.au/resources/publications/australian-national-breastfeeding-strategy-2019-and-beyond

Cornet M, Wu YW, Forquer H, et al. Maternal treatment with selective serotonin reuptake inhibitors during pregnancy and delayed neonatal adaptation: a population-based cohort study. Arch Dis Childhood – Fetal Neonatal Ed. 2024 Apr;109(3):294-300. doi: 10.1136/archdischild-2023-326049

Crepinsek MA, Taylor EA, Michener K, et al. Interventions for preventing mastitis after childbirth. Cochrane Database Syst Rev. 2020;9:CD007239.

Datta P, Baker T, Hale T. Balancing the use of medications while maintaining breastfeeding. Clin Perinatol. 2019;46(2):367-82. doi.org/10.1016/j.clp.2019.02.007 (accessed 6 February 2024)

Drugs and Lactation Database (LactMed®) [Internet]. Bethesda (MD): National Institute of Child Health and Human Development; 2006. Oxycodone. [Updated 2024 Feb 15]. Available from: https://www.ncbi.nlm.nih.gov/books/NBK501245/ (accessed 1 April 2024)

Drugs and Lactation Database (LactMed®) [Internet]. Bethesda (MD): National Institute of Child Health and Human Development; 2006. Codeine. [Updated 2023 Dec 15]. Available from: https://www.ncbi.nlm.nih.gov/books/NBK501212/ (accessed 1 April 2024)

Gardiner S, Begg E. Drug safety in lactation. Prescriber Update. 2001 May; 21:10-23. https://www.medsafe.govt.nz/Profs/PUarticles/lactation.htm (accessed 6 February 2024)

Gibson CM, Davis S, Thompson KA. Potential consequences of codeine use in lactating mothers. Hospital Pharmacy. 2016;51(2):107-109. doi.org/10.1310/hpj5102-10

Hale TW, Krutsch K. Hale's Medications & Mothers' Milk (20th edn). Springer Publishing, 2023.

Hale T. Drug entry into human milk. Infant Risk Centre, September 22, 2015. https://www.infantrisk.com/content/drug-entry-human-milk (accessed 1 April 2024)

Hotham N, Hotham E. Drugs in breastfeeding. Aust Presc. 2015;38(5):156. doi.org/10.1186/1746-4358-6-11 (accessed 30 November 2023)

Illamola SM, Bucci-Rechtweg C, Costantine MM, et al. Inclusion of pregnant and breastfeeding women in research – efforts and initiatives. Br J Clin Pharmacol. 2018 Feb;84(2): 215-222. doi: 10.1111/bcp.13438. Epub 2017 Oct 22. PMID: 28925019; PMCID: PMC5777434 (accessed 6 February 2024)

Jones W. How to advise women on the safe use of medicines while breastfeeding. Pharmaceutical J. 23 June 2023[Online]. https://pharmaceutical-journal.com/article/ld/how-to-advise-women-on-the-safe-use-of-medicines-while-breastfeeding

Jordan S, Bromley R, Damase-Michel C, et al. Breastfeeding, pregnancy, medicines, neurodevelopment, and population databases: the information desert. Int Breastfeed J. 2022;17;55. doi.org/10.1186/s13006-022-00494-5

Khan YS, Fakoya AO, Sajjad H. Anatomy, thorax, mammary gland. [Updated 2023 Dec 10]. In: StatPearls [Internet]. Treasure Island (FL): StatPearls Publishing; 2024 Jan. https://www.ncbi.nlm.nih.gov/books/NBK547666/

Kirkegaard H, Bliddal M, Støvring H, et al. Breastfeeding and later maternal risk of hypertension and cardiovascular disease – the role of overall and abdominal obesity. Prev Med. 2018;114:140-148. doi:10.1016/j.ypmed.2018.06.014

Krzyzaniak N, Bajorek B. Medication safety in neonatal care: a review of medication errors among neonates. Ther Adv Drug Saf. 2016 Jun;7(3):102-19. doi: 10.1177/2042098616642231. Epub 2016 Apr 1. PMID: 27298721; PMCID: PMC4892407.

LactMed® Drugs and Lactation Database. Bethesda (MD): National Institute of Child Health and Human Development; 2006. https://www.ncbi.nlm.nih.gov/books/NBK501922/

Lynch MM, Squiers LB, Kosa KM, et al. Making decisions about medication use during pregnancy: implications for communication strategies. Matern Child Health J. 2018;22(1):92-100. doi: 10.1007/s10995-017-2358-0

Mauvais-Jarvis F, Berthold HK, Campesi I, et al. Sex- and gender-based pharmacological response to drugs. Pharmacol Rev. 2021;73(2):730-762. doi.org/10.1124/pharmrev.120.000206 (accessed 6 February 2024)

McClatchey AK, Shield A, Cheong LH, et al. Why does the need for medication become a barrier to breastfeeding? A narrative review. Women Birth. 2018 Oct;31(5):362-366. doi: 10.1016/j.wombi.2017.12.004. Epub 2017 Dec 16. PMID: 29258800 (accessed 30 November 2023)

McGuire T. Safe use of drugs while breastfeeding. In W Brodribb (Ed.), Breastfeeding Management in Australia (5th edn, pp. 279-323). Australian Breastfeeding Association 2019.

McGuire TM. Drugs affecting milk supply during lactation. Aust Prescr. 2018;41:7-9. doi.org/10.18773/austprescr.2018.002 (accessed 6 February 2024)

Mitchell KB, Johnson HM, Rodriguez JM, et al. Academy of Breastfeeding Medicine Clinical Protocol #36: The Mastitis Spectrum, Revised 2022. https://www.bfmed.org/assets/ABM%20Protocol%20%2336.pdf

Molenaar N, Kamperman A, Boyce P, et al. Guidelines on treatment of perinatal depression with antidepressants: an international review. Aust N Z J Psychiatry. 2018 Apr;52(4):320-327. doi.org/10.1177/0004867418762057

Navarrete F, García-Gutiérrez MS, Gasparyan A, et al. Cannabis use in pregnant and breastfeeding women: behavioral and neurobiological consequences. Front Psychiatry. 2020 Nov 2;11:586447. doi: 10.3389/fpsyt.2020.586447. PMID: 33240134; PMCID: PMC7667667.

National Health and Medical Research Council. Infant Feeding Guidelines: information for health workers. NHMRC, Australian Government, 2013. https://www.nhmrc.gov.au/about-us/publications/infant-feeding-guidelines-information-health-workers (accessed 6 February 2024).

Quinn P, Tanis SL. Attitudes, perceptions, and knowledge of breastfeeding among professional caregivers in a community hospital. Nurs Womens Health. 2020 Apr;24(2):77-83. doi: 10.1016/j.nwh.2020.01.010. Epub 2020 Feb 27. PMID: 32112725 (accessed 6 February 2024)

Saha MR, Ryan K, Amir LH. Postpartum women's use of medicines and breastfeeding practices: a systematic review. Int Breastfeed J. 2015;10:28. doi.org/10.1186/s13006-015-0053-6

Scime NV, Metcalfe A, Nettel-Aguirre A, et al. Association of postpartum medication practices with early breastfeeding cessation among mothers with chronic conditions: a prospective cohort study. Acta Obstet Gynecol Scand. 2023;102:420-429. doi.org/10.1111/aogs.14516

Stephens A, Brodribb W, McGuire T, et al. Breastfeeding questions to medicines call centres from the Australian public and health professionals. Aust J Prim Health. 2018 Nov;24(5):409-416. doi: 10.1071/PY18010. PMID: 30086825 (accessed 6 February 2024)

Stordal B. Breastfeeding reduces the risk of breast cancer: a call for action in high-income countries with low rates of breastfeeding. Cancer Med. 2023;12(4):4616-4625. doi: 10.1002/cam4.5288

Victora CG, Bahl R, Barros AJD, et al. Breastfeeding in the 21st century: epidemiology, mechanisms, and lifelong effect. Lancet. 2016 Jan;387(10017):475-490. doi: 10.1016/S0140-6736(15)01024-7

Wang J, Johnson T, Sahin L, et al. Evaluation of the safety of drugs and biological products used during lactation: workshop summary. Clin Pharmacol Ther. 2017 Jun;101(6):736-744. doi: 10.1002/cpt.676. PMID: 28510297; PMCID: PMC5591026

Weld ED, Bailey TC, Waitt C. Ethical issues in therapeutic use and research in pregnant and breastfeeding women. Br J Clin Pharmacol. 2022;88(1):7-21. https://doi.org/10.1111/bcp.14914 (accessed 6 February 2024)

Zik JB, Roberts DL. The many faces of oxytocin: implications for psychiatry. Psychiatry Res. 2015;226(1):31-37.

ONLINE RESOURCES

Australian Breastfeeding Association. Resources: https://www.breastfeeding.asn.au/resources (accessed 6 February 2024)

Academy of Breastfeeding Medicine (2019): https://www.bfmed.org/ (accessed 6 February 2024)

Australian Institute of Health and Welfare. Australia's mothers and babies: Breastfeeding, 29 June 2023: https://www.aihw.gov.au/reports/mothers-babies/breastfeeding-practices (accessed 6 February 2024)

Australian Medicines Handbook: https://amhonline.amh.net.au/auth

Australian Medicines Handbook, Children's Dosing Companion (2024): https://childrens.amh.net.au/auth

Best Practice Advocacy Centre NZ (BPAC). Antibiotics: Choices for Common Infections. Updated March 2021: https://bpac.org.nz/antibiotics/guide.aspx

Toronto Public Health. Breastfeeding Protocols for health Providers, Protocol #16 Drugs and Breastfeeding: https://www.toronto.ca/wp-content/uploads/2017/11/967e-tph-breastfeeding-protocol-16-drugs-2013.pdf

Australian Breastfeeding Association. Breastfeeding and medicines: https://www.breastfeeding.asn.au/resources/breastfeeding-and-medicines

COAG Australian National Breastfeeding Strategy: 2019 and Beyond: https://www.health.gov.au/sites/default/files/documents/2022/03/australian-national-breastfeeding-strategy-2019-and-beyond.pdf

Hales Medications and Mothers' Milk (2022): https://www.halesmeds.com/

Infant Risk Centre website: https://www.infantrisk.com/ (accessed 25 March 2024)

LactMed Database: https://www.ncbi.nlm.nih.gov/books/NBK501922/ (accessed 25 March 2024)

MEDSAFE: New Zealand Medicines and Medical Devices Safety Authority: https://www.medsafe.govt.nz/ (accessed 25 March 2024)

Medicines Information Australia: www.1300medicine.com.au (accessed 25 March 2024)

MotherSafe – Royal Hospital for Women, Randwick: https://www.seslhd.health.nsw.gov.au/royal-hospital-for-women/services-clinics/directory/mothersafe (accessed 25 March 2024)

New Zealand Formulary: http://nzformulary.org/ (accessed 11 March 2024)

NPS Medicinewise: https://www.nps.org.au/ (accessed 25 March 2024)

PHARMAC, Pharmaceutical Management Agency of New Zealand. Online access to New Zealand Pharmaceutical Schedule detailing which pharmaceuticals attract subsidy: http://www.pharmac.govt.nz/ (accessed 25 March 2024)

Queensland Clinical Guidelines, Neonatal Medicines (2019): https://www.health.qld.gov.au/__data/assets/pdf_file/0043/859678/g-neomed.pdf

The Royal Women's Hospital (Melbourne) – Pregnancy and breastfeeding medicines guide: https://thewomenspbmg.org.au/ (requires a subscription)

Therapeutic Goods Administration. Prescribing medicines in pregnancy database: https://www.tga.gov.au/products/medicines/find-information-about-medicine/prescribing-medicines-pregnancy-database (accessed 4 October 2023)

Phone resources (Australia)

1300 MEDICINE (1300 633 424) or Poisons Information Centre on 13 11 26 (all states & territories)

National Breastfeeding Helpline (1800 686 268)

—CHAPTER 11—

VACCINATIONS IN PREGNANCY AND RECOMMENDED SCHEDULE FOR NEWBORNS

Michelle Gray, Roslyn Donnellan-Fernandez, Kirsten Small

Key Abbreviations

DNA	deoxyribonucleic acid
DTPa	diphtheria-tetanus acellular pertussis vaccine (paediatric formulation)
dTpa	diphtheria-tetanus vaccine acellular pertussis vaccine (reduced antigen formulation)
Hib	Haemophilus influenzae type b
HPV	human papillomavirus
Ig	immunoglobulin
IM	intramuscular
IPV	inactivated poliovirus
mRNA	messenger ribonucleic acid
RNA	ribonucleic acid
SARS-CoV-2	severe acute respiratory syndrome coronavirus 2
SC	subcutaneous
VLP	virus-like particle

Key Terms

adjuvant 222
adsorbed 222
antibody 214
antigen 213
cell-mediated immunity 215
conjugate polysaccharide vaccine 223
humoral immunity 213
live attenuated vaccine 220
primary series 220
pure polysaccharide vaccine 223
recombinant vaccine 224
toxoid 223

Chapter Focus

This chapter provides an overview of the immune system, passive and active immunisation, vaccine immunology, and clinical considerations specifically related to pregnancy. It outlines the different types of vaccines and how they work to elicit an immune response.

A vaccine is a biological preparation that contains antigens (or ANTIbody GENerating substances) that are derived from a disease-causing microorganism. When introduced into the body, a vaccine confers acquired immunity to a specific disease.

Vaccines are considered one of the greatest achievements in modern medicine. Globally, it is estimated that each year they prevent more than three million deaths (WHO 2024). All health professionals play a vital role in vaccine advocacy and education. Appropriately trained and qualified health professionals may administer vaccines; however, the midwife and general practitioner are both ideally focused on providing women with advice and evidence-based information related to optimising immune function during the childbearing continuum. This includes the role of vaccination in the prevention of disease for mothers and babies.

Understanding how different types of vaccines work enables health professionals to appreciate the rationale behind vaccine schedules (e.g. number of primary and booster doses), contraindications, common adverse effects following immunisation, and why some vaccines are recommended during pregnancy and others are not.

If women enter pregnancy fully vaccinated, they optimise their chance of being protected from infection and also provide antibodies to their fetus via the placenta. Pre-conception care provides an opportunity to encourage women to ensure their vaccinations are up to date before becoming pregnant. Vaccinations for rubella or varicella are live attenuated vaccines and they are contraindicated during pregnancy.

Key Drug Groups

Whole pathogen:

- Live attenuated vaccines
- *Measles, mumps, rubella*
- Inactivated or killed vaccines
- Whole cell
- *Pertussis*
- split virion
- *Influenza*

Subunit vaccines (pieces of pathogen):

- Recombinant vaccines
- Protein
- *Hepatitis B*
- Virus-like particles
- *Human papillomavirus vaccine*
- Polysaccharide vaccines
- Pure polysaccharide
- Conjugate vaccines

- *Meningococcal vaccines*
- Toxoid vaccines
- *Diphtheria, tetanus vaccines*
- Nucleic acid vaccines

- mRNA vaccines
- COVID-19 vaccine
- Viral vector vaccines

Learning Outcomes

- Understand the difference between active and passive immunisation.
- Describe the aims and clinical considerations of vaccination related to pregnancy.
- Understand the distinction between vaccination and immunisation.
- Outline the role of the midwife in relation to vaccination for mothers and babies.
- Demonstrate awareness of vaccinations recommended in Australia across the childbearing continuum for women and their babies.
- Critically appraise woman-centred approaches to the ethical management of issues associated with challenges such as vaccine hesitancy and adverse reactions.

CRITICAL THINKING SCENARIO

The SARS-CoV-2 international pandemic put the lives of the vulnerable at risk. Pregnancy is a vulnerable state due to the reduced immunological response. Rebecca is a healthy 19-year-old and received the recommended COVID-19 vaccinations. She also followed the recommended practices of mask wearing, use of hand gel and personal distancing when directed by national health policy. At 16 weeks pregnant with her first child, Rebecca worked as a salesperson in a department store.

1   Does Rebecca require another vaccination against COVID-19 during pregnancy?

2   If so, what gestation is recommended for vaccination?

3   Which type of vaccination is the safest for use during pregnancy?

4   What advice can you offer Rebecca to help her protect herself during exposure with the general public?

Rebecca gave birth to her baby, Sam, and before being discharged from the maternity ward, Sam was administered the hepatitis B vaccine. Today, 2 months on, Rebecca is attending an appointment with her son at the community health centre, for the community nurse to administer recommended vaccines. Sam is given two injections and one vaccine orally. One injection contained antigens to protect against six infections (diphtheria, tetanus, pertussis, hepatitis B, polio, and *Haemophilus influenzae* type b). The other injection aims to protect against pneumococcal infection, while the oral vaccine aims to provide protection against rotavirus. The injections were administered into the mid-anterolateral thigh (vastus lateralis muscle).

5   How do these vaccines work to protect Sam from natural infections? How long will it take for Sam to develop antibodies to the antigens present in the vaccines?

6   Describe and explain the different types of vaccines Sam has had administered.

7   Which of the vaccines contained adjuvants to improve their immunogenicity? What is meant by a conjugated vaccine? Which of the administered vaccines was conjugated?

8   Which of the vaccines are part of a primary series? Which of them require booster doses to maintain protection?

9   Discuss some of the common side effects of vaccines. Why might they occur?

Introduction

A vaccine is a biological preparation that confers acquired immunity to an infectious disease when introduced into the body. The first vaccine, Dr Edward Jenner's smallpox vaccine, was introduced in 1796. Today, 29 infectious diseases can be prevented through vaccination, including cholera, COVID-19, dengue fever, diphtheria, Ebola virus, *Haemophilus influenzae* type b (Hib), hepatitis A, B and E, herpes zoster (shingles), human papillomavirus (HPV) infection, influenza, Japanese encephalitis, malaria, measles, meningococcal disease, mumps, pneumococcal disease, pertussis, poliomyelitis, Q fever, rabies, rotavirus, rubella (German measles), varicella (chickenpox), and yellow fever.

Calculating the exact number of deaths that vaccines have prevented is impossible. However, the World Health Organization (WHO) estimates that globally, each year, vaccination prevents at least 3 million deaths (WHO 2024). Because of vaccination, smallpox – a highly infectious disease that killed one-third of those infected and left those who survived with permanent scarring – was declared globally eradicated in 1980. Today, once common childhood diseases such as measles and poliomyelitis are controlled in most parts of the world.

The global COVID-19 pandemic, estimated to be responsible for the deaths of more than 5 million people, resulted in rapid response efforts around the world to develop effective vaccines that would reduce both mortality and longer-term co-morbidities that are now being linked to this disease.

Most vaccines are administered intramuscularly (IM) via an injection; however, they can also be administered subcutaneously (SC), intradermally, intranasally, and orally. There is a range of vaccine types, and broadly they can be divided into whole-cell and subunit vaccines. Whole-cell vaccines contain the whole pathogen (bacteria or virus) and include live attenuated and whole-cell killed or inactivated vaccines. Subunit vaccines contain only a piece or multiple pieces of the pathogen and include toxoid, pure polysaccharide, conjugated polysaccharide, recombinant protein, virus-like particle, nucleic acid, and viral vector vaccines.

The different types of vaccines work differently to elicit an immune response in the vaccinated person. When an immune response is stimulated and sufficient antibodies and memory have been produced, it is said that the person is immunised.

11.1 The immune system

Our bodies are exposed to millions of potential pathogens (disease-causing microorganisms such as bacteria, viruses, and fungi) each day. When a pathogen is introduced into the body, the immune system responds.

Broadly the immune system is classified into two subtypes:

- innate immune system (or natural, non-specific)
- adaptive immune system (or acquired, specific).

The immune system is also divided into first, second, and third line defences. The first and second line of defence are part of the innate immune system, while the third line of defence is part of the adaptive immune system.

Innate immunity

Innate immunity comprises the body's first two lines of defence. It is rapid, non-specific, and has no memory. The body's first line of defence are barriers or broad external defences that prevent pathogens from gaining entry. It includes physical barriers (e.g. skin, hairs, cilia and tears, and during pregnancy a thickening of mucosal linings), chemical barriers (e.g. the acidity pH of the vagina increases during pregnancy, enzymes) and reflexes (e.g. airway defences such as the sneeze and cough). If the pathogen breaks through the first line of defence it encounters the second line of defence. The second line of defence includes physiological changes (fever, inflammation), protein (interferon, complement, acute-phase protein) and cellular defences (e.g. granulocytes [neutrophils, basophils, eosinophils, mast cells], natural killer cells, macrophages). The second line works quickly to prevent the spread of pathogens in the body and fight infection.

The innate response may eradicate the pathogens independently or it may call in the adaptive immune response for assistance using antigen-presenting cells (macrophages and dendritic cells). Together, both arms of the immune system will now work to remove pathogens from the body and restore health.

Adaptive immunity

Adaptive immunity, also known as acquired immunity, is specific to a particular pathogen. Pathogens have unique **antigens** (proteins, peptides, or polysaccharides) usually on their surface. Simply put, an antigen is any substance that causes the immune system to GENerate ANTIbodies (also known as immunoglobulins) against it.

There are two main types of adaptive immunity: humoral and cellular immunity.

Humoral immunity

As the name suggests, **humoral immunity**, also known as antibody-mediated immunity, deals with antigens that are circulating freely in the humors (or body fluid – blood, plasma, lymph).

On first exposure to an antigen, antigen-presenting cells (macrophages, dendritic cells) of the innate immune system will engulf, break down, and process the antigen, then 'present' a component of it on a structure on the surface of the antigen-presenting cells known as the major histocompatibility complex II (MHC-II).

Presenting the antigen on the MHC-II complex is like the cell flying a flag saying, 'I'm infected with antigen! Help!' Enter the T helper cell. On the surface of T helper cells is a T-cell receptor. T-cell receptors recognise and bind to antigens presented on the MHC-II. If the T-cell has never seen the pathogen before, it is called a naïve T helper cell. When the processed antigen on the MHC-II binds with a corresponding T-cell receptor, the T helper cell is activated and becomes an effector cell. T helper cells are characterised by a CD4 marker or co-receptor on their surface; for this reason you may see them referred to as CD4 cells, CD4+ T-cells or T4 cells. T helper cells make up approximately 13% of circulating white blood cells.

During pregnancy there is an overall increase in total white cell count which commences in the first trimester, peaks at 30 weeks then plateaus until birth. This is mainly due to an increased percentage of neutrophils thought to be the result of impaired neutrophil apoptosis. While the maternal immune system may tolerate fetal antigens through suppression of cell-mediated immunity, evidence indicates normal humoral immunity is retained (Mutua et al 2018).

T helper cells coordinate both the humoral and cellular immune response (Fig 11.1). Specifically, on first exposure to an antigen, in humoral immunity T helper cells stimulate and enable naïve B-cells to differentiate into plasma B-cells (the effector cell). Plasma B-cells are **antibody** factories, and once activated they produce antigen-specific antibodies. Antibodies are Y-shaped proteins that bind to antigens and neutralise, agglutinate (clump together), and trigger their destruction (by lysis or phagocytosis). Antibodies are antigen-specific, much like a lock and key. For each antigen (key), there is only one type of antibody (lock) – they are highly specific. The

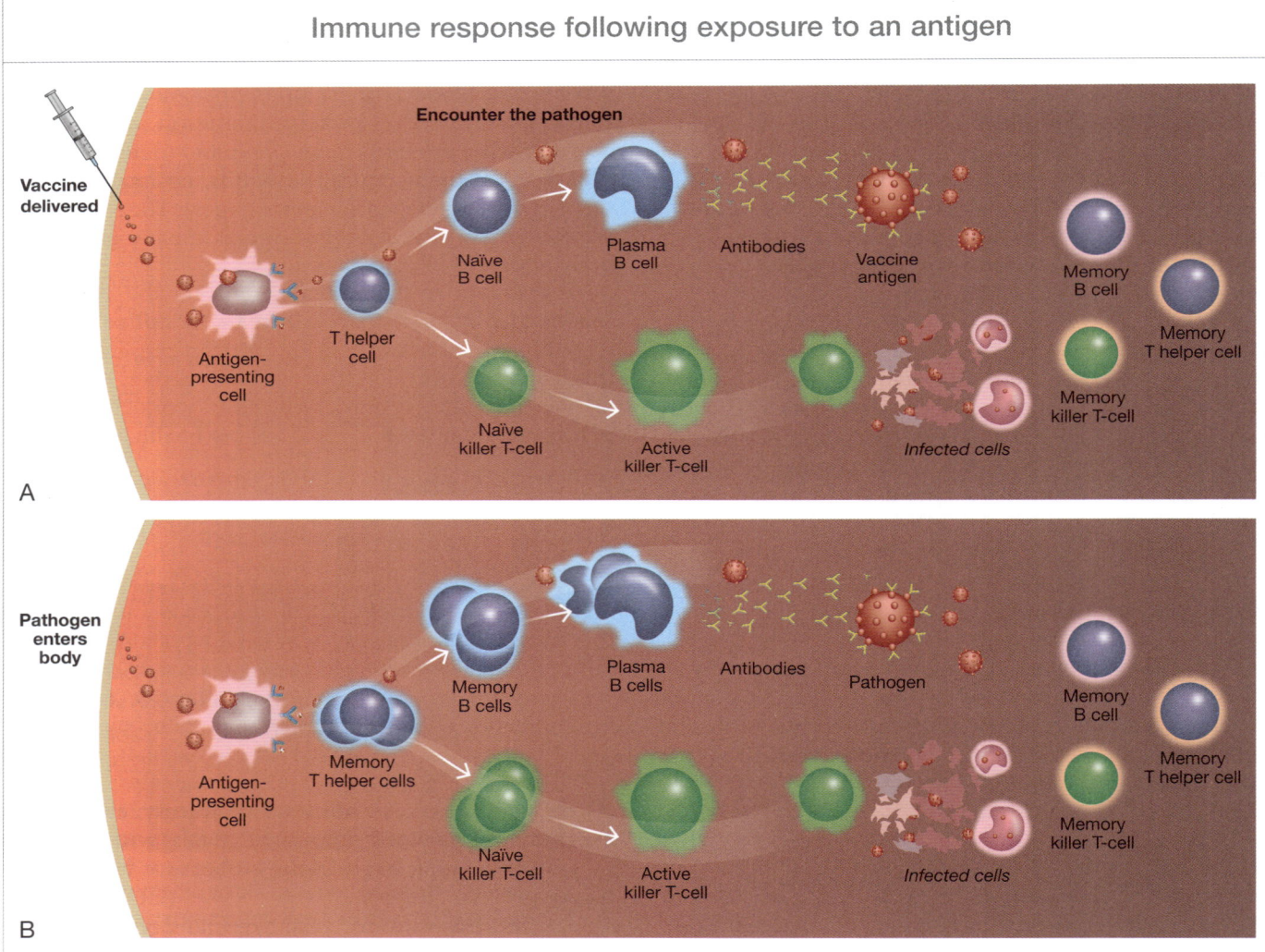

FIGURE 11.1 A Immune response following first exposure to an antigen; **B** Immune response following subsequent exposure to an antigen

location of the antigen that binds to the antibody is known as the epitope or antigenic determinant.

The humoral immune response cannot destroy an antigen that has already entered and infected host cells (i.e. the antigen is no longer in the humors).

Cell-mediated immunity

Cell-mediated immunity does not involve antibodies. Cell-mediated immunity refers to the production of antigen-specific T-cytotoxic cells that enable the destruction of infected host cells. On first exposure to an antigen, activated T helper cells release cytokines (signalling molecules) that lead to naïve T-cells binding to the infected cell's MHC antigen complex, enabling the T-cell to differentiate into either T-cytotoxic or T helper cells.

As the name suggests, T-cytotoxic cells kill infected cells, by a process known as lysis (disintegration or rupture of the cell). Cytotoxic T helper cells secrete more cytokines that attract neutrophils and macrophages, which further assist in destroying the pathogen. Both memory T helper and memory T-cytotoxic cells are generated after exposure to an antigen (Fig 11.1). These antigen-specific memory cells locate themselves in lymph nodes and the spleen. On subsequent exposure, these cells proliferate rapidly, enabling a more immediate and robust immune response to the antigen.

During pregnancy there is a change in cell-mediated immunity. Lymphocyte numbers remain the same, but cytotoxic T helper cell numbers decline in relation to the T-cytotoxic-killer cells. Specifically, regulatory T-cells are key in preventing fetal rejection by the maternal immune system. Different anti- and pro-tolerogenic factors such as cytokines, pregnancy hormones, seminal fluid and decidual (d)-NK and -CD14$^+$ cells can modulate the number and the functions of regulatory T-cells.

Most T-cell activity consists of T-cytotoxic cells which attack cells infected by microorganisms or cancerous cells. They will attack tissue transplanted from another person (like a kidney). The fetus has the potential to be attacked due to the expression of paternal antigens; however, changes to the immune system in pregnancy described mean that potential reactions to fetal antigens are suppressed (Rocca et al 2014). The exception to this is women with autoimmune conditions – such as systemic lupus erythematosus – who are more likely to produce antibodies that may attack the fetus, which can increase the risk of spontaneous recurrent abortion.

Primary immune response and immunological memory

When the body is exposed to an antigen (i.e. pathogen) for the first time, the primary immune response, or primary immunisation, occurs. This response is slow and limited (Fig 11.2). Depending on the type of pathogen, the primary infection can take up to 14 days to resolve, after which immunological memory has developed.

Secondary immune response

On subsequent exposure to the same antigen, the existence of antigen-specific lymphocytes (T and B memory cells) created during the primary immune

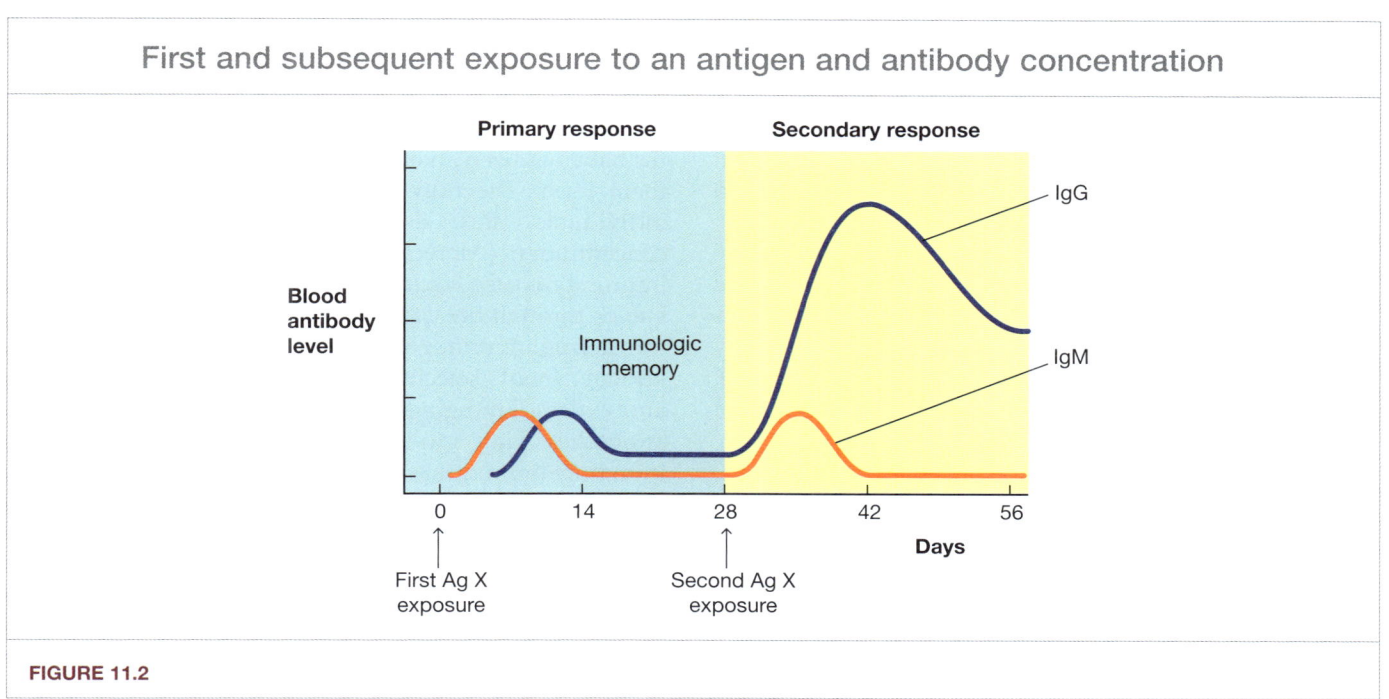

First and subsequent exposure to an antigen and antibody concentration

FIGURE 11.2

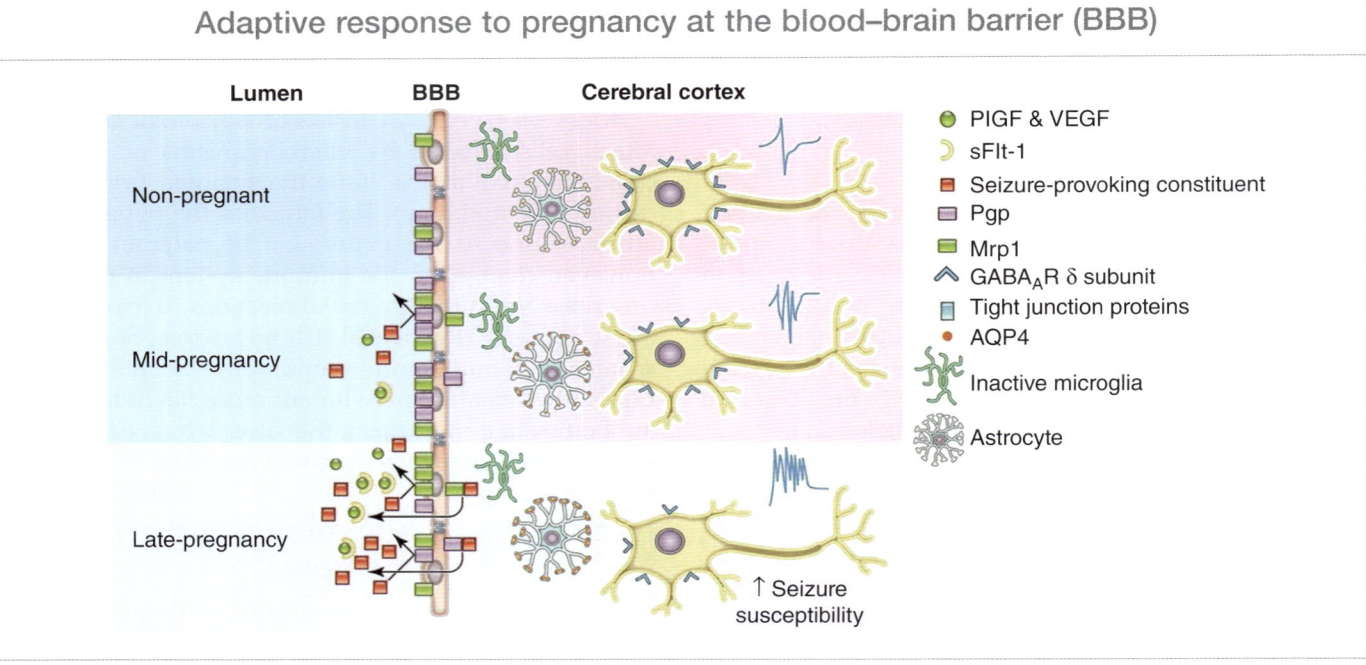

Adaptive response to pregnancy at the blood–brain barrier (BBB)

FIGURE 11.3

Source: Reproduced from: Johnson AC, Cipolla MJ 2015. The cerebral circulation during pregnancy: adapting to preserve normalcy. Physiology (Bethesda), 30, 139–147.

response enables the immune system to respond rapidly and effectively. The hallmark of the adaptive immune response is the clonal expansion of antigen-specific lymphocytes (Adams et al 2020). Clonal expansion is the rapid proliferation of T- and B-cells from a few clonal cells to millions in a short time. Each T- and B-cell clone is specific for the same antigen as the original clone (parent cell). Memory cells are also specific for a particular antigen and are long-lasting. Memory cells are what sustain the adaptive immune response long term, and they form the biological basis of vaccination.

On successive exposure to a pathogen the immune pathways are preexisting (there is immunological memory). Reactivation of the immune pathway is immediate, and specific antibodies (predominantly immunoglobulins [Ig] G and M) are rapidly produced, neutralising the antigen, often with the absence of symptoms (Fig 11.3).

Active vs artificially acquired immunity

Active immunity occurs when the person develops antibodies and memory to a specific disease. This is different from passive immunity, which is when antibodies (natural or synthetic) are administered to someone. Passive immunity provides short-term protection, and immunological memory is not developed – for example,

the transfer of maternal antibodies in breast milk to the feeding baby, or the parenteral administration of monoclonal antibodies (e.g. sotrovimab) to treat and prevent COVID-19. In the case of transplacental passive immunity, during the last three months of pregnancy, antibodies are passed from mothers to their unborn babies, providing a protective shield from pathogen-mediated disease. The type of immunity is passive because the baby has been given the antibodies rather than making them itself. The number of antibodies differs between individuals and depends on maternal antibody concentration (Albrecht et al 2020). Lactational passive immunity is also conferred by mothers to their newborn babies through breast milk. While the role of placentally transferred immunoglobulin G (IgG) is established, less is known about selection and transfer of breast milk antibodies. Emerging evidence suggests breast milk antibodies play multi-faceted roles in protecting the immature immune system of the baby. These roles include prevention of infection, supporting selection of bacterial commensals, and boosting the baby's immune tolerance (Atyeo et al 2021).

For a woman, active immunity must be acquired prior to becoming pregnant to ensure the woman has the greatest protection from infectious diseases. The principle behind vaccination is to intentionally introduce an antigen, derived from or synthetically designed to mimic an antigenic component of a disease-causing microorganism. The antigenic component should stimulate the adaptive immune system and immunological memory, but not cause disease. New vaccine technologies (e.g. mRNA; see section below) introduce genetic material that codes for an antigen, so the host essentially makes the vaccine (the antigen) in situ. The national schedule of vaccination (Fig 11.4) outlines the recommended inoculations from birth to adulthood. Evidence suggests women newly arrived from overseas can be missing some recommended scheduled vaccinations. Therefore, while pre-conception advice for all women may contribute to optimising vaccination status, pre-conceptional advice may be especially beneficial for women new to the Australian and New Zealand health systems. Artificially acquired immunity is the body's first exposure to the pathogen, so on subsequent exposure the body already has memory.

Memory cells are not generated immediately after the administration of a vaccine. That is why women should be advised to complete recommended vaccinations prior to conception. The current *Australian Immunisation Handbook* recommends women planning for pregnancy consider vaccination for hepatitis B, measles, mumps, rubella, varicella, and influenza as part of their pre-conception health check. Women with additional risk factors for pneumococcal disease, including smokers, and Aboriginal and Torres Strait Islander women, should also be assessed for pneumococcal vaccination. Women who receive live vaccines should avoid pregnancy within 28 days of vaccination. Pregnant women are routinely recommended to receive influenza vaccine at any time during pregnancy, and pertussis-containing vaccine (dTpa – reduced antigen diphtheria-tetanus-acellular pertussis) between mid-second trimester and early third trimester (Australian Government 2023).

FIGURE 11.4

Source: (a) National Immunisation Program schedule. For the most up-to-date information, access the online version available at: https://www.health. gov.au/topics/immunisation?language=und

Continued

National Immunisation Program Schedule *(continued)*

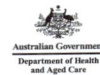 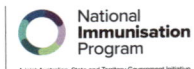

Australian Government
Department of Health and Aged Care

National Immunisation Program
A joint Australian, State and Territory Government initiative

Adult vaccination

(also see vaccination for people with medical risk conditions)

Age	Diseases	Vaccine Brand	Notes
All ages	Influenza (adults with specified medical risk conditions) Influenza (Aboriginal and Torres Strait Islander adults) Pneumococcal (adults with specified medical risk conditions) Shingles (herpes zoster) (adults with specified medical risk conditions)	Age appropriate Age appropriate Prevenar 13® and Pneumovax 23® Shingrix®	Influenza vaccine: Administer annually. For information on age appropriate vaccines or specified medical risk conditions refer to the Immunisation Handbook or the annual ATAGI advice on seasonal influenza vaccines. Pneumococcal vaccine: For people with specified medical risk conditions administer a dose of 13vPCV at diagnosis followed by 2 doses of 23vPPV. Refer to the Immunisation Handbook for dose intervals. Shingles vaccine: For immunocompromised people aged 18 and older with specified medical risk conditions administer 2 doses. Refer to the Immunisation Handbook for dose intervals.
50 years and over	Pneumococcal (Aboriginal and Torres Strait Islander adults) Shingles (herpes zoster) (Aboriginal and Torres Strait Islander adults)	Prevenar 13® and Pneumovax 23® Shingrix®	Administer a dose of 13vPCV, followed by first dose of 23vPPV 12 months later (2–12 months acceptable), then second dose of 23vPPV at least 5 years later. Shingles vaccine: For Aboriginal and Torres Strait Islander people 50 years and older administer 2 doses. Refer to the Immunisation Handbook for dose intervals.
65 years and over	Influenza (annually) (non-Aboriginal and Torres Strait Islander adults) Shingles (herpes zoster) (non-Aboriginal and Torres Strait Islander adults)	Age appropriate Shingrix®	Influenza vaccine: Administer annually. The adjuvanted influenza vaccine is recommended in preference to standard influenza vaccine. For information on age appropriate vaccines refer to the Immunisation Handbook or the annual ATAGI advice on seasonal influenza vaccines. Shingles vaccine: For people 65 years and older administer 2 doses. Refer to the Immunisation Handbook for dose intervals.
70 years and over	Pneumococcal (non-Aboriginal and Torres Strait Islander adults)	Prevenar 13®	
Pregnant women	Pertussis (whooping cough) Influenza	Boostrix® or Adacel® Age appropriate	Pertussis vaccine: Single dose recommended each pregnancy, ideally between 20–32 weeks, but may be given up until delivery. Influenza vaccine: In each pregnancy, at any stage of pregnancy.

Additional vaccination for people with medical risk conditions

Age	Diseases	Vaccine Brand	Notes
All ages	Meningococcal ACWY Meningococcal B	Nimenrix® Bexsero®	For people with asplenia, hyposplenia, complement deficiency and those undergoing treatment with eculizumab. Refer to the Immunisation Handbook for dosing schedule. The number of doses required varies with age.
≥ 6 months (annually)	Influenza	Age appropriate	For people with specified medical risk conditions that increases their risk of complications from influenza. Refer to the Immunisation Handbook for information on age appropriate vaccines.
<12 months	Pneumococcal	Prevenar 13® and Pneumovax 23®	For people with specified medical risk conditions that increase their risk of pneumococcal disease, an additional (3rd) dose of 13vPCV in infancy, followed by a routine booster dose at age 12 months (as with other healthy children), then followed by 2 doses of 23vPPV. Refer to the Immunisation Handbook.
≥12 months	Pneumococcal	Prevenar 13® and Pneumovax 23®	For people with specified medical risk conditions that increase their risk of pneumococcal disease, administer a dose of 13vPCV at diagnosis followed by 2 doses of 23vPPV. Refer to the Immunisation Handbook for dose intervals.
≥5 years	Haemophilus influenzae type b (Hib)	Act-Hib®	For people with asplenia or hyposplenia, a single dose is required if the person was not vaccinated in infancy or incompletely vaccinated. (Note that all children aged <5 years are recommended to complete Hib vaccination regardless of asplenia or hyposplenia).

State and territory health departments may also fund additional vaccines. Check the immunisation schedule for your area.

State/Territory	Contact Information
Australian Capital Territory	(02) 5124 9800
New South Wales	1300 066 055
Northern Territory	(08) 8922 8044
Queensland	13 HEALTH (13 4325 84)
South Australia	1300 232 272
Tasmania	1800 671 738
Victoria	immunisation@health.vic.gov.au
Western Australia	(08) 9321 1312

- The National Immunisation Program (NIP) provides the above routine vaccinations free to infants, children, adolescents and adults who have, or are eligible for a Medicare card.
- All Aboriginal and Torres Strait Islander children aged 6 months to less than 2 years of age are eligible for meningococcal B vaccines if missed at the recommended schedule points. Refer to the Immunisation Handbook for timing of doses.
- All people (including refugees and humanitarian entrants) less than 20 years of age are eligible for the NIP vaccines missed in childhood, except for HPV which is available free up to and including age 25. The number and range of vaccines and doses that are eligible for the NIP funded catch-up is different for people aged less than 10 years and those aged 10-19 years. Refer to the Immunisation Handbook for timing of doses.
- Refugees and humanitarian entrants aged 20 years and over are eligible for the following vaccines if they were missed: diphtheria-tetanus-pertussis, chickenpox, poliomyelitis, measles-mumps-rubella and hepatitis B, as well as HPV (up to and including age 25). Refer to the Immunisation Handbook for timing of doses.
- National Immunisation Program Schedule current from 1 November 2023.
- *If individuals have received Zostavax® through the NIP, they will need to wait 5 years before accessing Shingrix® for free. If individuals have received Zostavax® privately, they are eligible for Shingrix®. An interval of 12 months is recommended from the date of Zostavax® vaccination.

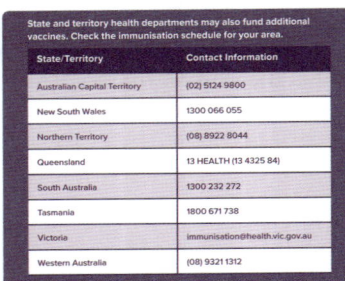

MORE INFORMATION: ● health.gov.au/immunisation ● immunisationhandbook.health.gov.au

A2

National Immunisation Schedule

Antigen(s) Brand name	DTaP-IPV-HepB/Hib Infanrixhexa	PCV13 Prevenar 13	MenB Bexsero	RV1 Rotarix	MMR Priorix	Hib Hiberix	VV Varilrix	DTaP-IPV Infanrix-IPV	Tdap Boostrix	HPV9 Gardasil 9	Influenza Afluria Quad	rZV Shingrix
Pregnancy									Tdap		Influenza	
6 weeks	DTaP-IPV-HepB/Hib	PCV13 ᵃ		RV1								
3 months	DTaP-IPV-HepB/Hib		MenB ᵇ	RV1								
5 months	DTaP-IPV-HepB/Hib	PCV13	MenB									
12 months		PCV13	MenB		MMR							
15 months					MMR	Hib	VV					
4 years								DTaP-IPV				
11 or 12 years									Tdap	HPV9 (2 doses)		
45 years									Tdap			
65 years									Tdap		Influenza (annually)	rZV (2 doses)

Key:

D = diphtheria; T = tetanus; aP = acellular pertussis; IPV = inactivated polio vaccine; HepB = hepatitis B; Hib = *Haemophilus influenzae* type b; PCV13 = 13-valent pneumococcal conjugate vaccine; RV1 = rotavirus vaccine (monovalent); MenB = meningococcal B vaccine; MMR = measles, mumps and rubella; VV = varicella vaccine; d = adult diphtheria; ap = adult acellular pertussis; HPV9 = human papillomavirus (9 serotypes); rZV = herpes zoster vaccine.

a. For children at high risk of pneumococcal disease, an additional dose of PCV13 is given at age 3 months.

b. An alternative approved schedule for MenB given at 8 weeks (2 months), 4 months and 12 months is available.

All individuals aged from 5 years are eligible to receive two doses of a COVID-19 vaccine. Additional doses and booster doses are also available to different groups.

B

FIGURE 11.4, cont'd

Source: (b) New Zealand: https://www.health.govt.nz/our-work/preventative-health-wellness/immunisation/new-zealand-immunisation-schedule

The immune system

- The immune system can be divided into two subsystems: the innate (non-specific) and the adaptive system (specific). Both systems continually interact with each other to elicit an immune response.

- There are two main types of adaptive immunity: humoral (B-cells) and cell-mediated immunity (T-cells). Humoral immunity is antibody mediated. Cell-mediated immunity does not involve antibodies. Instead, cell-mediated immunity activates cytotoxic T-cells to kill infected cells.

- An important outcome of the adaptive immune response is the development of immunological memory. Whether via natural or artificial infection (vaccination), people exposed to an antigen acquire long-term protection from the disease. This state of protection is due to immunological memory.

- Pregnancy is a state of reduced immunological response.

11.2 Vaccines given during pregnancy

During pregnancy the immune system undergoes minor alterations in both primary and secondary defence mechanisms. There is a third T-cell group, called suppressor T-cells. These cells control the suppression of damage to the body by limiting the body's ability to attack its own cells. During the processing of T-cells in the bone marrow and thymus, clones capable of damaging the body's own tissues are destroyed before they can colonise the tissues.

Pregnancy is characterised by immune suppression and consequently a period of increased risk of bacterial and viral infection (Mor et al 2017). While a successful organ transplant requires constant immunosuppression, successful pregnancy requires a robust, dynamic, and responsive immune system. The immune response associated with placental viral infections can affect maternal and fetal survival. Maternal inflammation due to viral or bacterial infections has detrimental consequences for fetal development (Mor et al 2017).

Types of vaccine

Not all vaccines use the same technology to stimulate an immune response, hence there are different types of vaccines. Conventional vaccine types include live attenuated vaccines, inactivated (killed whole antigen), and subunit (purified antigen) vaccines. Over recent decades, a better understanding of the genomes of pathogens, coupled with enhanced laboratory and computer technologies, has led to new types of vaccines. New vaccine types include nucleic acid vaccines (e.g. mRNA) and viral vector vaccines. The COVID-19 global pandemic, and the urgent need for the widespread use of an effective vaccine, resulted in novel vaccine types being used extensively in humans for the first time (Iwasaki et al 2020).

Types of vaccine include:

Whole cell

  a. Live attenuated
    i. viral
    ii. bacterial
  b. Inactivated
    i. split

Subunit (fractional) vaccines

  c. protein-based recombinant protein
    i. DNA recombinant
    ii. virus-like particles (VLPs)
  d. toxoid
  e. polysaccharide (sugars)
    i. pure
    ii. conjugate
  f. nucleic acid (genetically engineered)
    i. mRNA
    ii. DNA
  g. viral vector vaccines.

Live attenuated viral vaccines such as MMR, rotavirus and varicella are contraindicated in pregnant women due to the hypothetical risk of harm if the virus replicates in the fetus. Women need counselling about the potential (but very unlikely) risk of adverse effects on the fetus if they are pregnant and were inadvertently given a live attenuated viral vaccine, or they became pregnant within 28 days of receiving a live attenuated viral vaccine. Other than influenza, and diphtheria-, tetanus- and pertussis-containing vaccines, many inactivated vaccines also are not routinely recommended during pregnancy as a precaution against fever. Pregnant women are only recommended to receive inactivated bacterial or inactivated viral vaccines when the benefits of protection outweigh the risks. Inadvertent administration of a vaccine contraindicated in pregnancy should be reported to the Therapeutic Goods Administration (TGA). While limited data is available on use of immunoglobulins during pregnancy, and they are not routinely recommended, susceptible pregnant women at risk of exposure to vaccine-preventable diseases can receive immunoglobulins. It is rare that vaccination is contraindicated in breastfeeding women. For most vaccines, infant immune response to vaccination in relation to breastfeeding has been considered. Breastfeeding does not adversely affect immunisation, and

DRUG MONOGRAPH 11.1
Pertussis vaccine

Pertussis (whooping cough) is a highly contagious respiratory infection caused by the bacterium *Bordetella pertussis*, both in children and adults. Pertussis can cause serious complications including brain damage, pneumonia, and sometimes death. The most effective way to protect newborn infants is for pregnant women to be vaccinated when they are between 20 and 32 weeks gestation. Vaccination during pregnancy reduces whooping cough in babies aged less than 3 months by over 90%. The pertussis vaccine is an acellular vaccine. It contains various pertussis antigens (subunits) including pertussis filamentous haemagglutinin (adherence protein), pertussis fimbriae 2 + 3 and pertussis toxoid. It is not available as a single-antigen vaccine. It comes in combination with diphtheria and tetanus toxoids, with or without other antigens such as hepatitis B, inactivated poliomyelitis, and Hib.

Indications

To reduce the risk of being infected with pertussis, children should be vaccinated against pertussis according to the National Immunisation Program Schedule and receive a three-dose **primary series** (at 2, 4 and 6 months). This is followed by two booster doses (at 18 months and 4 years), which contain the same amount of antigen as the primary series. Adolescents are administered one reduced antigen pertussis-containing vaccine. The recommended age of administration for the adolescent dose differs between jurisdictions. Vaccination with dTpa is recommended for any adult who wishes to reduce the risk of being infected with pertussis, particularly people (family, carers) who have close contact with newborn babies.

Pharmacokinetics immunogenicity

The three-dose vaccine DTPa primary inoculation results in 84% protective efficacy against severe pertussis. Natural infection with pertussis or a primary series of pertussis vaccination does not confer lifelong protection against reinfection. Protective immunity after pertussis vaccination wanes after 4–6 years, while naturally acquired immunity wanes after 4–20 years. Booster doses of pertussis are needed to increase antibodies and combat waning pertussis immunity.

Drug interactions

Immunosuppressant medicines such as corticosteroids, chemotherapy alkylating agents, antimetabolites, and radiation may reduce the effectiveness of the vaccine. The pertussis vaccine can be given at the same time as other vaccines.

Adverse reactions

Local reactions are common and include pain and tenderness at the injection site. Irritability and drowsiness are also common.

Warnings and contraindications

History of anaphylaxis following a previous dose of a pertussis-containing vaccine or to any vaccine component is a contraindication for further doses.

Dosage and administration

The dose of all pertussis-containing vaccines is 0.5 mL administered by IM injection.

---

breastfeeding is not a contraindication for any vaccines recommended for infants (Australian Government 2023).

Whole-cell vaccines
Live attenuated vaccines

Live attenuated vaccines contain a weakened or altered version of the whole pathogen (virus or bacteria). Weakening, but not killing, the pathogen means that while it can replicate, it has lost significant pathogenicity, and cannot cause serious disease in people with a healthy immune system. Live attenuated vaccines that can replicate in the human host provide continuous antigenic stimulation and confer longer and stronger immunity than most other types of vaccines. They activate both humoral (B-cells) and cellular immunity (T-cells). Examples of live attenuated vaccines include bacille Calmette-Guérin (tuberculosis), measles, mumps, rubella, varicella, poliomyelitis, yellow fever, rotavirus, rabies, herpes zoster, Japanese encephalitis, and influenza (intranasal formulation only). The first vaccine that provided protection against smallpox was also a live vaccine. Smallpox was a serious infectious disease caused by the variola virus, thought to be eradicated globally due to a successful immunisation campaign. However, a recently emerged virus – monkeypox, a rare infectious disease caused by the monkeypox virus – has been found to be related to the virus that causes smallpox. Monkeypox is mostly found in tropical rainforest areas of Central and West Africa. It is linked to travellers who spread the infection when they leave the area, with the first cases reported in Australia in 2022. Monkeypox is usually a mild disease that resolves in 2–4 weeks but can potentially be a serious illness. The risk of more severe symptoms is higher in children or people with reduced immunity. While a vaccine has been developed, this is currently restricted for higher risk groups which do not include pregnant women (Fig 11.5).

Live attenuated vaccines.

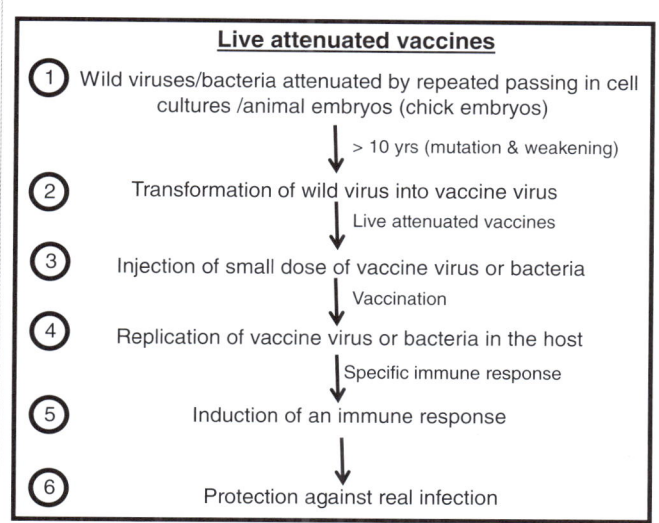

Live attenuated vaccines

1. Wild viruses/bacteria attenuated by repeated passing in cell cultures /animal embryos (chick embryos)

↓ > 10 yrs (mutation & weakening)

2. Transformation of wild virus into vaccine virus

↓ Live attenuated vaccines

3. Injection of small dose of vaccine virus or bacteria

↓ Vaccination

4. Replication of vaccine virus or bacteria in the host

↓ Specific immune response

5. Induction of an immune response

↓

6. Protection against real infection

FIGURE 11.5

Source: Verma, AS, Singh, A (2020). Animal biotechnology: Models in Discovery and Translation. Academic Press.

Live attenuated vaccines are generally contraindicated in pregnant women due to a theoretical risk of harm to the fetus. It is recommended that women avoid conceiving for 28 days after having a live attenuated vaccine. Pregnant women who contract rubella are at increased risk for miscarriage or stillbirth, and the developing baby is at increased risk for severe birth defects including deafness, blindness, heart defects and infection, especially during the first 3 months of pregnancy. Where rubella IgG antibody titre is either negative or below recommended titre level, vaccination will be recommended during the postnatal period to ensure immunity before any subsequent pregnancy.

Live vaccines are also contraindicated in immunocompromised people. That is, all people with congenital (e.g. congenital agammaglobulinemia, congenital IgA deficiency), acquired (e.g. HIV/AIDS) and pharmacological (e.g. chemotherapy, radiotherapy, immunosuppressive therapy) immune-deficient states should not be given live attenuated vaccines. In such people, an attenuated vaccine pathogen may replicate too much, causing disease – the risks outweigh the benefits of the vaccine. Immunocompromised people rely on herd immunity to protect them from vaccine-preventable

---

DRUG MONOGRAPH 11.2
Measles vaccine

The measles vaccine is a live attenuated vaccine. Measles vaccine is not available as a single-antigen vaccine. It is only available in combination with mumps and rubella virus (MMR) or measles, mumps, and varicella virus (MMRV).

Indications

Vaccination against measles is recommended in the National Immunisation Program Schedule with a two-dose primary series (12, 18 months). Due to gaps in past immunisation policies, there is a group of adults who are at risk of measles. In Australia, the second dose of the measles vaccine was not routinely given until the 1990s. People born between 1966 and 1994 may not be fully protected against measles. Those born before 1966 were likely infected with the measles virus itself and are low risk.

Pharmacokinetics immunogenicity

Antibodies for the measles virus appear several days following vaccination, with the greatest protection after 2 or 3 weeks. One dose of measles-containing vaccine provides long-term immunity in approximately 95% of people. After a second vaccine dose, about 99% of people have seroconverted and are protected against measles. The minimum interval between the first and second dose of a measles-containing vaccine is 4 weeks (28 days). After two doses the person should have lifelong immunity.

Drug interactions

Because it is a live attenuated vaccine, it should be given 1 month before or after administration of other vaccines.
* People who have received or are receiving immunoglobulin or a blood product (should wait 3–11 months before vaccine administration).
* People who are taking high doses of corticosteroid (should wait > 1 month before vaccine administration).

Adverse reaction

Local reactions are common (17–30%), for example, pain and tenderness at the injection site (usually resolves within 3 days). Systemic reactions may also occur (5–15% of vaccine recipients), usually between days 7 and 12, and last 1 or 2 days. A generalised rash that lasts for about 2 days occurs in 2–5% of people.

Warnings and contraindications

History of anaphylaxis following a previous dose of MMR vaccine or to any vaccine component. The MMR vaccine should not be given to pregnant or immunocompromised people. It should not be given to someone who is febrile, or who has active untreated tuberculosis. Precaution should be taken in people with a history of low platelet count.

Dosage and administration

The measles vaccine should be administered via IM or SC injection. See specific vaccine product information.

diseases. Thus, people who can be vaccinated should be encouraged to do so for the greater good of society.

Inactivated whole-cell vaccines

Inactivated vaccines are made from whole pathogens (e.g. virus, bacteria) that have been killed by chemicals, or inactivated through heat or radiation. The inactivated pathogens are then used to make vaccines. Many will contain an **adjuvant** (immune enhancer), a substance that helps elicit a more robust immune response (Table 11.1).

When a vaccine contains an adjuvant, we say it is **adsorbed**. Because the pathogens used to make the vaccine are inactivated or dead, they cannot replicate, and they cannot cause disease. However, this also means that they cannot mount a strong, lasting immune response, and booster (multiple) doses are required. Examples of inactivated whole-cell killed vaccines include the inactivated poliovirus (IPV) vaccine, the inactivated influenza vaccine, adsorbed inactivated Japanese encephalitis virus, and the inactivated whole-cell oral

TABLE 11.1 Types of vaccines

	VACCINE TYPE	VACCINE	VIRUS/ BACTERIA	PATHOGEN	ADSORBED OR CONJUGATED	PRIMARY SERIES BOOSTER	ROUTE
Whole cell	Live attenuated Not recommended during pregnancy	Bacille Calmette-Guérin Measles Mumps Rubella Varicella Japanese encephalitis Rotavirus Typhoid Yellow fever Zoster	Bacteria Virus Virus Virus Virus Virus Bacteria Virus Virus	*Mycobacterium bovis* Measles morbillivirus (DM 11.1) Mumps virus Rubella virus Varicella zoster virus Japanese encephalitis Rotavirus *Salmonella typhi* Yellow fever virus Herpes virus	No No No No No No No No No	No Booster Booster Booster Booster No No No No	Intracutaneously or ID SC or IM SC or IM SC or IM SC or IM Imojev SC Oral Vivotif Oral SC or IM
Whole cell	Inactivated (inactivated bacteria are also called killed antigen vaccines – viruses that were never alive to begin with)	Cholera Hepatitis A Q fever (killed) Influenza Japanese encephalitis (IM) Poliomyelitis (IPV) Rabies	Bacteria Virus Bacteria Virus Virus Virus	*Vibrio cholerae* Hepatitis A virus *Coxiella burnetii* Influenza A or B Japanese encephalitis Poliovirus *Rabies lyssavirus*	No Adsorbed No Adsorbed Adsorbed No No	Primary series + booster Primary series + booster Single dose (do not revaccinate) Annual Primary series + booster Primary series + booster Primary series + booster	Oral IM SC IM JEspect IM SC IM
Subunit	Toxoid (inactivated toxin)	Diphtheria	Bacteria	*Corynebacterium diphtheriae* secretes diphtheria toxin	Adsorbed	Primary series + booster	IM
		Tetanus	Bacteria	*Clostridium tetani* secretes tetanospasmin, a neurotoxin	Adsorbed	Primary series + booster	IM
Subunit	Recombinant subunit	COVID-19 Pertussis (acellular) (DM 11.2) Hepatitis B (recombinant DNA hepatitis b surface antigen) Meningococcal B (recombinant)	Virus Bacteria Virus Bacteria	Severe acute respiratory syndrome coronavirus 2 *Bordetella pertussis* Hepatitis B virus *Neisseria meningitidis*	Adsorbed Combination only dTPa Adsorbed Adsorbed not conjugated	Primary series + booster Primary series + booster Primary series Primary series	IM IM IM IM

TABLE 11.1 Types of vaccines—cont'd

VACCINE TYPE	VACCINE	VIRUS/ BACTERIA	PATHOGEN	ADSORBED OR CONJUGATED	PRIMARY SERIES BOOSTER	ROUTE
Subunit	Virus-like particles (VLPs)	HPV (recombinant HPV capsid [L1] protein)	Virus	HPV Malaria	Adsorbed	Primary series	IM
Subunit	Conjugate/ polysaccharide	Hib Meningococcal C Meningococcal ACWY Pneumococcal 13vPCV Pneumococcal 23vPPV (not conjugated) Typhoid	Bacteria Bacteria Bacteria Bacteria Bacteria Bacteria	Hib *Neisseria meningitidis* *Neisseria meningitidis* *Streptococcus pneumoniae* *Streptococcus pneumoniae* *Salmonella typhi*	Conjugated Conjugated Conjugated Conjugated Not conjugated Conjugated	Primary series Primary series Primary series	IM IM IM IM IM IM or SC Typhim Vi IM
Nucleic acid	Messenger ribonucleic acid (mRNA)	COVID-19	Virus	Severe acute respiratory syndrome coronavirus 2	No	Primary series + booster	IM
Vector	Viral vector	COVID-19	Virus	Severe acute respiratory syndrome coronavirus 2	No	Primary series + booster	IM

cholera vaccine. Inactivated whole-cell vaccines are safe in pregnant women and in immunocompromised people. However, an immunocompromised person may require additional doses of inactivated vaccine to mount an immune response comparable to that seen in a healthy person.

Subunit vaccines

Subunit vaccines (sometimes called acellular vaccines) contain only the antigenic components/pieces of the pathogen (e.g. a surface antigen). Specifically, they contain the parts of the pathogen required to elicit an immune response. Because they are only 'parts' of the pathogen, they are not 'live'. All subunit vaccines are, by their nature, inactivated. When compared with live or nucleic acid vaccines, most subunit vaccines do not elicit strong immune responses. They generally require repeated doses initially (priming series) and boosters to maintain immunity. Adjuvants are often used in subunit vaccines (Table 11.1). Adjuvants are non-antigen vaccine components that are pro-inflammatory and increase the activity of antigen-presenting cells, which activate further innate (e.g. natural killer cells) and adaptive immune responses (B-cells and T-cells). Aluminium salts and toll-like receptor agonists are currently used in vaccines as adjuvants. A downside is that vaccines that contain adjuvants are associated with increased local reactions such as a sore arm.

There are several types of subunit vaccines:

- pure polysaccharide
- conjugate polysaccharide
- toxoid
- recombinant protein
- virus-like particles.

Pure polysaccharide vaccines

To date, there are polysaccharide vaccines for pneumococcal and meningococcal diseases, Hib and *Salmonella typhi*. **Pure polysaccharide vaccines** trigger a T-cell independent response and therefore cannot generate a robust and long-lasting immune response (Fig 11.6).

Conjugate polysaccharide vaccines

Polysaccharides can also be covalently linked (or chemically combined) to a protein carrier. This process results in a **conjugate polysaccharide vaccine** and greatly increases the immunogenicity of the polysaccharide vaccine. This is because conjugated polysaccharide vaccines can stimulate a T-cell dependent immune response, and subsequent T-cell memory. Most polysaccharide vaccines are conjugated (Table 11.1). For example, the Hib vaccine is conjugated with the tetanus toxoid.

Toxoid vaccines

Some bacteria, such as diphtheria, tetanus, botulism and cholera, cause disease by secreting a toxin. For example, the tetanus **toxoid** vaccine is manufactured by growing the highly toxigenic strain *Clostridium tetani*. The *Clostridium tetani* bacteria secrete the toxin in the laboratory environment, in large quantities. The toxin is then

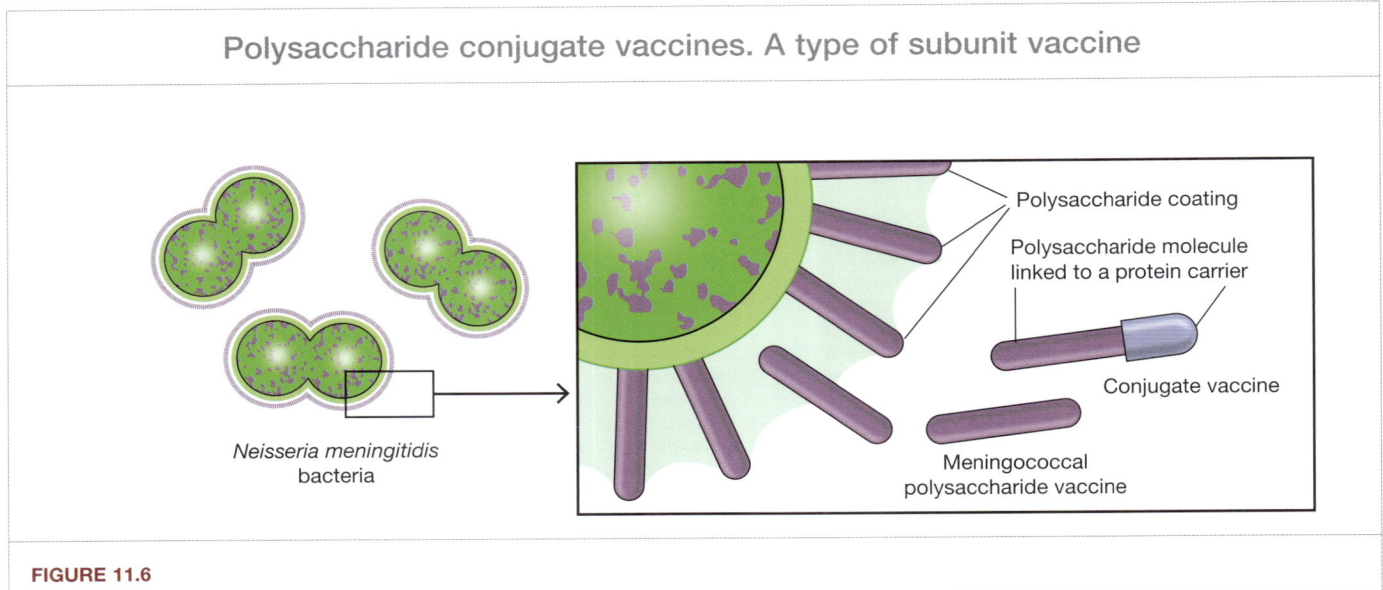

Polysaccharide conjugate vaccines. A type of subunit vaccine

Polysaccharide coating

Polysaccharide molecule linked to a protein carrier

Conjugate vaccine

Meningococcal polysaccharide vaccine

Neisseria meningitidis bacteria

FIGURE 11.6

chemically denatured by formaldehyde to produce a tetanus toxoid. The toxoid is physiochemically like the toxin, enabling the generation of antibodies and subsequent immunity; however, it is different enough to be non-toxigenic and unable to cause the disease itself. The other toxoid vaccines are produced in a similar way. They generally cannot mount a strong immune response unless given in multiple doses (primary series) and booster doses. To strengthen their immunogenicity, they contain adjuvants (i.e. they are adsorbed).

Recombinant protein vaccines

Recombinant vaccines use DNA technology in their manufacture. In the laboratory, a small piece of DNA is taken from a virus or bacterium that immunity is sought from. This small piece (subunit) of DNA is the gene or genetic code for an antigen. For example, the hepatitis B vaccine uses the DNA that codes for the hepatitis B surface antigen (HBsAg). This piece of DNA is then inserted into an expression vector (a harmless host such as yeast or bacteria).

The first recombinant protein vaccine was the hepatitis B vaccine, first marketed in the late 1980s. To date, there are three recombinant vaccines marketed in Australia:

- hepatitis B vaccine (adsorbed recombinant DNA surface antigen)
- meningococcal B recombinant vaccines
- HPV vaccine (adsorbed recombinant HPV capsid [L1] protein). (This vaccine is also known as a virus-like particle vaccine and is discussed in more detail below.)

Virus-like particles

VLPs are assembled from viral proteins and are therefore structurally like viruses; however, they do not contain viral genetic material (DNA or RNA). Because they do not contain genetic material, they cannot replicate and therefore are not infectious when used as vaccines. The HPV vaccine is an example of a recombinant vaccine and a VLP vaccine.

So, while it characteristically 'looks' like the real virus, it is not a virus; it is 'virus-like'.

When the HPV VLPs are introduced into the body via vaccination, the body recognises them as foreign, triggering an immune response. Despite being a subunit vaccine, the VLPs used in the HPV vaccine are highly immunogenic and efficacious. They elicit a robust immune response and stimulate both the antibody and cell-mediated arms of the adaptive immune system. On subsequent exposure to the real virus, the body mounts a strong and immediate secondary immune response.

Viral vector vaccines

Viral vector vaccines use the vaccinated person's own body cells to produce the antigen, which confers immunity. So how does this happen? The name of the vaccine tells us that this technology employs the use of 'viral vectors'. When most people think of a 'vector' they think of an animal such as a mosquito or tick that transmits a disease from one animal to another – for example, mosquitoes are vectors for malaria. Essentially, the vector is a host or a delivery system that enables the transmission of disease. We can extrapolate this logic to viral vector vaccines. In this case, the vector (or the host that carries and enables the transfer of disease) is a live, harmless, modified virus. Its cargo is a piece of genetic material from another virus, the one that protection is sought from, that codes for an antigen.

Viruses are non-living and must be taken into a host cell to replicate. Viral vector vaccines exploit this process, so both the vector and the genetic material (usually

DNA) it is carrying are taken into the human cells. Because the viral vector is genetically modified, it cannot cause disease. Consistent with how viruses obtain entry to a human cell, the viral vector attaches to the host cell and injects the genetic material. The human cell then transcribes the DNA into mRNA, which generates the protein antigen. The antigens are then presented on the infected host cell's surface, eliciting a robust immune response that generates both humoral and cell-mediated immunity. Viral vectors can be categorised into replicating and non-replicating viral vectors.

The Ebola vaccine and the Oxford AstraZeneca COVID-19 vaccine (Vaxzevria) are viral vector vaccines. The viral vector used in Vaxzevria is an adenovirus, a chimpanzee common cold pathogen, ChAdOx1. The genetic material or DNA is carried inside the vector codes for the severe acute respiratory syndrome coronavirus 2 (SARS-CoV-2) protein spike, a key antigen of the COVID-19 virus. Because there is only a piece of the SARS-CoV-2 genetic material (only the code for the protein spike), it cannot assemble the entire SARS-CoV-2 virus, and therefore cannot cause COVID-19. Viral vector vaccines are safe in immunocompromised people and pregnant women.

One limitation of viral vector vaccines is that people may already have preexisting immunity to the vector. When this happens, the body will mount an immune response against the viral vector, clearing it from the body, before it has played its role and delivered the genetic material to the host cell that codes for an antigen. For this reason, the Oxford AstraZeneca COVID-19 vaccine used a chimpanzee common cold virus that was not a common infection in humans as the viral vector, improving the vaccine's efficacy.

New vaccine type: Nucleic acid vaccines

Although scientists had been working on nucleic acid vaccines since the late 1980s, the first nucleic acid vaccine was not approved for human use until 2020. It was a COVID-19 vaccine. There are two types of nucleic acid vaccines:

- mRNA vaccines
- plasmid DNA vaccines.

To date, outside clinical trials, no DNA vaccine has been approved for human use.

New vaccine type: mRNA vaccines

Once the genome for a pathogen has been sequenced, mRNA vaccines can be chemically synthesised in a laboratory from a template. When producing the vaccine, there is no need for pathogen cells. The key immunogenic component of mRNA vaccines is the mRNA that encodes for the pathogen of interest's protein antigen. For example, the Pfizer-BioNTech COVID-19 vaccine (Comirnaty) contained the mRNA that encoded for the protein spike of the SARS-CoV-2 virus (Polack et al 2020).

mRNA alone is very fragile and degrades easily when introduced into the body. It is also difficult for mRNA alone to enter host cells because the cell membrane acts as a barrier. To stimulate an immune response, the mRNA must cross the host cell membrane to reach the cytoplasm. Therefore, to prevent degradation and enable entry into host cells, the mRNA is enclosed in a delivery system.

These delivery systems protect the mRNA from degradation. By a process known as endocytosis, the delivery system with the enclosed mRNA is taken into the host cell cytoplasm. The mRNA is read at the ribosomes and results in the synthesis of translated protein antigens. The host has effectively created the 'vaccine' in situ. The antigens that have been produced are then displayed on the cell membrane, triggering an immune response. Because the antigen has been taken into the host cells, it activates both humoral and cellular immunity (Sahin 2020). The result is a robust immune response. Because mRNA does not enter the host cell's nucleus, it cannot integrate into the host cell genome (and cannot alter human DNA). The mRNA is transiently expressed and eventually destroyed by the host cell.

mRNA vaccines are quicker, easier, and cheaper to produce than more traditional vaccine technologies. They can also be modified easily to provide protection against rapidly mutating pathogens. Pregnant women afflicted with COVID-19 are at an elevated risk of premature rupture of membranes, acute kidney injury, acute respiratory distress syndrome, multi-organ failure, preterm labour, intrauterine death; requiring admission to an intensive care unit, oxygen therapy and mechanical ventilation (Juan et al 2020; Liang et al 2020; Shimabukuro 2021). The Pfizer-BioNTech and Moderna mRNA vaccines have been designed to elicit a cellular and humoral immune response providing the genetic information that initiates the biosynthesis of a viral spike protein as an immunogen (Heinz et al 2021). In doing so, recipients can form defensive antibodies that mediate viral entry into the host of SARS-CoV-2 S glycoproteins (Kalafat et al 2021; Ou et al 2020; Yadav et al 2020). Moreover, mRNA cannot influence human DNA, as the injected mRNA is translated and quickly degraded by the cell's ribosomes and is thus unable to enter the nucleus of the recipient's cell (Labdi 2021). In comparison, the safety and efficacy of Novavax and AstraZeneca COVID-19 vaccines are yet to be established in pregnancy.

Vaccine hesitancy in pregnancy was initially attributed to the accelerated speed of COVID-19 vaccine development and fear for the safety of neonates from long-term effects due to a lack of data because pregnant women were excluded from the clinical trials (Craig et al 2021). COVID-19 vaccine hesitancy – defined as reluctance to receive vaccines and reductions in vaccine uptake during the perinatal period have been observed (Puri et al 2020; Skirrow et al 2022), with a greater level of hesitancy observed in ethnic minority communities (Hanif et al 2020), despite evidence that Pfizer-BioNTech and Moderna vaccines have provided safe and robust protective efficacy to pregnant women (Riley 2021; Shimabukuro 2021). The WHO has recognised the global significance of COVID-19 vaccine hesitancy, citing it as one of the greatest risks to life (WHO 2019).

The perceived risks of COVID-19 disease and vaccinations have raised prenatal anxiety and fears (Basu et al 2021). However, much of the early fear was roused by social media misconceptions regarding COVID-19 vaccinations' safety during pregnancy (Puri et al 2020) and a lack of trust in healthcare providers and government authorities (Castillo et al 2021).

Recent studies undertaken to determine the frequency and nature of significant health events among pregnant females who received COVID-19 mRNA vaccine have established a good safety profile in pregnancy (Sadarangani et al 2022).

KEY POINTS

Vaccines given during pregnancy

- Measles is a live attenuated vaccine administered as part of the MMR vaccine.
- Inactivated whole-cell vaccines have had the bacteria inactivated through heat, chemicals, or radiation.
- Viral vector vaccines stimulate a reaction from the body's own defence system to achieve immunity.
- Subunit vaccines do not contain the live vaccines. Only part of the pathogen required to elicit a response is used. Repeat vaccination is required.
- Polysaccharide vaccines trigger a T-cell independent response.
- Conjugated polysaccharide vaccines can stimulate a T-cell dependent immune response and subsequent T-cell memory.
- Toxoid vaccines are physiochemically similar the original toxin but has been deactivated.
- Recombinant protein vaccines are created from a small piece of DNA inserted into a harmless host, such as yeast, to grow the vaccine.
- Virus-like particles structurally replicate the virus but they are not 'real' and therefore are safe for use during pregnancy.
- New vaccine types – mRNA and plasmid DNA vaccines – target the COVID-19 infection. While traditionally vaccines have been contraindicated in pregnancy, the benefits of protection outweigh the risks of non-vaccination.

11.3 Vaccine schedules

Vaccine schedules are based on an understanding of how the different types of vaccine work and epidemiological research. Schedules are constantly being reviewed by immunisation experts to ensure people are best protected against vaccine-preventable diseases. The National Immunisation Program Schedule (Australia) and the New Zealand Immunisation Schedule (New Zealand) outline the vaccines recommended across the life span. Both countries offer these vaccines free to citizens. When examining the vaccine schedules, it is evident that some vaccines are given as a primary series, and then in booster doses.

Primary series

In a primary series, a series of vaccine doses (usually 2–4) is required to achieve full vaccine effectiveness. For example, in New Zealand the diphtheria, tetanus, pertussis, polio, hepatitis B, and Hib are all given at the age of 6 weeks, 3 months, and 5 months. In Australia, these vaccines are given at 2, 4, and 6 months of age. Both schedules are examples of a primary series.

Boosters

Excluding several live attenuated vaccines, most vaccines require booster doses to ensure protection (Table 11.1). Booster doses are given months or years after the primary dose/series. They 'boost' the immune system and protect against waning immunity. For example, two booster doses are recommended for diphtheria, tetanus, and whooping cough in childhood. The first booster is given at 18 months of age and the second at 4 years of age. Another booster is given in adolescence at roughly 12–13 years, and is then recommended for adults who wish to reduce their risk of becoming ill or transmitting the infection to others (e.g. people caring for a newborn).

When planning a pregnancy, women are advised to review the vaccine schedule and arrange to catch up on any vaccines or vaccine doses they may not have previously completed.

Annual influenza vaccine

Influenza is not just a cold. Influenza is a highly contagious, acute respiratory infection caused by an influenza virus. It is a serious disease for pregnant women and the developing and newborn baby. Changes to immune, heart, and lung function make pregnant women more vulnerable to severe illness from influenza. Pregnant women are more than twice as likely to be admitted to hospital as other people with influenza. In Australia in 2019 (pre-pandemic) there were 313,033 laboratory-confirmed cases and 902 influenza deaths. It is estimated that globally influenza causes 389,000 deaths (uncertainty range 294,000–518,000) each year (Paget et al 2019). Influenza viruses are constantly evolving and changing, and different strains can circulate in the population. This is the rationale behind changing the influenza vaccine composition each year. To provide the greatest protection, the vaccine should contain viruses that are a 'match' or are antigenically like those currently circulating. Each year, the WHO recommends the strains to be included in influenza vaccines. This recommendation is based on knowledge of the circulating strains in the opposite hemisphere's influenza season (usually winter). That is, the southern hemisphere looks to the northern hemisphere (and vice versa) to inform vaccine composition. The influenza vaccine comes in both quadrivalent (two influenza A subtypes and two influenza B lineages) and trivalent (two influenza A subtypes and one influenza B lineage) formulations.

Vaccine efficacy of the influenza vaccine varies by year but is generally less than 60% in healthy adults, well below the efficacy of other vaccines. This is, in part, attributed to the difficulty of predicting the circulated strains.

There are two types of influenza vaccine: the live attenuated (LAIV) and the inactivated (IIV). In Australia, however, the LAIV is yet to be marketed. There are two types of IIV split virion or subunit vaccines. Split virion influenza vaccines report a greater vaccine efficacy than subunit vaccines (Talbot et al 2015).

Pregnant women are recommended to be given the inactivated vaccine annually. If the woman received the vaccine before becoming pregnant, she should have the vaccine repeated during the second or third trimester of pregnancy during flu season to protect the fetus.

Herd immunity

Vaccines have both an individual and collective benefit. The person who is administered a vaccine will likely go on to develop immunity and individual protection against the vaccine-preventable disease. The collective benefit arises when a significant number of people (often called the critical mass threshold) within the population have developed immunity either naturally or by vaccination, reducing the number of susceptible hosts and the spread of the disease. This provides protection to those without individual immunity (e.g. unvaccinated). The critical proportion of the population that must be immune to provide herd immunity varies by the disease. For example, to provide adequate measles protection for the whole population, approximately 95% of the population needs to have active immunity. Given that measles is a live attenuated vaccine, and is contraindicated in people who are immunocompromised, such people rely on the 'herd' to get vaccinated to protect them. With such a high critical mass threshold, there have been several sporadic and small outbreaks of measles in Australia in recent times.

Vaccines are victims of their own success. Because people do not have a lived experience of the morbidity and mortality caused by now vaccine-preventable diseases, they become more concerned about vaccine safety. Ongoing education concerning the risks of vaccine-preventable disease is important. Vaccine hesitancy or reduced vaccine uptake is a barrier to achieving herd immunity, leaving those who cannot, or choose not to be, vaccinated at greater risk. A recent example of this occurred in Samoa in 2019 when routine measles immunisation rates fell to 31% which led to a measles outbreak and a national emergency with 5707 cases reported, resulting in 83 deaths; 87% of these were children less than 5 years old (Craig et al 2020).

KEY POINTS

Vaccine schedules

- A primary series of vaccinations (2–4) is required to achieve full immunity.

- Boosters are required months or years after the initial course to maintain immunity.

- Annual influenza is highly contagious, requiring annual vaccinations to respond to the latest strain of bacteria.

- Herd immunity protects immunosuppressed members of society. Herd immunity can only be achieved if everyone who is able to be vaccinated maintains the recommended vaccination schedules.

11.4 Clinical considerations

Vaccine cold chain management

Vaccines are temperature-sensitive. To ensure potency, they must be stored in a predetermined cold chain from initial manufacture, during transportation and storage through to administration. This process is known as cold chain management. Breaches in the vaccine cold chain may result in the administration of vaccines that cannot elicit an immune response and therefore leave the person and community at risk of vaccine-preventable diseases. Most vaccines need to be stored between 2°C and 8°C, and exposure to freezing temperatures is likely to cause irreversible loss of vaccine potency. However, the new mRNA vaccines (e.g. COVID-19) need to be stored at ultra-cold temperatures during initial transport and storage (between –90°C and –60°C). Keeping mRNA vaccines at such ultra-low temperatures has been one of the great logistical challenges during the COVID-19 vaccine rollout. It is important that health professionals ensure vaccines are always maintained within the cold chain and that suspected or actual breaches in vaccine cold chain are reported.

Vaccine administration technique

Injury related to vaccine administration is a very rare, preventable complication that occurs when a vaccine is administered incorrectly. Vaccinators should use appropriate landmarking techniques, helping to identify key anatomical landmarks to determine a safe injecting zone. It is important that vaccinators use the correct injection site, technique and equipment when vaccinating. This includes selecting the correct gauge (needle thickness) and needle length. Needles used for IM injections generally have a lower gauge (i.e. wider) than those used for SC injections. A needle with a wider bore helps to dissipate the vaccine over a wider area, reducing localised inflammation at the injection site. IM injections need to go deeper into the body tissues than SC injections, and therefore IM needles are longer (usually 25 mm) and inserted at a 90° angle. SC vaccines are inserted on a 45° angle (Fig 11.7). While administered deeper into the body tissues, IM vaccines tend to cause fewer local reactions such as irritation and inflammation than SC injections.

Vaccines that are administered IM deposit the antigen into the muscle fascia, which has an abundant blood supply. In comparison, the SC layer does not have a rich blood supply. Administering a vaccine into the SC layer, when is it is intended for the muscle fascia, may delay the presentation of the antigen to the immune cells and result in a reduction in immunogenicity or even vaccine failure.

Using body landmarks to administer intramuscular vaccines

Two anatomical sites are routinely used to administer vaccines: the anterolateral thigh and the deltoid (upper arm) muscle. The ventrogluteal (side of hip) area may also be used as an alternative. The anatomical site selected for vaccine administration depends on the person's age. In general, infants up to 12 months of age will receive vaccines in the anterolateral thigh, and people aged over 12 months will have vaccines administered into the deltoid. Vaccinators should use anatomical markers or landmarking techniques when administering vaccines to ensure appropriate vaccine administration. Common landmarking techniques are described below. Further

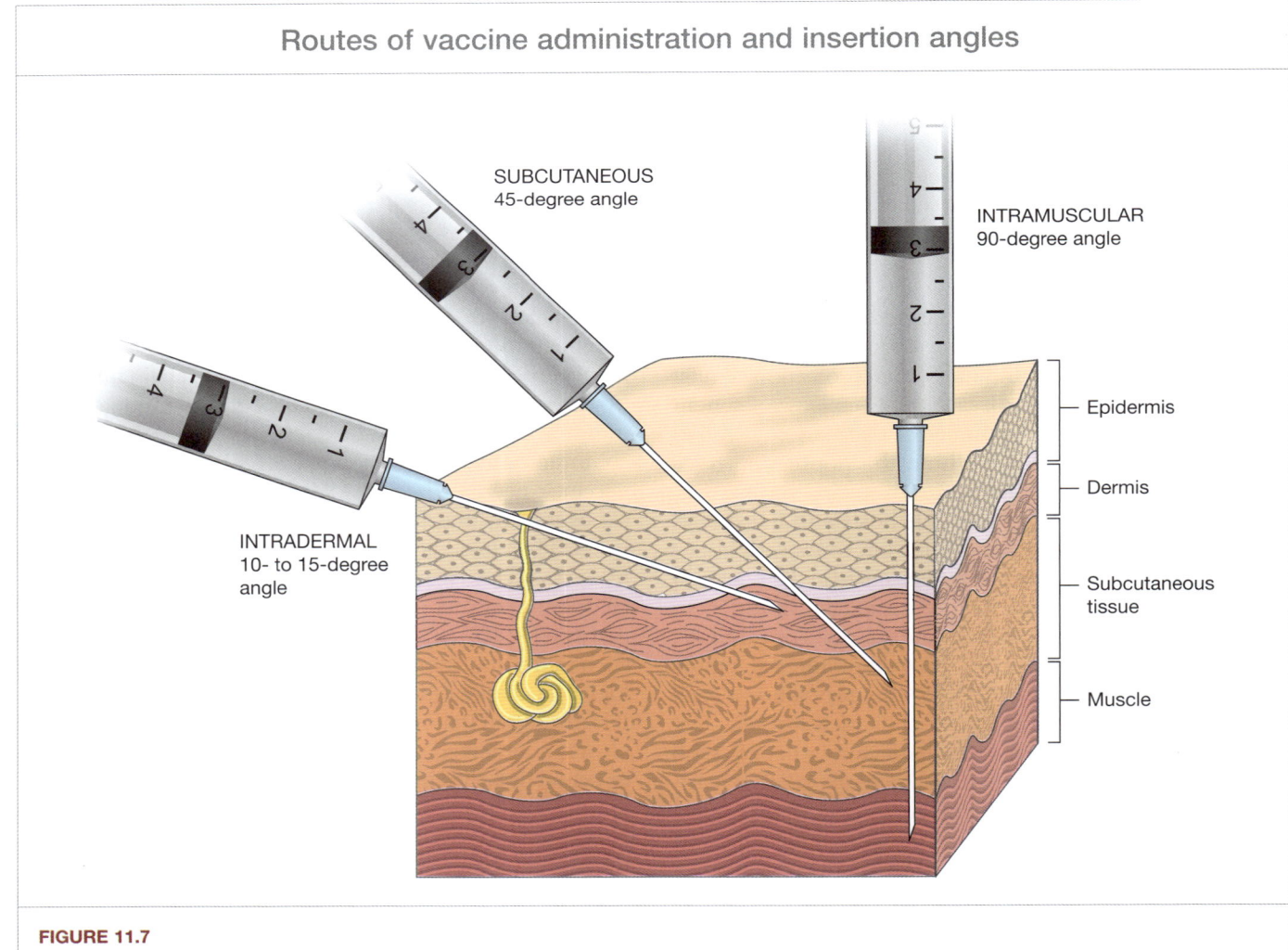

Routes of vaccine administration and insertion angles

SUBCUTANEOUS
45-degree angle

INTRAMUSCULAR
90-degree angle

INTRADERMAL
10- to 15-degree angle

Epidermis

Dermis

Subcutaneous tissue

Muscle

FIGURE 11.7

information can be found in the *Australian Immunisation Handbook* (see Online resources).

Administering a vaccine into the vastus lateralis (anterolateral thigh)

The vastus lateralis (VL) or anterolateral thigh muscle is the preferred anatomical site for vaccines in infants aged under 12 months. Vaccines should be administered into the outer side of the middle third of the VL muscle. To locate the site of the injection, the vaccinator should landmark the femur (greater trochanter) and the knee (patella) and draw an imaginary line between the two landmarks down the front of the thigh (dividing the thigh into sides). Then they should draw two imaginary lines dividing the thigh across into thirds. The vaccines should be administered in the middle third and on the outer side. It is recommended to remove the infant's nappy to locate the anatomical landmarks and administer the vaccine. If two vaccines are to be administered at the one appointment, both VLs should be used. When more than two vaccines are to be administered, up to two vaccines may be administered into a single VL; however, they should be spaced 2.5 cm apart.

Administering a vaccine into the deltoid

The deltoid is a triangular shaped muscle located on the upper arm (Fig 11.8). It sits on top of the clavicle, scapular and humerus bones. IM vaccines should be administered into the middle (or bulkiest part) of the deltoid. The *Australian Immunisation Handbook* recommends vaccinators landmark using both the acromion process (shoulder tip) and deltoid tuberosity (deltoid muscle insertion point roughly in the middle of the humerus bone). The vaccinator should measure two to three fingerbreadths below the acromion process; the fingers form the top of an imaginary inverted triangle, preventing the vaccine being injected into the shoulder bursae. Anywhere within this inverted triangle area is an appropriate site for IM vaccination.

When administering an IM injection, the vaccinator should:

- use a needle 22–25 in gauge
- for infants (> 2 months), children or adults, use a needle 25 mm in length
- insert the needle on a 90° angle to the skin
- insert the needle all the way to the hub
- withdraw the needle on the same angle as it was inserted (i.e. 90° angle).

When administering a vaccine to a very large person, a 38 mm needle may be used to ensure the antigen is delivered into the muscle layer. Using a needle this length on a small or thin person may result in the needle 'hitting the bone' and may cause osteonecrosis. Therefore, it is important the vaccinator uses a needle of an appropriate length.

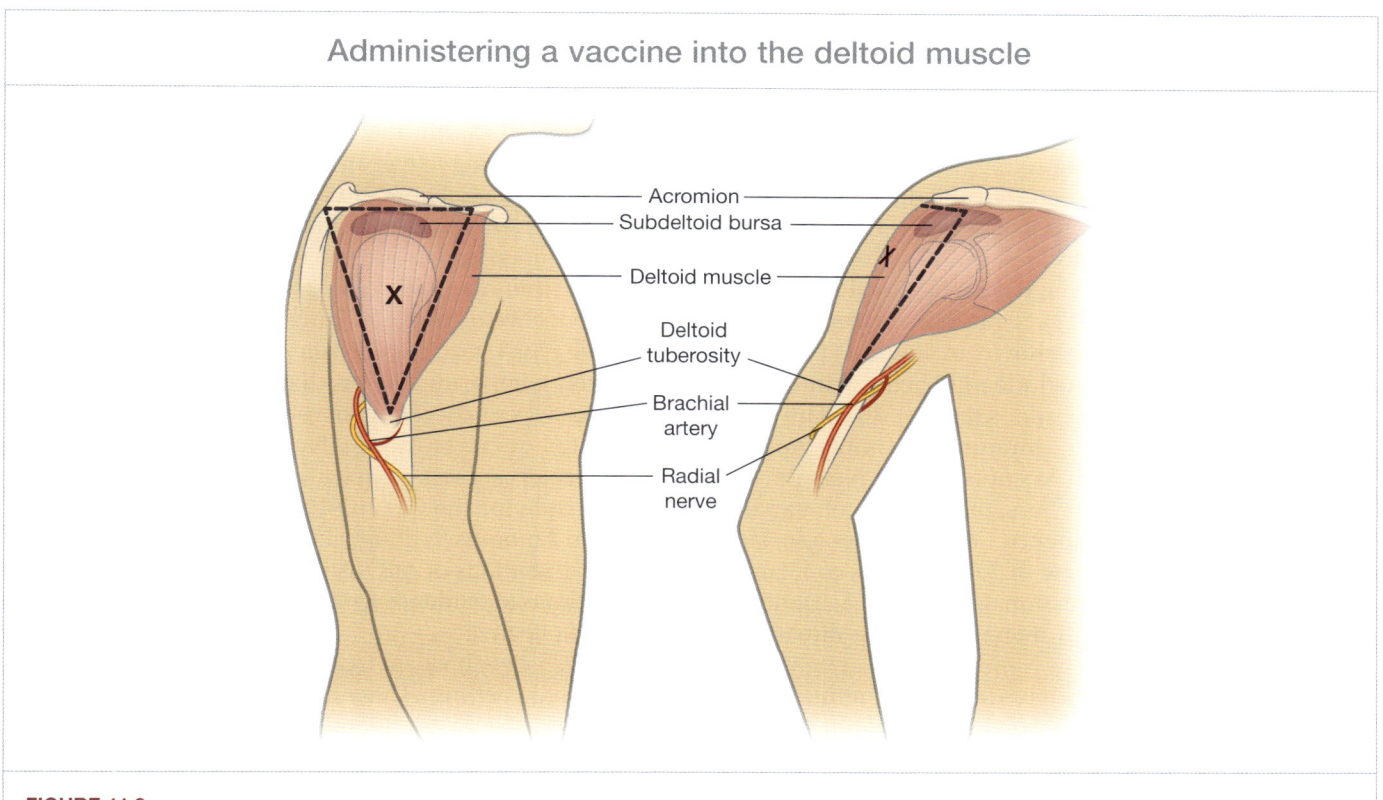

Administering a vaccine into the deltoid muscle

Acromion
Subdeltoid bursa
Deltoid muscle
Deltoid tuberosity
Brachial artery
Radial nerve

FIGURE 11.8

When administering an SC injection, the vaccinator should:

- use a needle 25–27 in gauge
- use a needle 16 mm in length.
- insert the needle on a 45° angle to the skin plane
- insert the needle all the way to the hub
- withdraw the needle on the same angle as it was inserted (i.e. 45° angle).

Reporting vaccinations to national registers

In Australia, health professionals should upload the details of every vaccine administered to the Australian Immunisation Register at the time of vaccination. This enables an accurate real-time vaccination record to be kept for individuals. It also enables vaccination coverage to be determined at the population level. Health professionals can view a person's vaccination history to recommend vaccines to be administered. During the COVID-19 pandemic, people needed a record of their vaccination status for work and travel.

As outlined in the *Australian Immunisation Register Act 2015*, there is specific information that should be uploaded to the Australian Immunisation Register after vaccination, including mandatory reporting of specific vaccines such as COVID-19 vaccinations.

Vaccine side effects

While vaccines have an excellent safety profile, all vaccines have potential side effects (Dudley et al 2020). By their mechanism of action, vaccines stimulate an immune response, and therefore it is not surprising that many people experience the signs and symptoms of inflammation such as pain, redness, and swelling at the injection site. This could be interpreted as a good thing because it is an indication that the vaccine has stimulated an immune response. Vaccines can also have systemic adverse effects such as fever, headache, myalgia, rash, or fatigue (Hervé et al 2019). Common adverse events following vaccination are shown in Figure 11.9. Other very rare adverse events include mild acute arthralgia or arthritis, encephalitis, febrile seizures, Guillain-Barré syndrome, herpes zoster, immune thrombocytopenic purpura, meningitis, and syncope. Such adverse events are estimated to occur in less than 0.01% of vaccines administered. The incidence of vaccine-associated anaphylaxis is less than one in 1,000,000 doses for most vaccines. All health professionals should be trained to administer adrenaline and manage this life-threatening event.

All suspected adverse events following immunisation should be reported. In Australia, this is via a National Adverse Events Following Immunisation reporting form submitted to the TGA (see Online resources).

KEY POINTS

Clinical considerations

- Vaccines are temperature-sensitive and must be stored in a predetermined cold chain from initial manufacture, during transportation and storage through to administration.

- Using the correct administration technique for the given vaccine helps to optimise immunogenicity and reduce the local side effects.

- IM injections are inserted on a 90° angle to the skin plane. SC vaccines are inserted on a 45° angle.

- The anterolateral thigh and the deltoid muscle are the most common anatomical sites for vaccine administration.

- All vaccinations should be recorded, and information uploaded to the national immunisation register.

CONCLUSION: THE FUTURE OF VACCINES

When the deadly COVID-19 pandemic hit, the world needed a vaccine, and scientists across the globe put efforts into vaccine development. More than 500 vaccines entered clinical trials. Some vaccines used traditional (e.g. protein subunit, inactivated), and some used new vaccine technology (e.g. mRNA, viral vector). Prior to COVID-19, no nucleic acid vaccine had been licensed for human use. However, the first COVID-19 vaccine that was developed and approved was an mRNA vaccine. So how did this happen? Well, for a start the technology had been 30 years in the making and there were safe and effective DNA vaccines for veterinary use.

When comparing the production of more traditional vaccines where the antigens need to be inactivated or attenuated or created through recombination, producing nucleic acid vaccines is faster, easier, and safer. Once the genetic code for the COVID-19 virus was known, it took less than 2 months to design and create an mRNA vaccine. Now with billions of mRNA vaccines administered, there is a plethora of evidence to show that mRNA vaccines are safe and effective.

By 2023, new bivalent COVID-19 vaccines had replaced the original vaccines. These newer vaccines offered better protection against the Omicron strain of SARS-CoV-2 (Australian Government 2023). It is expected that the future of vaccine technology will continue to gain momentum.

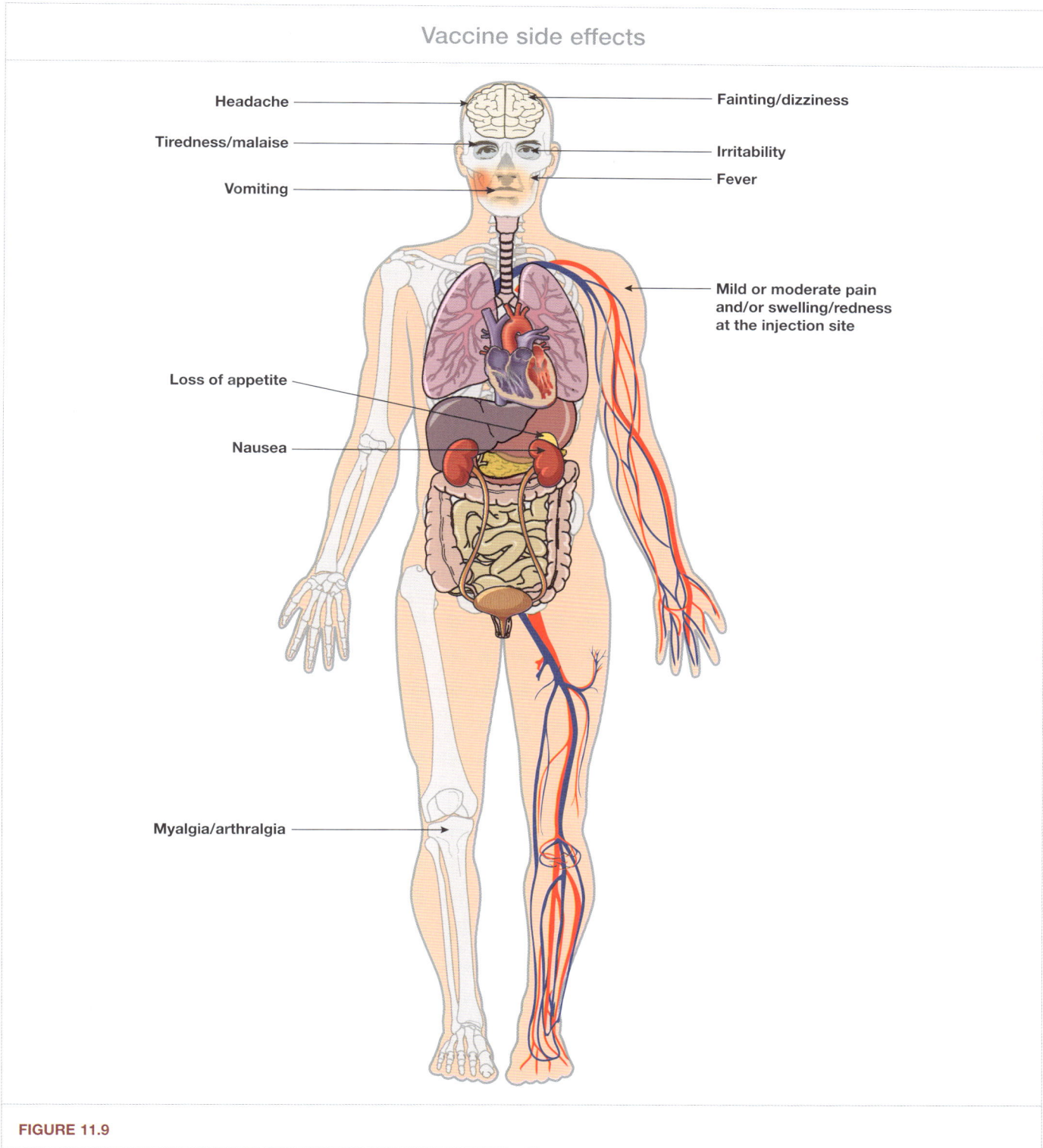

Vaccine side effects

FIGURE 11.9

REVIEW EXERCISES

1 Amelia is a 19-year-old woman who moved from Somalia to Australia 2 years ago. This is her first pregnancy. Her blood results show she is not immune to rubella. Can she receive rubella vaccination during pregnancy? What type of vaccine is the rubella vaccine? What would you recommend for future pregnancies?

2 Madeleine is 23 years old and pregnant with her second child. She is hesitant to receive any COVID-19 vaccinations during pregnancy. What information can you provide her about the different types and their safety during pregnancy?

3 Tonya is attending her antenatal appointment after completing her anomaly scan. No concerns were identified, and she is fit and well. What health promotion advice could you deliver at this appointment with regards to scheduled vaccinations?

4 When a woman has a conscientious objection to receiving vaccination during pregnancy, what is the recommended approach to information sharing and care for her midwife? Discuss relevant ethical principles and professional standards.

REFERENCES

Australian Government. National immunisation program schedule – July 2023. https://www.health.gov.au/health-topics/immunisation/when-to-get-vaccinated/national-immunisation-program-schedule

Adams NM, Grassmann S, Sun JC. Clonal expansion of innate and adaptive lymphocytes. Nat Rev Immunol. 2020;20(11): 694-707.

Albrecht M, Arck PC. Vertically transferred immunity in neonates: mothers, mechanisms and mediators. Front Immunol. 2020 Mar;11:555. doi.org/10.3389/fimmu.2020.00555

Atyeo C, Alter G. The multifaceted roles of breast milk antibodies. Cell. 2021 Mar;184:1486-1499. doi.org/10.1016/j.cell.2021.02.031

Basu A, Kim HH, Basaldua R, et al. A cross-national study of factors associated with women's perinatal mental health and wellbeing during the COVID-19 pandemic. PLoS One. 2021;16(4);e0249780. doi.org/10.1371/journal.pone.0249780

Castillo E, Patey A, Macdonald N. Vaccination in pregnancy: challenges and evidence-based solutions. Best Pract Res Clin Obstet Gynaecol. 2021;76:83-95. doi.org/10.1016/j.bpobgyn.2021.03.008

Craig AM, Hughes BL, Swamy GK. Coronavirus disease 2019 vaccines in pregnancy. Am J Obstet Gynecol MFM. 2021;3(2):100295. doi.org/10.1016/j.ajogmf.2020.10029

Craig AT, Heywood AE, Worth H. Measles epidemic in Samoa and other Pacific islands. The Lancet Infect Dis. 2020 Mar;20(3):273-275. doi.org/10.1016/S1473-3099(20)30053-0

Dudley MZ, Halsey NA, Omer SB, et al. The state of vaccine safety science: systematic reviews of the evidence. Lancet Infect Dis. 2020 May 1;20(5):e80-89.

Hanif W, Ali SN, Patel K, et al. Cultural competence in covid-19 vaccine rollout. BMJ. 2020;371:m4845. doi.org/10.1136/bmj.m4845

Hervé C, Laupèze B, Del Giudice G, et al. The how's and what's of vaccine reactogenicity. NPJ Vaccines. 2019 Sep;4(1):39.

Iwasaki A, Omer SB. Why and how vaccines work. Cell. 2020;183(2):290-295.

Juan J, Gil M, Rong M, et al. Effect of coronavirus disease 2019 (COVID-19) on maternal, perinatal and neonatal outcome: systematic review. Ultrasound Obstet Gynecol. 2020;56(1): 15-27. doi.org/10.1002/uog.22088

Liang H, Acharya G. Novel corona virus disease (COVID-19) in pregnancy: what clinical recommendations to follow? Acta Obstetricia et Gynecologica Scandinavica. 2020; 99(4), 439-442. doi.org/10.1111/aogs.13836

Mutua DN, Njagi ENM, Orinda GO. Hematological profile of normal pregnant women. J Blood Lymph. 2018;8:220. doi:10.4172/2165-7831.1000220

Paget J, Spreeuwenberg P, Charu V, et al. Global mortality associated with seasonal influenza epidemics: new burden estimates and predictors from the GLaMOR Project. J Global Health. 2019;9(2):020421-020421.

Polack FP, Thomas SJ, Kitchin N, et al. Safety and efficacy of the BNT162b2 mRNA Covid-19 vaccine. N Engl J Med. 2020;383(27):2603-2615.

Puri N, Coomes EA, Haghbayan H, Gunaratne K. Social media and vaccine hesitancy: new updates for the era of COVID-19 and globalized infectious diseases. Hum Vaccin Immunother. 2020 Nov;16(11):2586-2593. doi.org/10.1080/21645515.2020.1780846

Riley LE. mRNA Covid-19 vaccines in pregnant women. N Engl J Med. 2021;384(24):2342-2343. doi.org/10.1056/nejme2107070

Rocca Cl, Carbone F, Longobard S, Matarese, G. The immunology of pregnancy: regulatory T cells control maternal immune tolerance toward the fetus. Immunol Lett. 2014;162(1):41-48. doi.org/10.1016/j.imlet.2014.06.013

Sadarangani M, Soe P, Shulha HP, et al. Safety of COVID-19 vaccines in pregnancy: a Canadian National Vaccine Safety (CANVAS) network cohort study. Lancet. 2022 Nov;22(11): 1553-1564. doi.org/10.1016/S1473-3099(22)00426-1

Sahin U, Muik A, Derhovanessian E, et al. COVID-19 vaccine BNT162b1 elicits human antibody and TH1 T cell responses. Nature. 2020;586(7830):594-599.

Shimabukuro T, Kim T, Myers SY, et al. Preliminary findings of mRNA Covid-19 vaccine safety in pregnant persons. N Engl J Med. 2021 Jun 17;384(24):2273-2282. doi:10.1056/NEJMoa2104983

Skirrow H, Barnett S, Bell S, et al. Women's views on accepting COVID-19 vaccination during and after pregnancy, and for their babies: a multi-methods study in the UK. BMC Pregnancy and Childbirth. 2022;22(1). doi.org/10.1186/s12884-021-04321-3

Talbot HK, Nian H, Zhu Y, et al. Clinical effectiveness of split-virion versus subunit trivalent influenza vaccines in older adults. Clin Infect Dis. 2015;60(8):1170-1175.

World Health Organization. Ten threats to global health, 2019. https://www.who.int/news-room/spotlight/ten-threats-to-global-health-in-2019

World Health Organization. Vaccines and immunization, 2024. https://www.who.int/health-topics/vaccines-and-immunization#tab=tab_1

ONLINE RESOURCES

Australian Government. Covid 19 vaccination decision guide for women who are pregnant, breastfeeding or planning pregnancy, 2023: https://www.health.gov.au/sites/default/files/2023-06/covid-19-vaccination-shared-decision-making-guide-for-women-who-are-pregnant-breastfeeding-or-planning-pregnancy.pdf https://www.health.gov.au/sites/default/files/2023-06/covid-19-vaccination-shared-decision-making-guide-for-women-who-are-pregnant-breastfeeding-or-planning-pregnancy.pdf (accessed 22 August 2023)

Australian Immunisation Handbook: https://immunisationhandbook.health.gov.au/ (accessed 22 August 2023)

Australian Immunisation Register for health professionals: https://www.servicesaustralia.gov.au/australian-immunisation-register-for-health-professionals (accessed 22 August 2023)

National Centre for Immunisation Research and Surveillance (NCIRS): https://www.ncirs.org.au/health-professionals (accessed 22 August 2023)

National Immunisation Program Schedule: https://www.health.gov.au/health-topics/immunisation/when-to-get-vaccinated/national-immunisation-program-schedule (accessed 22 August 2023)

New Zealand Ministry of Health: New Zealand Immunisation Schedule, March 2023: https://www.health.govt.nz/our-work/preventative-health-wellness/immunisation/new-zealand-immunisation-schedule (accessed 22 August 2023)

NSW Health immunisation programs: https://www.health.nsw.gov.au/immunisation/Pages/default.aspx (accessed 22 August 2023)

World Health Organization – Vaccines and immunisation: https://www.who.int/health-topics/vaccines-and-immunization (accessed 22 August 2023)

—CHAPTER 12—

INFECTION AND SEPSIS – MATERNAL AND NEONATAL

Michelle Gray, Roslyn Donnellan-Fernandez

Key Abbreviations

CMV	cytomegalovirus
E coli	Escherichia coli
GAS	group A beta-haemolytic streptococcus
GBS	group B streptococcus
HIV	human immunodeficiency virus
HSV	herpes simplex virus
IVAB	intravenous antibiotics
MMR	measles mumps rubella
PPROM	preterm premature rupture of membranes
PROM	premature rupture of membranes
STDs	sexually transmitted diseases
UTI	urinary tract infection

Key Terms

antimicrobial 244
antibacterial 244
anti-infectives 234
antiviral 243
bacteriostatic 244
chlamydia 240
colonisation 236
concentrations 246
flora 237
gonorrhoea 241
half-life 245
microbes 236
microbiome 248
microorganisms 248
pathogens 235
sepsis (sometimes referred to as septicaemia) 236
susceptible 235
syphilis 240
varicella 240

Chapter Focus

This chapter focuses on the pharmacological treatments used to treat infection during pregnancy, childbirth, the puerperium and in the neonate. The aetiology of local and systemic infections common during the childbearing period is considered. Immunological response is covered in Chapter 11. Infection during pregnancy must be treated promptly to prevent serious complications for the mother and infant that could lead to sepsis and other adverse outcomes. This chapter identifies the role of the midwife in assessing signs and symptoms that necessitate investigation, assessment, and treatment of infection. Contemporary pharmacological treatments commonly recommended as safe for use during pregnancy are explained.

Key Drug Groups

Antibacterials:
- aminoglycosides
- beta-lactam antibiotics; cephalosporins
- topical antibiotics
- macrolides
- nitrofurantoin
- trimethoprim
- metronidazole

Anti-infectives:
- penicillins; amoxicillin

- cefalexin

Anti-mycobacterials:
- rifampicin
- isoniazid

Antivirals:
- acyclovir
- valacyclovir

Learning Outcomes

- Understand the aetiology of infection during pregnancy, birth, puerperium, and infection in the infant.
- Recognise the signs and symptoms of infection and the potential impact on pregnancy outcomes.
- Describe the six causes of infection and how to reduce their incidence.
- Discuss methods of screening and diagnosis of infection type to ensure correct treatment including the role of the midwife in antibiotic stewardship to prevent antibiotic resistance.
- Determine appropriate pharmacological treatment approaches and apply these.
- Understand the midwife's scope of practice and responsibility for timely consultation and referral when required.

CRITICAL THINKING SCENARIOS

Mother

Melinda attends the clinic for her antenatal appointment at 28 weeks. It is a hot day outside, at 32°C. Melinda is G1P0, rhesus positive. She appears hot and sweaty. Melinda reports that she has been experiencing flu-like symptoms for 2 weeks now and has not taken any medication to resolve her symptoms of snuffiness, lethargy, aches, and pains. She states she has increased her daily fluid intake, which includes warm lemon and honey drinks. She has also been ingesting up to five cloves of raw garlic per day and several 'extra' vitamin C tablets to 'boost' her natural immune response but now worries that these measures may not be sufficient. Her blood pressure is 130/70, pulse is 98 bpm and respirations are 20. On abdominal palpation her fundal height equals the expected height and equates to her gestational dates. The fetal heart rate is heard at 145 bpm.

1 What potential infections may she be suffering from based on her symptoms?

2 What are your next actions to assess for further objective data, including relevant history?

3 What is the latest guidance on over-the-counter self-medications for flu-like symptoms during pregnancy?

4 What advice should the midwife offer Melinda based on the symptoms presented?

Infant

Baby Jaydon is 7 days old. He has a yellow sticky discharge oozing from his left eye, which is only partially open.

5 What investigation will you perform to determine any bacterial cause of the infection?

6 What are the potential causes of the infection, and which of these is the most likely?

7 What is the preferred choice of immediate treatment while you wait for the microscopy result?

8 Jaydon's mother questions you regarding the evidence base for direct application of breast milk into his sticky eye, as her own mother, a midwife, has advised this will effectively resolve the problem without a need to resort to the use of pharmaceuticals. What is your response?

Introduction

Normal flora and external and internal defences protect the body from invasive microbes. The skin is the largest organ and the first barrier when healthy and intact. The skin barrier provides protection against bacterial microbes, fungi, and viruses. Secondary defences include cellular and chemical barriers that protect the ports of entry to the body.

Possible entry ports for infection include orifices such as the ear, nose, and throat, whose ports of entry are protected by fine cilia hair and secretions, which form a physical and chemical barrier. For example, the nasal passages contain nasal hairs and secretions to trap foreign bodies from being inhaled into the respiratory system. The gastrointestinal tract is protected by gastric acid which can destroy bacteria in food and render it harmless. However, during pregnancy women are susceptible to food-borne **pathogens** such as salmonella and listeriosis, the latter of which can result in miscarriage, premature birth, and stillbirth. This example illustrates the serious potential adverse consequences of infective processes, not all of which respond to pharmaceutical

treatment. The midwife's role in education – as well as in the early detection, assessment, investigation, and implementation of pharmacological management where appropriate – is critical.

12.1 Aetiology of infection

Significant systemic immunological adaptation occurs during a healthy pregnancy. The immunological response to the invasion of bacteria and the subsequent creation of antibodies is covered in Chapter 11. Despite a plethora of scientific literature on this topic, a clear understanding of how these changes modulate the risk of infection is lacking (Abu-Raya et al 2020). Pregnancy is a period where a woman may be more **susceptible** to a variety of infections, which has implications both for her and her unborn baby. Sepsis, the body's extreme response to an infection, is a medical emergency, with heightened morbidity and mortality for both infant and mother (CFB 12.1). While prudent use of pharmacological drugs in treating infection in childbearing women and babies is essential and can be lifesaving, in 2021 sepsis continued to comprise one of the leading causes of maternal mortality in Australia (11%) and New Zealand (5%) (AIHW 2023).

Where **microbes** successfully breach the external body barriers, an immunological response to infection results in a cascade of swelling to reduce the mobility of the microbes and limit their ability to spread further. A rise in temperature affects the optimal environment, preventing cell division and thus inhibiting the ability of the microbes to multiply. Deterioration of the invasive pathogen renders it inactive while leucocytes (macrophages and lymphocytes) clean up the debris and microbes (Justiz-Vaillant et al 2022).

Physiological and anatomical changes during pregnancy, birth, and the puerperium can exacerbate the risk of contracting an infection, and then cause challenges for optimum healing. During pregnancy women are more susceptible to urinary tract infections (UTI) due to structural changes in the ureters. The impact of hormones such as progesterone and relaxin mean that the ureters can distort and kink, leading to urine being trapped. Stagnant urine that is not able to drain from the obstruction caused by the occlusion can result in the trapped urine becoming a medium for bacterial growth. The link between recurrent UTI in pregnancy and premature labour and birth is well established, and although evidence for optimal pharmacological management remains limited (Schneeberger et al 2015), 25–30% of pregnant women with asymptomatic bacteriuria will develop a symptomatic UTI, including pyelonephritis with risk reduction of 70–80% if the bacteriuria is eradicated (see Online resources: Therapeutic Guidelines).

The single biggest risk factor for postpartum maternal infection is caesarean section. Medical interventions experienced during childbirth involving abdominal surgeries, such as emergency and elective caesarean section surgery, create wound sites that pose specific additional risks for infective process, even where evidence-based prophylactic antibiotic therapy is routinely practised as part of these procedures (Smaill & Grivell 2014). Following vaginal birth, perineal trauma within the vulva and perineum also presents a challenging site for optimum healing as the warm moist area is the perfect site for bacterial growth. During the postnatal period, vascular engorgement can increase intracellular pressure within breast tissue structures leading to mastitis, as can secondary infection through **colonisation** of the organisms *Pasteurella haemolytica* and *Staphylococcus aureus* (Blackmon et al 2024). Methicillin-resistant *S. aureus* (MRSA) has become an increasingly frequent cause of mastitis (see Chapters 9 and 10), highlighting the importance of antibiotic stewardship for all health professionals (see Online resources: National Centre for Antimicrobial Stewardship).

CLINICAL FOCUS BOX 12.1

Sepsis

Sepsis is the escalation of an infection that overpowers the body's defences and attacks the body systems. Most viral infections resolve themselves as the body's own defence system fights the virus. However, sepsis which develops from an infection such as a sore throat, vomiting and diarrhoea, pneumonia or a UTI progresses to a multi-organ dysfunction. Group A beta-haemolytic streptococcus (GAS) infection is the most common cause of sepsis (Bowyer et al 2017). Thirty percent of people who get sepsis do not survive (Sepsis Alliance 2022), with 25% of maternal deaths in Australia caused by sepsis. Sepsis is a major cause of mortality among Aboriginal and Torres Strait Islander peoples (ACSQHC 2024). (See Online resources: ACSQHC, National Sepsis Program).

Signs and symptoms can initially be nondescript, presenting with vague fever. Early detection is essential in achieving a favourable outcome. Deterioration can be rapid, and one assessment tool that has been reported as useful in screening and diagnosing sepsis is the obstetrically modified qSOFA (quick Sequential [sepsis related] Organ Failure Assessment score) tool.

Identification of sepsis should occur as soon as possible. The woman should be transferred to a high dependency facility where she can receive intensive care from a multi-disciplinary team. Treatment involves taking samples from potential sources of infection; throat, vaginal, wound swabs, and blood cultures for pathology; however, treatment should not be delayed for the results. Instead, a combination of broad spectrum antibiotics should be commenced immediately. Figure 12.1 illustrates the SOMANZ recommendations for management of sepsis. The first-line investigations recommended for sepsis are shown in Table 12.1.

KEY POINTS

Aetiology of infection in pregnancy

- Pregnancy is a period during which a woman may be more susceptible to infections due to changes in the immune system response.
- Physiological and anatomical changes during pregnancy, birth and the puerperium can increase the likelihood of contracting an infection, and then cause challenges for optimum healing.

12.2 Pathogens

There are six main types of microorganisms: bacteria, viruses, fungi, parasites, protozoa, and algae. The last three are not common in Australia (Gordon et al 2012).

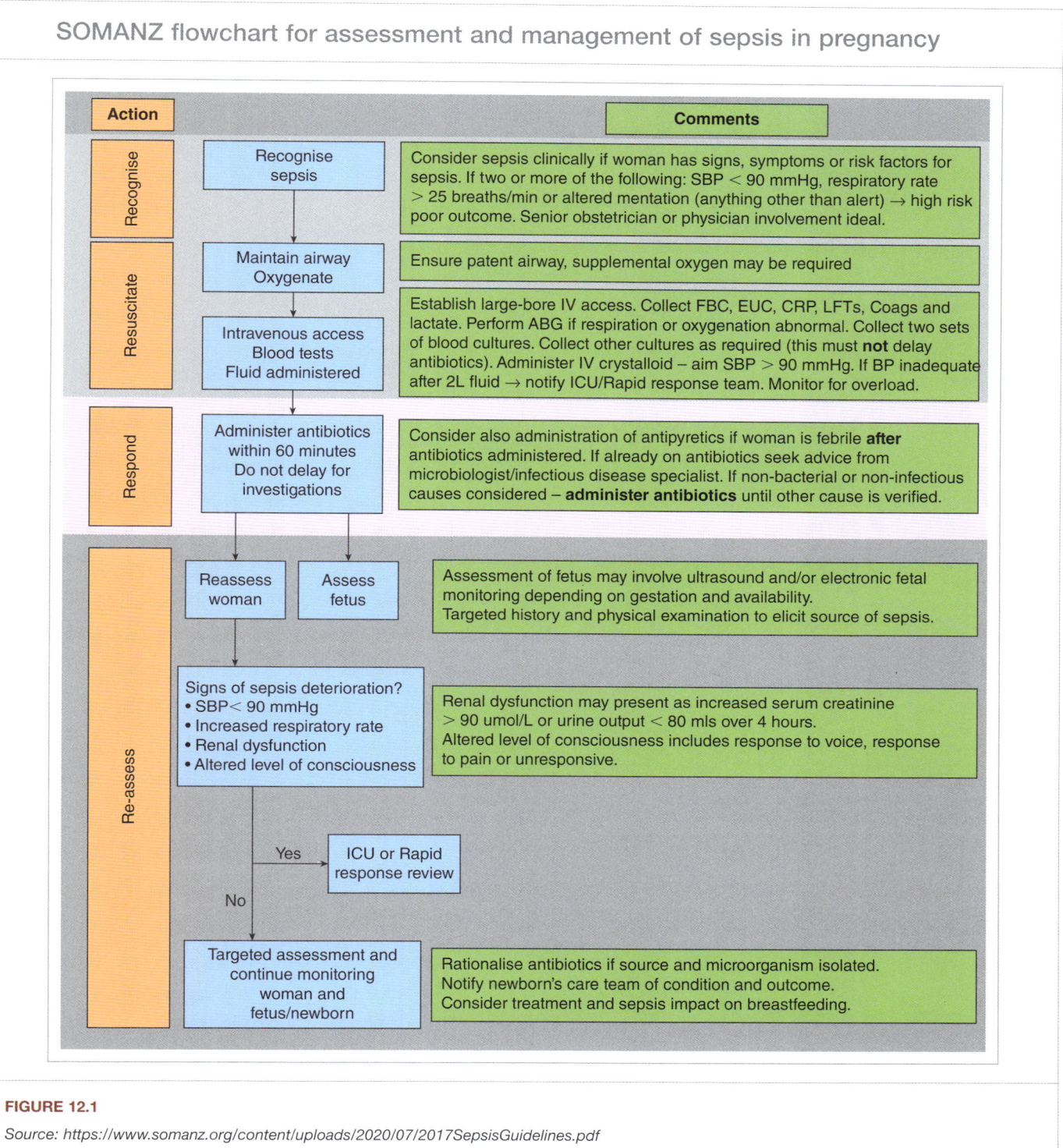

SOMANZ flowchart for assessment and management of sepsis in pregnancy

FIGURE 12.1

Source: https://www.somanz.org/content/uploads/2020/07/2017SepsisGuidelines.pdf

Bacteria

Bacteria are relatively small and usually harmless to humans. Healthy bacteria exist in the body and assist in digestion and maintaining gut **flora**. They also assist in fighting cancer and infection from bad bacteria within the mucous membranes and secretions, as well as in the eyes, mouth and nose. However, bacteria have been known to be resistant and exist outside the human body for long periods. 'Fossilized records show that bacteria have existed for about 3.5 billion years, and bacteria can survive in different environments, including extreme heat and cold, radioactive waste, and the human body' (Ansorge 2021, NP)

TABLE 12.1 First-line investigations recommended for suspected sepsis

INVESTIGATION[2–5]	RESULTS IN NON-OBSTETRIC SEPSIS[2–5]	OBSTETRIC REFERENCE RANGE (if relevant)[1]
Blood cultures • At least two sets, prior to antibiotic commencement as long as there is no delay. Obtain samples from different sites Cultures should also be obtained from IV access devices	May be positive for organism	
Other cultures • Obtain cultures of additional sites as clinically indicated and as soon as possible E.g. urine MCS, wound swab – episiotomy, caesarean, placental swabs, amniotic fluid, sputum MCS, naso-pharyngeal aspirate/swab, cerebrospinal fluid, vaginal swabs, stool culture	May be positive for organism	
Arterial blood gases • detect acidosis, hypoxaemia, lactate as below		PaO_2: 1st trimester: 93–100 mmHg 2nd trimester: 90–98mmHg 3rd trimester: 92–107mmHg $PaCO_2$: 25–33mmHg, Arterial pH: 7.4–7.47 HCO3 16–22mmol/L
Lactate • elevated levels in sepsis relate to tissue hypoperfusion and are associated with an increased sepsis mortality risk	$\geq$ 2 mmol/L associated with increased mortality	0.6–1.8 mmol/L
Full blood count	WCC > 12 ×109/L or < 4 x 10^9/L Normal WCC count with > 10% immature forms Thrombocytopenia is a severe sign of sepsis (platelet count < 100 x 10^9/L indicates organ dysfunction)	WCC 6–17 × 10^9/L WCC in hours post-delivery between 9–15 × 10^9 (steroids also increase WCC) Platelets – lower limit of normal 150–420 x 10^9/L
Coagulation studies	May be abnormal in sepsis with INR > 1.5, APTT > 60 secs and indicating organ dysfunction	No change
Creatinine urea and electrolytes Measure at baseline and until the patient improves Elevated creatinine is a sign of severe sepsis Abnormal electrolytes and elevated urea may be seen in sepsis	Sepsis is severe if[6]: Creatinine > 120 µmol/L (presuming premorbid baseline renal function was normal)	Creatinine varies with gestation (reference ranges): 1st trimester 35–62 µmol/L 2nd trimester 35–71 µmol/L 3rd trimester 35–80 µmol/L
Liver function tests Baseline test May be elevated if sepsis source is from hepatic or perihepatic infections May be elevated due to septic shock affecting hepatic blood flow and metabolism	Plasma total bilirubin > 70 µmol/L indicates organ dysfunction	AST 3–33 U/L ALT 2–33 U/L Alkaline phosphatase 17–229 U/L GGT 2–26 U/L Total bilirubin 1.7–19 µmol/L
CXR	May show evidence of infection such as consolidation or pleural effusion	May show evidence of infection such as consolidation or pleural effusion. Diaphragm elevation may be distorted by fundus, cardiac axis rotated in pregnancy
Fetal assessment – CTG and/or fetal ultrasound		A non-reassuring CTG suggests inadequate uteroplacental perfusion and may reflect maternal organ hypoperfusion

1. Abbassi-Ghanavati M, Cunningham FG. Pregnancy and laboratory studies: a reference table for clinicians. Obstet Gynecol. 2009;114:1326–1331.
2. RCOG Royal College of Obstetrics and Gynecology. Bacterial sepsis following pregnancy. Green-top guideline. 2012:64b.
3. RCOG Royal College of Obstetrics and Gynecology. Bacterial sepsis in pregnancy. Green-top guideline. 2013:64a.
4. Ford JM, Scholefield H. Sepsis in obstetrics: cause, prevention, and treatment. Curr Opin Anaesthesiol. 2014;27:253–258.
5. Dellinger RP LM, Rhodes A, Annane D, et al. Surviving sepsis campaign: international guidelines for management of severe sepsis and septic shock: 2012. Crit Care Med. 2013;41:580–637.
5. Rivers E NB, Havstad S, Ressler J, et al. Early goal-directed therapy in the treatment of severe sepsis and septic shock. N Engl J Med. 2001;345:1368–1377.
Source: Bowyer L, Robinson H, Barrett H, Crozier T, Giles M, Idel I, Lowe S, Lust K, Marnoch C, Morton M, Said J, Wong M and Makris A. SOMANZ Guidelines for sepsis in pregnancy, 2017. Society of Obstetric Medicine Australia and New Zealand.

The presence of good bacteria can revert from protecting the body to infecting the body if bacteria is relocated to different parts of the body. For instance, if bacteria from faeces is transported on hands after using the toilet to the mouth or an open wound, this could cause the growth of microorganisms that then cause infection in the new location. During pregnancy and infancy bacteria can be harmful due to these immunosuppressed states and can cause severe illness and even death through sepsis.

Bacteria can take many forms. They can be mobile or non-mobile and aerobic or non-aerobic. The shape and mobility of bacteria aids in the identification of infection under the microscope. Staining of bacteria that has been collected and smeared onto a glass microscope slide can determine if bacteria is gram-negative or gram-positive. This information helps determine antibiotic selection.

Viruses

Viruses are the smallest and most common pathogen. They are tinier than bacteria; the largest virus is smaller than the smallest bacteria. Viruses are prevalent in the community but are surprisingly weak and easy to kill. Viruses cannot survive outside the human body and are easily destroyed through hand washing with hot soapy water (Fig 12.2).

All viruses have a protein coat and a core of genetic material: either ribonucleic acid (RNA) or deoxyribonucleic acid (DNA). Viruses reprogram the cell's DNA or RNA to replicate themselves to make new viruses. During multiplication the original host cell swells, bursts and then dies. Viruses are responsible for changing normal cells into malignant or cancerous cells. Unlike bacteria, most viruses do not cause disease. Viruses are specific about which cells they attack: the liver, respiratory system, or blood. In some cases, viruses target bacteria.

Fungi

Fungi is the largest microorganism, and diseases caused by fungi are called myoses (Gordon et al 2012). Fungal skin infections are the most common infections in humans, affecting more than 20–25% of the world's population and can be classified as superficial, cutaneous, or subcutaneous mycoses (Patel et al 2021). Fungi are part of the normal flora of the body and only cause problems when the individual is susceptible to infection, such as during pregnancy. For example, *Candida albicans* is part of the normal body flora; however, changes in skin integrity, friction, moisture, or the use of antibiotics can result in pH changes which can destroy normal flora and increase fungal growth in skin folds, the genitalia, mouth, or nipple and breast tissues.

Listeriosis is contracted by eating contaminated food such as soft cheeses and some ice cream. During the first trimester listeriosis can cause miscarriage, premature birth, and stillbirth.

Parasites

A parasite is an organism that lives on a host and relies on the host for nutrition. There are three types of parasites

Hand Hygiene Australia:
5 Moments for Hand Hygiene

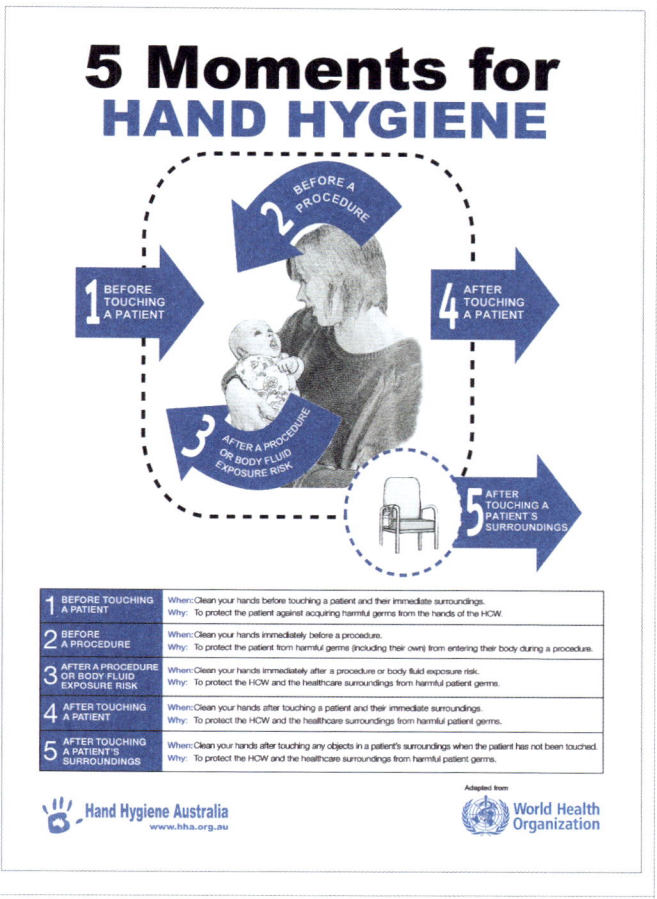

FIGURE 12.2

Source: 5 Moments for Hand Hygiene, Hand Hygiene Australia (HHA). Retrieved from: https://www.hha.org.au/component/jdownloads/send/34-posters/72-poster7.

found in humans: protozoa, helminths, and ectoparasites (CDC 2022):

- *Protozoa* – These are one-cell organisms invisible to the naked eye. Protozoa that live in the blood or tissue of humans are transmitted to other humans through the bite of a mosquito or sand fly. These organisms are also transmitted through the faecal–oral route from contaminated water or food. Ho (2019) of Western Sydney University wrote that, 'protozoa giardia has a two-stage life cycle. In the first stage, called trophozoite, the parasite swims around and consumes nutrients from the small bowel. In the second stage it develops into a non-moving cyst. Cysts excreted in faeces can contaminate the water supply and ingesting contaminated food or water results in transmission. Close human-to-human contact and unsanitary living conditions can promote transmission. Symptoms of giardia can include severe or chronic diarrhoea, abdominal cramps, fatigue, weakness and weight loss' (NP). Once diagnosed through a stool specimen, treatment should be initiated quickly during pregnancy as prolonged diarrhoea can cause premature labour.

- *Helminths* – There are several types of intestinal worms. The most common include tapeworm and roundworms. These are normally visible to the naked eye within the stool sample. They can live in the intestines for a long time and can be parasitic in nature or free living. Diagnosis is through stool samples.
- *Ectoparasites* – This term is used to cover ticks, fleas, scabies, and head lice. Ectoparasites burrow or attach to the skin and source nutrition from their host (Ho 2019). Infestations of scabies and head lice are more likely in highly populated living conditions where close contact is a perfect transmission environment. Scabies is characterised by the itchy raised red spots on the skin. Scabies is very contagious, and bedding, towels and clothing should not be shared until treatment is completed. Head lice attach to the shaft of the hair. Unable to fly they are transferred on shared hairbrushes or by head-to-head contact.

Algae

Some blue green algae (cyanobacteria) can cause illness in humans. Toxins from blue green algae can cause sickness such as nausea and vomiting, diarrhoea, skin, eye and throat irritation, allergic reactions, and breathing difficulties. Pregnant women should be cautioned against eating shellfish and crustaceans from recreational waters. Contaminated products with toxins can also be transferred to an infant during pregnancy or through breast milk.

KEY POINTS

Pathogens

- There are six main types of microorganisms: bacteria, viruses, fungi, parasites, protozoa, and algae.
- Viruses cannot survive outside the human body and are easily destroyed through hand washing with hot soapy water.

12.3 Infections during pregnancy

Pregnancy is a state of increased immunosuppression, thus women are susceptible to contracting infections which they would normally fight off. Some of the different types of bacteria that cause a potential risk during pregnancy include **syphilis**, gastro, **chlamydia**,

conjunctivitis, parvovirus, **varicella**, urogenital infections, chorionic amnionitis, and candida. Listed below are the most common occurring bacterial infections contracted during pregnancy.

Note that bacterial and viral infections are dissimilar in many ways due to their size, shape and structure, and in other important aspects, for instance most of them respond to medications in different ways.

Bacterial infection

Asymptomatic bacteria

Asymptomatic bacterial infection occurs in about 10% of the population, and thus all pregnant women are recommended to have a mid-stream specimen of urine sent for bacterial examination. Approximately 25–30% of pregnant women will experience a UTI which increases their risk of premature labour, premature rupture of membranes and if left untreated, pyelonephritis.

A result of greater than 108 CFU/L contamination of bacteria in a urine sample requires treatment to prevent cystitis, pyelonephritis, premature labour, and birth. The identified bacterial growth should be treated with the appropriate treatment for at least 5 days minimum and then followed, post-treatment, by repeated urine analysis 48 hours after completion of the antibacterial treatment (see Online resources: Therapeutic Guidelines). Due to the high possibility of reinfection a microscopy of the woman's urine sample should be repeated at each antenatal appointment.

Bacterial vaginosis

Bacterial infections of the vagina (such as bacterial vaginosis) can be asymptomatic, however lead to premature birth, low birth weight, or premature rupture of membranes (Giannella et al 2023). Routine screening is not recommended (see Online resources: Australian Pregnancy Care Guidelines). However, symptoms of increased vaginal discharge with a distinctive 'fishy smell' (Brocklehurst et al 2013) should be treated with antibiotics.

Chorioamnionitis (intra-amniotic infection)

Chorioamnionitis is a gestational infection in the membranes, amniotic fluid, placenta, or decidua that can be passed to the fetus in utero. Ascending infection through the cervicovaginal passage can involve one or many pathogens which can enter as the result of prolonged ruptured membranes.

Symptoms may initially be nondescript, but antenatal assessment will determine a fever, tachycardia, uterine tenderness, and possibly offensive liquor. Left untreated, chorioamnionitis can cause premature birth with morbidity and mortality, and in the mother, endometritis. A small number of babies can develop sepsis following birth. Risk factors for neonatal sepsis include maternal history of invasive group B strep with previous baby, current group B strep, PROM and PPROM > 18 hours in preterm birth.

Endometritis

Endometritis is an inflammation of the endometrial lining and may involve the myometrium. Suspected chorioamnionitis can be confirmed by a maternal fever over 38 degrees. The mother needs treatment with intravenous antibiotics for confirmed or suspected bacterial infection in labour, or 24 hours prior to or after birth. Postpartum endometrial infection has been reported to be polymicrobial, involving both aerobic and anaerobic bacteria (Taylor et al 2024), including:

- *Gram-positive cocci:* groups A and B Streptococci, Staphylococcus, Enterococcus
- *Gram-negative bacilli:* Escherichia coli, Klebsiella pneumoniae, Proteus
- *Anaerobic organisms:* Bacteroides, Peptostreptococcus, Peptococcus, Prevotella, and Clostridium.

Group B streptococcal (GBS)

Group B streptococcal is a beta-haemolytic gram-positive aerobic coccobacillus bacterium which is usually found in the urethra or vagina in the genital tract, or in the gastrointestinal tract. The symptoms can be diverse between adults and infants. For instance, approximately 35% of women carry the bacteria with no adverse effects; however, for people with existing co-morbidities such as diabetes the consequences can include serious illnesses such as meningitis.

During pregnancy, GBS can be detected on a urine culture; heavy growth is indicative of GBS colonisation of the vagina. Women will also be offered screening towards the end of pregnancy (around 36 weeks) to determine if GBS is detected prior to birth. Transplacental or vertical transmission to the infant is a risk, with over half of neonatal infections attributed to GBS.

Intrapartum antibiotic prophylaxis can provide some protection to women who are confirmed to have a GBS positive screening result. GBS infection has been found to occur early – after birth or later. Antibiotics reduce the incidence of early onset sepsis but do not prevent late onset GBS that can occur for up to 6 weeks.

With newborns, there is early onset and late onset GBS disease:

- *Early onset* – The infection (meningitis, sepsis, pneumonia) begins within 7 days of birth. Exposure to GBS in the birth canal or other contact with the birthing parent in delivery is usually the cause.
- *Late onset* – The infection, which is typically meningitis, begins a week to a few months after birth. Exposure to GBS from the mother or any other person who carries it can cause late onset GBS infection. (See Online resources: Healthline, Meningitis.)

Escherichia coli (E coli)

Escherichia coli bacteria live in the intestines of healthy people and assist with good gut flora and digestion. However, certain strains ingested through dirty water, unwashed fruit and vegetables or contaminated soil can cause serious illness in those who have a lowered immunological response or are susceptible to the development of complications.

Listeriosis

Listeriosis is a bacterial infection contracted from eating soft cheeses, pate, and unpasteurised milk, ice cream or yoghurt. Maternal ingestion of bacteria from food then causes placentitis, meconium before 34 weeks gestation, and increases the chance of miscarriage, stillbirth, or preterm labour. Listeriosis can be transmitted from mother to child transplacentally or perinatally.

Newborns may be born with listeriosis and be extremely unwell. The American College of Obstetricians and Gynaecologists reports that listeriosis can cause lifelong health problems for the infant, including intellectual disability, paralysis, seizures, blindness, or problems with the brain, kidneys, or heart (see Online resources: ACOG, Listeria and pregnancy). However, symptoms may be delayed until after the first week after birth. Listeriosis has a high morbidity and mortality rate in newborns.

Bacterial sexually transmitted diseases (STDs)

STDs can lead to premature labour and premature birth. **Gonorrhoea** and chlamydia can both cause conjunctivitis. Genital herpes can be transmitted to the baby during vaginal delivery.

Chlamydia trachomatis

The incidence of chlamydia is prevalent, thus all young women under the age of 30 years are recommended to be screened in the first trimester if living in a high incidence area (see Online resources: STI Guidelines Australia).

Chlamydia is contracted from genital contact and if caught during pregnancy, and not treated, can cause intrauterine growth retardation and premature birth (Rours et al 2011). The possible long-term impacts of chlamydia for the woman include infertility, pelvic inflammatory disease, ectopic pregnancy, and pelvic pain.

If the infection is active at the time of birth it can cause eye infections or pneumonia in the infant. Antibiotic eye ointment can be used shortly after birth. This treatment can prevent blindness.

Syphilis

Syphilis is a sexually transmitted disease caused by *Treponema pallidum* (ACSQHC 2024). It is recommended that all women are screened for syphilis during their first prenatal visit. Women considered to be high risk should be screened again in the third trimester. Syphilis may pass from an infected mother to her fetus during pregnancy. The infection has been linked to congenital syphilis, preterm birth, stillbirth, and, in some cases, death shortly after birth (Homer 2022). Untreated infants who survive tend to develop problems in many organs, including the brain, eyes, ears, heart, skin, teeth, and bones. Syphilis can cause permanent impairment or disability. Penicillin is very effective in eradicating the disease.

Viral infection

Viral infections are caused by microorganisms that replicate themselves quickly after entering the body. Viruses do not survive outside the host's body as they need optimum conditions of warmth and moisture to multiply and spread. Examples of viruses include the common cold, flu, Ebola, COVID-19 and HIV.

Congenital cytomegalovirus (CMV)

CMV is part of the herpes family and is prevalent in young children's saliva and urine; therefore, women working in childcare centres with a likelihood of increased exposure are recommended to be tested early in their pregnancy (CDC 2020). It is highly infectious and is spread through saliva and during close contact, such as kissing or sharing of utensils. The host may not be aware they are a carrier of the infection. CMV may not present any symptoms or cause any health problems and can lie dormant in the body for years until a time of immunological susceptibility, such as pregnancy (Table 12.2).

During pregnancy the virus can cross the placenta causing congenital CMV infection in the fetus/neonate. CMV is particularly dangerous to the fetus as it can restrict growth, damage the fetus's liver and lead to deafness and brain damage. Researchers are searching for solutions to prevent the transmission of CMV during pregnancy, such as vaccinations, viral treatments (Esposito et al 2021).

An infant may be born asymptomatic. Current practice is that routine screening is not recommended. However, some infants have health problems such as hearing or vision loss, seizures, or intellectual disabilities

TABLE 12.2 Intrauterine viral transmission

VIRUS	MODE/RATE OF TRANSMISSION
Cytomegalovirus (CMV) – a member of the herpes virus family.	Prenatal infection affects 1–2% of live births. Virus replicates in the uterus, infects the placenta, and then is transmitted to the fetus. Transmission rate is approx. 50% in women with primary infection. It remains latent in the host after primary infection and may become active again, particularly during times of immune compromise.
Herpes simplex virus (HSV-2) – a virus causing painful sores of the anus or genitals that may lie dormant in nerve tissue. Not to be confused with HSV-1, a virus that causes cold sores.	Infrequent prenatal infection. Transmission occurs primarily at the time of birth (80%) and also possibly through an ascending infection after the membranes rupture.
Human immunodeficiency virus (HIV) – infection with HIV begins with an asymptomatic stage with gradual compromise of immune function, eventually leading to acquired immunodeficiency syndrome (AIDS).	Transmission primarily at the time of birth. Isolated cytotrophoblasts infected in vitro. (The most common way to diagnose HIV infection is by a test for antibodies against HIV-1 and HIV-2. HIV antibodies are detectable in at least 95% of patients within 3 months of infection.)
Hepatitis B virus (HBV) – a virus that affects the liver. It has an incubation period of 6 weeks to 6 months, and is excreted in various bodily fluids including blood, saliva, vaginal fluid and breast milk; these fluids may be highly infectious.	Transmission primarily perinatal. Some intrauterine infection from maternal blood (5%).
Hepatitis C virus (HCV) – a virus known to be one of the major causes of liver cirrhosis, hepatocellular carcinoma and liver failure; HCV is a major public health concern.	Intrauterine infection and at birth (2–12%).
Human parvovirus B19 – a viral infection transmitted from animals. Infection during pregnancy can result in fetal hydrops and death.	Placental infection associated with inflammatory cytokines. Complications in early gestation.
Rubella virus – the pathogenic agent of the disease rubella and the cause of congenital rubella syndrome when infection occurs during the first weeks of pregnancy. Humans are the only known host of this virus.	Placental infection during primary maternal infection. Transmission in first trimester (80%) and second trimester (25%).
Human papillomavirus (HPV) – a viral infection spread through skin-to-skin contact. HPV is a group of more than 100 different viruses. It causes genital warts and plays a causative role in cervical dysplasia and cervical cancer.	Infection via maternal genital secretions at birth.
Varicella zoster virus – a virus in the herpes family that causes chickenpox during childhood and may reactivate later in life to cause shingles in immunosuppressed individuals.	Congenital infection low (2%). Transmission during primary infection in late gestation (25–50%).

Source: Pereira K, Maidji E, McDonagh S, et al. Insights into viral transmission at the uterine-placental interface. Trends Microbiol. 2005;13(4):164-174.

that are apparent at birth or develop later during infancy or childhood. Congenital CMV infection can be diagnosed by testing a neonate's saliva, urine, or blood. Treatment with **antiviral** drugs may decrease the risk of health problems and hearing loss in some infected infants.

Human immunodeficiency virus (HIV)

'HIV is one of the few microorganisms that directly attacks the central processes involved in the development of an immune response' (Gordon et al 2012). HIV infection can be transmitted from mother to child transplacentally or perinatally. When the mother is not treated, the risk of transmission at birth is about 25–35% (see Online resources: CDC).

Rubella (German measles)

Healthcare providers recommend that women are vaccinated against rubella before they become pregnant because contracting rubella (sometimes called German measles) during pregnancy can cause problems with the pregnancy as well as birth defects in the infant. Rubella can cause inadequate growth before birth (small for gestational age), cataracts, birth defects of the heart, hearing loss or profound deafness, and delayed development. MMR vaccine is available for infants and adults.

Varicella (chickenpox)

Varicella, or chickenpox, is caused by the *Varicella zoster* virus. Chickenpox during pregnancy increases the risk of a miscarriage. It may damage the eyes of the fetus or cause defects of the limbs, blindness, or intellectual disability. The fetus's head may be smaller than normal (microcephaly).

Herpes simplex virus (HSV)

HSV-1, commonly referred to as cold sores, is characterised by sores and blisters around or in the mouth. It is very infectious. 'An estimated 3.7 billion people under age 50 (67%) globally have herpes simplex virus type 1 (HSV-1) infection, the main cause of oral herpes' (WHO 2023). HSV-1 can be passed to the genital area and cause HSV-2 genital herpes.

Herpes simplex virus types 1 and 2 can be transmitted to the fetus and neonate. Harris and Holmes (2017) estimate that 3000–20,000 live births are affected by HSV and state that transmission to the neonate can occur 'via four methods: delivery through infected genital tract, ascending HSV exposure through ruptured amniotic membranes, intrauterine HSV exposures, or postnatal exposure from an infected caregiver' but that 'intrauterine transmission is rare'.

Hepatitis B virus (HBV)

The initial infection of hepatitis is normally acute, with an incubation period of 6 weeks to 6 months. HBV is normally transmitted through body fluids as the virus is excreted in the urine, blood, saliva, vaginal secretions, and breast milk. It is recommended that all women are tested for HBV at the first antenatal visit. After infection, women can become carriers and pass the virus on to their fetus. It can also be transmitted from mother to baby during birth. Hepatitis in a pregnant woman can increase the risk of premature birth. Following the birth, immediate treatment can reduce the impact of transmission (see Chapter 11).

Zika virus

Mosquito bites are the main source in the transmission of Zika virus, but it can also be spread through direct genitalia contact. Although symptoms are usually mild, Zika infection during pregnancy can cause pregnancy loss and other pregnancy complications, as well as birth defects, facial distortion, microcephaly, hyperactivity, and severe irritability for the infant (Wheeler 2018). Diagnosis is with enzyme-linked immunosorbent assay or reverse transcriptase–polymerase chain reaction (RT-PCR). Treatment is supportive.

Hepatitis C

It is recommended that all women are screened for hepatitis C in early pregnancy. The hepatitis C virus can cause liver cirrhosis, liver failure and hepatocellular carcinoma (Homer 2022). There is no effective treatment to prevent transfer from mother to fetus; however, direct acting antiviral agents are recommended postnatally.

Parasitic infection

Protozoa

Common protozoan infectious diseases include malaria, giardia, and toxoplasmosis. As this chapter focuses on pregnancy, only toxoplasmosis is covered here. Toxoplasmosis is dangerous in pregnancy as the parasite can cross the placenta and infect the unborn baby.

Toxoplasmosis is a protozoal infection caused by the *Toxoplasma gondii* parasite. In humans, the disease is usually mild, and is often mistaken for a common cold; lifelong antibodies are produced. However, in pregnant women the parasite may pass to the fetus and cause complications such as serious birth defects including damage to the brain, liver and eyes, and preterm birth.

Toxoplasma gondii can infect any mammal or bird, and people across all continents are affected. Once infected, a person carries *Toxoplasma* for life. Globally, estimates are that 30–50% of people are infected with *Toxoplasma* – and infections may be increasing. In Australia, for instance, a survey of studies conducted at blood banks and pregnancy clinics across the country in the 1970s put the infection rate at 30%. However, a recent Western Australian community-based study found 66% of people were infected (Justine Smith and João Furtado Conversation 2022).

One source of exposure to *Toxoplasma gondii* infection is from cat faeces or used cat litter, as cats get the parasite from eating small animals or birds. Toxoplasmosis can also be contracted during pregnancy from the dirt on fruit and vegetables. Education should include warning pregnant women to avoid touching cat litter trays and gardening without gloves. All fruit and vegetables should be washed and thoroughly cooked before eating.

Helminths (worms)

Intestinal worms will not cause any significant harm to the woman or the fetus, and thus treatment can be delayed until the second trimester. However, treatment is highly recommended from the second trimester to reduce anaemia in the mother (Salam et al 2021) and low birth weight.

Pediculosis (lice)

There are three types of lice: head, body and pubic lice. The female lice can lay up to 300 eggs in their lifetime. Nits hatch in 7–10 days. Body lice infestations usually cause minimal problems; however, they can cause discomfort and embarrassment, sometimes leading to secondary infections due to skin irritation and inflammation if left untreated.

Scabies

Sarcoptes scabiei is a microscopic mite that is contracted from infected sources of clothing, bedding or towels. Highly infected areas include highly populated residences, such as childcare centres and aged care homes. Aboriginal and Torres Strait Islander peoples are a susceptible group and this can be exacerbated if close living conditions exist.

Crusted scabies (Norwegian scabies) is a contagious variant. This variant of scabies often occurs in immunosuppressed people who are unable to mount attack from the T-helper 2 cells.

KEY POINTS

Parasitic infections during pregnancy

- Parasites can occur during pregnancy and can be embarrassing to the woman.
- The midwife should be respectful and supportive in providing appropriate referral for treatment.

12.4 Treatments

Viral infections do not require antibiotic treatments. Instead, the body needs to be encouraged to fight the infection using its own defences. In cases where the infected person may be immunocompromised, **bacteriostatic** drugs can be prescribed as they hinder bacterial growth, giving the body a longer period to mobilise its own defences (Loree et al 2023).

Antimicrobials destroy or prevent the proliferation of microorganisms; however, antibiotics should only be used to treat bacterial infection (CFB 12.2). Other microbials include antivirals, antifungals and anti-mycobacterials. Bactericidal microbials destroy the organism (Hunter & Davis 2019).

Antibiotics have a specific scope of effectiveness. Antibiotics that treat a broad range of organisms are said to have a broad spectrum of activity. Broad spectrum antibiotics include amoxicillin, co-amoxiclav, ciprofloxacin, and doxycycline, and are used when there are several bacteria involved or when the bacteria is unknown and test results are awaited.

Narrow spectrum antibiotics include azithromycin, clarithromycin, erythromycin and clindamycin. Antibiotics with a narrow range of effectiveness are selected to treat and eradicate specific pathogens. They may treat gram-positive or gram-negative pathogens but not both.

CLINICAL FOCUS BOX 12.2

Antimicrobial resistance

When antimicrobial treatments lose their effectiveness against viruses, bacteria, parasites, and fungus infections, the options for treatment become limited. This increases the risk of morbidity in the general population and as a result, the overprescribing of antibiotics is a significant problem that is currently being addressed through national guidelines such as Antimicrobial Stewardship in Australian Healthcare (ACSQHC 2023).

Narrow spectrum beta-lactamase resistant penicillins are one example of how antibiotics can lose their ability to destroy bacteria. Where antibiotic resistance was becoming problematic, the solution has been to extend the spectrum of penicillin using a beta-lactamase inhibitor. The addition of clavulanic acid or tazobactam makes the following antibiotics effective against otherwise resistant strains of *S. aureus*: amoxicillin/clavulanic acid; piperacillin/tazobactran; and ticarcillin/clavulanic acid. The addition of beta-lactamase inhibitor binds to the beta-lactamase, enabling the active penicillin to work. Piperacillin and ticarcillin have the widest range of action against gram-negative organisms (Brant et al 2015).

Antibacterial medications

Antimicrobial medications include antiviral, antifungal, and anti-mycobacterial treatments. It is important to avoid giving **antibacterial** treatments to pregnant women unless there is strong evidence of a bacterial infection. Use of any antibacterial during pregnancy should be based on whether benefits outweigh risk, which varies by trimester (NICE Guidelines 2017). Severity of the infection and other options for treatment are also considered. Aminoglycosides may be used during pregnancy to treat pyelonephritis and chorioamnionitis, but treatment should be carefully monitored to avoid maternal or fetal damage. This is because these medications all readily cross the placenta, although the mechanisms for transport for some medications are not always known.

Adverse reactions

Adverse reactions to antibiotics can range from a mild rash, diarrhoea, or nausea to a fever and anaphylaxis (see Chapter 6). Any reaction to medication should be recorded in detail as there is a marked difference between sensitivity and adverse anaphylaxis. Documentation that includes a thorough health history and medication review with specific details of a previous reaction to the medication is critical to differentiate severity of response. In cases of sensitivity medications should be discontinued. Approximately 10% of people are allergic to penicillin and 7% of these also have reactions to other antibiotics (Devchand & Trubiano 2019).

Penicillins G and V

Penicillins are grouped as benzyl penicillins (Pen G [IV]) or phenoxymethylpenicillin (Pen V [oral]). Although penicillins are generally considered safe during pregnancy they are prescribed selectively, as penicillin crosses the placenta and is found in breast milk. Penicillin binds to plasma proteins, and is partially metabolised to its inactive metabolites in the kidneys. Due to increased clearance rates during pregnancy, doses need to be high to extend the **half-life** – alternatively, the medication can be administered more frequently. Two examples of prophylactic use of penicillin are in women with group B streptococcus or a history of cardiac conditions (Hunter & Davis 2019).

Drug types include ampicillin, amoxicillin and ticarcillin (only 16% of the drug is metabolised; the majority is eliminated via the kidneys) (Momper & Brooke 2022). Thus, IV amoxicillin studies recommend a 2 gram dose during labour and preterm rupture of membranes; followed by 1 gram every 4 hours.

Amoxicillin 500 mg every 8 hours is suitable for asymptomatic bacteria urea when determined from a culture result. Fifty percent of E. coli bacteria are resistant to amoxicillin.

Beta-lactam group antibiotics

Beta-lactam group antibiotics are a group of antibiotics with a molecular structure that contains a ring-like band of beta-lactam. Some bacteria have developed the ability to break this ring down using an enzyme called beta-lactamase, resulting in antibiotic resistance. The group of beta-lactam antibiotics includes penicillins, cephalosporins, monobactams, carbapenems, and beta-lactamase inhibitors.

Flucloxacillin (beta-lactamase resistant antibiotic) is useful for treating S. aureus. Flucloxacillin and dicloxacillin are the antibiotics of choice as first-line antibiotic treatment of mastitis, including for breast abscess. Where there is a history of penicillin hypersensitivity, clindamycin or vancomycin may be indicated. In the case of community-acquired methicillin-resistant staphylococcus aureus (MRSA), clindamycin or trimethoprim + sulfamethoxazole may be indicated.

Sulphonamide

Sulphonamides are usually safe during pregnancy. However, long-acting sulphonamides cross the placenta and can displace bilirubin from binding sites. These drugs are often avoided after 34 weeks gestation because neonatal kernicterus is a risk.

Tetracyclines

Tetracyclines are not recommended during pregnancy as they pose an increased risk for maternal hepatotoxicity, cross the placenta and bind in high concentration as deposits in fetal bones and teeth causing staining. Use of tetracycline should be avoided during pregnancy, particularly from the middle to end of the pregnancy. Research undertaken by Warner et al (2022) indicates that tetracyclines retained in bone may have lasting effects on skeletal metabolism, and the impact of this medication on skeletal maturation and homeostasis is poorly understood, including mechanisms of action on bone cells and role of gut microbiota. Tetracyclines are excreted in the faeces and urine.

Macrolide antibiotics

Macrolides are generally considered safe in pregnancy. These broad spectrum antibiotics include erythromycin and azithromycin, which are useful for the treatment of infections where penicillin cannot be used.

'Erythromycin estolate is contraindicated in pregnancy, because of drug-related hepatotoxicity. Erythromycin ethylsuccinate is compatible for pregnancy' (Wilmer et al 2016 cited in Hunter & Davis 2019). Azithromycin can be used for both gram-negative and gram-positive bacteria and is recommended for use to treat chlamydia (Wiffen et al 2012).

Trimethoprim

Trimethoprim is typically the first choice of antibiotic for the treatment of UTI but is contraindicated in the first trimester of pregnancy. However, a study reported in 2017 in the United Kingdom has found that a third of urine samples in the laboratory are resistant to the antibiotic trimethoprim (NICE 2017) (ESPAUR report). When used, trimethoprim 300 mg at night for 3 days is recommended by Cochrane. However, the treatment of choice now is nitrofurantoin (see Online resources: Therapeutic Guidelines).

Nitrofurantoin

Nitrofurantoin has been used for decades for the treatment of UTI. As a bactericide it alters the bacteria's ribosomal proteins and other cell molecules. It is a broad spectrum antibiotic that is not known to cause congenital malformations as the placental exposure is low. Some of the drug is metabolised in the liver but it is mostly excreted unchanged. Reports of antibiotic resistance are limited to 3% (NICE 2017).

It is contraindicated in women with glucose-6-phosphate dehydrogenase (G6PD) and all women near term due to the risk of haemolytic reactions (anaemia) in mothers and infants (Therapeutic Guidelines 2023). Nitrofurantoin should not be prescribed for mothers breastfeeding infants less than 1 month old as the medication has been detected in breast milk and can cause haemolysis in the newborn (Toxnet 2017, cited in Hunter & Davis 2019).

Absorption of nitrofurantoin is increased when taken with food. However, antacids and urine alkalinisers all interfere with the normal absorption of nitrofurantoin. Antacids have the potential to impair absorption, while nitrofurantoin is more effective in an acid environment. The medication will cause the urine to have a brownish discolouration and can also cause drowsiness and dizziness; therefore, education should be included as part of ongoing medication review and prior to prescription of the drug regarding these and other side effects.

Metronidazole

Metronidazole is a category B2 medication used to treat anaerobic bacteria such as bacterial vaginitis or trichomonal infections (Hunter & Davis 2019). Metronidazole use during the first trimester used to be considered controversial; however, in multiple studies, no teratogenic or mutagenic effects have been seen (see Online resources: CDC–Trichomoniasis). Thus, the New Zealand Sexual Health Society (NASHZ 2015) recommends the use of metronidazole in all trimesters to eradicate trichomonal infection. One dose is advised. Couples should then abstain from sex or wear a condom for 7 days. Lactating mothers should avoid breastfeeding for 24–48 hours as metronidazole has been found in breast milk and causes an unpleasant metallic taste. Infants may also experience nausea, vomiting, stomach cramps or diarrhoea where abstinence of feeding for 24–48 hours is not observed.

Cephalosporins

Cephalosporins are generally considered safe during pregnancy as they tend to have a shorter half-life, lower serum levels, increased distribution, and clearance, suggesting the need for higher dosage or more frequent medication. Cephalosporins are broad spectrum antibiotics. They all cross the placenta and small amounts are found in breast milk; 60–90% is protein bound in the plasma (Momper & Brooke 2022).

Cephalosporins should not be used in women with sensitivity to penicillin. Cephalosporins are classified into different generations which define when they were created. Each generation has a specific effect on different bacteria (Hunter & Davis 2019).

- *First generation* – gram-positive bacteria: cephalexin, cephradine, cefazolin, cefadroxil.

Cephalothin requires no dose change as 10–40% is metabolised and the remainder is excreted by the kidneys. Cephradine and cefazolin have increased clearance in pregnancy, higher distribution volumes, decreased urine **concentrations** and shorter half-lives (Momper & Brooke 2022).

- *Second generation* – gram-negative bacteria: cefaclor, cefprozil, cefuroxime, cefoxitin, cefotetan, cefaclor, axetil.

Second-generation agents are generally excreted unchanged in the urine. Cefuroxime has a shorter half-life after 21 weeks and has lower plasma concentrations.

- *Third and fourth generation* – longer acting, gram-negative and beta-lactamase producing organisms: cefotaxime, ceftazidime, ceftriaxone, ceftizoxime, cefixime, cefditoren, cefdinir, cefpodoxime, ceftibuten, cefepime, ceftaroline.

Oral cephalosporins are used to treat *S. aureus* or streptococcal infections on the skin or in wounds. While they are useful as an alternative to penicillins, they should not be used to treat people who have reported serious reactions to penicillin as the adverse reactions are similar (see Online resources: Australian Medicines Handbook).

Chloramphenicol

Chloramphenicol is a synthetic antibiotic available as eye drops and eye ointment used to treat bacterial conjunctivitis – a bacterial infection involving the mucous membrane on the surface of the eye. Given to the mother, even in large doses, it does not appear to harm the fetus; however, neonates cannot adequately metabolise chloramphenicol, and the resulting high blood levels may lead to circulatory collapse (grey baby syndrome). Chloramphenicol binds to plasma proteins in high quantities (60%) especially in the placenta and is well absorbed. It is generally considered safe during pregnancy if taken as directed.

Aminoglycosides

Aminoglycosides are prescribed for gram-negative infections and work by inhibiting protein synthesis (Hunter & Davis 2019). This group of medications includes gentamicin, neomycin, netilmicin, streptomycin, and tobramycin. The therapeutic range of these medications is quite narrow, and careful observation is required to avoid adverse reactions which could include renal and neurological damage, and ototoxicity. If treatment is prescribed for more than 72 hours, blood serum levels and renal function testing is recommended as part of safe medication monitoring practice (Bryant & Knight 2015).

Antivirals

Treatment of women infected with viral conditions during pregnancy is essential to prevent transmission to the fetus. Herpes simplex virus and HIV are two examples of conditions that can cause central nervous system damage and death. Thus, optimising treatment management during pregnancy is vital to ensure a good outcome for the infant. Management of HSV includes reducing neonatal transmission, treating acute infections, and limiting adverse neurodevelopmental damage as part of ongoing antenatal prophylaxis if the woman acquires HSV for the first time in pregnancy (primary occurrence), or secondary outbreak (Straface et al 2012). Transmission to the fetus will be influenced by route of birth and whether maternal suppressive therapy has been taken (Harris & Holmes 2017).

Harris and Holmes report that neonatal HSV infections are divided into three categories: localised skin, eyes, or mouth; localised central nervous system; or disseminated infections. Maternal treatment with acyclovir is the treatment of choice. Antiviral treatment is self-administered by the woman.

Oral acyclovir may be used as suppressive therapy after acute treatment completion in specific neonatal populations, reducing long-term adverse neurodevelopmental outcomes and future skin eruptions. However, dosage strategies and durations of therapy may vary based on disease state severity, presentation, and patient characteristics. The mother should be advised that reoccurrences of HSV-1 lesions can be asymptomatic. The infant mortality rate remains high, even with treatment (Harris & Holmes 2017).

COVID-19 antiviral therapy

The National Clinical Evidence Taskforce (NCET) Guidelines specify recommendations for the use of anti-SARS-CoV-2 monoclonal antibodies and antivirals in adults, and children and adolescents (aged over 12 years) in Australia, based on available evidence for prophylaxis or for the treatment of patients in the early phase of infection with COVID-19 who are at risk of progression to severe disease. The antivirals must be given as early as possible, preferably before 5–7 days of onset to limit the spread beyond the respiratory system (NCET 2023).

DRUGS AT A GLANCE
Drugs used in the treatment of infection

PHARMACOLOGICAL GROUP AND EFFECT	KEY EXAMPLES	CLINICAL USE
Antibacterials	amoxycillins ampicillin cephalosporins;1st and 2nd generations macrolides (erythromycin) chloramphenicol tetracyclines	gram-pos/some gram-neg gram-neg orgs gram-pos/gram-neg gram-pos orgs bacterial conjunctivitis broad spectrum
Antifungals	clotrimazole (Canesten) econazole miconazole terbinafine (Lamisil) fluconazole (Diflucan) ketoconazole (Daktarin) nystatin (Nystan) amphotericin	vaginal candidiasis fungal/yeast infections candidiasis dermatophytes systemic candida oral candida oral candida systemic fungal infection HSV-1
Antivirals	acyclovir	
Parasitic infections	tapeworm – Niclosamide	herpes simplex virus 1

Antifungals

There are four main classes of antifungal drugs: polyenes, azoles, allylamines, and echinocandins.

Antifungal antibiotics can be occasionally administered topically in the form of creams, ointments, and tinctures. Antibiotics should only be used in the case of infection. Caution should be exercised in selection and use of this medication in the first trimester where fungal skin infections require systemic antifungal therapy, since safety data for use in early pregnancy is limited.

Vaginal candidiasis is a common infection experienced during pregnancy, and is related to increased levels of estrogen and vaginal glycogen production. Treatment is indicated as vaginal candidiasis can elevate the risks for preterm rupture of membranes, preterm labour, chorioamnionitis, and candidiasis infection in the newborn. Topical azoles and terbinafine are the preferred antifungal medication considered safest during pregnancy (Patel & Patel 2021). Topical antifungal antibiotics commonly used in the treatment of candidiasis in Australia and New Zealand include chlotrimazole, nystatin, miconazole, and fluconazole. Use of these oral and topical preparations extends to the postnatal period for both mother and infant.

Neonatal infections

To treat skin conditions, sticky eyes, and umbilical cord stumps:

- clotrimazole (Canesten)
- econazole
- miconazole
- terbinafine (Lamisil)
- fluconazole (Diflucan)
- ketoconazole (Daktarin)
- nystatin (Nystan)
- amphotericin.

Parasitic infection treatment

Toxoplasmosis

There is no treatment for toxoplasmosis. To date there is no drug that can eradicate the *Toxoplasma gondii* parasite from the body and no vaccine is approved for use in humans.

Pediculosis (head, pubic and body lice)

Treatment for head lice is a topical application of anti-parasitics permethrin (Quellada) and benzyl benzoate. While anecdotal data suggest these preparations may be used during pregnancy there is a lack of evidence-based safety data that conclusively supports this, and some publications suggest otherwise. For example, Elston (2023) advises that benzyl benzoate should not be used during pregnancy or in lactating women, infants, or children under 2 years of age because of the risk of neurotoxicity. Treatment of pubic and body lice requires clothing and bedding to be washed in hot water.

Helminths (worms)

Intestinal worm infections are generally treated with medicines that kill the parasite without harming the person, as they are not significantly absorbed by the GI tract.

Praziquantel, currently category B by the US FDA, is an anthelminthic drug classed as safe during pregnancy for the treatment of parasitic infections. Mebendazole (Vermox) is recommended as safe from the second trimester (de Silva et al 1999), and Ivermectin is a

category C and should not be used during pregnancy. Albendazole is not recommended for use during the first trimester of pregnancy.

Scabies

Treatment is topical permethrin preparations such as Lyclear Scabies Cream, Quellada lotion or benzyl benzoate 25% (Ascabiol or Benzemul 25%).

12.5 The microbiome and complementary and alternative medicine (CAM) considerations

The **microbiome** is a combination of healthy **microorganisms** that exist in our bodies (Dietert 2021). Our microbiome makeup is influenced by genetics, nutrition, age, BMI, medications, and health status. Pickard et al 2017 identified that this healthy balance of bacteria is composed of fungi, viruses, bacteria, and protozoa that exists without harm to the host (Fig 12.3).

Giannella et al (2023) identify three key areas of the female body where microbiota changes in pregnancy are linked with other pregnancy complications related to hypertensive disorders, gestational diabetes, preterm birth and recurrent miscarriage. These are the oral microbiome, the vaginal microbiome, and the gut microbiome.

During vaginal birth the mother transfers her microbiome to the infant from the genital tract (Jenkins et al 2019); thus, infants born via caesarean section are at a disadvantage as they are not exposed to the natural maternal microbiome. Rutayisire et al (2016) has reported lower bacterial diversity in infants born by caesarean section. This can be rectified by skin-to-skin and breastfeeding (Liu et al 2019) and vaginal seeding (Cunnington et al 2016; Haahr et al 2018. Plus, parents should be encouraged to delay bathing their baby for 24 hours.

International studies have reported that stimulus of the immune system in early life encourages activation of the T cells. Exposure to an environment rich in the family's microbes via the skin, respiratory tract and gut provides a positive activation of the infant's immune system to build tolerance to their environment.

CAM considerations

During pregnancy women should be advised to avoid all pharmacological medications not prescribed by a doctor or midwife. Caution is required with complementary therapies as there is no evidence to support many self-help remedies. The following information addresses the use of CAMs during pregnancy and breastfeeding for infections such as colds and flu, sore throats, bites and

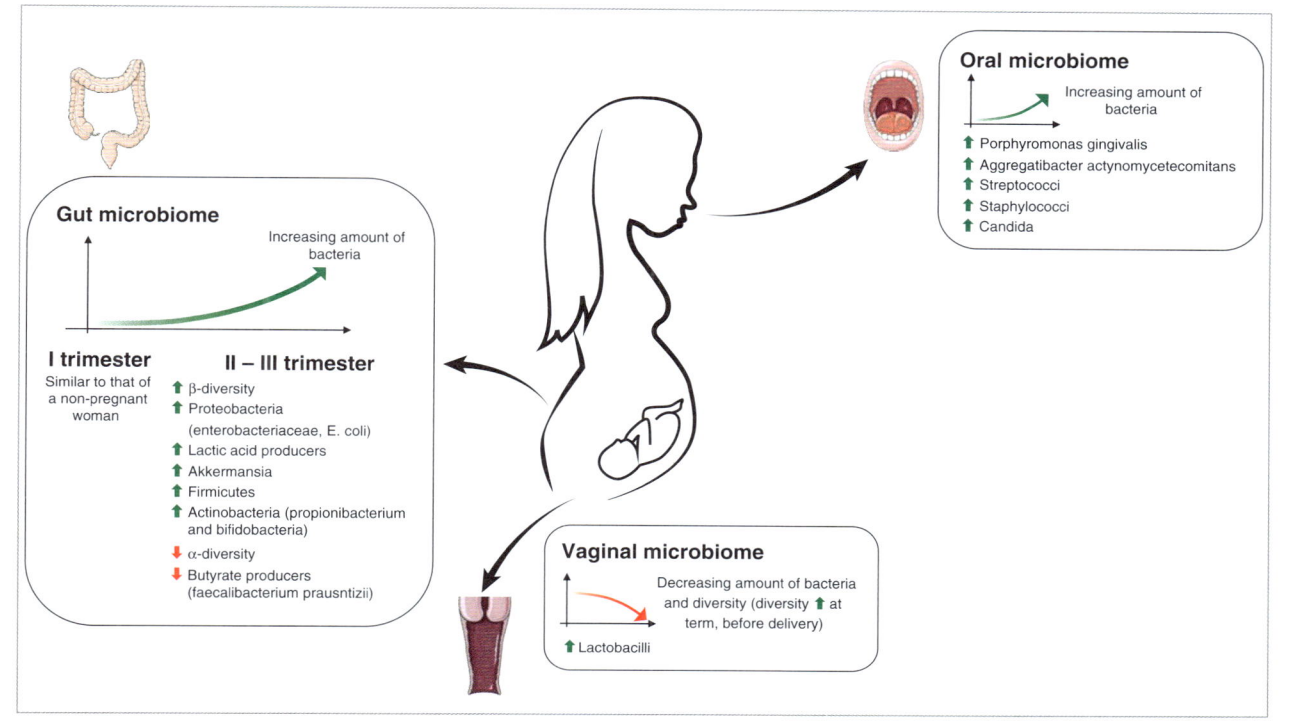

FIGURE 12.3

Source: Giannella L, Grelloni C, Quintili D, et al. Microbiome changes in pregnancy disorders. Antioxidants. 2023;12(2):463. https://doi.org/10.3390/antiox12020463

bee stings. Many treatments are complementary and recommended for use alongside pharmacological prescriptions. Some are recognised/recommended as alternative sources of treatment.

Influenza

During pregnancy it is recommended that cold and flu pharmacological remedies are avoided, and this includes paracetamol. Nutritional supplements can 'enhance or depress the immune function depending on the nutrients and level of intake' (Kotsirilos et al 2011). A deficiency in nutrients can impact the T-cell mediated response, further increasing susceptibility to infection. A synergy of all complete vitamins and trace elements will assist in reducing the incidence of influenza.

Perineal wound healing

Level 1 evidence purports that honey may improve healing of wounds. Cochrane and others report shorter healing times (Jull et al 2015). However, honey has not been found to have any impact on perineal pain (Geros et al 2022).

Historically, people have used plant resources to treat wounds based on empirical observations without any scientific knowledge. Research on albino mice suggests that seaweed can assist in wound healing (Premarathna et al 2021).

The medicinal and antibacterial properties of both manuka honey and seaweed have been applied to promote its use in assisting perineal wound healing post childbirth.

Bites and bee stings

Evidence-based results from RCTs are limited; however, some studies have found positive results in the use of tea tree oil for acne and for reducing histamine reactions in the skin (Kotsirilos et al 2011), such as insect bites. Tea tree oil has been reported to have significant antibacterial properties *in vitro* against a range of microorganisms such as *S. aureus*, *E. coli* and candida. While tea tree oil has been found to be effective for the topical treatment of skin, bacterial and fungal infections, no essential oils should be used in the first trimester of pregnancy (Tiran 2000).

CONCLUSION

This chapter introduced the midwife to the six types of infections most common in humans. Not all of these are seen frequently during pregnancy but when such infections do occur during pregnancy, treatments (both pharmaceutical and complementary) must consider the safety of the fetus. Not all infections require medication and can be resolved by good hygiene and the use of non-pharmacological self-help treatments such as good nutrition, rest and fluids. Over-the-counter purchase of treatments should be in consultation with a pharmacist, and complementary and alternative therapies should only be used under the guidance of a qualified practitioner. The midwife must remember their scope of practice and facilitate referral to a pharmacologist or naturopath, homeopathist or aromatherapist when required.

REFLECTIVE THINKING EXERCISES

1   Have you or a family member ever had a viral infection and sought antibiotics from your doctor?

2   What prompted you to seek antibiotics? How were you feeling?

3   What response did you receive?

4   What is your understanding of the difference between a virus and bacterial pathogen?

CRITICAL THINKING EXERCISES

Complete the following table by inserting the organisms responsible for infections experienced during pregnancy. Add the most appropriate advice that should be provided by the midwife and any recommended treatment.

Condition	Midwife's advice	Treatment
Influenza – blocked nose, mild fever, aches, and pains		
Sinusitis		
Frequency of micturition, dysuria, urgency		
'Thrush' Candidiasis		
Neonatal sticky eye		
Red umbilical stump		

REVIEW QUESTIONS

1   Describe the different physical barriers that protect the woman and infant from infection from microbes.

2   Which evidence-based resources would you consult to determine the safety profile of medication recommended to women in the first trimester of pregnancy when considering treatment options for a range of infections?

3   Describe and differentiate the assessment, diagnostic investigations and transfer/referral processes that should be initiated by the midwife for timely diagnosis and treatment of suspected sepsis in a pregnant woman, parturient mother, or newborn infant.

REFERENCES

Abu-Raya B, Michalski C, Sadarangani M, et al. Maternal immunological adaptation during normal pregnancy. Front Immunol. 2020;11:575197. doi: 10.3389/fimmu.2020.575197 (accessed 26 February 2024)

Australian Government Department of Health. Infectious syphilis outbreak, 2021. https://www1.health.gov.au/internet/main/publishing.nsf/Content/ohp-infectious-syphilis-outbreak.htm

Australian Commission on Safety and Quality in Health Care. National Sepsis Program, 2024. https://www.safetyandquality.gov.au/our-work/national-sepsis-program#:~:text=The%20Australian%20Sepsis%20NetworkExternal,as%20a%20result%20of%20sepsis

Australian Commission on Safety and Quality in Health Care. Antimicrobial stewardship in Australian healthcare, 2023. https://www.safetyandquality.gov.au/publications-and-resources/resource-library/antimicrobial-stewardship-australian-health-care

American College of Obstetricians and Gynecologists. HIV and pregnancy, 2012. http://www.acog.org/Patients/FAQs/HIV-and-Pregnancy (accessed 18 January 2017)

Ansorge, R. Bacterial and viral infections, 2021. WebMD. https://www.webmd.com/a-to-z-guides/bacterial-and-viral-infections

Australian Institute of Health and Welfare. Australia's mothers and babies: maternal deaths 2023. https://www.aihw.gov.au/reports/mothers-babies/maternal-deaths-australia

Baghel RS, Choudhary B, Pandey S, et al. Rehashing our insight of seaweeds as a potential source of foods, nutraceuticals, and pharmaceuticals. Foods. 2023; 12(19):3642. doi.org/10.3390/foods12193642 (accessed 11 March 2024)

Blackmon MM, Nguyen H, Mukherji P. Acute mastitis. [Updated 21 July 2023]. In: StatPearls [Internet]. Treasure Island (FL): StatPearls Publishing; 2024 Jan. (accessed 27 February 2024)

Bowyer L, Robinson H, Barrett H, et al. SOMANZ Guidelines for sepsis in pregnancy, 2017. Society of Obstetric Medicine Australia and New Zealand. doi.org/101111ajo.12646.

Centers for Disease Control and Prevention. STDs during pregnancy – CDC fact sheet (detailed), 2023. https://www.cdc.gov/std/pregnancy/stdfact-pregnancy-detailed.htm (accessed 11 March 2024)

Centers for Disease Control and Prevention. About parasites, 2022. https://www.cdc.gov/parasites/about.html

Centers for Disease Control and Prevention. Cytomegalovirus (CMV) and congenital CMV infection, 2020. https://www.cdc.gov/cmv/resources/pregnant-women-parents.html (accessed 11 March 2024)

Centers for Disease Control and Prevention. Trichomoniasis, 2022. https://www.cdc.gov/std/treatment-guidelines/trichomoniasis.htm (accessed 12 March 2024)

Cunnington AJ, Sim K, Deierl A, et al. 'Vaginal seeding' of infants born by caesarean section. BMJ. 2016 Feb;352:i227. doi: 10.1136/bmj.i227. PMID:26906151 (accessed 11 March 2024)

De Silva NR, Sirisena JL, Gunasekera DP, et al. Effect of mebendazole therapy during pregnancy on birth outcome. Lancet (London, England). 1999;353(9159):1145-1149. doi.org/10.1016/s0140-6736(98)06308-9

Devchand M, Trubiano JA. Penicillin allergy: a practical approach to assessment and prescribing. Aust Prescr. 2019;42:192–199. doi.org/10.18773/austprescr.2019.065

Dietert RR. Microbiome first medicine in health and safety. Biomedicines. 2021 Aug;9(9):1099. doi: 10.3390/biomedicines9091099. PMID:34572284; PMCID:PMC8468398 (accessed 11 March 2024)

Elston D. 257 ectoparasites (lice and scabies). In: Principles and practice of pediatric infectious diseases. 6th edn. 2023:e1324-1328. doi.org/10.1016/B978-0-323-75608-2.00257-3

Esposito S, Chiopris G, Messina G, et al. Prevention of congenital cytomegalovirus infection with vaccines: state of the art. Vaccines (Basel). 2021 May;9(5):523. doi: 10.3390/vaccines9050523. PMID:34069321; PMCID:PMC8158681 (accessed 11 March 2024)

Gerosa D, Santagata M, Martinez de Tejada B, et al. Application of honey to reduce perineal laceration pain during the postpartum period: a randomized controlled trial. Healthcare (Basel). 2022 Aug;10(8):1515. doi: 10.3390/healthcare10081515. PMID:36011172; PMCID:PMC9408762 (accessed 11 March 2024)

Giakoumelou S, Wheelhouse N, Cuschieri K, et al. The role of infection in miscarriage. Hum Reprod Update. 2016 Jan-Feb;22(1):116-33. doi: 10.1093/humupd/dmv041. Epub 2015 Sep 19. PMID:26386469

Giannella L, Grelloni C, Quintili D, et al. Microbiome changes in pregnancy disorders. Antioxidants. 2023;12(2):463. doi.org/10.3390/antiox12020463 (accessed 11 March 2024)

Haahr T, Glavind J, Axelsson P, et al. Vaginal seeding or vaginal microbial transfer from the mother to the caesarean-born neonate: a commentary regarding clinical management. BJOG. 2018 Apr;125(5):533-536. doi: 10.1111/1471-0528.14792. Epub 2017 Aug 22. PMID:28626982 (accessed 11 March 2024)

Harris JB, Holmes AP. Neonatal herpes simplex viral infections and acyclovir: an update. JPPT. 2017;22(2):88-93. doi.org/10.5863/1551-6776-22.2.88

Homer C. Screening and assessment. In: Pairman S, Tracy SK, Dahlen HG, Dixon L (eds). Midwifery; preparation for practice. 5th edn. Elsevier, 2022.

Ho V. What are parasites and how do they make us sick? The Conversation. 18 November 2019. https://theconversation.com/what-are-parasites-and-how-do-they-make-us-sick-121489

Hunter M, Davis D. Pharmacology and prescribing. In: Pairman S, Tracy SK, Dahlen HG, Dixon L (eds). Midwifery; preparation for practice. 5th edn. Elsevier, 2019. (accessed 11 March 2024).

Jenkins H, Hyde M. The microbiome relating to labour and birth. In: Downe S, Byrom S (eds). Squaring the circle. London: Pinter & Martin Ltd, 2019.

Jull AB, Cullum N, Dumville JC, et al. Honey as a topical treatment for wounds. The Cochrane Library. Hoboken, NJ: John Wiley & Sons Ltd, 2015.

Justiz Vaillant AA, Sabir S, Jan A. Physiology, immune response. [Updated 26 Sep 2022]. In: StatPearls [Internet]. Treasure Island (FL): StatPearls Publishing; 2024 Jan. https://www.ncbi.nlm.nih.gov/books/NBK539801/ (accessed 26 February 2024)

Kotsirilos V, Vitetta L, Sali A. A guide to evidence based integrative and complementary medicine. Elsevier, 2011.

Liu Y, Qin S, Song Y, et al. The perturbation of infant gut microbiota caused by caesarean delivery is partially restored by exclusive breastfeeding. Front Microbiol. 2019 Mar;10:598. doi: 10.3389/fmicb.2019.00598. PMID: 30972048; PMCID: PMC6443713. https://pubmed.ncbi.nlm.nih.gov/30972048/ (accessed 11 March 2024)

Lokugamage AU, Pathberiya SDC. The microbiome seeding debate – let's frame it around women-centred care. Reprod Health. 2019;16:91. doi.org/10.1186/s12978-019-0747-0 (accessed 11 March 2024)

Momper JD, Brooke MB. Chapter 12 – Clinical pharmacology of anti-infectives during pregnancy. In: Clin Pharmacol During Pregnancy (2nd edn, p. 177–202). Elsevier, 2022. doi.org/10.1016/B978-0-12-818902-3.

National Clinical Evidence Taskforce Living Guidelines [internet]. NCET: Melbourne; 2021 [accessed 7 February 2022]. Available from: https://covid19evidence.net.au/#living-guidelines

National Institute of Clinical Excellence (NICE) (2017). Antibiotic resistance is now common in urinary tract infections. https://www.nice.org.uk/news/article/antibiotic-resistance-is-now-common-in-urinary-tract-infections

National Institute of Clinical Excellence. The English surveillance programme for anti-microbial utilisation and resistance (ESPAUR report). NICE, 2017. https://www.gov.uk/government/publications/english-surveillance-programme-antimicrobial-utilisation-and-resistance-espaur-report#ESPAUR%20report%202022%20to%202023

The National Clinical Evidence Taskforce. Guidance for the use of anti-SARS-CoV-2 monoclonal antibiotics and antiviral agents as prophylaxis or to prevent severe infection from COVID-19 in NSW. NCET, 2023.

New Zealand Sexual Health Society. Best Practice Guidelines 2015. NASHZ, 2015. http://www.nzshs.org/docman/guidelines

Patel MA, Aliporewala VM, Patel DA. Common antifungal drugs in pregnancy: risks and precautions. J Obstet Gynaecol India. 2021;71(6):577-582. doi.org/10.1007/s13224-021-01586-8 (accessed 11 March 2024)

Premarathna AD, Wijesekerac SK, Jayasooriyad AP, et al. In vitro and in vivo evaluation of the wound healing properties and safety assessment of two seaweeds (Sargassum ilicifolium and Ulva lactuca) BB Reports. 2021;26(2021):100986. https://www.sciencedirect.com/science/article/pii/S2405580821000807#:~:text=The%20seaweeds%20can%20also%20be,process%20%5B7%2C16%5D

Rours GI, Duijts L, Moll HA, et al. Chlamydia trachomatis infection during pregnancy associated with preterm delivery: a population-based prospective cohort study. Eur J Epidemiol. 2011;26(6):493-502. https://www.ncbi.nlm.nih.gov/pubmed/21538042 (accessed 18 January 2017)

Salam RA, Das JK, Bhutta ZA. Effect of mass deworming with antihelminthics for soil-transmitted helminths during pregnancy. Cochrane Database Syst Rev. 2021;5(5):CD005547. doi.org/10.1002/14651858.CD005547.pub4

Schneeberger C, Geerlings SE, Middleton P, Crowther CA. Interventions for preventing recurrent urinary tract infection during pregnancy. Cochrane Database Syst Rev. 2015;7:CD009279. doi: 10.1002/14651858.CD009279.pub3 (accessed 27 February 2024)

Sepsis Alliance. Sepsis and viral infections. Sepsis Alliance 2022. https://www.sepsis.org/sepsisand/viral-infections/

Smaill FM, Grivell RM. Antibiotic prophylaxis versus no prophylaxis for preventing infection after cesarean section. Cochrane Database Syst Rev. 2014;10:CD007482. doi: 10.1002/14651858.CD007482.pub3 (accessed 27 February 2024)

Smith JR, Furtado, JM. One in three people are infected with Toxoplasma parasite – and the clue could be in our eyes. The Conversation, 2022. https://theconversation.com/one-in-three-people-are-infected-with-toxoplasma-parasite-and-the-clue-could-be-in-our-eyes-182418 (accessed 11 March 2024)

Straface G, Selmin A, Zanardo V, De Santis M, Ercoli A, Scambia G. Herpes simplex virus infection in pregnancy. Infect Dis Obstet Gynecol. 2012;2012:385697. doi: 10.1155/2012/385697. Epub 2012 Apr 11. PMID:22566740; PMCID: PMC3332182 (accessed 11 March 2024).

Taylor M, Jenkins SM, Pillarisetty LS. Endometritis. [Updated 26 Oct 2023]. In: StatPearls [Internet]. Treasure Island (FL): StatPearls Publishing; 2024 Jan. https://www.ncbi.nlm.nih.gov/books/NBK553124/ (accessed 23 March 2024)

Tiran D. Complementary therapies for pregnancy and childbirth. 2nd edn. Balliere Tindall, 2000.

Warner AJ, Hathaway-Schrader JD, Lubker R, et al. Tetracyclines and bone: unclear actions with potentially lasting effects. Bone. 2022 Jun;159:116377. doi: 10.1016/j.bone.2022.116377. Epub 2022 Mar 3. PMID: 35248788; PMCID:PMC9035080 (accessed 11 March 2024)

Wiffen P, Mitchell M, Snelling M, et al. Oxford handbook of clinical pharmacy, 2nd edn. Oxford UK; Oxford University Press, 2012.

Wheeler AC. Development of infants with congenital Zika syndrome: what do we know and what can we expect? Pediatrics. 2018 Feb;141(Suppl 2):S154-S160. doi: 10.1542/peds.2017-2038D. PMID:29437048; PMCID:PMC5795516 (accessed 11 March 2024)

World Health Organization. Herpes simplex virus. WHO, 2023. https://www.who.int/news-room/fact-sheets/detail/herpes-simplex-virus (accessed 11 March 2024)

ONLINE RESOURCES

Australian Institute of Health and Welfare (AIHW). Australia's mothers and babies: https://www.aihw.gov.au/reports/mothers-babies/maternal-deaths-australia (accessed 26 February 2024)

American College of Obstetricians and Gynaecologists (ACOG). Listeria and pregnancy: https://www.acog.org/womens-health/faqs/listeria-and-pregnancy#:~:text=Babies%20born%20with%20listeriosis%20may,can%20cause%20death%20in%20newborns (accessed 23 March 2024)

American College of Obstetricians and Gynecologists (ACOG). Hepatitis B and hepatitis C in pregnancy, FAQ093: https://www.acog.org/womens-health/faqs/hepatitis-b-and-hepatitis-c-in-pregnancy (accessed 30 December 2020)

Australian Commission on Safety and Quality in Health Care (ACSQHC). National Sepsis Program: https://www.safetyandquality.gov.au/our-work/national-sepsis-program#:~:text=The%20Australian%20Sepsis%20NetworkExternal,as%20a%20result%20of%20sepsis

Australian Medicines Handbook: https://amhonline.amh.net.au/auth (accessed 11 March 2024)

Australian Pregnancy Care Guidelines – Australian Living Evidence Collaboration: https://app.magicapp.org/?language=bi#/guideline/jm83PE (accessed 11 March 2024).

Australian STI Management Guidelines for use in primary care. Pregnant people | STI Guidelines Australia: https://sti.guidelines.org.au/populations-and-situations/pregnant-people/

Centers for Disease Control (CDC). For information on infections during pregnancy and sexually transmitted infections (STIs) and pregnancy. Division of HIV Prevention, National Center for HIV, Viral Hepatitis, STD, and TB Prevention, Centers for Disease Control and Prevention: https://www.cdc.gov/hiv/group/pregnant-people/index.html?CDC_AA_refVal=https%3A%2F%2Fwww.cdc.gov%2Fhiv%2Fgroup%2Fgender%2Fpregnantwomen%2Findex.html (accessed March 11 2024)

Healthline. Meningitis: https://www.healthline.com/health/meningitis/gbs-meningitis#risk-factors

Medline Plus. Genital herpes: http://www.nlm.nih.gov/medlineplus/ency/article/000857.htm (accessed 18 January 2017)

MSD. MSD manual, ZIKA virus: https://www.msdmanuals.com/en-au/professional/searchresults?query=zika%20virus

MSD. MSD manual, Infectious disease in pregnancy: https://www.msdmanuals.com/en-au/professional/gynecology-and-obstetrics/pregnancy-complicated-by-disease/infectious-disease-in-pregnancy

National Centre for Antimicrobial Stewardship, Australia: https://www.ncas-australia.org/about-us (accessed 27 February 2024)

New Zealand: National Women's Health: https://www.nationalwomenshealth.adhb.govt.nz/assets/Womens-health/

Documents/Policies-and-guidelines/Sepsis-During-Pregnancy-and-Postpartum.pdf (accessed 26 February 2024)

Therapeutic Guidelines. Urinary tract infection and bacteriuria in pregnancy: www.tg.org.au (accessed 11 March 2024)

The UK Sepsis Trust: https://sepsistrust.org/

Sepsis Alliance: https://www.sepsis.org/

Healthline. Marcin A. Group B Streptococcal (GBS) meningitis: symptoms, treatment, outlook, and more: https://www.healthline.com/health/meningitis/gbs-meningitis#risk-factors

CHAPTER 13

DIABETES IN PREGNANCY AND ITS MANAGEMENT

Maryam Bazargan, Kirsten Small, Roslyn Donnellan-Fernandez

Key Abbreviations

BGL	blood glucose level
DPP4	dipeptidyl peptidase-4
GDM	gestational diabetes mellitus
GLP	glucagon-like peptide
GLUT-4	principal glucose transporter protein
GTT	glucose tolerance test
HPL	human placental lactogen
IGF	insulin-like growth factors
NIDDM	non-insulin-dependent diabetes mellitus
NPH	neutral protamine Hagedorn
OCTs	organic cation transporters
OHA	oral hypoglycaemic agent
SGLT2	sodium-glucose co-transporter 2

Key Terms

antihyperglycaemic drugs 259
basal release 256
blood glucose level 261
euglycaemia 260
gestational diabetes mellitus 257
glucagon 256
gluconeogenesis 256
glycogenolysis 256
glycosuria 256
hyperglycaemia 256
hypoglycaemia 269
incretins 268
insulin 256
islets of Langerhans 256
ketoacidosis 257
ketogenesis 256
lipolysis 256
macrosomia 256
polydipsia 257
polyphagia 257
polyuria 257
somatostatin 256
type 1/type 2 diabetes 256

Chapter Focus

Insulin and glucagon, hormones secreted by the pancreas, have major roles in the regulation of blood glucose levels (BGLs) and nutrient storage. Inadequate production of insulin and/or resistance to insulin cause diabetes mellitus, a disorder of carbohydrate metabolism affecting approximately 8.5% of the adult population. Gestational diabetes impacts approximately 14% of pregnant women worldwide. Complications of diabetes in pregnancy can impact maternal and neonatal outcomes.

Women with type 1 or type 2 diabetes do experience pregnancy, and some women without preexisting glucose intolerance will develop gestational diabetes mellitus (GDM) during pregnancy. Women with type 1 diabetes are dependent on parental insulin (injections, pumps). Many formulations of human and bovine insulin are available. Type 2 diabetes may be managed with lifestyle modifications, such as diet and exercise, and/or treated with antihyperglycaemic drugs. Many women with type 2 diabetes find insulin improves their glucose control.

Management of GDM involves controlling blood glucose through diet, exercise and, if necessary, oral antihyperglycaemic medications like metformin and/or insulin (Wu et al 2024). Postpartum, both mother and neonate benefit from monitoring of BGL. By maintaining a healthy lifestyle, women with a history of GDM may reduce the risk of future type 2 diabetes and other metabolic disorders.

Hypoglycaemia is a potential adverse effect of insulin use and most antihyperglycaemic drugs. Hypoglycaemia can be treated with hyperglycaemic medications such as glucose or glucagon.

Key Drug Groups

- **Glucagon**
- **Insulins:**
  - Human insulin (DM 13.1)
  - Insulin lispro, insulin isophane, insulin glargine

Oral hypoglycaemic agents (OHAs):
- Metformin (DM 13.2)

Learning Outcomes

- Understand the different types of diabetes, including risk factors, and how they may impact pregnancy and birth for mother and neonate.
- Understand non-pharmacological and pharmacological management of all types of diabetes in pregnancy, labour, and the early postpartum period.
- Describe the mechanism of action of oral hyperglycaemic (metformin) and parenteral insulin.

- Describe how over-the-counter and social drugs can affect blood glucose levels and alter diabetic control, leading to potential for drug interactions with insulin and other antihyperglycaemic medication.
- Critically apply knowledge of hyperglycaemia and hypoglycaemia management to the care of the woman and her infant.

CRITICAL THINKING SCENARIO

Smitha is pregnant with her second baby. Having had GDM in her first pregnancy, she opted for an early oral glucose tolerance test (OGTT) test and was diagnosed with GDM at 14 weeks of gestation (fasting BGL was 5.4 mmol/L and one-hour OGTT was 10 mmol/L). Smitha commenced managing her GDM with lifestyle/diet modification. When glycaemic control was not achieved after one month, metformin was prescribed.

Smitha's BGL responded well to metformin. At her 30-week appointment, Smitha's midwife became concerned that her current treatment plan was no longer effective, with several high fasting BGLs and a HbA1c of 7.8%. After further review, her endocrinologist added insulin to her treatment regimen alongside her metformin. Her BGLs normalised once again.

1 What are the recommended BGLs for both before (i.e. fasting) and 2 hours after meals (i.e. post-prandial) in pregnancy?

2 Why is good blood glucose control more difficult to maintain with advancing gestation?

3 What are the potential fetal consequences of prolonged maternal hyperglycaemia?

4 What implications can these consequences have for labour/birth and the early postnatal period for the woman and her baby?

Smitha is now 37 weeks pregnant and over the last 3 days has developed symptoms of a urinary tract infection. This has included nausea and loss of appetite. As a result, her oral intake has fallen yet she continued her metformin and insulin. You are seeing Smitha for a routine antenatal visit and you notice she looks unwell. She reports episodes of dizziness, headaches, and sweating over the past few days and has put this down to the infection.

During the appointment she suddenly faints and remains unconscious.

1 Explain what was happening physiologically for Smitha when she became dizzy, sweating, and had headaches.

2 What treatment changes would you recommend she make to reduce her symptoms?

3 To treat this episode of loss of consciousness, what treatment(s) would you administer? Ensure you consider appropriate routes of administration.

4 Discuss your considerations for fetal wellbeing during the loss of consciousness episode. How would you respond to these?

Introduction

The endocrine tissue of the pancreas – the islets of Langerhans – consists of clumps of cells scattered throughout the organ. The islets produce hormones (insulin, glucagon, and somatostatin) that control blood glucose levels and some gastrointestinal functions. Insulin is produced by beta (or B) cells, glucagon by alpha (or A) cells, and somatostatin by delta (or D) cells. Pathologies of pancreatic endocrine function cause widespread and serious disorders including diabetes mellitus and metabolic syndrome.

Pregnancy is associated with significant adaptation in carbohydrate metabolism. Placental hormones, including human placental lactogen (HPL), progesterone, and cortisol decrease the responsiveness to insulin (increase resistance to insulin in peripheral tissue). This adaptation (diabetogenic effect of pregnancy) increases the availability of glucose to be transferred to the fetus. Insulin resistance is often exaggerated in overweight and obese women.

Growth and development of the fetus is dependent on the availability of a constant supply of glucose from mother through the placenta. Glucose is transported across the placenta from mother to the fetus via facilitated diffusion; however, maternal insulin cannot cross the placenta. The fetus produces its own insulin. The major regulators of fetal growth are insulin-like growth factors (IGF 1 and 2). Chronic (long-term) hyperglycaemia in the mother with diabetes results in long-term fetal hyperglycaemia (since there is a linear relationship between maternal and fetal glucose level), which augments fetal insulin secretion and suppresses glucagon. Since insulin is a fetal growth hormone, fetal hyperinsulinemic states are associated with fetal and neonatal **macrosomia**.

13.1 Pancreatic hormones and diabetes mellitus

Insulin from the pancreas

Insulin is a protein hormone consisting of two polypeptide chains joined by disulfide bridges. Insulin was the first protein for which the amino acid sequence was determined, and the first synthesised by genetic engineering technologies, showing its importance in healthcare.

Insulin release and circulation

There is a low **basal release** of insulin in pulses every 15–30 minutes into the portal circulation to the liver. Release is increased within 30–60 seconds after absorption of glucose from a meal, with a rapid initial rise due to release of stored insulin, then a slower delayed phase over 60–90 minutes as newly synthesised insulin is also released.

Insulin release is inhibited by falling BGLs, fasting, **somatostatin**, adrenaline (epinephrine; via α_2-receptors) and drugs such as the thiazide diuretics. Deficiencies of release occur in the pancreatic disorders diabetes mellitus, pancreatitis, and tumours.

Insulin circulates bound to a β-globulin. As a protein, insulin is rapidly digested in the gut if given orally, with a half-life of only a few minutes, so it must be administered parenterally when used therapeutically. Its biological duration of action is longer than the half-life would suggest at 2–4 hours, as it is bound to receptors in tissues where it acts preventing its metabolism.

Insulin actions and mechanism

Insulin facilitates removal of glucose from the blood into muscle and fat cells via biochemical reactions affecting uptake, utilisation, and storage of carbohydrates, fats, and amino acids in liver, adipose, and muscle cells. Insulin controls intermediary metabolism, promotes the anabolic state (building up), and has long-term effects on cell proliferation and growth regulation.

Mechanism of action

Insulin binds to specific membrane receptors on target cells. This initiates a cascade of reactions in the cell which results in fusion of intracellular vesicles containing a glucose transporter (GLUT-4) with the plasma membrane and a rapid 10- to 30-fold increase in glucose uptake into the cell. Cells in the brain, exercising muscle and liver are not dependent on insulin-mediated glucose uptake.

Glucagon is a 29-amino-acid polypeptide hormone secreted by alpha cells of the **islets of Langerhans** in response to hypoglycaemia and high-protein meals, and is also stimulated by exercise, stress, and infection. It is a fuel-mobilising hormone and has been called an 'anti-insulin'. Its actions include:

- stimulating hepatic **glycogenolysis, gluconeogenesis** (the conversion of glycerol and amino acids to glucose), **lipolysis** and **ketogenesis**
- inhibiting glycogen synthesis
- stimulating release of catecholamines, hence inhibiting tone and motility in GIT smooth muscle, plus other sympathomimetic effects
- increasing release of growth hormone and ACTH, and (paradoxically) of insulin.

Secretion is inhibited by insulin, hyperglycaemia, and incretins. In diabetes, the lack of insulin leads to increased release of glucagon, which contributes to raised BGLs and eventually to the state of ketosis. Glucagon is used clinically to treat hypoglycaemia, including in neonates and when excessive insulin has been administered.

Diabetes mellitus

Diabetes mellitus is characterised by polyuria associated with a chronic disorder of carbohydrate and lipid metabolism and an inappropriate rise in glucose level in the blood, due to defects in insulin secretion, insulin action, or both. The two main types of diabetes are **type 1** (formerly known as insulin-dependent diabetes mellitus, IDDM, or juvenile-onset), in which there is complete lack of insulin; and **type 2** (non-insulin-dependent diabetes mellitus, NIDDM, maturity-onset), where there is a relative lack of insulin or defects of the insulin receptors. Gestational diabetes mellitus (GDM) is like type 2 diabetes, with placental hormones creating insulin resistance, which will usually rectify following the birth of the placenta.

Features of different types of diabetes are summarised in Table 13.1.

Pathologies

Lack of insulin or resistance to insulin produces a complex disorder of carbohydrate, fat, and protein metabolism.

General aspects of diabetes include:

- *Hyperglycaemia*: Lack of or resistance to insulin means glucose cannot be taken up into cells. Without treatment, BGLs rise rapidly (hyperglycaemia), and excess glucose is secreted by the kidneys (**glycosuria**).

TABLE 13.1 Features of type 1, type 2, and gestational diabetes

FEATURE	TYPE 1	TYPE 2	GDM
Synonyms (former)	Insulin-dependent diabetes, juvenile-onset	Non-insulin-dependent diabetes, maturity-onset	Non-insulin-dependent diabetes, pregnancy-onset
Age of onset	Usually < 20 years	Usually > 35 years	Usually > 28 weeks gestation
Onset of symptoms	Sudden (symptomatic)	Gradual	Gradual
Body weight	Usually non-obese	Obese (80%)	Independent, although obesity is a risk factor
Aetiology	Predisposition inherited; viral infection may cause auto-immune onset	Family history often positive. Risk factors: advancing age, obesity, cardiovascular disease, metabolic syndrome, tobacco use	Developing insulin resistance due to placental hormones. Risk factors: obesity, ethnicity, multiple pregnancy, advanced maternal age, polycystic ovarian syndrome, tobacco use, gestational hypertension
Incidence (% all diabetes)	5%	90–95%	14% of pregnant women worldwide, 17.9% in Australia
Insulin levels	Low, then absent	May be low, normal or high (insulin resistance)	Normal
Insulin-dependent	Yes	Usually not (may progress to be)	Usually not (may need insulin to manage glucose levels more precisely)
Insulin resistance	No	Yes	Yes
Insulin receptors	Normal	Usually low or defective	Normal, but resistant
Complications	Frequent	Frequent	Low
Ketoacidosis	Prone to	Rare	Rare
Dietary modifications	Mandatory	Mandatory	Helpful
Treatment	Insulin essential	Diet, exercise, antihyperglycaemic drugs, possibly insulin	Diet, exercise, metformin (oral antihyperglycaemic), insulin for moderate-to-severe GDM

In GDM, excess glucose will be readily available to the fetus via placental diffusion (facilitated diffusion)

- *Signs and symptoms of diabetes:* These include increased appetite (**polyphagia**), thirst (**polydipsia**), increased urine output (**polyuria**), fruity breath odour (ketosis), anorexia and weight loss, abdominal pain, nausea and vomiting, dry mouth, rapid deep breathing, weakness (fatigue), and recurrent infections
- *Diagnosis of diabetes outside of pregnancy:* Diagnosis is by signs and symptoms, by measurement of high BGL (random > 11.1 mmol/L, fasting > 7.0 mmol/L), by oral glucose tolerance testing (OGTT), 75 gram of glucose administered orally, after overnight fasting (fasting glucose ≥ 7.0 mmol/L or 2 hr glucose ≥ 11.1 mmol/L), and/or by glycated haemoglobin levels (HbA1c ≥ 6.5%; 48 mmol/mol) (see Online resources: Diabetes Australia)
- *Type 1 diabetes:* Type 1 usually occurs before the age of 20 years. High breakdown of proteins and fats causes ketone bodies (acetoacetic acid, acetone, and

β-hydroxybutyric acid) to accumulate, resulting in ketosis and acidosis. Diabetic **ketoacidosis** with associated cerebral oedema is a medical emergency. Regular injections of exogenous insulin are required lifelong for survival
- *Type 2 diabetes:* People with type 2 diabetes generally have some functioning islet cells. There is impaired insulin secretion (especially the early phase after glucose load) and/or insulin resistance because of receptor and post-receptor defects
- *Gestational diabetes mellitus:* This category includes women in whom diabetes or impaired glucose tolerance is first detected during pregnancy. In GDM, the function of pancreatic islet cells is unaffected and insulin production in pregnancy is increased compared to a non-pregnant person. There is reduced sensitivity to insulin or insulin resistance (the body does not respond to insulin effectively) because of receptor and post-receptor function alterations due to placental hormones. Insulin resistance is a normal physiological adjustment to

prioritise nutrient supply to the growing fetus. Placental hormones, mainly human placental lactogen and human placental growth hormone, induce insulin resistance to ensure sufficient glucose, which constitutes 80% of the fetus's energy source for proper growth, will go to the fetus through the placenta. Diagnosis is by OGTT, at 28 weeks (or at 14 weeks for women with risk factors) if fasting glucose $\geq$ 5.1 mmol/L or 1 hr glucose $\geq$ 10 and 2 hr glucose $\geq$ 8.5 mmol/L and/or by glycated haemoglobin levels (HbA1c $\geq$ 6.5%; 48 mmol/mol) (see Online resources: Diabetes Australia, Diagnostic testing 2020).

Insulin resistance sufficient to cause GDM develops during the second and third trimesters in approximately one in six pregnant women, notably in older women. Prolonged high BGLs in pregnancy lead to fetal hyperinsulinism; this may cause increased fetal growth leading to macrosomia, organomegaly, and neonatal hypoglycaemia. If BGL cannot be controlled with diet and exercise, mild GDM may be treated first with metformin, then insulin added or substituted as required. Moderate–severe GDM is best managed with immediate insulin therapy. Following childbirth, maternal impaired glucose tolerance resolves, though women with previously undiagnosed type 2 diabetes will continue to have high glucose levels. All women receiving a diagnosis of GDM should be followed up postnatally for education regarding increased risk, including ongoing screening for developing diabetes later in life.

Risks associated with diabetes in pregnancy

The risks associated with diabetes in pregnancy are significant and extend to both the mother and the baby. Several studies have established a clear link between hyperglycaemia during pregnancy and adverse outcomes (Shah et al 2020). Therefore, optimal BGL control during pregnancy can improve maternal and neonatal outcomes. However, the controversy surrounding diagnosis and management of GDM persists. Although there is correlation between OGTT glucose levels and adverse pregnancy outcomes, further research into the real determinants of adverse pregnancy outcomes is required. The current management is not able to normalise diabetic pregnancy outcomes even when achieving current glucose therapeutic targets or by using continuous glucose monitoring tools throughout pregnancy (Carreiro et al 2018).

The adverse maternal outcomes include preeclampsia, caesarean section, birth trauma, and breastfeeding difficulties. Adverse infant outcomes include stillbirth, macrosomia or being small for gestational age, premature birth, and long-term effects like childhood overweight and metabolic factors that may increase the risk of type 2 diabetes and cardiovascular disease as the child matures into adulthood. Babies born to mothers with diabetes, particularly those with high birth weight, are at risk of complications such as shoulder dystocia, jaundice, and long-term health issues such as obesity and glucose intolerance (Buchanan et al 2012). In Australia, women with preexisting type 1 or type 2 diabetes, gestational diabetes, and Aboriginal and Torres Strait Islander mothers with diabetes face higher risks of various adverse outcomes such as caesarean section and preeclampsia, highlighting the need for careful monitoring and management (see Online resources: Australian Pregnancy Care Guidelines).

Risk factors for GDM

Identifying women at risk of GDM during pregnancy enables maternity professionals to offer timely screening for the condition. Factors contributing to an increased risk of GDM include increased maternal age, increased weight (especially increased BMI), polycystic ovarian syndrome, previous history of gestational diabetes or high birth weight, family history of diabetes (especially maternal family history), ethnic origin (with higher risk in certain ethnic groups such as Indian subcontinent) and migration status (being a migrant is associated with increased risk) (Seghieri et al 2020).

Screening for GDM

There is variability among guidelines on whether to test all pregnant women or only those with risk factors for hyperglycaemia. However, in Australia and New Zealand, the Australasian Diabetes in Pregnancy Society (ADIPS) recommends universal testing of all women for GDM at 24–28 weeks gestation (see Nankervis et al 2014; Online resources).

In New Zealand and Australia, a two-stage approach to testing is advised, adding first-trimester testing for hyperglycaemia for women with risk factors (Tieu et al 2017). Glycated haemoglobin (HbA1c) and fasting blood glucose are suitable tests in the first trimester. Suggested thresholds for identifying hyperglycaemia in early pregnancy are HbA1c $\geq$ 41 mmol/mol (5.9%) and fasting plasma glucose of 6.1 to 6.9 mmol/L. The implementation of this first-trimester screening has demonstrated that early detection and management of hyperglycaemia is associated with decreased risk of preeclampsia (Ryan et al 2018). However, Lowe et al's 2012 Hypoglycemia and Hyperglycemia and Adverse Pregnancy Outcome (HAPO) study demonstrated that glucose values is a better indicator for adverse outcomes such as neonatal birth weight (> 90%) compared to HbA1c in GDM.

Between 24 and 28 weeks gestation, testing for hyperglycaemia is advised for all women. Repeat testing is recommended for women tested early due to risk factors who had a normal result initially.

The diagnostic thresholds for diabetes and gestation diabetes in Australia are based on the World Health Organization (WHO) and International Association of Diabetes and Pregnancy Study Groups (IADPSG)

TABLE 13.2 WHO/IADPSG criteria for diagnosis of diabetes in pregnancy

WHO/IADPSG criteria	mmol/ml/dl dose (diabetes)
Fasting plasma glucose	≥ 7.0 mmol/l (126 mg/dl)
2-hour plasma glucose	≥ 11.1 mmol/l (200 mg/dl) following a 75 g oral glucose load
Random plasma glucose	≥ 11.1 mmol/l (200 mg/ dl) in the presence of diabetes symptoms

WHO/IADPSG criteria	mmol/ml/dl dose (gestational diabetes)
Fasting plasma glucose	5.1–6.9 mmol/l (92–125 mg/dl)
1-hour plasma glucose	≥ 10.0 mmol/l (180 mg/dl) following a 75 g oral glucose load
2-hour plasma glucose	8.5–11.0 mmol/l (153–199 mg/dl) following a 75 g oral glucose load

recommendation (IADPSG 2010; Carreiro et al 2018) (Table 13.2).

Management approaches for diabetes in pregnancy

The general aims of treatment of all types of diabetes are to maintain glucose at physiological levels using insulin, **antihyperglycaemic drugs**, or exercise and dietary regimens; and to avoid or delay acute symptoms and long-term complications.

Standard pharmacological treatment plans are:

Type 1: daily insulin, with regimen and doses determined by monitored BGLs

Type 2: dietary and weight control and/or an antihyperglycaemic drug with insulin as necessary

GDM: dietary and exercise, and/or an antihyperglycaemic drug (typically metformin) with insulin as necessary. People with diabetes need to be taught to self-monitor BGL and to self-administer insulin and/or antihyperglycaemic drug(s).

Treatment for diabetes preferably involves a multidisciplinary team, including an endocrinologist, pharmacist, podiatrist, optometrist, diabetes educator, obstetrician, midwife, and dietitian as required. Regular monitoring is recommended of eyes, blood pressure, feet, blood lipids and kidney functions, and specialised care is required during concurrent illness, surgery, travel, and other stressful times.

Management of hyperglycaemia during pregnancy (due to preexisting diabetes or GDM) is crucial for the wellbeing of both the mother and the baby. The primary goal is to maintain BGLs within target ranges to prevent adverse outcomes. Diabetes Australia has specified maximum levels for fasting BGL (6–8 mmol/L) and glycated haemoglobin (6.5–7.5%) in non-pregnant people (see Online resources). In pregnancy, the target glycaemic goals for women with GDM are to keep the fasting glucose ≤ 5–5.3 mmol/l (90–95 mg/dl), and either 1-hour post-meal ≤ 7.8 mmol/l (140 mg/dl), or 2 hours post-meal ≤ 6.7 mmol/l (120 mg/dl) (Alfadhli 2015).

In addition to managing BGLs during pregnancy, it is important to monitor fetal growth and wellbeing. Women with any form of diabetes are at an increased risk of developing preeclampsia. Regular blood pressure monitoring, urine tests, and clinical assessments during prenatal visits help detect and manage preeclampsia early. Discussions about the optimal timing, place, and mode of birth should occur in the antenatal period and be personalised to the woman's specific context. The healthcare team will consider factors such as blood glucose control, fetal growth, the history of any previous births, and the overall health of both the mother and the fetus when making recommendations.

To women with type 1 or type 2 diabetes, ADIPS recommends the following to reduce the risk of preeclampsia:

- aspirin 100–150 mg daily with evening meal (unless contraindicated) from 12 weeks gestation and ceased at 36 weeks gestation
- calcium supplementation (total 1.5 g daily including dietary calcium) from 12 weeks gestation
- blood pressure measurement and urinalysis at each antenatal visit (Rudland 2020).

During labour and birth (including planned CS), it is important to closely monitor BGLs. Any hyperglycaemia during labour and birth should be managed by insulin.

Postnatal management

After the birth of the placenta, the physiological insulin resistance typically diminishes as the placental hormones are no longer present. Consequently, the demand for insulin in the postnatal period tends to decrease, but it is important to monitor the mother for any signs of hypoglycaemia. In women with GDM, insulin and oral hypoglycaemics are ceased at birth. During the early postnatal period, the woman may be required to monitor her BGLs for one day, or follow the internal protocol of her birthing place, which may involve taking a random BGL measurement. However, OGTT should be repeated at 6 weeks postnatal to assess whether they return to normal levels. Women with GDM have a higher risk for later development of diabetes, especially diabetes type 2.

For the woman with type 1 or 2 diabetes, it is important to continue blood glucose monitoring and adjustment of her treatment accordingly, as dosage reductions in insulin and/or oral hypoglycaemic agents after the birth will be required. Schedule postnatal check-ups to assess the mother's overall health, including diet and weight, medication review and stabilisation/return of BGL to pre-pregnancy levels, breastfeeding, exercise levels and mental health. Note that lactation onset occurs later in women with type 1 diabetes, and there is an even greater delay in those with poor glucose control. However, once established, lactation persists. Insulin requirements therefore are generally lower in women who breastfeed, most likely due to glucose being used for milk production.

A comprehensive postnatal review should be planned for 6 weeks. Additionally, women who have had GDM should be screened for type 2 diabetes within 6 weeks to 6 months postpartum, with a 2-hour 75 g OGTT; before a future pregnancy; and every 3 years or more often, depending on the presence of other risk factors for type 2 diabetes. The latter group are at a higher risk of developing diabetes and cardiovascular disorders later in life.

Blood glucose monitoring

Large-scale trials have shown that tight control of BGLs reduces microvascular risks of retinopathy, nephropathy and neuropathy, and other cardiovascular complications. Due to the relatively short period of pregnancy, microvascular risks are negligible in GDM or at least there are no reports in this area. However, tight BGL monitoring is vital to decrease the risk associated with gestation such as preeclampsia. To maintain **euglycaemia**, BGLs are regularly determined by blood glucose monitoring (self-monitored blood glucose), by test strips and blood glucose meters. Historically, urine glucose levels were monitored but this is considered inadequate for good management.

Continuous glucose monitoring is a novel way of recording BGLs without constant finger pricks. Instead, a disposable sensor inserted under the skin, which measures the BGLs in the interstitial fluid. The person can then make necessary adjustments to their medication, diet, and exercise.

Prescribed, over-the-counter, and social drugs can all affect BGL and alter diabetic control (Table 13.3), leading to many potential drug interactions with insulin and antihyperglycaemic agent(s).

TABLE 13.3 Some drugs reported to cause hyperglycaemia or hypoglycaemia

HYPERGLYCAEMIA	HYPOGLYCAEMIA
(Hence, insulin requirements may need to be increased)	*(Hence, insulin requirements may need to be reduced)*
Antipsychotics (some)	α-blockers
Tricyclic antidepressants	Aspirin (analgesic doses)
Glucagon	β-blockers (non-selective)
Glucocorticosteroids	Disopyramide
Progestogens (oral contraceptives)	Insulins
Protease inhibitors	Monoamine oxidase inhibitors
Sympathomimetics (adrenaline [epinephrine], high-dose salbutamol)	Oral hypoglycaemics (OHA)
Thyroid hormones	Quinine
Social drugs: amphetamines, cocaine, psychedelics, caffeine drinks (large amounts), marijuana, tobacco/nicotine	Sulfonamides
	Social drugs: ethanol (alcohol)

Note: β-blockers may mask the symptoms of hypoglycaemia.
Sources: Australian Medicines Handbook 2021; MIMS Annual Online (see Online resources).

CLINICAL FOCUS BOX 13.1

Insulin in pregnancy

Morgan is a 32-year-old woman having her third child. She had GDM in her second pregnancy 3 years ago, and following that pregnancy was diagnosed with type 2 diabetes. Prior to pregnancy she used metformin 500 mg daily with her evening meal and has continued with this so far. Up to 32 weeks gestation, her BGL remained within the desired range (< 5.5 mmol/L fasting sugar first thing in the morning, and < 6.7 mmol/L 2 hours after each meal). However, her BGLs started to increase above the recommended ranges, so low-dose insulin was commenced at 33 weeks gestation: 4 units of NovoRapid (insulin aspart) with each meal and 20 units of Protophane (isophane) at night.

Morgan's labour was induced at 39 weeks and resulted in a forceps-assisted birth of a healthy 3.8 kg baby boy, Dylan, who was observed for hypoglycaemia. Morgan is advised to breastfeed Dylan more regularly to avoid hypoglycaemia risk in the baby.

(See Online resources: ADIPS.)

KEY POINTS

Pancreatic hormones and diabetes mellitus

- Maintaining BGLs within target ranges during pregnancy is vital to avoid complications like preeclampsia and ensure the wellbeing of both mother and baby.

- After the birth, a follow-up oral glucose tolerance test at 6 weeks postpartum is recommended. Continuous BGL monitoring and treatment adjustment are essential for women with type 1 or type 2 diabetes, focusing on overall health, breastfeeding, and long-term diabetes risk.

13.2 Management of gestational diabetes

In GDM, the first management approach is diet and exercise to maintain **blood glucose levels** at normal physiological levels. If it is not possible to maintain BGLs within the normal range, there might be a need for pharmacotherapy with oral metformin and/or parenteral insulin (Simmons et al 2023).

Drugs for gestational diabetes

Metformin is recommended as second-line therapy when management with diet and exercise has not consistently achieved the desired BGL targets. If glycaemic management is not achieved by metformin, insulin is advised (DMs 13.1, 13.2).

Insulin

By the time type 1 diabetes is diagnosed, people usually have no functioning pancreatic islet tissue remaining, and so are dependent on an exogenous source of insulin as lifesaving, lifelong therapy (hence the term 'insulin-dependent diabetes mellitus'). While other anti-hyperglycaemics may be used as first-line management for people with type 2 diabetes and GDM, exogenous insulin may be advised to achieve BGLs in target ranges. Some guidelines recommend insulin as the first-line therapy in GDM.

Insulin formulations

Early sources of insulin were beef (bovine) or pig (porcine) pancreas. Preparations available in Australia now are either human insulin (synthesised by chemical alteration of porcine insulin or by recombinant DNA technology) or bovine insulin (rarely used now), which differs from human insulin by three amino acids. Insulins produced by recombinant DNA technology are identical to insulin produced by the human pancreas (DM 13.1).

DRUG MONOGRAPH 13.1
Human insulin

Indications

People with type 1 diabetes require lifelong insulin replacement. Outcomes are best when BGL, diet and lifestyle factors are controlled, and a multidisciplinary clinical team is advised when available.

Various formulations of human or bovine insulins are available, with differing pharmacokinetic characteristics. The dosage regimen is determined by results of self-monitored BGLs.

Dosing needs to be regularly altered to accommodate changes in health status, activity levels, diet, and the stage of pregnancy. Insulin is indicated in type 1 diabetes, and in type 2 diabetes during emergencies, in stress situations, or as an adjunct to treatment with oral hypoglycaemic agents (OHAs). In GDM, insulin is indicated if BGLs have not been managed with diet and/or metformin. The wide variety of insulins available (including combination mixtures) allows titration of dose to achieve tight BGL control depending on the woman's needs and lifestyle.

Pharmacokinetics

The onset, time to peak, and duration of action depend on types and proportions of insulin used. Insulin injected SC is gradually leached from the injection site into the bloodstream and will circulate to tissues where it acts, especially in liver, muscles, and fat. Insulin is metabolised and inactivated rapidly in most tissues of the body. The disulfide bonds are cleaved, then the peptide chains are broken down into amino acids. However, biological activity continues much longer.

Drug interactions

Many drugs (prescribed, OTC, and social) can affect BGL and thus interact with insulin and impair diabetes control – in particular, corticosteroids and β-blockers (Table 13.3). Dosage adjustments of insulin may be necessary. β-blockers can mask the symptoms of hypoglycaemia and prolong it by blocking gluconeogenesis. The use of corticosteroids for lung maturation in preterm babies is common practice, necessitating consideration of associated hyperglycaemia and its impact on the management of hyperglycaemia in pregnant women when receiving them. β-blockers are also commonly used in pregnancy for managing hypertension. It is recommended to consider maternal and neonatal glycaemic control if the mother is on β-blockers.

Continued

DRUG MONOGRAPH 13.1
Human insulin—cont'd

Adverse reactions

Rare with human insulin. Allergic reactions and lipodystrophy (breakdown of subcutaneous fat) can occur. Overdose is indicated by symptoms of hypoglycaemia: faintness, sweating, and tremor.

Warnings and contraindications

Insulin requirements may increase in acute trauma or illness and during prolonged surgery. Insulin is contraindicated with hypoglycaemia or hypersensitivity to human insulin solutions. Changes in type, brand, or species of insulin should be made cautiously. Insulin is considered safe during pregnancy and breastfeeding. Numerous studies and clinical guidelines support the safety and effectiveness of insulin use during pregnancy (Amigó et al 2022).

Dosage and administration

Dosage depends on the person's weight, diet, and activity levels, and on the type of insulin and regimen used. Dosage is individualised by monitoring BGLs.

Time-course of formulations

Insulins have been formulated in different ways to alter their pharmacokinetic properties. In the very-short-acting and new long-acting analogues, minor changes are made in the amino acid sequences of the protein (Fig 13.1). The pharmacodynamic actions and mechanisms are unaltered. Most ampoules contain 100 IU/mL. The range of formulations available allows titration of dosage to optimise BGL control and minimise fluctuations

(Table 13.4). Insulin lispro, aspart, and detemir are approved for use in pregnancy.

Formulations are described as very-short-acting or ultra-short-acting (or rapid), short-acting, intermediate-acting, or long-acting, as follows:

- *Ultra-short-acting synthetic analogues:* Insulin lispro, insulin aspart, and insulin glulisine. These are also called 'post-prandial', very-short, or rapid. They are administered as a 'bolus' immediately before or after

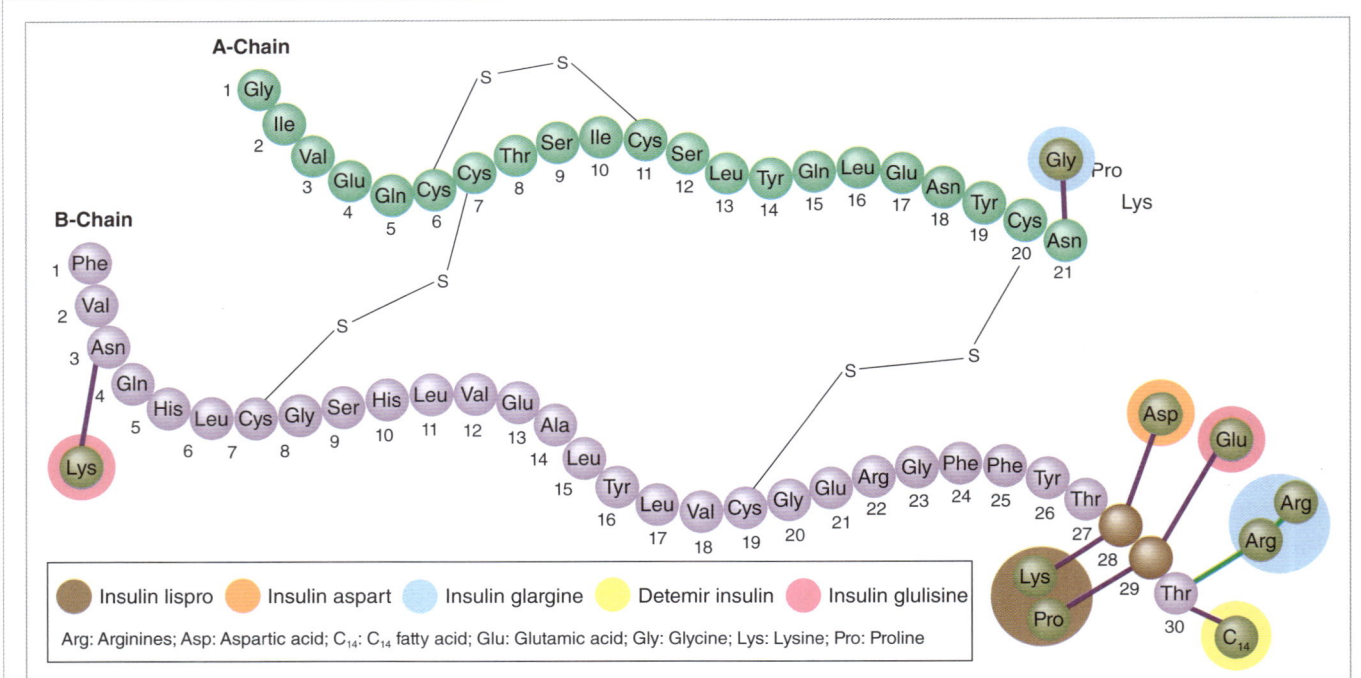

Structure of human insulin, and modifications to make insulin analogues

● Insulin lispro ● Insulin aspart ● Insulin glargine ● Detemir insulin ● Insulin glulisine

Arg: Arginines; Asp: Aspartic acid; C₁₄: C₁₄ fatty acid; Glu: Glutamic acid; Gly: Glycine; Lys: Lysine; Pro: Proline

FIGURE 13.1 Purple line denotes substitution of an amino acid; green line denotes addition.

Source: Adapted from Heile & Schneider 2012.

TABLE 13.4 Characteristics of insulin preparations after subcutaneous administration

INSULINS	ONSET (h)	PEAK EFFECT (h)	DURATION OF ACTION (h)
Ultra-short-acting (rapid)[a]			
Insulin lispro and insulin aspart	0.25	1–3	3–5
Insulin glulisine	0.25	1	3–5
Short-acting[a]			
Neutral insulin	0.5	2–3	6–8
Intermediate-acting			
Isophane insulin (NPH insulin)	1–2.5	4–12	16–24
Long-acting			
Insulin glargine (basal insulin analogue) (100 IU/mL)	1–2	(no peak)	24
Insulin glargine (basal insulin analogue) (300 IU/mL)	1–6	(no peak)	24–36
Insulin detemir	1–2	3–14	12–24
Typical combination[#]			
Neutral human insulin (30%) and isophane insulin (70%) (Humulin 30/70)	0.5–1	2–12	16–24

[a] These soluble insulins may be administered IV under medical supervision. Intravenously, the onset of action is within 10–30 minutes, peak effect is within 15–30 minutes, and duration of action is 30–60 minutes. # Other combinations have properties combining those of the constituents.
Note that the time-course of action may vary among individuals, or at different times in the same person, and is dependent on site of injection, blood supply, body temperature, physical activity, etc.
Note **insulin lispro, aspart, and detemir** are approved for use in pregnancy.
Sources: Australian Medicines Handbook 2021; MIMS Annual Online (see Online resources); product information from Novo Nordisk.

a meal. Short duration of action (3–5 hours). People with type 1 diabetes usually require concurrent use of an intermediate- or long-acting product to provide basal insulin activity

- *Short- and intermediate-acting (the early insulins):* Neutral insulin, insulin zinc suspension, isophane insulin (also known as neutral protamine Hagedorn, NPH)
- *'Basal'/long-acting insulins:* Their long, flat absorption profiles give them a more reproducible effect than older formulations. *Insulin glargine* has a slightly different amino acid sequence – after injection, microcrystals form in the tissues and insulin is slowly released. It may cause pain on injection and must not be mixed with other insulins. *Insulin detemir* has a fatty acid compound attached to the insulin molecule, providing slow release. Detemir

formulations may cause local reactions but are less likely than other insulins to cause weight gain

- *Pre-mixed commercial combination formulations:* These are 30/70 or 50/50 mixtures of short-acting plus intermediate-acting insulins, or ultra-short plus long-acting insulins, providing varying pharmacokinetic characteristics dependent on proportions in the mixture. They suffer the disadvantage of all fixed-dose combinations, namely that the dose of an individual component cannot be varied when needed.

Insulin administration

Routes of administration

Insulins are supplied in vials, usually 100 IU/mL, for use with a syringe, or prepacked in cartridge 'pens', facilitating

---

CLINICAL FOCUS BOX 13.2

Insulin formulations for use in pregnancy
Rapid-acting insulin (Novorapid, Humalog)

- A safe starting dose is 4 units after meals.
- Increase the dose by 2–4 units once or twice a week until the post-meal BGL is below 7.4 mmol/L.
- It is best to give the dose 15–30 minutes before the meal, so the peak effect coincides with the glucose peak from the absorbed carbohydrate.

Pre-mixed insulin (Novomix 30, Humalog Mix 25, Humalog Mix 50, Mixtard 30/70)

This insulin is a combination of rapid-acting insulin and a slower acting insulin.

- A safe starting dose is 4 or 6 units once or twice a day.
- Increase the dose by 2–4 units once a week until the pre-breakfast and post-meal BGLs are below 5.0 mmol/L and 7.4 mmol/L respectively.
- It is best to give the dose 15–30 minutes before the meal, so the peak effect coincides with the glucose peak from the absorbed carbohydrate.

Long-acting insulin (Protaphane, Lantus, Levemir)

These insulins have a duration of action of up to 24 hours and control the pre-meal BGLs.

- A safe starting dose is 4 or 6 units at bedtime or twice a day.
- Increase the dose by 2–4 units once a week until the pre-breakfast glucose levels are below 5.0 mmol/L
  1. **Lantus** has a flat, reliable absorption profile which lasts 24 hours. It is administered once daily, best given at bedtime.
  2. **Levemir** is a reliably absorbed insulin that lasts 20–22 hours. It is given at bedtime.
  3. **Protaphane** lasts for 16 hours and is less reliable in its absorption than Lantus. It is given at bedtime.

Source: Adapted from Diabetes Hub, https://www.diabeteshub.com.au/info-for-medical-professionals/outpatient-care-general-practice/gestational/insulin

injection and improving convenience and adherence. Vials or cartridges of insoluble preparations should be rotated and inverted gently before a dose is withdrawn, to resuspend the protein. Vigorous shaking or freezing could denature the protein. Insulin stocks not in use should be refrigerated (2–8°C), but the vial or cartridge currently in use is stable at room temperature (Khurana et al 2019). The older-type insulin formulations were all chemically compatible and could be mixed, but some newer forms cannot, especially insulins detemir and glargine.

Insulin (short-acting) is usually administered 'ac, SC' – that is, before meals (15–30 minutes before), subcutaneously. Injection sites are alternated, rotating around the abdomen and thighs, to minimise adverse local effects from injections. In an emergency (diabetic ketoacidosis), short-acting insulins can be administered IV by infusion or IM.

Portable battery-operated, computer-programmed pumps delivering insulin via an implanted SC catheter may improve diabetic control. The insulin pump does not monitor the BGL but is programmed based on the person's estimated daily insulin needs, diet, and physical exercise. Pumps are expensive, subject to mechanical failure and require careful maintenance. Since June 2022, the National Diabetes Services Scheme provides access to subsidised continuous glucose monitoring (CGM) and flash glucose monitoring (Flash GM) products for eligible individuals (all people with type 1 diabetes). Additionally, pregnant women can access subsidies for blood glucose monitoring and management equipment (see Online resources). Women on insulin can get insulin needles for free from the pharmacy.

Insulin dosage and regimens

There is no standard dose of insulin. People are taught to carry out self-monitoring of blood glucose, and to adjust their insulin doses to avoid hypoglycaemia or hyperglycaemia. A typical daily dose might be in the order of 0.7 IU/kg (reflecting the average pancreatic production of about 50 IU per day) split into 2–4 injections and, possibly, two or three different types of insulin in a non-pregnant individual. Treatment programs need to be reviewed and adjusted regularly, depending on gestational age, illness, surgery, development of anti-insulin antibodies, concomitant administration of drugs, changes in lifestyle, missing a meal, or doing unexpected exercise. Regimens are as follows:

- *Basal–bolus regimen:* A bolus dose of short-acting insulin is given before each meal, plus some intermediate- or long-acting insulin at bedtime. This regimen is preferred. While it is demanding, requiring multiple daily injections, it mimics well the body's natural rhythms of insulin release.
- *Split–mixed regimen:* The total daily dose in units is estimated, and this is split between 1/3 short-acting and 2/3 intermediate- or long-acting insulins, with 2/3 of the total mixture given before breakfast and the other 1/3 before the evening meal.

Dosage in altered circumstances

As well as regular self-monitoring of BGL and subsequent adjustment of insulin dosage, there are many clinical situations in which dosage is altered:

- *After birth:* Insulin requirements may drop for 24–72 hours postpartum and slowly return to pre-pregnancy levels in about 6 weeks (CFB 13.2)
- *Exercising:* Requires increased caloric intake and/or reduced insulin dose
- *Other illnesses:* Metabolic instability can lead to hyperglycaemia and diabetic ketoacidosis; insulin requirements usually increase by 15–20%

DRUGS AT A GLANCE
Antihyperglycaemic drugs in pregnancy

PHARMACOLOGICAL GROUP AND EFFECT	KEY EXAMPLES	CLINICAL USE
Insulins Increase the uptake of glucose into cells = increased glucose metabolism Decrease the body's production of glucose Decrease lipolysis	Ultra-short-acting -aspart, -lispro	Treat type 1, type 2 diabetes mellitus, and GDM Control blood glucose concentration
	Short-acting -neutral	
	Intermediate-acting -isophane	
	Long-acting (basal) - detemir, -glargine	
	Biphasic insulins (mixed) combinations with various ratios of ultra-short/neutral/isophane insulins	
Biguanide Decreases glucose production in the liver Increases peripheral utilisation of glucose	Metformin	Treat type 2 diabetes mellitus and GDM

- *Vomiting:* Sugary drinks should replace solid food; if vomiting lasts more than 6 hours, offer admission for hospital care
- *Fasting, including for surgery:* Some basal insulin is still required, plus some IV or SC glucose
- *International travel:* People on insulin are advised to take copies of prescriptions and medical records, plus double their anticipated insulin needs and carbohydrate snacks.

KEY POINTS

Management of GDM

- In GDM, the first management approach is diet and exercise to maintain blood glucose levels at normal physiological levels.

- Insulin is the preferred drug by clinicians/guidelines for management of GDM, and metformin is recommended as the second-line therapy.

13.3 Management of type 2 diabetes

In Australia, almost 1.2 million (4.6%) people have type 2 diabetes and the ratio of men to women is equal (AIHW 2021). The prevalence of type 2 diabetes is higher in Aboriginal and Torres Strait Islander people and in 2018–19, it was about 10.7% (51,900). Prior to pregnancy, 1–2 % of women have a diagnosis of diabetes with 30–50% being due to type 2 diabetes (Wang et al 2022).

In type 2 diabetes, generally some functioning pancreatic islet cells are available. There is reduced insulin production and secretion (especially the early phase after glucose load) and/or insulin resistance (the body does not respond to insulin effectively) because of receptor and post-receptor defects.

Risk factors for type 2 diabetes, as discussed previously, include age, obesity, family history, cardiovascular disease, hypokalaemia following the use of thiazide diuretics, and polycystic ovary syndrome. Being Aboriginal and Torres Strait Islander, low socioeconomic status, having GDM in a previous pregnancy, and hypertension are among the risk factors for women of reproductive age. The condition comes on gradually, with glucose intolerance often associated with hypertension and hyperlipidaemia (called metabolic syndrome). People with type 2 diabetes are at risk of long-term complications and of hyperosmolar coma, but diabetic ketoacidosis is rare.

Drugs for type 2 diabetes

In women with pregestational type 2 diabetes, during pregnancy, insulin is the drug of choice. However, usually metformin is recommended as OHA therapy unless contraindicated (as in renal, hepatic, or cardiac impairment). If glycaemic control is not achieved, insulin is the appropriate second-line agent during pregnancy. Antiglycaemic treatments for type 2 diabetes include sulfonylureas, DPP4 inhibitor, GLP-1 analogues, SGLT2 inhibitors, acarbose and pioglitazone. Combination products with two antihyperglycaemic drugs are available.

Metformin

Metformin, a biguanide, is the first-line treatment of type 2 diabetes (DM 13.2) either alone or in combination with other antidiabetic medications, including insulin. Metformin is usually continued lifelong in patients with type 2 diabetes unless contraindicated. Movement of metformin in the body during absorption in the GI tract, tissue distribution and renal elimination is mainly mediated by organic cation transporters (OCTs), which are Na+-independent electrogenic channels located in plasma membranes. OCTs are widely expressed in fetal and placental tissues, resulting in exposure of the fetus to metformin at the same plasma level of the mother. However, expression of OCTs at embryo is limited and therefore the use of metformin in first trimester is considered safe. It has been categorised as C by the TGA within the Australian categories for prescribing medicines (see Online resources). Currently there is lack of consensus for the use of metformin in pregnancy for treatment of type 2 diabetes or GDM. There have not been reports of teratogenicity of metformin use in pregnancy and in conclusion it has been considered an acceptable treatment for women with GDM in pregnancy (Tocci et al 2023).

Actions, mechanisms, and indications

Metformin's mechanism of action is not completely understood; however, it is known to:

- increase glucose uptake and utilisation in skeletal muscle (thus reducing insulin resistance)
- reduce glucose production in the liver (gluconeogenesis)
- reduce low- and very-low-density lipoproteins
- increase insulin sensitivity, via increased number of receptors and affinity for receptors.

Metformin does not affect the pancreatic B cells, so it does not increase insulin release and is unlikely to cause hypoglycaemia.

DRUG MONOGRAPH 13.2
Metformin

Metformin is a biguanide, an OHA. (For actions and mechanisms, see text.) It rarely causes hypoglycaemia or weight gain.

Indications

Metformin is indicated for treating uncomplicated type 2 diabetes, when diabetes is not controlled by diet and exercise. It may be given together with insulin or another OHA. It reduces the risk of diabetes-associated complications or mortality. It is also used to treat anovulation and cycle irregularity due to polycystic ovary syndrome. Despite the debates on metformin use in pregnancy, it has been considered safe in pregnancy and lactation and is used for managing GDM/diabetes in pregnancy by itself or in combination with insulin. Metformin could significantly decrease gestational weight gain for women with no significant reduction in neonatal birth weight.

There have been reports of higher therapeutic failure with metformin, requiring additional insulin treatment to maintain the maternal BGL at the recommended levels (Tocci et al 2023; Elmaraezy et al 2017). The use of metformin is not recommended when the mother has some risks of exposure to an ischaemic environment, such as gestational hypertension or preeclampsia, as it may contribute to growth restriction or acidosis (Tocci et al 2023). It has been reported that children exposed to metformin had a greater MBI z-score which may increase the risk of cardiometabolic problems over the course of life. It is therefore suggested that metformin is to be used with caution in pregnancy (Hanem et al 2019).

Pharmacokinetics

Metformin is absorbed after an oral dose along the length of the GIT. It has a short half-life (5–10 hours) and is excreted unchanged in the urine (Table 13.5).

Drug interactions

Drug interactions occur with alcohol (increased risk of lactic acidosis), and any drugs that impair glucose tolerance, cause hyper- or hypoglycaemia, or reduce clearance of metformin (including cimetidine, dolutegravir, topiramate, trimethoprim, and warfarin). BGLs should be monitored whenever another drug is introduced, as dosage adjustment may be necessary (see also Table 13.3).

Adverse reactions

Adverse reactions include gastrointestinal upsets such as nausea, vomiting, anorexia, and diarrhoea (common) and, rarely, lactic acidosis, acute hepatitis, or vitamin B12-deficiency anaemia.

Warnings and contraindications

Use with caution in people with renal or GIT problems and conditions affecting BGLs. Use is avoided in people with metformin hypersensitivity, severe liver or kidney disease, lactic acidosis, cardiac disorders, severe burns, dehydration, or severe infections, in people in diabetic coma or with ketoacidosis, and in those who have recently had major surgery or trauma. The Australian Pregnancy Safety classification is C; and it is a class B in America. However, research has demonstrated safety and efficacy of metformin in managing GDM in pregnancy (Bastian et al 2022).

The amount of metformin in breast milk is between 0.18% and 1.08% of the mother's dose, and this dose is much less than the usual 10% level of concern.

Dosage and administration

Doses are taken orally with meals; dosage is individualised and based on BGL. Initial dosage is low to minimise GIT adverse effects: 500 mg once or twice daily, gradually increasing to 1 g three times daily if necessary; or extended-release form once daily, increasing to maximum of 2 g/day.

Currently, metformin is contraindicated in people at risk of lactic acidosis – that is, those with liver disease, acidosis, and those taking alcohol or drugs that raise metformin levels. It can be administered cautiously in low doses to people with mild renal disease provided treatment is closely monitored.

OHAs not used in pregnancy

The following are oral hypoglycaemic medications used for type 2 diabetes which are not considered suitable in pregnancy. There are not enough data on the safety of these medications in pregnancy. Metformin, glyburide, and glipizide appear to be compatible with breastfeeding.

Sulfonylureas

Glibenclamide, glipizide, gliclazide, and glimepiride are sulfonylureas drugs. Their mechanism of action is to bind to receptors and block ATP-sensitive potassium channels (K-ATP), thus blocking potassium efflux and causing cell depolarisation, calcium entry and insulin secretion from pancreatic B cells. Sulfonylureas also increase the number of insulin receptors, decrease insulin uptake by peripheral tissues, and reduce hepatic glycogenolysis.

TABLE 13.5   Antihyperglycaemic drugs: Pharmacokinetics and usual adult doses

DRUG	ROUTE	PEAK IN PLASMA (h)	HALF-LIFE (h)	PROTEIN BINDING	USUAL ADULT MAINTENANCE DOSE[a]	COMMENTS
Biguanide						
Metformin	Oral	2–3	3	Not bound	500–1000 mg bd or tid	Risk of lactic acidosis. Take with food to reduce nausea and vomiting. (R) Not metabolised
Sulfonylureas						
Glibenclamide	Oral	2–6	2–10	99%	2.5–20 mg/day	(H) (R) (A)
Gliclazide	Oral	4–6	12	94%	30–320 mg/day (max single dose 160 mg)	(H) (R)
Glimepiride	Oral	2.5	5–8	> 99%	1–4 mg once/day	(R) (A)
Glipizide	Oral	2	2–4	98%	5–40 mg before meals in divided doses	(H) (R)
Dipeptidylpeptidase-4 (DPP-4) inhibitors (gliptins)						
Alogliptin	Oral	1–2	21	20%	25 mg/day	Used in combination with other antihyperglyceamic agents or as monotherapy; lower dose in moderate-to-severe renal failure (A: saxagliptin)
Linagliptin	Oral	1.5	3-phase	90%	5 mg/day	
Saxagliptin	Oral	2	2.5	Not bound	5 mg/day	
Sitagliptin	Oral	1–4	12.4	Low (38%)	100 mg/day	
Vildagliptin	Oral	1.75	2–3	9%	50–100 mg/day	
Glucagon-like peptide-1 (GLP-1) receptor agonists						
Dulaglutide	Subcutaneous	48 h	120	N/A	1.5 mg once weekly	Used in combination with other antihyperglycaemic agents; avoid in severe kidney impairment
Exenatide	Subcutaneous	2.1	2.4	N/A	5–10 microgram bd, or 2 mg once weekly	
Liraglutide	Subcutaneous	8–12	13	98%	0.6–1.8 mg/day SC	
Thiazolidinediones (TZD)						
Pioglitazone	Oral	2–4	5–23	> 99%	15–45 mg/day	
Sodium-glucose co-transporter 2 (SGLT2) inhibitors						
Dapagliflozin	Oral	2	13	91%	10 mg once daily with or without meals	Efficacy is reduced in renal impairment
Empagliflozin	Oral	1.3–3	21	20%	10–25 mg/day	
Ertugliflozin	Oral	0.5–1.5	11–17	94–96%	5–15 mg daily	
Alpha 1 glucosidase inhibitor						
Acarbose	Oral	1	2	< 2% absorbed	50–200 mg tid with meals	Most effective if given with high-fibre diet

A = active metabolites; bd = twice daily; H = hepatic impairment leads to increased risk of hypoglycaemia; N/A = not available or not applicable; R = renal impairment leads to increased risk of hypoglycaemia; tid = three times daily.
A = May be given as divided doses.
Source: Adapted from data in Medsafe website and Australian Medicines Handbook 2021. Product information sheets should be consulted for detailed dosing advice.

Common adverse effects include hypoglycaemia, weight gain, GIT and taste disturbances, and rashes. Serious blood disorders and allergic reactions occur rarely. Interactions are common with drugs involved with CYP2C9 metabolic pathways (see Australian Medicines Handbook 2021, Table D1-4 Drugs and CYP enzymes), alcohol, drugs that compete for protein-binding sites, and drugs affecting BGL.

All sulfonylurea drugs have the potential to induce severe hypoglycaemia. Animal studies have reported teratogenic effects. No teratogenic effects have been observed in neonates born to mothers who were using a sulfonylurea drug at the time of delivery; nor severe hypoglycaemia (4–10 days postnatal).

Incretin-based antihyperglycaemic agents

Incretins are peptide hormones that are released from the GIT in response to food; those currently known are GIP and GLP-1. People with type 2 diabetes have a markedly lowered response to incretins, so drugs such as sitagliptin, linagliptin, saxagliptin, vildagliptin and alogliptin that enhance incretin actions provide a different mode of action. In Australia they are currently only approved as add-on therapy, usually with metformin. Due to limited data, they are not recommended for use in pregnancy or lactation. The use of incretin-based antihyperglycaemic agents might be considered as a potential option; however, they may lead to fetal hypertrophy, which may cause several perinatal complications as well as neonatal hypoglycaemia (Lende et al 2020).

Thiazolidinediones (glitazones)

Pioglitazone is a thiazolidinedione. Its mechanism of action is via activation of the peroxisome proliferator-activated (PPAR)-gamma receptor, a nuclear receptor that regulates gene transcription, especially in adipocytes, via proteins including GLUT-4 (the principal glucose transporter protein), lipoprotein lipase and transporter, and binding proteins for fatty acids. They enhance the sensitivity of peripheral tissues and the liver to insulin and thus reduce insulin resistance. Circulating free fatty acid levels and hepatic glucose output are reduced.

Adverse effects include anaemia, peripheral oedema, weight gain and increased risk of heart failure and peripheral limb fractures; liver enzymes should be monitored. Pioglitazone appears to be safer with respect to cardiovascular risk factors, but prolonged use may be associated with increased risk of bladder cancer. Thiazolidinediones are pregnancy class C drugs with teratogenic potential, as PPAR-gamma is necessary for terminal differentiation of the trophoblast and placental vascularisation.

Alpha-glucosidase inhibitor: Acarbose

Acarbose is an oligosaccharide that inhibits α-glucosidase and thus delays digestion and absorption of carbohydrates in the small intestine, reducing glucose load. It is indicated as an adjunct to diet for the treatment of type 2 diabetes.

Drug interactions occur particularly with drugs that affect absorption in the intestine, such as digestive enzymes and cholestyramine. The most frequent adverse reactions are disturbed gut functions. If hypoglycaemia occurs, it should be treated with glucose rather than sucrose, as the absorption of sucrose will be impaired by the drug. As the drug is relatively new, use in pregnancy and renal impairment is not advised due to limited safety data (Table 13.5).

SGLT2 inhibitors: ('-flozin')

Dapagliflozin, empagliflozin and ertugliflozin are selective, reversible inhibitors of the sodium-glucose co-transporter 2 (SGLT2). SGLT2 causes reabsorption of glucose in the renal tubules. Inhibiting SGLT2 produces glycosuria (excess sugar in the urine) and osmotic diuresis, reduces hyperglycaemia, and reduces weight and fluid load. SGLT2 inhibitor actions affect renal function and do not depend on insulin secretion or sensitivity. Potential risks include urinary and genital tract infections, thirst, hypovolaemia, increased haematocrit, and bone fractures risks.

Hypoglycaemia

Hypoglycaemia in adults

Hypoglycaemia (BGL < 3.5 mmol/L) can occur rapidly from excess insulin and is also a common adverse effect of treatment with a sulfonylurea or dipeptidyl peptidase-4 (DPP4) inhibitor (Amiel et al 2019). Hypoglycaemia can also occur from unexpectedly high levels of exercise, inadequate food intake, or as an adverse effect of various drugs (Table 13.3). The early symptoms of a 'hypo' are faintness, anxiety, blurred vision, cold sweating, pallor, confusion, difficulty in concentrating, drowsiness, headache, nausea, increased pulse rate, shakiness, weakness, and increased appetite. Unless treated with an oral rapidly absorbed glucose source, this can lead to coma and death.

Treatment is with hyperglycaemic agents:

- In mild-to-moderate hypoglycaemia, a readily available sugar source such as jellybeans, honey or a sweet drink can be administered, followed by slowly absorbed complex carbohydrates such as bread or dried fruit.
- Glucose can be administered orally, in adults 10–20 g, repeated in 10 minutes if necessary.
- In severe hypoglycaemia, if the person is unconscious or cannot take oral glucose, glucagon is administered SC or IM.
- People at risk of developing hypoglycaemia may carry a glucagon injection kit, and their families or carers should know how to administer it. Glucagon is

commonly carried in ambulances and administered by paramedics.

- Glucose 50% solution may also be administered IV into the antecubital vein.

Unconscious people with hypoglycaemia should wake within 5–10 minutes of these therapies.

Hypoglycaemia in neonates

Postnatally, monitoring BGLs in the neonate is a crucial aspect of midwifery care. Neonatal BGLs reflect the balance between glucose supply and utilisation, and deviations from the normal range can have significant implications for the newborn's health. Neonates undergo physiological adaptations during the transition from the intrauterine to extrauterine environment, involving the switch from a continuous glucose supply from the placenta to the intermittent oral intake of nutrients. Infants born to mothers with diabetes/GDM (particularly when there has been persistent hyperglycaemia during pregnancy) are at an increased risk of hypoglycaemia due to excessive insulin production, with additional risk factors such as preterm birth, low birth weight, and macrosomia. Routine screening of BGL is conducted for at-risk infants. Other indications for monitoring of BGL in neonates include symptoms of hypoglycaemia, such as jitteriness, irritability, poor feeding, lethargy, or seizures.

Hypoglycaemia (BGL < 2.6 mmol/L) can occur in neonates. Maternal GDM and pre-pregnancy diabetes (type 1 and 2) are the main predisposing factors for neonatal hypoglycaemia. Other risk factors for neonatal hypoglycaemia are:

- prematurity
- large for gestational age (LGA) babies
- small for gestational age (SGA) babies
- other maternal medications such as beta-blockers
- birth trauma
- respiratory distress
- infection
- congenital metabolic disorders
- maternal substance abuse due to intrauterine growth restriction or other complications.

Interventions for neonatal hypoglycaemia may include early and frequent feeding, oral glucose gel (applied buccally) or, in cases of severe or persistent hypoglycaemia, intravenous administration of glucose. Untreated hypoglycaemia in the neonatal period can lead to adverse neurodevelopmental outcomes, including cognitive impairments and an increased risk of neurodevelopmental disorders.

KEY POINTS

Pharmacological management of hyperglycaemia in pregnancy

- Type 2 diabetes in a non-pregnant person is managed by lifestyle modification (diet and weight reduction) and, if necessary, OHA drugs.

- People with type 2 diabetes may require insulin at some stage.

- OHAs acting by different mechanisms are available: metformin, sulfonylureas, incretin mimetics and enhancers, and SGLT2 inhibitors; thiazolidinediones ('glitazones') and acarbose.

- Metformin is the only OHA used in pregnancy.

- Management of preexisting type 2 diabetes in pregnancy is by insulin and/or metformin.

- Insulin is the recommended drug for management of preexisting hyperglycaemia in pregnancy.

REVIEW EXERCISES

Fiona is pregnant for the first time and has just been diagnosed with GDM. Fiona would like you, her midwife, to describe how her diabetes may impact her pregnancy and understand any risks to herself and her baby.

1 How would you discuss with Fiona the complications that could occur from poorly managed GDM in her pregnancy, labour, and birth, and to her unborn baby?

2 What does a HbA1c of 7.8% at 30 weeks gestation mean? How would you explain the significance of this result to Fiona, including the options for ongoing pharmacological management?

3 At 32 weeks, Fiona started using insulin (Novarapid 4 units pre-meal and 6 units of Protaphane at bedtime). What is the mechanism of action of insulin in treating GDM? What are some common drug interactions and adverse reactions you should be aware of when counselling about this drug?

4 After the birth, you encourage Fiona to breastfeed her baby more regularly and to keep her warm. Why are frequent feeds and temperature regulation important? You also discuss with her the need for BGL checks of her baby and the threshold for treating hypoglycaemia. How do you administer glucose gel?

5 What specific advantages related to glycaemic stability may there be for both woman and infant related to initiation of breastfeeding immediately post birth? Discuss the related physiology and effects on glycaemic control for both, including the impact on pharmacological treatment.

REFERENCES

Alfadhli EM. Gestational diabetes mellitus. Saudi Med J. 2015 Apr;36(4):399-406. doi: 10.15537/smj.2015.4.10307. PMID: 25828275; PMCID: PMC4404472.

Amiel SA, Frier BM, Heller SR, et al. Hypoglycaemia, cardiovascular disease, and mortality in diabetes: epidemiology, pathogenesis, and management. Lancet Diabetes Endocrinol. 2019;7(5):385-396. doi: 10.1016/S2213-8587(18)30315-2.

Amigó J, Corcoy R. Type 1 diabetes and pregnancy: an update on glucose monitoring and insulin treatment. Endocrinol Diabetes Nutr. 2022;69:433-441. https://doi.org/10.1016/j.endien.2022.06.008 (accessed 19 March 2024)

Australian Medicines Handbook 2021. Australian Medicines Handbook, Adelaide: AMH.

Bastian B, Smithers LG, Davis W, et al. Metformin: a promising option for the management of gestational diabetes mellitus – exploring the benefits, challenges and clinical needs in the current management of gestational diabetes mellitus. Aust N Z J Obstet Gynaecol. 2022 Jun;62(3):453-456. doi: 10.1111/ajo.13513. Epub 2022 Apr 1. PMID: 35362563; PMCID: PMC9542201.

Buchanan T, Xiang A, Page K. Gestational diabetes mellitus: risks and management during and after pregnancy. Nat Rev Endocrinol. 2012;8:639–649. https://doi.org/10.1038/nrendo.2012.96 (accessed 19 March 2024)

Carreiro MP, Nogueira AI, Ribeiro-Oliveira A. Controversies and advances in gestational diabetes – an update in the era of continuous glucose monitoring. J Clin Med. 2018 Jan 25;7(2):11. doi: 10.3390/jcm7020011. PMID: 29370080; PMCID: PMC5852427.

Elmaraezy A, Abushouk AI, Emara A, et al. Effect of metformin on maternal and neonatal outcomes in pregnant obese non-diabetic women: a meta-analysis. Int J Reprod Biomed. 2017 Aug;15(8):461-470. PMID: 29082364; PMCID: PMC5653907.

Hanem LG, Salvesen Ø, Juliusson PB et al. Intrauterine metformin exposure and offspring cardiometabolic risk factors at 5–10 year follow-up: The PedMet Study (October 18, 2018). Lancet Child Adolesc Health. 2019 Mar;3(3):166-174. doi: 10.1016/S2352-4642(18)30385-7.

Heile M, Schneider D The evolution of insulin therapy in diabetes mellitus. J Family Practice. 2012;61(Suppl 5):S6–S12.

International Association of Diabetes and Pregnancy Study Groups Consensus Panel; Metzger BE, Gabbe SG, Persson B, et al. International association of diabetes and pregnancy study groups recommendations on the diagnosis and classification of hyperglycemia in pregnancy. Diabetes Care. 2010 Mar;33(3):676-682. doi: 10.2337/dc09-1848. PMID: 20190296; PMCID: PMC2827530.

Khurana G, Gupta V. Effect on insulin upon storage in extreme climatic conditions (temperature and pressure) and their preventive measures. J Soc Health Diabetes. 2019;7(01):006-010.

Lende M, Rijhsinghani A. Gestational diabetes: overview with emphasis on medical management. Int J Environ Res Public Health. 2020 Dec 21;17(24):9573. doi: 10.3390/ijerph17249573. PMID: 33371325; PMCID: PMC7767324. (accessed 19 March 2024) 2022, https://doi.org/10.1111/ajo.13513

Nankervis A, McIntyre H, Moses R, et al. ADIPS consensus guidelines for the testing and diagnosis of hyperglycaemia in pregnancy in Australia and New Zealand. 2014. https://www.adips.org/information-for-health-care-providersapproved.asp

Rudland VL, Price AL, Callaway L. ADIPS position paper on pre-existing diabetes and pregnancy. 2020. https://obgyn.onlinelibrary.wiley.com/doi/full/10.1111/ajo.13266

Ryan DK, Haddow L, Ramaesh A, et al. Early screening and treatment of gestational diabetes in high-risk women improves maternal and neonatal outcomes: a retrospective clinical audit. Diabetes Res Clin Pract. 2018 Oct;144:294-301. doi:10.1016/j.diabres.2018.09.013. Epub 2018 Sep 21. PMID: 30244050: 294-301.

Seghieri G, Di Cianni G, Seghieri M, et al. Risk and adverse outcomes of gestational diabetes in migrants: a population cohort study. Diabetes Res Clin Pract. 2020 May;163:108128. doi: 10.1016/j.diabres.2020.108128. Epub 2020 Apr 4. PMID: 32259610.

Shah BR, Sharifi F. Perinatal outcomes for untreated women with gestational diabetes by IADPSG criteria: a population-based study. BJOG. 2020 Jan;127(1):116–122. https://doi.org/10.1111/1471-0528.15964

Simmons D, Immanuel J, Hague WM, et al. TOBOGM Research Group. Treatment of gestational diabetes mellitus diagnosed early in pregnancy. N Engl J Med. 2023 Jun 8;388(23):2132-2144. doi: 10.1056/NEJMoa2214956. Epub 2023 May 5. PMID: 37144983.

Tieu J, McPhee AJ, Crowther CA, et al. Screening for gestational diabetes mellitus based on different risk profiles and settings for improving maternal and infant health. Cochrane Database Syst Rev. 2017;8(8):CD007222. https://doi.org/10.1002/14651858.CD007222.pub4

Tocci V, Mirabelli M, Salatino A, et al. Metformin in gestational diabetes mellitus: to use or not to use, that is the question. Pharmaceuticals. 2023 Sep;16(9):1318. https://doi.org/10.3390/ph16091318

Wang H, Li N, Chivese T, et al. IDF Diabetes Atlas: estimation of global and regional gestational diabetes mellitus prevalence for 2021 by International Association of Diabetes in pregnancy study group's criteria. Diabetes Res Clin Pract. 2022;183:109050.doi: 10.1016/j.diabres.2021.109050.

Wu R, Zhang Q, Li Z. A meta-analysis of metformin and insulin on maternal outcome and neonatal outcome in patients with gestational diabetes mellitus. J Matern Fetal Neonatal Med. 2024 Dec;37(1):2295809. doi:10.1080/14767058.2023.2295809

ONLINE RESOURCES

Australasian Diabetes in Pregnancy Society: http://adips.org (accessed 14 May 2021)

Australian Institute of Health and Welfare: https://www.aihw.gov.au/reports-statistics/health-conditions-disability-deaths/diabetes/overview (accessed 14 May 2021)

Australian Institute of Health and Welfare, Pregnancy care guidelines, Hyperglycaemia: https://www.health.gov.au/resources/pregnancy-care-guidelines/part-f-routine-maternal-health-tests/hyperglycaemia

Australian Diabetes Society, Type 2 diabetes management algorithm: https://diabetessociety.com.au/20200908%20T2D%20Management%20Algorithm%2003092020.pdf (accessed 14 May 2021)

Australian Government Department of Health and Aged Care, Australian Pregnancy Care Guidelines: https://www.health.gov.au/pregnancy-care-guidelines/hyperglycaemia.

Australian Medicines Handbook (2021): https://amhonline.amh.net.au/auth

Diabetes Australia: https://www.diabetesaustralia.com.au/ (accessed 24 January 2024)

Diabetes Australia, Best practice guidelines: www.diabetesaustralia.com.au/for-health-professionals/best-practice-guidelines (accessed 14 May 2021)

Diabetes Australia, ADIPS, ADS, ADEA: Diagnostic testing for gestational diabetes during COVID-19: https://www.diabetesaustralia.com.au/wp-content/uploads/Diagnostic-Testing-for-Gestational-Diabetes-during-COVID-19-advice.pdf (updated 7 May 2020)

MIMS Annual Online: https://www.mims.com.au/index.php/products/mims-annual (accessed 14 May 2021)

National Diabetes Services Scheme (NDSS): https://www.diabetessociety.com.au/national-diabetes-services-scheme-ndss/ (accessed 19 March 2024)

New Zealand Health Survey 2016–17: https://www.health.govt.nz/publication/annual-update-key-results-2016-17-new-zealand-health-survey (accessed 14 May 2021)

New Zealand Medicines and Medical Devices Safety Authority: https://www.medsafe.govt.nz/ (accessed 14 May 2021)

Therapeutic Goods Administration, Prescribing medicines in pregnancy database: https://www.tga.gov.au/products/medicines/find-information-about-medicine/prescribing-medicines-pregnancy-database (accessed 19 March 2023).

World Health Organization: https://www.who.int/news-room/fact-sheets/detail/diabetes (accessed 14 May 2021)

Australian Institute of Health and Welfare, Incidence of GDM in Australia: https://www.aihw.gov.au/reports/diabetes/incidence-of-gestational-diabetes-in-australia/contents/testing-and-diagnosis

— CHAPTER 14 —

THE THYROID

Kirsten Small, Maryam Bazargan

Key Abbreviations

hCG	human chorionic gonadotropin
T_3	tri-iodothyronine (liothyronine)
T_4	tetra-iodothyronine (thyroxine)
TRH	thyrotrophin-releasing hormone
TSH	thyroid-stimulating hormone (thyrotrophin)

Key Terms

antithyroid antibodies 279
goitre 278
hyperthyroidism 281
hypothyroidism 278
thyroglobulin 275
thyroid-stimulating hormone 274
thyrotrophin-releasing hormone 274
thyroxine 273
tri-iodothyronine 273

Chapter Focus

The thyroid gland performs roles that are central to normal physiological processes in many organ systems. The thyroid hormones thyroxine and tri-iodothyronine increase oxygen consumption and basal metabolic rate; accelerate carbohydrate, lipid and protein metabolism; increase sensitivity to sympathetic stimulation and promote growth; and are required for normal development of the central nervous system. Thyroid disorders are one of the more common medical complications in pregnancy and can complicate lactation. Replacement thyroid hormones are useful in treating hypothyroidism; and iodine (iodide ion), radioactive iodine, and antithyroid drugs are used to treat hyperthyroidism.

Key Drug Groups

Antithyroid drugs:
- thioureylenes: carbimazole (DM 14.2), propylthiouracil

Iodine:
- radioactive iodine

Thyroid hormones:
- thyroxine (DM 14.1), liothyronine

Learning Outcomes

- Describe the production, control, and effects of the thyroid hormones.
- Identify and describe common thyroid disorders and their impact on pregnancy and the neonate.
- Outline the therapeutic uses of thyroxine in pregnancy and the postnatal period.
- Describe the dose, frequency, monitoring, adverse effects, and storage requirements of thyroxine.
- List and discuss the use of antithyroid agents during pregnancy and lactation.
- Discuss considerations for collaborative multi-disciplinary care for a woman with a thyroid disorder.

CRITICAL THINKING SCENARIO

Alondra is a 28-year-old woman with a history of thyroid disease. This is Alondra's second pregnancy, and she is aware that effective management of her thyroid is crucial for the wellbeing of both herself and her baby. Alondra contacts her midwife at 8 weeks for advice as she is experiencing some worrying symptoms, including hyperemesis gravidarum and tachycardia. During her first pregnancy Alondra's thyrotoxicosis was successfully treated with low doses of antithyroid drugs.

1   What type of thyroid disorder do Alondra's symptoms suggest?

2   Related to this thyroid disorder, what other issues and symptoms might occur for Alondra in her first trimester and why?

3   What advice, testing, monitoring and medication should occur with respect to the management of Alondra's thyroid disorder and who should this involve?

4   What is the likely course during pregnancy and postnatally if Alondra's condition is well managed pharmacologically? Discuss the implications of being poorly managed for Alondra and her baby.

Introduction

The thyroid gland, one of the most richly vascularised tissues of the body, is in the anterior throat, in front of the trachea. It has right and left lateral lobes, linked by a narrow central section, the isthmus (Fig 14.1). The thyroid lobules contain follicles filled with a thick colloid containing thyroglobulin and lined with follicular cells, which produce the thyroid hormones **thyroxine** (tetra-iodothyronine [T_4]) and **tri-iodothyronine** (T_3). The thyroid also contains parafollicular (C) cells, which produce the hormone calcitonin. In 1914, the main thyroid hormone, T_4, was purified and crystallised, allowing detailed studies of its physiological actions. It was not until 1952, however, that T_3 was discovered.

T_4 and T_3 are essential for normal growth, development, and functioning of the central nervous system, starting in the fetal period, and continuing through life. The growth-promoting actions of thyroid hormones are said to be 'permissive' – that is, a normal T_4 level permits the cells of the body to function properly. Children who develop hypothyroidism after birth have increasingly slow bodily growth and delayed maturity. Additionally, thyroid hormone secretion determines basal metabolic rate by altering carbohydrate, lipid, and protein metabolism; promotes normal gastrointestinal tract (GIT), cardiovascular, reproductive, and temperature regulation functions; and increases sensitivity to sympathetic stimulation through increased expression of β-adrenoceptors.

14.1 Thyroid hormones

Synthesis, storage and secretion

T_4 and T_3 are amino acid hormones, being iodinated derivatives of tyrosine. The synthesis, storage, secretion,

and circulation of the hormones involve many sequential steps. During the process, the scene of action moves from the bloodstream into the follicle cell, then into the follicle lumen, back into the cell, and finally into the blood again. A summary of the processes involved is given below and in Figure 14.2.

1   *Iodide trapping:* Iodide is extracted from the blood by the sodium–iodide symporter and shifted into the thyroid follicular cells where it is concentrated to many times the level found in plasma. Thus, the thyroid gland normally contains virtually all the iodide in the body. Around 1 mg of iodine is required by an adult each week. Most of this is ingested in food, water, and iodised table salt. The ratio of iodide in the thyroid gland to that in the plasma is expressed as the T/S ratio. Normally, this ratio ranges from 20:1 to 39:1. In hypoactivity of the gland, the ratio may be 10:1. In hyperactivity, it may be as great as 250:1.

2   *Synthesis of thyroglobulin in follicle cells:* Thyroglobulin is a large glycoprotein with about 115 tyrosine residues per molecule of thyroglobulin. Once synthesised, it is released into the lumen of the follicle as the main component of the thick colloid gel.

3   *Oxidation of iodide (I^-) to iodine (I_2):* Oxidation occurs in the follicle cells and is catalysed by the enzyme thyroperoxidase, followed by transfer of iodine into the lumen.

4   *Iodination of tyrosine residues in thyroglobulin:* Initially, one or two iodine atoms bind to tyrosine residues (yielding mono- or di-iodinated tyrosine, MIT or DIT).

5   *Coupling of MIT and DIT:* These occur as pairs: MIT + DIT gives T_3; and MIT + MIT gives T_4. The thyroid hormones are thus incorporated into thyroglobulin molecules, about 90% as T_4.

Thyroid gland

Thyroid and parathyroid glands

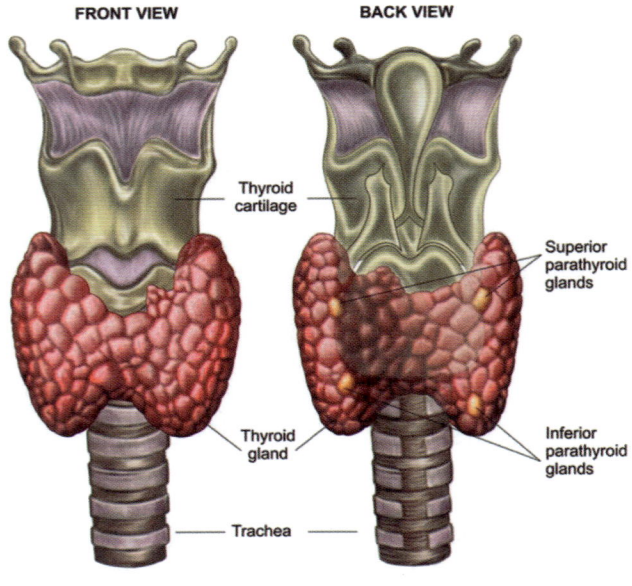

FRONT VIEW   BACK VIEW

Thyroid
cartilage

Superior
parathyroid
glands

Thyroid
gland

Inferior
parathyroid
glands

Trachea

FIGURE 14.1 The thyroid gland is located in the throat in front of the trachea, with the right and left lateral lobes linked by the isthmus. The small parathyroid glands are located on the posterior surface of each lobe of the thyroid gland.

Source: Getty Images/Stocktrek Images.

6   *Storage of T_3 and T_4:* T_3 and T_4 are stored in thyroglobulin in the lumen of the follicle. About 30% of the thyroid mass is thyroglobulin, which contains enough thyroid hormone to meet normal requirements for 2–3 months without any further synthesis.

7   *Release of active T_3 and T_4:* This is accomplished by proteolytic digestion of colloid in the follicle cells. The iodine, MIT, DIT, and peptide residues that remain are reused.

8   *Secretion of T_3 and T_4:* As lipid-soluble amino acids, these diffuse from thyroid cells into the bloodstream.

9   *Circulation:* T_4 is present as a large pool in the circulation, 99.95% protein-bound to thyroxine-binding globulin and other proteins. T_4 has a low turnover rate, with a half-life of about 6–7 days. As it circulates and enters cells, most T_4 is converted to

T_3. T_3 is present as a small pool, mainly stored intracellularly. T_3 is more potent than T_4, less strongly protein-bound, and has a faster turnover rate, with a half-life of about 2 days.

Regulation

High concentrations of circulating thyroid hormones activate typical negative-feedback loops, by inhibiting the synthesis of genes for both hypothalamic **thyrotrophin-releasing hormone** (TRH) and anterior pituitary **thyroid-stimulating hormone** (TSH, thyrotrophin) at the transcriptional level (Fig 14.3). This inhibits synthesis and release of TSH, thus overall reducing production of thyroid hormones. In contrast, low concentrations of circulating thyroid hormones increase the release of TSH from the pituitary gland and appear to influence the secretion of TRH from the hypothalamus.

Diagram of thyroid hormone synthesis and secretion, with the sites of action of drugs used in the treatment of thyroid disorders. Iodide in the blood is transported by carriers through the follicular cell and into the colloid-rich lumen, where it is incorporated into thyroglobulin under the influence of the thyroperoxidase enzyme. The hormones are produced by processing of the endocytosed thyroglobulin and exported into blood

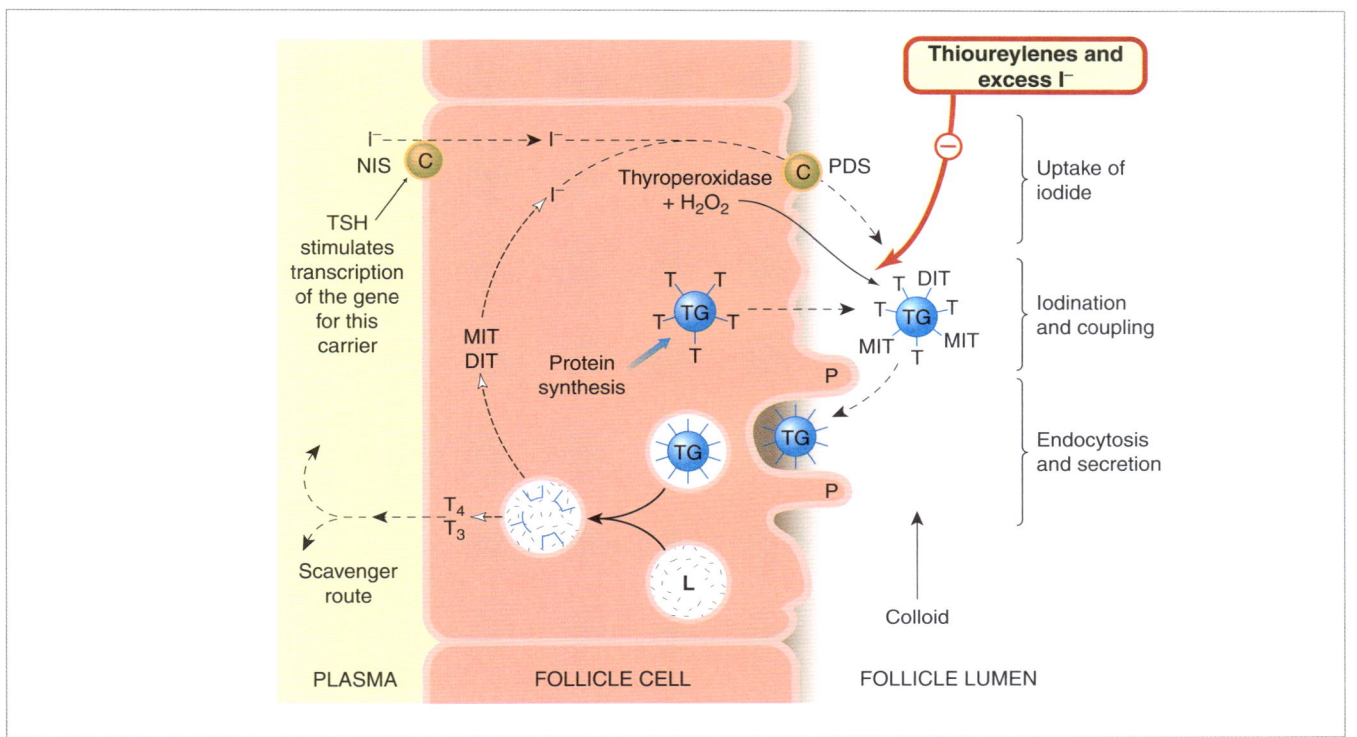

FIGURE 14.2 C= carrier; DIT = di-iodotyrosine; L = lysosome; MIT = monoiodotyrosine; P = pseudopod; T = tyrosine; T_3 = tri-iodothyronine; T_4 = thyroxine; TG = thyroglobulin; TSH = thyroid-stimulating hormone

Source: Adapted from Rang et al. 2012, Figure 33-1; reproduced with permission from Elsevier Churchill Livingstone.

TSH binds to TSH receptors on thyroid cells. These G-protein-coupled receptors, via activation of adenylyl cyclase and phosphorylation of enzymes, stimulate many aspects of thyroid gland function, including increasing:

- thyroid cell utilisation of glucose and oxygen
- blood flow to the thyroid gland
- iodide trapping by the gland
- iodination of thyroglobulin, thus increasing synthesis of hormones
- proteolysis of thyroglobulin and, hence, release of hormones.

In the long term, an increase in TSH leads to both thyroid hypertrophy (greater size of cells) and hyperplasia (greater number of cells). TSH is commonly measured in thyroid function tests to diagnose and monitor thyroid dysfunction (CFB 14.1).

Another factor regulating thyroid function is plasma iodide concentration. Reduced plasma iodide concentration reduces thyroid hormone synthesis and increases TSH secretion, while excessively high concentrations switch off production, via negative feedback and possibly by inhibiting the iodination of **thyroglobulin**.

CLINICAL FOCUS BOX 14.1

Thyroid function tests

Thyroid function tests are commonly carried out to determine the exact site of thyroid dysfunction, and to optimise therapy by monitoring treatment so dosage adjustment can be advised (Mortimer 2011). Note that many drugs can alter thyroid function test results and also affect thyroxine absorption and metabolism. Hormone

Secretion and control of thyroid hormones

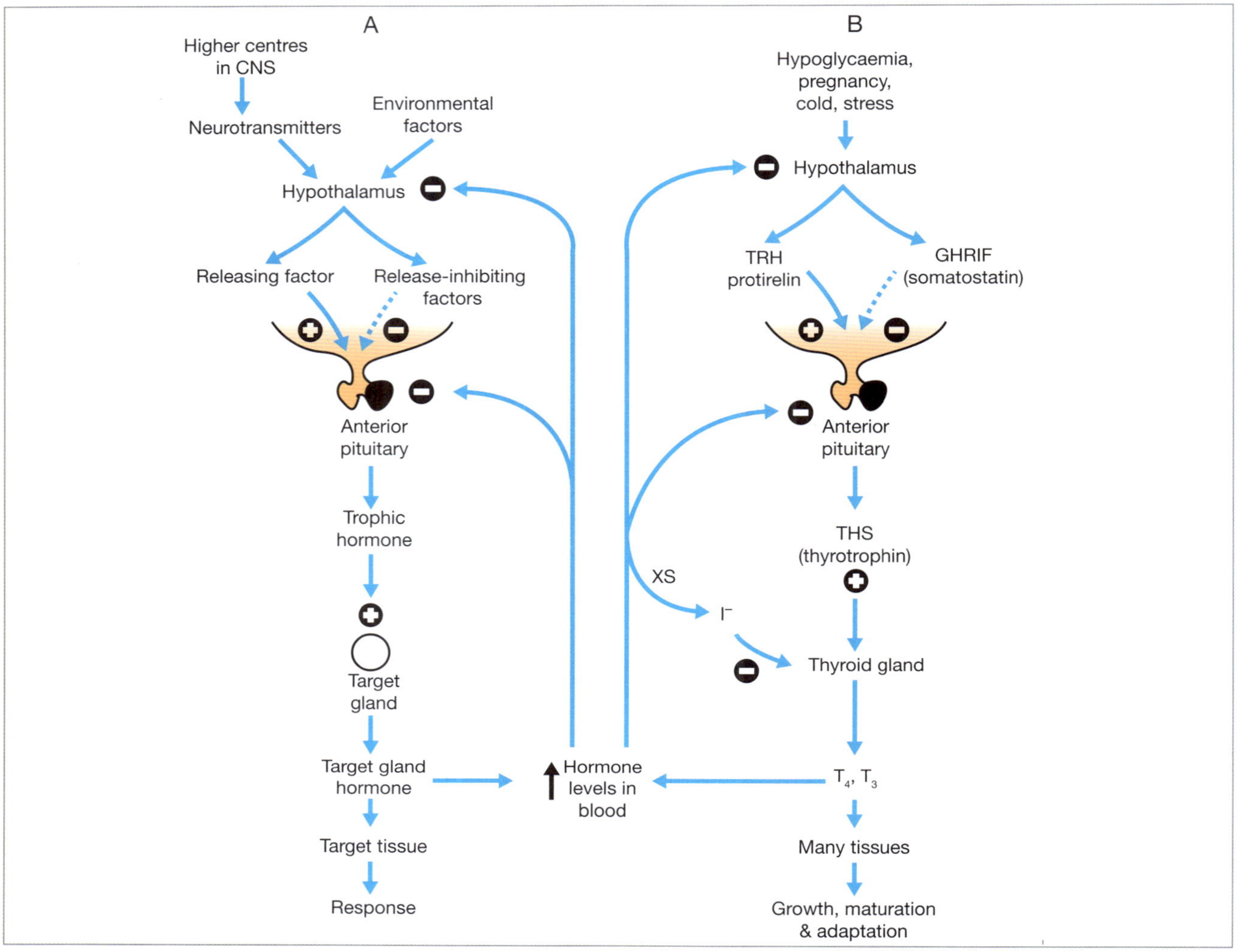

FIGURE 14.3 A General control mechanisms for hormone secretion. **B** Control mechanisms for thyroid hormone secretion. Environmental factors influence secretion of the hypothalamic factors thyrotrophin-releasing hormone (TRH) and growth hormone release-inhibiting factor (GHRIF, somatostatin) to increase or decrease release from the anterior pituitary of thyrotrophin (TSH), which stimulates production in the thyroid glands of thyroxine (T_4) and T_3.

levels vary during pregnancy so trimester-specific reference ranges should be used (Osinga et al 2022).

The hormone usually measured is TSH, a sensitive marker of thyroid function because it is influenced (inversely) by small changes in free T_4 concentration. A low TSH usually indicates hyperthyroidism. A raised TSH usually means primary hypothyroidism due to thyroid dysfunction. In this situation, TSH basal concentrations are raised, and the pituitary is hyper-reactive to TRH stimulation, but T_3 and T_4 concentrations remain low.

There are several other thyroid function tests, including the free T_4 index (FTI), free T_3 and T_3 resin uptake (T_3RU) tests, and thyroglobulin concentration, which may be useful in specific circumstances. The presence and concentration of thyroid-related autoantibodies can also be measured. Three types of thyroid autoantibodies can be tested: to thyroperoxidase (anti-TPO Ab), to thyroglobulin (anti-Tg Ab), or to the TSH receptor (TRAb). These autoantibodies play a role in both autoimmune diseases of the thyroid (such as Graves' disease and Hashimoto's thyroiditis). Thyroid autoantibodies are also present in some people with other autoimmune conditions, such as type I diabetes, rheumatoid arthritis, and coeliac disease. Anti-TPO and anti-Tg antibodies have been associated with female infertility, miscarriage, preterm labour, preeclampsia, and abruption (Frolich & Wahl 2017). All thyroid antibodies can cross the placenta, causing either stimulation or suppression of thyroid function depending on the antibody type.

Mechanism of thyroid hormone actions

T_4 (which is converted to T_3 on entering the cell) and T_3 enter the nucleus of target cells, where they bind to specific nuclear receptors. These then bind to thyroid response elements on genes. Transcription is then altered because of activation or repression of various genes. Hence, synthesis of specific proteins – for example, Na+–K+-ATPase – is altered. T_3 is more potent than T_4 and has a greater affinity for thyroid receptors.

KEY POINTS

The thyroid gland

- The thyroid gland has an important homeostatic role in growth and development, metabolism and energy balance, and cardiovascular and nervous system functions.

- Hormones produced by the thyroid gland include T_4, T_3, and calcitonin.

- Iodine is actively taken up from the circulation by the thyroid gland and incorporated in T_3 and T_4, which are stored in the thyroid follicles, bound in thyroglobulin.

- Synthesis, storage, and secretion of thyroid hormones is a multi-step process.

- High concentrations of circulating thyroid hormones activate negative-feedback loops by inhibiting the synthesis of genes for both hypothalamic TRH and anterior pituitary TSH at the transcriptional level, thus overall reducing production of thyroid hormones.

- Low concentrations of circulating thyroid hormones increase TSH release from the pituitary gland and appear to influence the secretion of TRH from the hypothalamus.

- T_4 and T_3 bind to nuclear receptors, altering transcription – and hence protein synthesis – by activation or repression of various genes.

14.2 Thyroid physiology and pregnancy

The thyroid gland increases in size and vascularity during pregnancy. Higher rates of renal glomerular filtration increase excretion of iodine, reducing circulating serum iodine concentration. Thyroid-binding globulin production is stimulated by high levels of oestrogen, so more thyroid hormone is bound during pregnancy. Human chorionic gonadotropin (hCG) molecules share similar chemical structure with the TSH molecule and can bind to and stimulate the TSH receptor. This stimulation results in higher levels of T_3 and T_4 and suppresses TSH release (Smith et al 2017). After birth, levels of T_3, T_4, and TBG fall rapidly, returning to

---

DRUG AT A GLANCE 14.1
Drugs affecting the thyroid

PHARMACOLOGICAL GROUP AND EFFECT	KEY EXAMPLES	CLINICAL USE
Thyroid hormones: • Control growth and development • Regulate metabolism and energy balance • Promote normal cardiovascular and nervous system functions	Levothyroxine (T_4)	Hypothyroidism Thyroid cancer Euthyroid goitre
	Liothyronine (T_3) not recommended for use in pregnancy	Severe hypothyroidism (e.g. myxoedema coma)
Iodine therapy: • Inhibition of thyroid hormone release	Iodine, iodine solution aqueous	Before surgery for Graves' disease
	I^{131} (radioiodine)	Hyperthyroidism Thyroid carcinoma Diagnostic thyroid function tests
Antithyroid agents: • Inhibit thyroid hormone synthesis • Inhibit peripheral conversion of T_4 to T_3 (propylthiouracil)	Carbimazole	Graves' disease Before thyroid surgery Before/after radioiodine Thyroid storm
	Propylthiouracil	

---

pre-pregnancy levels by 4–6 weeks postpartum (Ilias et al 2022). Adequate levels of T_3 and T_4 in the postnatal period support successful lactation.

During the first two trimesters of pregnancy, the fetus is entirely dependent on placental transfer of maternal T_4 for normal brain development. Iodine supply across the placenta and later in breast milk must be sufficient once the fetal thyroid begins to function in the third trimester to achieve normal fetal and early neonatal thyroid function (Ilias et al 2022). Since 2009, there has been mandatory fortification of bread with iodised salt with the expectation of consumption of three slices of bread/day. Pregnant and breastfeeding women are advised to achieve daily intake of 250 micrograms from dietary sources and supplements (Fig 14.4).

Pharmacotherapy of thyroid disorders

Iodine deficiency and simple (or non-toxic) goitre

Iodine deficiency is inevitably a result of inadequate dietary iodine intake, leading to insufficient synthesis of thyroid hormones and impairment of thyroid functions. Iodine is not abundant in most foods, except for fish and seafood. The World Health Organization (WHO) and UNESCO have therefore committed to a public health program of mandatory fortification of iodine in the food supply via staple dietary components. The recommendation is for the regular use of iodised salt (25–40 mg iodine per kilo salt), to provide about

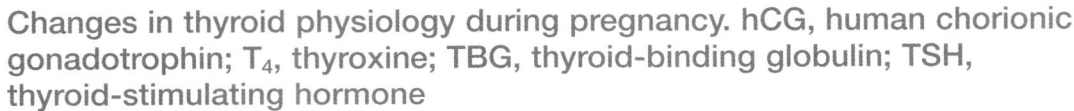

Changes in thyroid physiology during pregnancy. hCG, human chorionic gonadotrophin; T₄, thyroxine; TBG, thyroid-binding globulin; TSH, thyroid-stimulating hormone

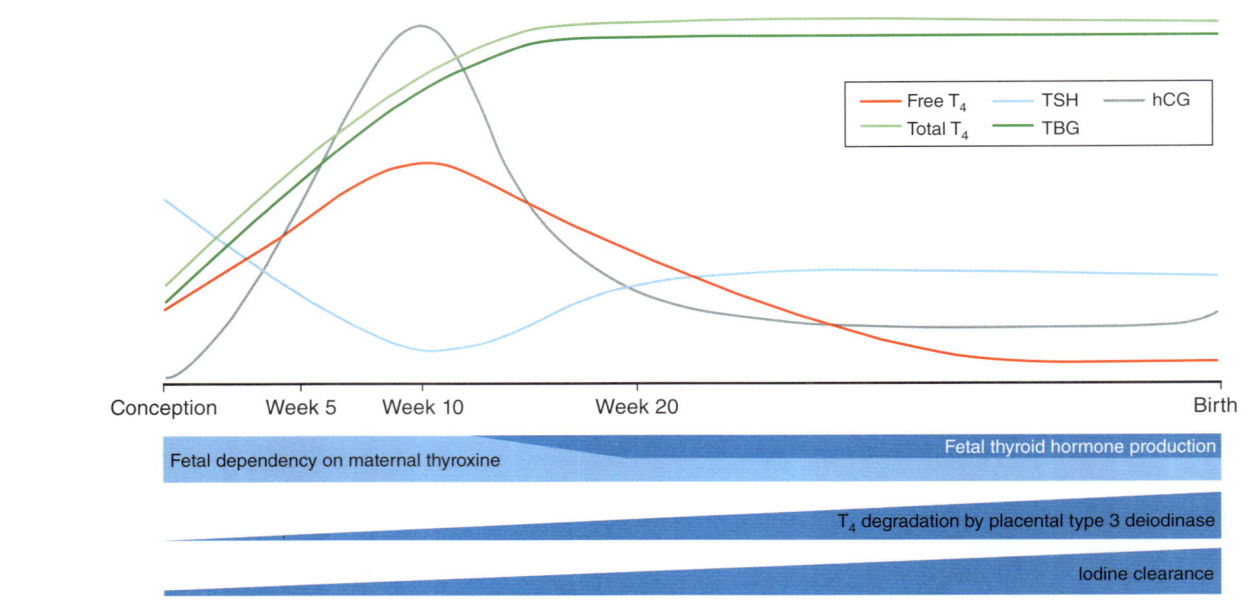

FIGURE 14.4

Source: Adapted from Korevaar TIM, Medici M, Visser TJ, Peeters RP. Thyroid disease in pregnancy: new insights in diagnosis and clinical management. Nat Rev Endocrinol. 2017 Oct;13(10):610–622

200 micrograms of iodine daily. The margin between too much iodine and too little is narrow, so excessive iodine-rich foods should not be eaten.

Endemic **goitre** is usually due to low soil iodine concentrations, especially common in inland hilly areas. Low soil iodine leads to prolonged low concentrations of iodine in the food chain and decreased synthesis of thyroid hormones. Compensatory increased hypothalamic TRH and pituitary TSH results in enlargement of the thyroid gland, known as a simple goitre. The enlarged thyroid scavenges residual traces of iodine from the blood. This type of goitre is prevented with an adequate supply of iodine. Note the presence of goitre is not necessarily diagnostic of simple goitre, as an enlarged thyroid gland may also be due to excessive stimulation of the gland in thyrotoxicosis.

Congenital hypothyroidism can arise from untreated iodine deficiency during pregnancy and the first few months of life. Congenital hypothyroidism is recognised by the WHO as the most common preventable cause of brain damage. Iodine supplements are sometimes thought of as complementary or alternate medicines, and there are other mineral and herbal compounds that are also used in managing thyroid conditions. Several of these are outlined in Clinical Focus Box 14.2.

CLINICAL FOCUS BOX 14.2

CAM considerations

- Iodine supplementation is recommended during pregnancy and lactation. Appropriate dosing is advised, as either too much or too little can lead to thyroid dysfunction.
- The mineral selenium is a component of several enzymes with roles in thyroid hormone production. Supplements have been used to support normal thyroid function and to assist in the management of several thyroid disorders.
- Several herbal compounds may be useful in managing thyroid conditions. These include: bugleweed (*Lycopus virginicus*), gypsywort (*Lycopus europaeus*), water horehound (*Lycopus lucidus* or *Lycopus americanus*), gromwell (*Lithospermum ruderale*), European gromwell (*Lithospermum officinale*), lemonbalm (Melissa officinalis), rosemary (*Rosmarinus officinalis*), sage (*Salvia officinalis*), and bladderwrack (*Fucus vesiculosus*) (Yarnell & Abascal 2006).

Hypothyroidism

Pathology

Hypothyroidism is estimated to be present in up to 2% of the population, and the incidence in pregnancy is similar. Hypothyroidism is associated with autoimmune disorders, previous Graves' disease (and antithyroid therapy), and is more common in people with Down syndrome. Aetiological factors include thyroidectomy or radiation therapy, iodine deficiency (simple non-toxic goitre), Hashimoto's thyroiditis (with autoantibodies to thyroglobulin and some components of thyroid tissue), use of antithyroid drugs, lithium, or amiodarone. People with primary hypothyroidism have low T_3 and T_4 concentrations despite an elevated TSH level. The condition can easily be missed, as it has variable and non-specific presentations with slow onset.

Screening for hypothyroidism in pregnancy

Universal screening of all pregnant women for hypothyroidism is not advised. Screening by testing TSH levels is currently advised for women with known risk factors (Australian Government 2019):

- History of thyroid dysfunction
- Symptoms or signs of thyroid dysfunction
- Presence of a goitre
- Known to have **antithyroid antibodies** (routine screening for these is not recommended)
- Age > 30 years
- Type 1 diabetes or other autoimmune conditions
- History of miscarriage, preterm birth, infertility
- Family history of thyroid dysfunction
- BMI > 40 kg/m2
- Use of amiodarone, lithium, or recent administration of iodinated radiological contrast
- Two or more prior pregnancies
- Living in an iodine-deficient area.

If TSH is elevated, further assessment with T_3 and T_4 levels and antithyroid antibody testing is advised to assist in making a diagnosis. Women with hypothyroidism during pregnancy (whether preexisting or newly diagnosed) should be offered multi-disciplinary management, including collaboration with an endocrinologist.

Clinical manifestations

Clinical manifestations are illustrated in Figure 14.5. Severe hypothyroidism in the adult is called myxoedema, referring to the thickened skin caused by acid mucopolysaccharide accumulation. In the last stage of longstanding, inadequately treated or untreated hypothyroidism, coma sets in accompanied by hypotension, hypoventilation, hypothermia, hyponatraemia, and hypoglycaemia.

Symptoms of hypothyroidism in pregnancy and lactation

There is some overlap in the usual symptoms of pregnancy and hypothyroidism, such as lethargy and constipation, that may lead to symptoms of hypothyroidism being missed during pregnancy. It is for this reason that screening women at risk for hypothyroidism has an important place in maternity care. Problems with lactation can be a manifestation of hypothyroidism. Consider hypothyroidism as a possibility in women with supply issues, particularly if this is associated with low energy, poor concentration, depressed mood, or hair loss.

Symptoms and consequences of hypothyroidism in infancy

Hypothyroidism in infancy is characterised by slowed physical and mental development, which leads to dwarfism and mental retardation. The condition may result from faulty development or atrophy of the thyroid gland during fetal life and may be caused by iodine deficiency during pregnancy. In congenital hypothyroidism, thyroid hormone concentrations equal to or above those required for the adult must be established immediately after birth to prevent permanent mental and physical retardation. The neonatal screening test performed a few days after birth routinely tests TSH levels and is recommended for all babies to facilitate early diagnosis and treatment of congenital hypothyroidism.

Treatment

The goal of treatment for people with hypothyroidism or myxoedema is to eliminate their symptoms and restore them to a normal physiological state (i.e. render them euthyroid). In pregnancy, therapy also aims to prevent congenital hypothyroidism. Therapy is simple. For lifelong hormone replacement, thyroid hormones are safe, stable, cheap, and available orally. Dosage regimens are adjusted in response to thyroid function test results. Thyroxine (levothyroxine, T_4; DM 14.1) is the drug of choice for replacement therapy. Initially 50–200 micrograms once daily orally on an empty stomach should be given. Dose changes should be considered only every 6–8 weeks, based on TSH results. Fine dosage adjustments can be achieved with alternating doses of 50, 75, 100, 125 or 200 microgram tablets. Liothyronine (T_3), preferred for emergency use, is not recommended in pregnancy because of the requirement of the fetal brain for T_4.

Clinical response is more important than blood hormone concentrations. Determination of TSH is used to assess adequacy and adherence to therapy. In infants with hypothyroidism, any delay in growth and maturity can be reversed by administration of T_4. There is a rapid catch-up growth spurt, and eventually the expected adult height is attained.

In women with hypothyroidism managed with thyroxine prior to pregnancy, a 30% dose increase once pregnancy is confirmed is advised. For women with a new diagnosis of hypothyroidism in pregnancy, a starting dose of 50 micrograms of thyroxine is advised. Response to treatment should be monitored with thyroid

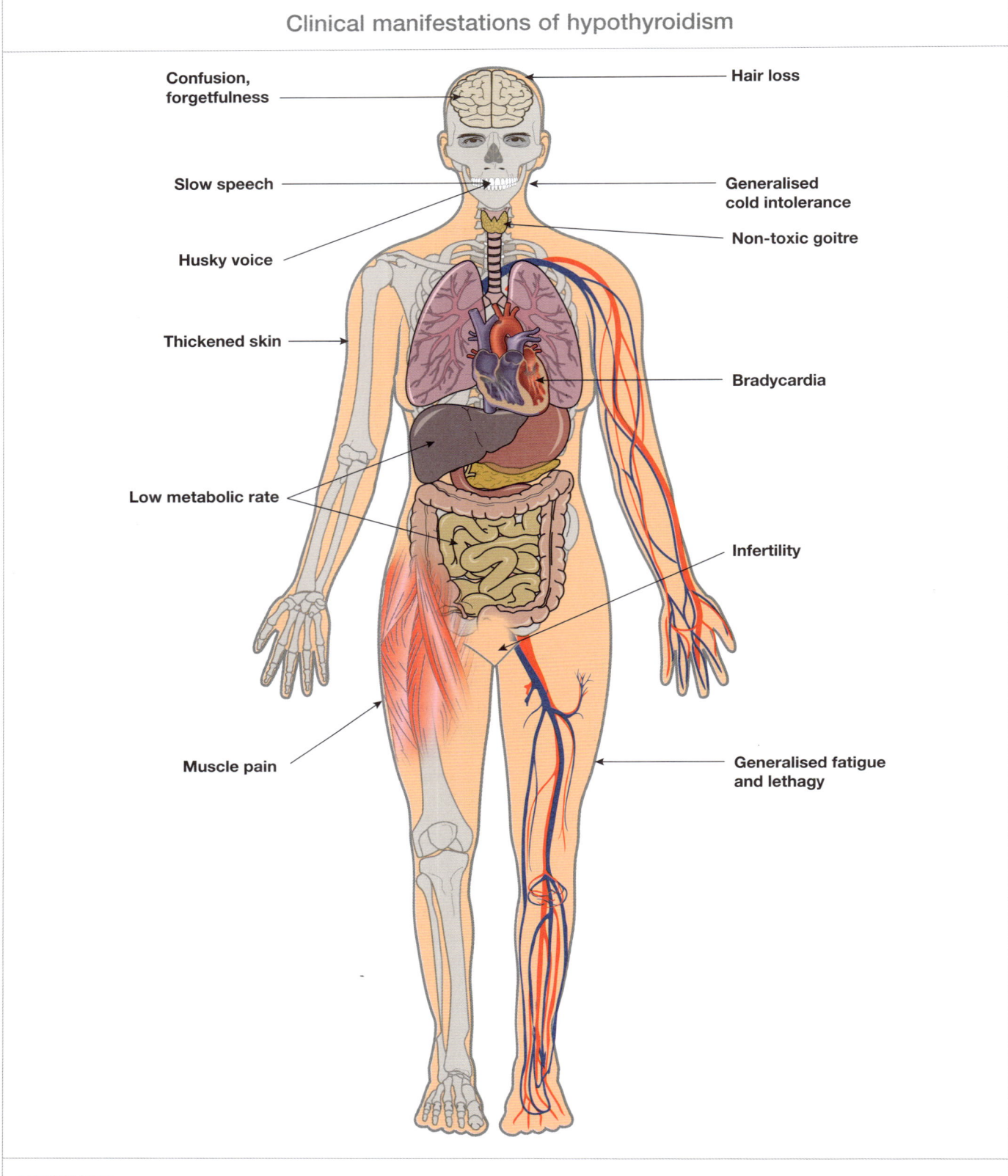

Clinical manifestations of hypothyroidism

Confusion, forgetfulness

Hair loss

Slow speech

Generalised cold intolerance

Husky voice

Non-toxic goitre

Thickened skin

Bradycardia

Low metabolic rate

Infertility

Muscle pain

Generalised fatigue and lethagy

FIGURE 14.5

function testing every 4 weeks in the first trimester, and every 6–8 weeks thereafter. During pregnancy the target TSH range is 0.5–2.5 mIU/L, and when not pregnant 0.4–5 mIU/L. The lower target range ensures adequate levels of T₄ for normal fetal brain development. The dose can be reduced to the pre-pregnancy level after birth (or by 30% for women diagnosed during pregnancy) and thyroid function tested at 6 weeks postpartum. Women with hypothyroidism are best managed during pregnancy in collaboration with an endocrinologist.

Hyperthyroidism (thyrotoxicosis)

Pathology

Excessive formation of the thyroid hormones and their release into the circulation results in thyrotoxicosis. This occurs in conditions such as multinodular goitre, toxic hot nodule (adenoma), Graves' disease, and subacute thyroiditis. Thyrotoxicosis can also occur as an adverse reaction to some drugs (iatrogenic causes), including thyroid hormones, excess iodine, lithium, and amiodarone.

Overt **hyperthyroidism** occurs in 0.2–0.6% of pregnant women, with around 85% of cases being due to Graves' disease. Graves' disease, or autoimmune hyperthyroidism, is the most common type of hyperthyroidism in people under age 40, affecting about 0.4% of the population, women more often than men, and can cause 'exophthalmic goitre'. Smoking exacerbates Graves' disease. The first symptoms noticed may be fullness in the neck, difficulty doing up buttons at the neck, and grittiness in the eyes. Other signs and symptoms are as described for hyperthyroidism. The

---

DRUG MONOGRAPH 14.1
Levothyroxine sodium

Synthetic levothyroxine (thyroxine) has all the chemical and pharmacological properties of natural thyroxine.

Indications

Thyroid hormone replacement is indicated for the treatment of hypothyroidism; treatment and prevention of goitre; replacement therapy after thyroid block in hyperthyroidism; and treatment of thyroiditis and thyroid carcinoma (where high doses are used for their suppressive effects). Thyroid hormones are also used as replacement therapy after thyroidectomy performed for thyroid cancers. In thyroid cancer, T₄ not only replaces the missing hormone but also activates the negative-feedback loop and thus suppresses pituitary release of TSH, which would stimulate any remaining thyroid cancer cells.

Pharmacokinetics

Levothyroxine is adequately absorbed from the GIT (48–80%) and is more than 99.9% bound in the circulation to thyroxine-binding globulin, thyroxine-binding prealbumin, and albumin. The plasma half-life of T₄ is 6–7 days and T₃ 1–2 days in euthyroid people. The duration of biological effect is much longer, so steady state may not be reached for 3–4 weeks. The physiological response to altered dosage is slow. T₄ is converted in the liver and kidney to T₃, and conjugated and de-iodinated metabolites are excreted in bile and urine. There is some enterohepatic recycling. Levothyroxine can be dosed once daily and is given on an empty stomach, usually before breakfast.

Drug interactions

The clearance of many drugs is reduced in hypothyroidism but not of anticoagulants, which may require higher doses. Current drug information sources should be consulted. (See Drug Interactions 14.1.)

Adverse reactions

- Adverse effects associated with excessive dosages generally correspond to symptoms of hyperthyroidism: tachycardia, elevated temperature, diarrhoea, hand tremors, increased irritability, weight loss, and insomnia.
- A rare adverse reaction is an allergic skin rash.
- Suppression of TSH by exogenous levothyroxine may reduce bone density and cause osteoporosis. Excessive doses may cause osteoporotic fractures, especially in the elderly.
- Adverse effects are dose-related and may occur more rapidly with T₃ than with T₄, as the former has a faster onset of action.
- Signs of under-dosage are those of hypothyroidism: coldness, dry skin, constipation, lethargy, headaches, drowsiness, tiredness, weight gain, and muscle aching. During the early period of treatment, hair loss may occur in children.
- To avoid either over- or under-treatment, individualised dosing is recommended, based on thyroid function testing.

Warnings and contraindications

Use with caution in people with diabetes mellitus, adrenocortical or pituitary insufficiency, cardiac disease, and malabsorption problems. Avoid use in people with hyperthyroidism, thyrotoxicosis, or thyroid hypersensitivity. Requirements increase during pregnancy, and dosage should be adjusted depending on TSH concentration, monitored during each trimester.

Dosage and administration

Levothyroxine tablets are available in a range of doses (25, 50, 75, 100, 125, and 200 micrograms) to allow easy dose adjustment. The stability of levothyroxine tablets is limited, and 'use-by' dates should be heeded. Except for Eltroxin, storage at 2–8°C is generally recommended. Not all brands are bioequivalent, so care should be exercised if changing brands.

DRUG INTERACTIONS 14.1
Thyroid hormone preparations

DRUG	POSSIBLE EFFECTS AND MANAGEMENT
Colestyramine, ciprofloxacin, calcium carbonate, ferrous sulfate, lanthanum, orlistat, proton pump inhibitors, raloxifene, sevelamer, simethicone, and sucralfate	These drugs reduce the absorption of levothyroxine from the GIT. A 4-hour interval is recommended between administration of these drugs and levothyroxine.
Imatinib, phenobarbital, phenytoin, rifampicin, ritonavir, and sunitinib	May increase metabolism of levothyroxine. Dose may need to be increased.
Warfarin	Thyroid hormones affect metabolism of clotting factors, thereby enhancing the therapeutic effects of warfarin. A lower oral anticoagulant dosage may be required. Monitor international normalised ratio.

classic sign, exophthalmos (i.e. protruding eyes), is due to fat deposition behind the eyeballs and oedema of the muscles controlling eye movements, leading to excessive fibrosis and eyelid retraction. Corneal ulceration can occur if the eyelids are unable to close. As well as therapy of the thyroid dysfunction to render the person euthyroid, immunosuppressants are used to minimise the autoimmune processes.

Autoantibodies against thyroid antigens can stimulate thyroid hormone release, which lead to the signs of hyperthyroidism and thyroid growth, hence leading to goitre. These autoantibodies are also able to cross the placenta, causing enlargement of the thyroid and hyperthyroidism in the fetus. Symptoms and signs of fetal hyperthyroidism slowly disappear after birth as maternal antibodies are cleared from the baby's circulation.

Primary hyperthyroidism is characterised by elevated concentrations of T_3 and T_4 despite a low TSH level. In pituitary (secondary) hyperthyroidism, high levels of T_3 and T_4 are secondary to high levels of TSH secretion in the pituitary.

Gestational thyrotoxicosis is a condition specifically limited to pregnancy, affecting 1–3% of pregnant women. High hCG levels stimulate the TSH receptor, so circulating levels of T_4 rise and TSH excretion is suppressed. Gestational thyrotoxicosis is more common in women with hyperemesis gravidarum, multiple pregnancy, or molar pregnancy.

Clinical manifestations

Hyperthyroidism leads to symptoms the opposite of those seen in myxoedema. Metabolic rate is increased, sometimes as much as 60% or more. Body temperature is frequently above normal, appetite increases, and body weight decreases. Other symptoms include restlessness,

anxiety, emotional instability, insomnia, muscle tremor and weakness, sweating, and exophthalmos. These symptoms can be overlooked in the postnatal period as some overlap with normal postnatal changes. Raised T_4 concentrations can cause cardiomegaly, dysrhythmias, congestive heart failure, and hepatic damage. Drug clearance may be increased, so doses of other drugs might need to be increased. Without treatment, women with hyperthyroidism are at increased risk for infertility, miscarriage, preeclampsia, preterm birth, or abruption.

A rare but serious complication of thyrotoxicosis is thyroid storm. A sudden onset of exaggerated hyperthyroid symptoms occurs, especially those affecting the nervous and cardiovascular systems, because of elevated T_4 concentrations. Thyroid storm is a life-threatening condition, potentially leading to heart failure and coma.

Treatment

The aims of treatment are to decrease thyroid hormone overproduction and block the peripheral effects of excess T_4. Before the advent of antithyroid drugs, treatment was surgical, by removal of most of the hyperactive gland. Antithyroid drugs lower the basal metabolic rate by interfering with the formation, release, or action of thyroid hormones. These include the thioureylene derivatives, iodine (iodide ion), and radioactive iodine. Beta-adrenoceptor antagonists (e.g. propranolol) are frequently used as adjunctive therapy to provide short-term relief of hyperthyroid symptoms due to the peripheral effects of excess T_4, including tachycardia, tremor, and sweating. Both cardioselective and non-selective β-blockers are effective. (These drugs are covered in more detail in Chapter 15.)

Women with Graves's disease are advised to discuss future pregnancy plans with their endocrinologist, prior to conception. Some women may consider surgery or radioiodine therapy to avoid the use of antithyroid agents and the associated risk of teratogenesis. Ideally, pregnancy should be planned once thyroid function tests have returned to normal and remained stable over several months. If radioiodine treatment has been used, pregnancy should be avoided for six months.

A multi-disciplinary approach is advised when caring for women with hyperthyroidism of any cause during pregnancy, with the involvement of obstetricians, endocrinologists, neonatologists, and midwives. Women using antithyroid drugs should be maintained on the lowest dose required to keep T_4 at or just above the reference range. TRAb concentration should be (re)assessed at the start of pregnancy. Elevated levels indicate fetal risk for thyrotoxicosis and additional ultrasound monitoring for fetal tachycardia, growth, and thyroid appearance is advised through the second half of pregnancy.

The management of gestational thyroxicosis is supportive, as symptoms can be expected to resolve as hCG levels begin to fall in mid-pregnancy. Beta-blockers can be used for symptom control if required.

Thioureylenes

The oral thioureylene drugs carbimazole (DM 14.2) and propylthiouracil inhibit thyroid hormone synthesis by competitively inhibiting the iodination of tyrosine residues in thyroglobulin. Propylthiouracil (but not carbimazole) also inhibits the conversion of T_4 to T_3 in peripheral tissues, which may make it more effective for treatment of thyroid storm. These drugs contain a sulfur–carbon–nitrogen linkage. They are closely related chemically to the sulfonamide antibacterials and the sulfonylurea hypoglycaemic agents. (Both of these drug groups may also interfere with thyroid function.)

High doses of thioureylenes are given initially to control severe hyperthyroidism, reducing the dose gradually after 3–4 weeks. A course of 12–18 months may be necessary for sustained remission of Graves' disease.

Of the two thioureylenes, propylthiouracil is the preferred agent in the first trimester of pregnancy as it has a lower risk of teratogenesis. Women whose Graves' disease has previously been well controlled on a low dose of their antithyroid drug may be able to successfully maintain normal thyroid function after ceasing treatment during early pregnancy (Hou et al 2022). However, regular monitoring of thyroid function is still recommended during pregnancy, and particularly in the early postnatal period when relapse is common.

Iodine/iodide

Iodine

Iodine, which is converted in the body to iodide (I^-), is the oldest antithyroid drug available. Although a small

---

DRUG MONOGRAPH 14.2
Carbimazole

Actions
Carbimazole acts as an antithyroid drug by inhibiting synthesis of the thyroid hormones.

Indications
The thioureylenes are indicated for the treatment of hyperthyroidism, either as a short course in thyroid storm, before surgery, or radiotherapy; or as a long course as adjunct therapy for the treatment of thyrotoxicosis.

Pharmacokinetics
Thioureylenes are readily absorbed from the GIT. Carbimazole is a prodrug. It is rapidly converted in the body to the active metabolite methimazole. The half-life of each drug is relatively short (2–6 hours); however, maximal effects may take some weeks to occur, as the body may already have large stores of preformed thyroid hormones. Thus, the peak effect occurs in about 7 weeks with carbimazole and 17 weeks with propylthiouracil. Metabolised in the liver and excreted by the kidneys, thioureylenes cross the placenta and can cause fetal hypothyroidism and goitre. As they are excreted in breast milk, the lowest effective doses with monitoring should be used during breastfeeding.

Drug interactions
Current drug information sources should be consulted. (See Drug Interactions 14.2.)

Adverse reactions
These include rash, pruritus, dizziness, loss of taste, nausea, vomiting, leucopaenia, paraesthesias, and stomach pain. Fever, mouth ulcers, and sore throat may be early indications of serious agranulocytosis, which necessitates cessation of the drug and appropriate antibiotic treatment. Overall, signs of thyrotoxicosis indicate inadequate dosing, and signs of hypothyroidism indicate possible overdosage.

Warnings and contraindications
Use with caution in individuals with a low leucocyte count. The lowest effective dose should be used during pregnancy, with regular monitoring. Avoid use in people with a history of carbimazole or propylthiouracil hypersensitivity or liver impairment. Regular blood tests and liver and thyroid function tests are recommended.

Dosage and administration
Dosage depends on usage: after an initial 3–4 weeks of high-dose antithyroid therapy, the dosage is either regularly adjusted to maintain euthyroid status, or high dosage is maintained, and thyroxine added to restore thyroid function to normal ('block-and-replace' regimen).
The carbimazole oral adult dosage is initially 10–45 mg daily (in severe cases, up to 60 mg daily) in divided doses, reducing to a usual maintenance dose of 5–15 mg daily (though this can vary from 2.5–40 mg daily). In the 'block-and-replace' regimen, the initial dose is continued with the addition of levothyroxine 100–150 micrograms if T_4 is in the normal range. Treatment is continued with monitoring for about 2 years, as remissions may occur. Relapse, however, is frequent.

DRUG INTERACTIONS 14.2
Thioureylene antithyroid drugs

DRUG	POSSIBLE EFFECTS AND MANAGEMENT
Anticoagulants (warfarin)	Treatment with carbimazole or propylthiouracil may alter metabolism of clotting factors and decrease the effective use of anticoagulants. Monitor closely and adjust dose based on international normalised ratio results.
Sodium iodide I^{131}	Thyroid uptake of I^{131} may be decreased by antithyroid agents. Antithyroid drug should be stopped at least 4 days before and for 3 days after I^{131} therapy.
Theophylline	May be metabolised faster in thyrotoxicosis. Theophylline concentration and effects should be monitored when either carbimazole or propylthiouracil are commenced, and the dose of theophylline adjusted if necessary.

amount of iodine is necessary for normal thyroid function and synthesis of thyroid hormones, large amounts of iodine depress TRH and TSH release (Fig 14.3), thus causing inhibition of thyroid hormone synthesis and release. High doses of iodides such as in Lugol's solution are generally used for 7–10 days before thyroid surgery to decrease the gland's size and vascularity, resulting in diminished blood loss and a less complicated surgical procedure (CFB 14.2).

CLINICAL FOCUS BOX 14.2

Lugol's solution

Lugol's solution, or iodine solution aqueous BP, was first documented in 1829. It is a mixture of 5% iodine and 10% potassium iodide in water; the total iodine content is 130 mg/mL. After oral administration, the iodine is converted to iodide in the GIT before systemic absorption. Iodine solution is indicated to protect the thyroid gland from radiation before and after the administration of radioactive isotopes of iodine or in radiation emergencies, and in people with hyperthyroidism, to suppress thyroid function and vascularity prior to thyroidectomy. The adult dose of Lugol's solution is 0.3–0.9 mL/day (in divided doses, administered in a full glass of water, fruit juice or milk) for 7 days immediately prior to thyroid surgery.

It is used with caution in people with tuberculosis, iodine or potassium iodide hypersensitivity, bronchitis, hyperkalaemia, or kidney impairment, and in pregnancy. Adverse reactions include diarrhoea, nausea, vomiting, stomach pain, rash, swelling of the salivary gland, and a metallic taste in the mouth.

Radioactive iodine

Radioactive iodine (radioiodine, I^{131}) is the preferred antithyroid drug for people who are unlikely to tolerate thyroid surgery, who have not responded adequately to antithyroid therapy, or with recurrent hyperthyroidism after surgery. The I^{131} radioactive isotope of iodine is chemically identical to iodine, so it has the same pharmacokinetic parameters. After oral administration, it is taken up actively by thyroid cells and accumulates in thyroid tissue, where the ionising beta-radiation emitted selectively damages thyroid cells. In the long term, definitive therapy that produces hypothyroidism, followed by replacement with adequate thyroxine ('block–replace'), better maintains the euthyroid state than antithyroid drugs. It may be appropriate prior to planned pregnancy. Radioiodine is not suitable for use during pregnancy as it readily crosses the placenta, leading to destruction of the fetal thyroid gland.

KEY POINTS

Pharmacotherapy of thyroid disorders

- Simple or non-toxic goitre is due to iodine deficiency, which leads to decreased synthesis of thyroid hormones. Compensatory increased hypothalamic TRH and pituitary TSH, and enlargement of the thyroid gland, is treated by increasing iodine intake – for example, iodised salt.
- Hypothyroidism characterised by decreased basal metabolic rate is treated by administration of oral levothyroxine, which mimics the actions of T_4.
- Hyperthyroidism (thyrotoxicosis) leads to increased basal metabolic rate.
- Pharmacotherapy of hyperthyroidism involves the use of oral drugs, including:
  - carbimazole and propylthiouracil, which reduce thyroid hormone synthesis by inhibiting iodination of thyroglobulin
  - I^{131}, which is sequestered by thyroid cells that are selectively damaged by the ionising beta-radiation emitted.
- Regular testing of thyroid function is required to monitor disease progression and therapy, and to optimise dosage regimens.

REVIEW EXERCISES

1   Dara, who is 33 years old, gave birth to twin girls by caesarean section 3 months ago. She has come to see her GP because of difficulty sleeping and higher levels of anxiety. Her GP notes that Dara is tachycardic and has a mild tremor. On further questioning, Dara explains

that a friend had suggested a herbal product, rich in kelp seaweed, to help her get back to her pre-pregnancy weight. Over the 2 months she had been taking it, Dara lost 6 kg in weight. Thyroid function testing is performed and her TSH is 0.05 microUI/mL (reference range 0.55–4.78 microUI/mL) and her free T_4 level is 3.06 nanograms/dL (reference range 0.89–1.76 nanograms/dL). What form of thyroid dysfunction does Dara have and what is the likely cause?

2 Lizzie gave birth to her third child 10 days ago. You visit her at home because of concerns about the baby's poor weight gain. Lizzie reports constant fatigue, low mood, feeling cold, and is worried that she does not have enough milk. She says it was nothing like this with her two previous births. Her mother is worried that Lizzie has postnatal depression. Could her symptoms be due to a thyroid disorder? Given her symptoms, what is the most likely diagnosis? What testing would be helpful? If thyroid disease is confirmed, what treatment(s) might be advised?

3 Tina is seeing you at her initial visit to your maternity service. She discloses a history of Hashimoto's thyroiditis, previously treated with thyroxine 150 micrograms daily. Tina stopped taking it 2 weeks ago as she was worried that it might not be safe in pregnancy. Discuss the safety of thyroxine in pregnancy, and the maternal and fetal risks of untreated hypothyroidism.

REFERENCES

Australian Government Department of Health and Aged Care. Pregnancy care guidelines: thyroid dysfunction. Published 2019. https://www.health.gov.au/resources/pregnancy-care-guidelines/part-g-targeted-maternal-health-tests/thyroid-dysfunction

Hou X, Guan H, Sun S, et al. Outcomes of early-pregnancy antithyroid drug withdrawal in Graves' disease: a preliminary prospective follow-up study. Thyroid. 2022;32(8):983-989. doi:10.1089/thy.2022.0088

Ilias I, Milionis C, Koukkou, E. Further understanding of thyroid function in pregnant women. In press. Expert Rev Endocrinol Metab. 2022 Jul;17(4):365-374. doi: 10.1080/17446651.2022.2099372

Mortimer RH. Thyroid function tests. Aust Prescr. 2011;34(1):12-15. doi.org/10.18773/austprescr.2011.011

Rang HP, Dale MM, Ritter JM, et al. Pharmacology. Edinburgh: Elsevier, 2012.

Smith A, Eccles-Smith J, d'Emden M, et al. Thyroid disorders in pregnancy and postpartum. Aust Prescr. 2017;40:214-219. doi: 10.18773/austprescr.2017.075

Osinga J, Derakshan A, Palomaki G, et al. TSH and FT4 reference intervals in pregnancy: a systematic review and individual participant data meta-analysis. J Clin Endocrinol Metab. 2022;107:2925-2933. https://doi.org/10.1210/clinem/dgac425

Yarnell E, Abascal, K. Botanical medicine for thyroid regulation. Alternative and Complementary Therapies. 2006 Jun;107-112.

ONLINE RESOURCES

Australian Prescriber: https://doi.org/10.18773/austprescr.2017.075

American Thyroid Association: https://www.thyroid.org/thyroid-disease-pregnancy/

Australian Thyroid Foundation: https://thyroidfoundation.org.au/pregnancy

CHAPTER 15

DRUGS AFFECTING THE HEART, VASCULAR SYSTEM AND BLOOD VOLUME

Maryam Bazargan, Kirsten Small

Key Abbreviations

AV	atrioventricular
CO	cardiac output
HR	heart rate
NA	noradrenaline
SA	sinoatrial
SV	stroke volume
ACE	angiotensin-converting enzyme
ARB	angiotensin-receptor blocker
NO	nitric oxide
RAAS	renin–angiotensin–aldosterone system

Key Terms

afterload 289
automaticity 294
diastole 289
dysrhythmia 303
heart failure 295
inotropic effect 299
preload 289
stroke volume 289
systole 289
aldosterone 291
angiotensin II 291
angiotensin-converting enzyme inhibitors 286
angiotensin-receptor antagonists 286
calcium channel blockers 296
centrally acting adrenergic inhibitors 303
potassium channel activators 298
renin–angiotensin–aldosterone system 292
vasodilator drugs 303

Chapter Focus

Knowledge of the anatomy and physiology of the heart, vascular system, haematological system, adrenal and renal system is essential for understanding the action and use of antihypertensive drugs in pregnancy. The focus of this chapter is on hypertension disorders in pregnancy and drugs that are suitable to use when managing this in women during pregnancy and lactation. Common antihypertensive drugs used in pregnancy produce relaxation of vascular smooth muscle by either a direct or indirect action. Some drugs act primarily on veins or arterioles, while others dilate both types of blood vessels. Antihypertensive drugs include calcium channel blockers, potassium channel activators, **angiotensin-converting enzyme inhibitors**, and **angiotensin-receptor antagonists**. These drugs are prescribed, either alone or in combination therapy when treating hypertension during pregnancy and lactation.

Key Drug Groups

Drugs for hypertension:

- aldosterone receptor antagonists: eplerenone, spironolactone
- angiotensin-converting enzyme (ACE) inhibitors: captopril, enalapril, fosinopril, lisinopril, perindopril, quinapril, ramipril, trandolapril
- angiotensin-receptor (AT_1) antagonists (also called angiotensin-receptor blockers [ARBs]): candesartan, eprosartan, irbesartan, losartan, olmesartan, telmisartan, valsartan

Calcium channel blockers:

- amlodipine, clevidipine, diltiazem, felodipine, lercanidipine, nifedipine (DM 15.1), nimodipine, verapamil

Centrally acting adrenergic inhibitors:

- clonidine, methyldopa (DM 15.3), moxonidine

Potassium channel activators:

- diazoxide, minoxidil

Adrenoreceptor antagonists:

- non-selective $\alpha 1$, $\beta 1$ and $\beta 2$ adrenoceptor antagonists: carvedilol, labetalol, propranolol, sotalol
- selective $\beta 1$ adrenoceptor antagonists: atenolol, bisoprolol, metoprolol, nebivolol
- non-selective $\beta 1$ and $\beta 2$ adrenoceptor antagonists: pindolol

Direct vasodilators:

- hydralazine (DM 15.2)

Learning Outcomes

- Understand hypertension disorders in pregnancy and differentiate between the states of gestational hypertension or pregnancy-induced hypertension, chronic hypertension, and preeclampsia.
- Describe the typical features of hypertension disorders in pregnancy, including implications for woman and baby if untreated.

- Discuss the key drug groups drugs that are suitable to use when managing hypertensive disorders in women during pregnancy and lactation, including indication, mechanism of action and effect.

- Consider the significance of the renin–angiotensin–aldosterone system and impact of drugs used on this system in the management of hypertensive disorders in relation to pregnancy.

- Outline the common adverse reactions and interactions, including contraindications/safety profile to use of specific antihypertensive drugs used singly or in combination during pregnancy and lactation, and/or special precautions.

CRITICAL THINKING SCENARIO

Sophie is a 32-year-old woman with essential hypertension. She also suffers from asthma and occasionally requires the use of reliever asthma puffers. Since her diagnosis at the age of 25, she has been managed well with two different antihypertensive medications. Her current medications include lisinopril dihydrate (an ACE inhibitor, 10 mg once per day) and nifedipine 5 mg (three times a day). She has been regularly monitoring her kidney and liver functions, and there have been no complications so far. Now, with the plan of pregnancy, Sophie is scheduled to visit her GP tomorrow.

1   Considering Sophie's plan for pregnancy, potential changes to her pharmacological hypertension management might be recommended. What are those and why?

2   During pregnancy, specific screening tests and considerations may differ for Sophie compared to those for a woman without these co-morbidities. What are these tests and considerations? Why are they different?

3   Is there any increased risk for preeclampsia during Sophie's pregnancy?

4   What are the recommendations for prophylactic aspirin intake?

15.1 Introduction: The heart

The heart, which lies in the mediastinum slightly to the left of the midline of the thoracic cavity, consists of four chambers – the upper right and left atria and the lower right and left ventricles. The heart wall consists of the external smooth epicardium, the middle layer of myocardium (or muscle tissue), and the inner endocardium, which lines the chambers of the heart and the valves. The pumping action of the heart depends on the ability of the cardiac muscle to contract. Contractility of the heart is energy-dependent, and the heart derives most of its energy from oxidative metabolism of fatty acids and lactate, which occurs in mitochondria and cardiac muscle cells (Fig 15.1a and b).

The myocardium is composed of interconnected branching muscle fibres, or cells, that form the walls of the atria and the ventricles. The atrial walls are thinner because the atria act more as delivery containers, whereas the ventricular walls are thicker because the ventricles forcibly contract and pump blood against resistance. The resistance of the pulmonary bed is low, so the wall of the right ventricle is not as thick as that of the left ventricle, which pumps blood to all parts of the body against total systemic vascular resistance.

Control by the autonomic nervous system

The cardiac conduction system possesses the inherent ability for spontaneous rhythmic initiation of the cardiac impulse, but the autonomic nervous system has an important role in regulating the rate, rhythm, and force of myocardial contraction of the heart. Postganglionic fibres of the sympathetic nervous system, which release noradrenaline (NA), innervate the sinoatrial (SA) node, atria, and ventricles. NA acts on $\beta1$ receptors located in both nodes and atrial/ventricular muscles to increase heart rate (HR) and force of contraction. Circulating adrenaline from the adrenal medulla also elicits cardiac responses – for example, tachycardia.

Vagal nerve fibres of the parasympathetic branch, which release acetylcholine, are found primarily in the SA and atrioventricular (AV) nodes and atrial muscle. Acetylcholine acts on muscarinic (M_2) receptors of the

A schematic diagram of the heart, blood flow and valves

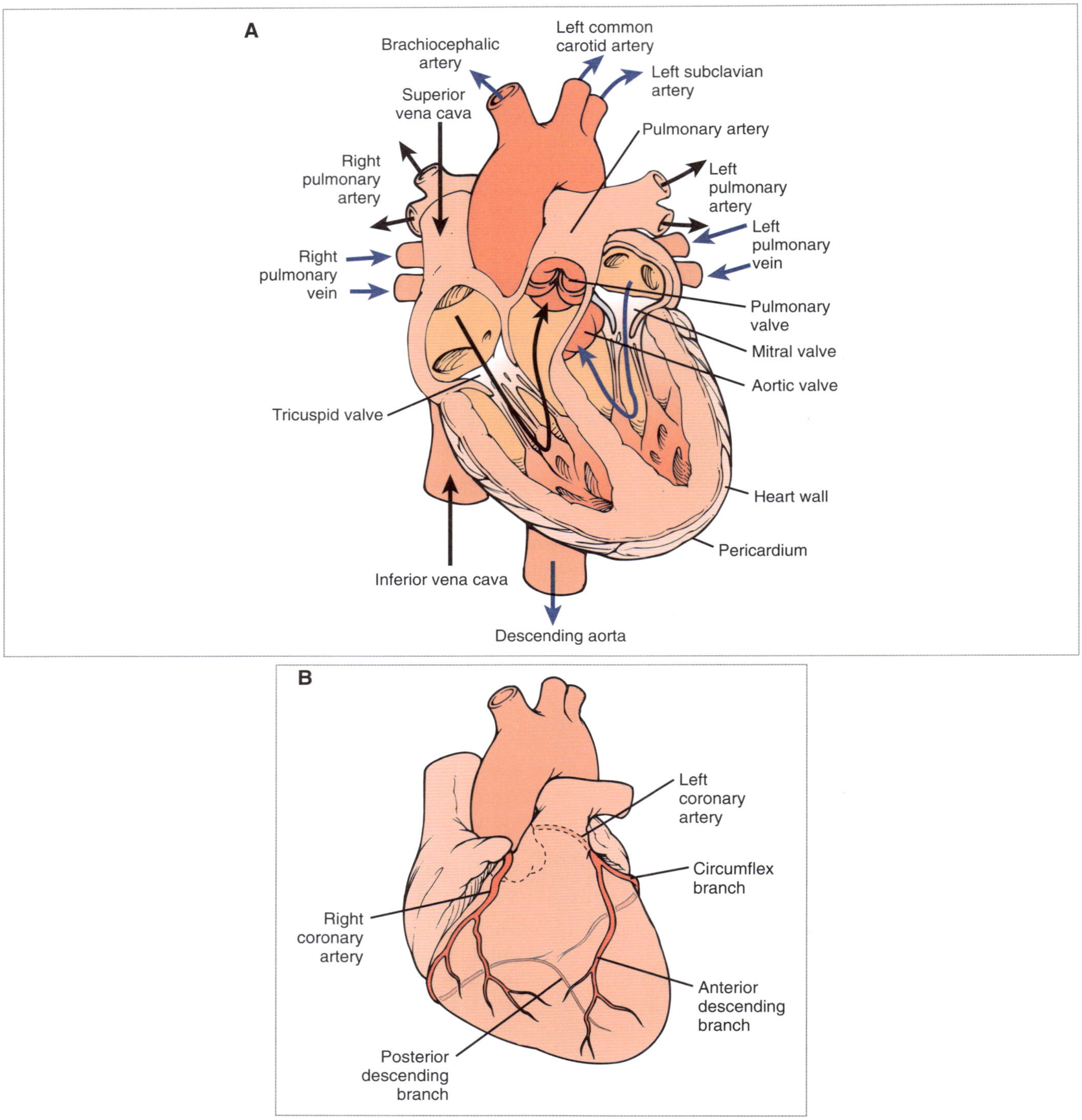

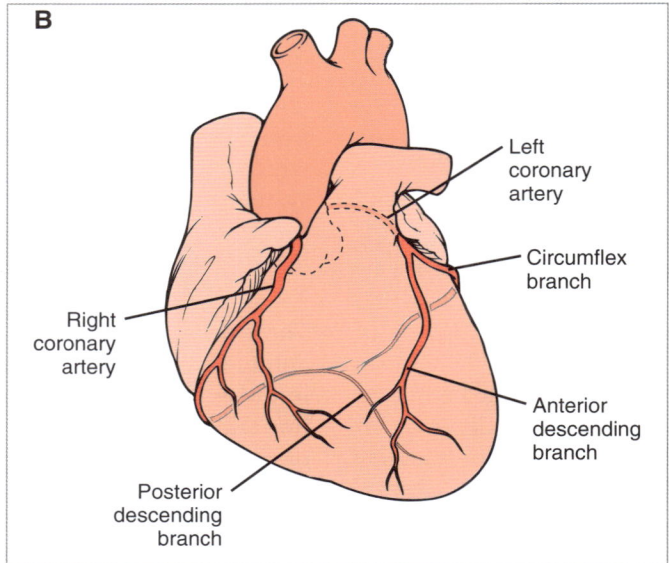

A

Brachiocephalic artery

Left common carotid artery

Left subclavian artery

Superior vena cava

Pulmonary artery

Right pulmonary artery

Left pulmonary artery

Left pulmonary vein

Right pulmonary vein

Pulmonary valve

Mitral valve

Aortic valve

Tricuspid valve

Heart wall

Pericardium

Inferior vena cava

Descending aorta

B

Left coronary artery

Circumflex branch

Right coronary artery

Anterior descending branch

Posterior descending branch

FIGURE 15.1 A Schematic diagram of the heart, valves, major blood vessels and blood flow. Black arrows indicate the direction of flow of deoxygenated blood, and blue arrows the flow of oxygenated blood. **B** Coronary blood supply to the heart. Dark-shaded vessels are those located on the external surface of the ventricles; light-shaded vessels show penetration of arterial branches towards the endocardial surface.

SA node to decrease HR and, to a limited extent, on the M_2 receptors on cardiac myocytes to reduce cardiac contractility. Control by the vagus nerve ensures the HR is regulated to approximately 75 beats/minute. In the absence of input from the vagus, the heart would contract at about 90–100 beats/minute, which is the normal automatic firing rate of the SA node. Normally, the HR is under the continuous influence of both parasympathetic and sympathetic nervous systems. The resting HR is the result of their opposing influences and at rest the firing rate of the sympathetic cardiac nerves is less than that of the vagus nerve.

The cardiac conduction system

Contraction of the heart depends on the regularity of events occurring in the cardiac cycle. Each cycle consists of a period of relaxation, **diastole**, followed by a period of contraction, **systole**. The rhythm and rate of the cardiac cycle are regulated by the conduction system, specialised cardiac cells that can initiate and transmit electrical impulses to stimulate cardiac muscle contraction.

The conduction system (Fig 15.2) comprises:

- the SA node
- internodal pathways
- the AV node
- the bundle of His
- right and left bundle branches
- Purkinje fibres.

The contractile mechanism

Activation of the actin filaments by calcium ions allows formation of the myosin cross-bridges. This interaction pulls the actin along the immobile myosin filaments towards the centre, shortening the sarcomere and producing muscle contraction (Fig 15.3). In this process, the lengths of individual filaments remain unchanged. The greater the quantity of calcium ions delivered to troponin, the greater the rate and numbers of interactions between actin and myosin. As a result of this response, the development of tension and contractility is increased.

Muscle relaxation depends on removing calcium ions from the sarcomere, thereby allowing the actin–myosin filaments of the sarcomere to return to their resting positions. This is achieved by a calcium ATPase (located in the walls of the sarcoplasmic reticulum), which actively returns some calcium ions to the sarcoplasmic reticulum while the remainder are removed from the cell by a Na^+–Ca^{2+} exchange protein that exchanges three sodium ions for every calcium ion.

Cardiac output

The primary function of the heart is to supply oxygenated blood to the body. When the body's requirement for oxygen increases (such as during physical activity and normal pregnancy), HR and cardiac output (CO) increase to meet demand. During pregnancy there is a 15% increase in the metabolic rate including a 20% increased consumption of oxygen (Soma-Pillay et al 2016). CO is a function of both the **stroke volume** (SV) and HR; that is:

$$CO = SV \times HR$$

SV is the volume of blood ejected during ventricular contraction. For example, in a healthy resting person, if SV was about 70 mL and HR 72 beats/minute, CO would equal 5040 mL/min. In women CO is 10–20% less than in men. Cardiovascular changes during pregnancy begin early. By eight weeks gestation the cardiac output has already increased by 20%. Maximum cardiac output is found at about 20–28 weeks gestation (Soma-Pillay et al 2016).

Factors regulating SV include the degree of stretch of heart fibres before contraction (**preload**), the force of contraction of the ventricles, and the pressure that must be overcome before the ventricles can eject the blood (**afterload**). The greater the preload, the stronger the contraction. This mechanism applies only when the muscle fibre is lengthened within physiological limits and is known as the Frank-Starling relation. The functional significance of the Frank-Starling relation is

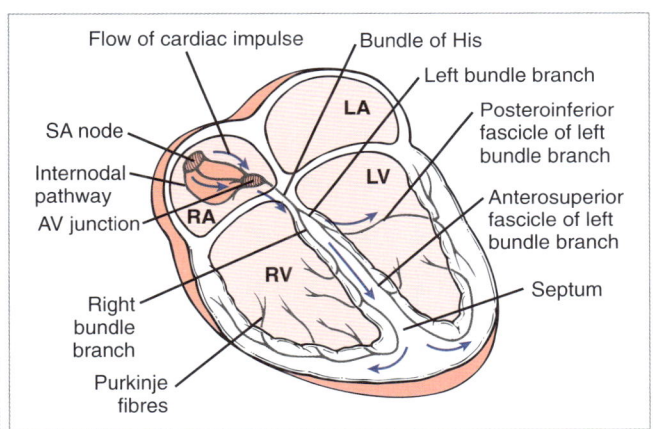

Cardiac conduction system

Flow of cardiac impulse — Bundle of His — Left bundle branch — LA — Posteroinferior fascicle of left bundle branch — SA node — LV — Internodal pathway — AV junction — RA — Anterosuperior fascicle of left bundle branch — RV — Septum — Right bundle branch — Purkinje fibres

FIGURE 15.2 Cardiac impulses are initiated at the SA node and transmitted through the internodal pathways to the two atria, resulting in atrial contraction. At the AV node, the electrical impulse is delayed. Conduction then speeds up at the bundle of His, with the impulse travelling through the right bundle branch and the left bundle branch and continuing through the posteroinferior fascicle and anterosuperior fascicle of the latter bundle branch. Finally, the arrival of impulses at the Purkinje fibres results in their distribution to all parts of both ventricles where, on excitation, ventricular contraction is produced. RA = right atrium; RV = right ventricle; LA = left atrium; LV = left ventricle; SA = sinoatrial

Source: Adapted from Salerno 1999, Figure 18.3; used with permission.

When contracted the sarcomere shortens so that the thick filaments approach the Z line and the width of the H zone between the thin filaments narrows. Calcium ions are required for contraction

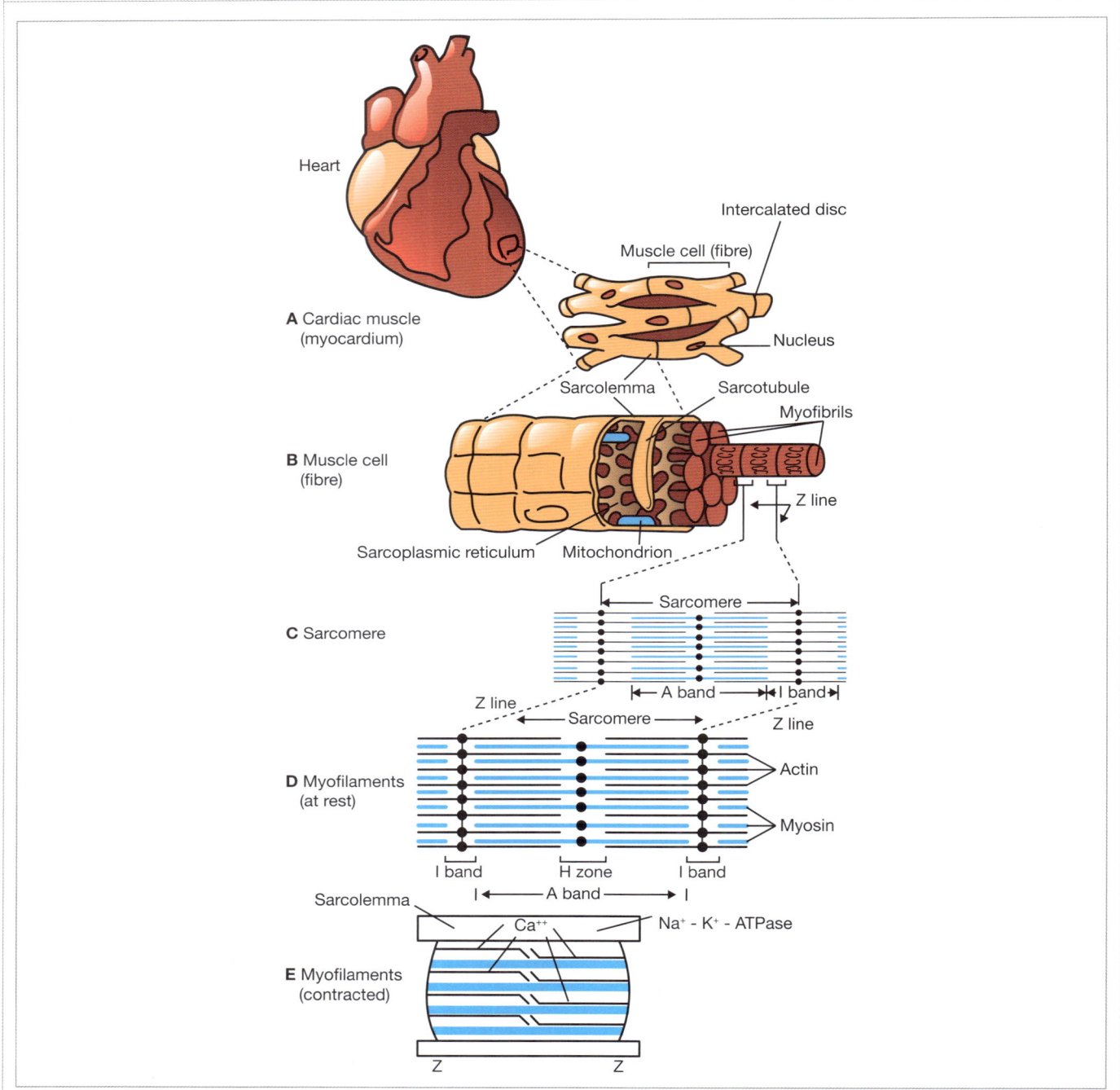

FIGURE 15.3

Source: Adapted from Salerno 1999; used with permission.

that effective CO can be brought about only by adequate relaxation and refilling of cardiac chambers after each myocardial contraction.

The vascular system

Once blood leaves the ventricles it enters the vascular system, comprised of arteries and arterioles, and venules and veins, that carry blood away from and back to the heart, respectively. Arterioles and capillaries are the main resistance vessels and regulate afterload, while the venules and veins are capacitance vessels, contributing to preload of the ventricles. The arterial wall consists of three layers: the inner (*tunica intima*), the middle (*tunica media*) and the outer (*tunica adventitia*). The middle (thickest) layer is composed of elastic and smooth muscle fibres, and the outer of elastic and collagen fibres.

The smooth muscle is arranged in a circular layer, and stimulation by the sympathetic nervous system causes contraction of the smooth muscle, which narrows the lumen of the vessel (vasoconstriction). In contrast, a diminution in sympathetic stimulation results in relaxation of the smooth muscle (vasodilation). The elastic properties of the arteries enable distension when the ventricles eject a volume of blood, and the elastic recoil aids in the forward propulsion of the blood.

Arteries branch to form arterioles and capillaries, the main resistance vessels, which play a key role in blood pressure regulation. Capillaries are the smallest of the arterial vessels and connect the arterioles to the venules. The combined resistance of the systemic blood vessels, but principally the arterioles, capillaries, and venules, is referred to as systemic vascular resistance (SVR) or total peripheral resistance.

Venules are the conduits through which blood flows from the capillaries to the veins. Unlike arteries, veins have a system of valves ensuring blood flows in a forward direction towards the heart.

The vascular endothelium

The luminal surface of the *tunica intima* is lined with a single layer of nucleated endothelial cells that are linked together laterally by tight junctions. Endothelial cells are a source of multiple endogenous mediators that influence vascular function through either vasodilation or vasoconstriction (Fig 15.4). An important mediator is nitric oxide (NO – not to be confused with the anaesthetic gas nitrous oxide, N_2O). The NO formed acts locally on the adjacent vascular smooth muscle cell where it decreases intracellular calcium, resulting in vascular relaxation (Fig 15.4). During pregnancy endothelium-dependent factors, including nitric oxide synthesis, upregulated by oestradiol and possibly vasodilatory prostaglandins (PGI2) result in increased peripheral vasodilation which in turn reduces systemic vascular resistance by 25–30%. To compensate, cardiac output increases by around 40% during pregnancy through increased stroke volume and sometimes increased heart rate (Some-Pillay et al 2016).

A rise in free calcium ion concentration is the primary event in triggering smooth muscle contraction and causing vasoconstriction. Activation of smooth muscle can reduce the calibre of small vessels markedly. Calcium channel-blocking drugs block calcium ion influx in the smooth muscle of blood vessels, thereby producing relaxation. Modulation of calcium concentration forms the basis for the actions of a range of drugs affecting the vascular system.

The renin–angiotensin–aldosterone system

The kidneys are by far the most important organs in the body for long-term regulation of blood pressure and, normally, excessive fluid retention is controlled by negative feedback mechanisms that operate to restore normal fluid and electrolyte balance. The RAAS regulates blood pressure by increasing or decreasing blood volume through modulation of renal function (Fig 15.5). Abnormal activation of the RAAS plays a key role in the development and pathophysiology of hypertension and cardiovascular disease and correlates directly with the incidence and extent of end-organ damage. The major effector molecules of the RAAS are renin, angiotensin II and the mineralocorticoid **aldosterone**. Additionally, it is now recognised that aldosterone is a proinflammatory molecule that plays a major role in the progression of ischaemic heart disease and that a raised aldosterone-to-renin ratio is common in patients with hypertension.

A reduction in blood flow through the kidneys decreases renal arterial pressure, which causes the release of renin into the circulation. Renin is secreted from the juxtaglomerular cells located in the afferent arteriolar walls of the nephron and catalyses the cleavage of angiotensinogen, a plasma globulin, to form angiotensin I, a weak vasoconstrictor. Subsequently, in endothelial cells, primarily in the lung, angiotensin I is converted by angiotensin-converting enzyme to angiotensin II. Arterial under-filling is a state unique to pregnancy, resulting from the fall in systematic vascular resistance that occurs from 6 weeks of pregnancy. Despite increased plasma volume SVR means that 85% of volume remains in the venous circulation. Other adaptive changes of pregnancy include specific placental hormonal effects, for example, relaxin, a peptide hormone, that regulates haemodynamic and water balance (Soma-Pillay et al 2016).

Angiotensin II, acting via AT_1 receptors, is one of the most potent vasoconstrictors known. It effectively constricts arterioles, which increases peripheral resistance and raises blood pressure. In addition, angiotensin II acts on the adrenal cortex to stimulate the secretion of aldosterone, which promotes reabsorption of sodium by the kidneys and the excretion of potassium. The increased

Endothelium-derived mediators

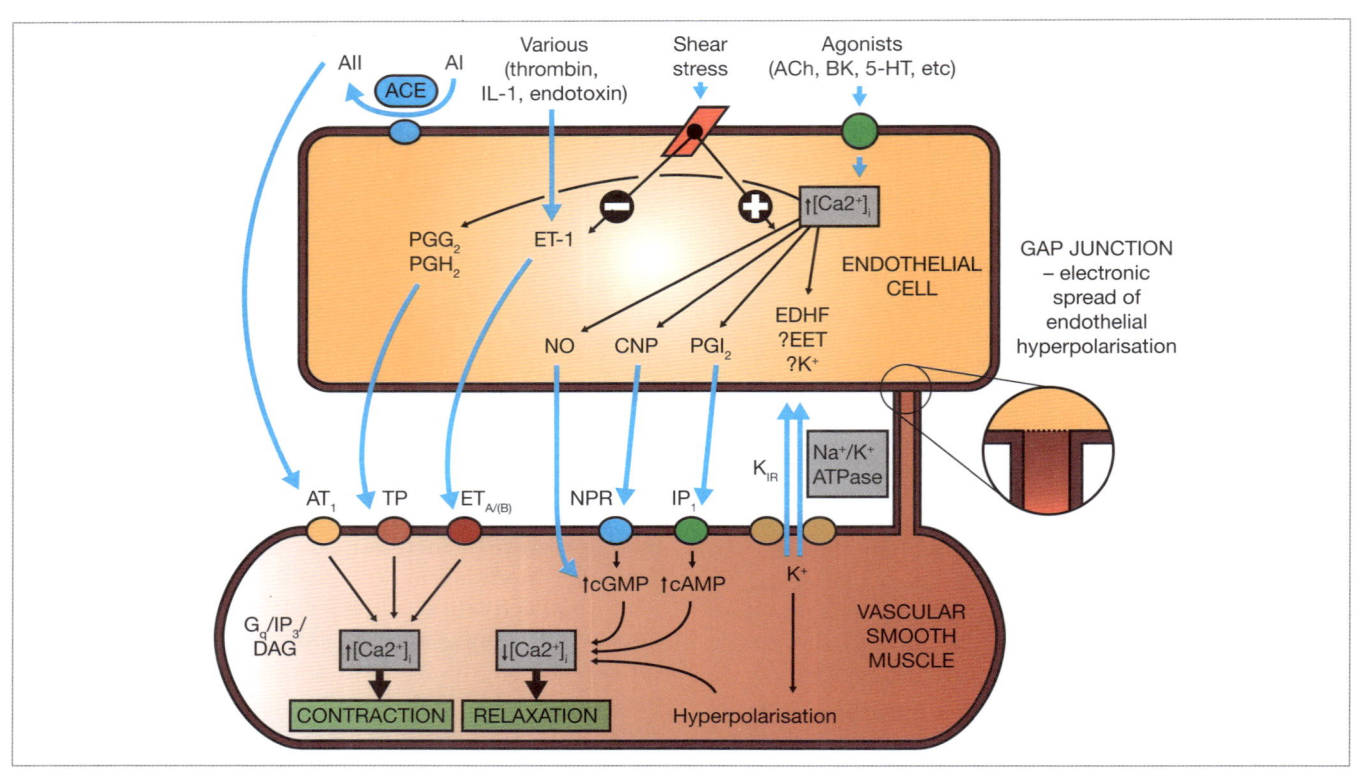

FIGURE 15.4 The schematic shows some of the more important endothelium-derived contracting and relaxing mediators; many (if not all) of the vasoconstrictors also cause smooth muscle mitogenesis, while vasodilators commonly inhibit mitogenesis. 5-HT = 5-hydroxytryptamine; A = angiotensin; ACE = angiotensin-converting enzyme; ACh = acetylcholine; AT1 = angiotensin AT1 receptor; BK = bradykinin; CNP = C-natriuretic peptide; DAG = diacylglycerol; EDHF = endothelium-derived hyperpolarising factor; EET = epoxyeicosatetraenoic acid; ET-1 = endothelin-1; ETA/(B) = endothelium A (and B) receptors; Gq = G-protein; IL-1 = interleukin-1; IP1 = prostanoid receptor; IP3 = inosinol 1,4,5-trisphosphate; K$_{IR}$ = inward rectifying potassium channel; Na+/K+ = ATPase electrogenic pump; NPR = natriuretic peptide receptor; PG = prostaglandin; TP = T prostanoid receptor

Source: Adapted from Rang et al 2012, Figure 22.1; used with permission.

sodium elevates the osmotic pressure of plasma, causing a release of antidiuretic hormone from the hypothalamus, leading to increased reabsorption of water from the renal tubules, which adds further to the rise in blood pressure. Angiotensin II itself also acts on the kidney tubules to promote reabsorption of water. Furthermore, activation of AT$_1$ receptors produces adverse effects on the cardiovascular system, including the promotion of vascular and cardiac hypertrophy, inflammation, and fibrosis. While the **renin–angiotensin–aldosterone system** is activated in early pregnancy, resistance to angiotensin II also develops to counterbalance the vasoconstrictive effect, enabling vasodilation. This resistance to angiotensin II is caused by the effects of progesterone and vascular endothelial growth as well as modification in the angiotensin I receptors during pregnancy. The placental vasodilators may be even more

important in maintaining vasodilation during the second half of pregnancy (Soma-Pillay et al 2016).

The sympathetic nervous system

The sympathetic (adrenergic) nervous system is the second major subdivision of the autonomic nervous system. This system acts in concert with the parasympathetic nervous system to regulate the heart, secretory glands and vascular and non-vascular smooth muscle (Table 15.1). Understanding the physiological responses mediated by adrenergic receptors aids in rationalising the pharmacological and adverse effects of drugs affecting noradrenergic transmission.

β-adrenoceptor antagonists

β-adrenoceptor antagonists, commonly referred to as β-blockers, competitively block the actions of

Interrelationship between renal perfusion, the renin–angiotensin–aldosterone system, hypertension and the sites of action of drugs targeting RAAS

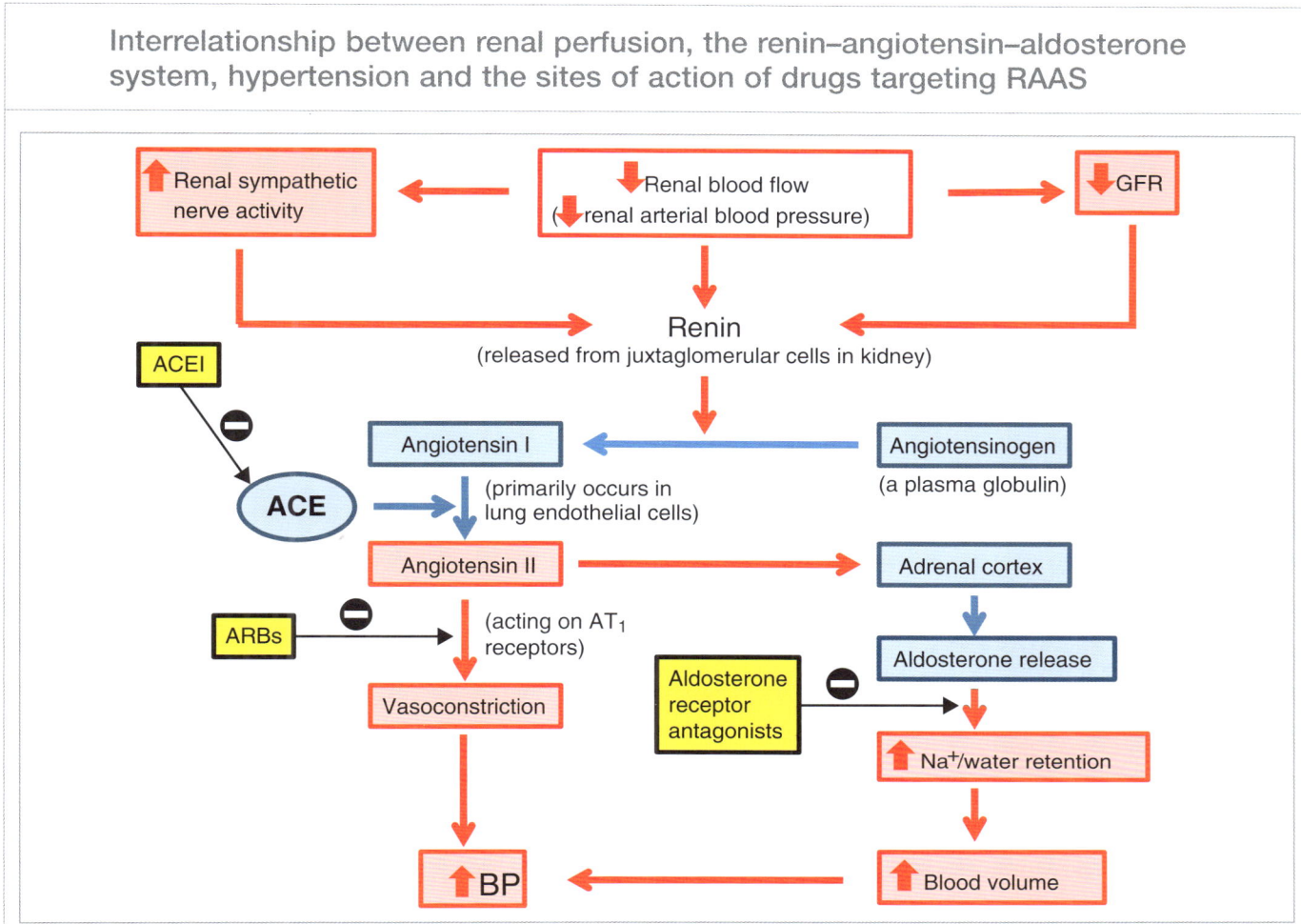

FIGURE 15.5 ACE = angiotensin-converting enzyme; ACEI = angiotensin-converting enzyme inhibitors; ARBs = angiotensin-receptor (AT1) antagonists; - = inhibitory effect

TABLE 15.1 Alpha and beta-adrenoceptor subtypes, examples of tissue localisation and dominant physiological response

LOCALISATION	α_{1A}	α_{1B}	α_{1D}	α_{2A}	α_{2B}	α_{2C}	β_1	β_2	β_3
Aorta			✓						
Brain	✓	✓	✓	✓		✓	✓	✓	
Blood vessels	✓	✓			✓			✓	
Coronary vessels			✓	✓					
Heart	✓						✓	✓	✓
Kidney		✓			✓		✓	✓	
Liver	✓				✓			✓	
Lung	✓	✓						✓	

Continued

TABLE 15.1 Alpha and beta-adrenoceptor subtypes, examples of tissue localisation and dominant physiological response—cont'd

LOCALISATION	α_{1A}	α_{1B}	α_{1D}	α_{2A}	α_{2B}	α_{2C}	β_1	β_2	β_3
Platelets			✓	✓	✓				
Prostate	✓		✓						
Smooth muscle (e.g. bladder, airways, uterus)	✓							✓	✓
Sympathetic neurons				✓					
Skeletal muscle							✓		✓

Dominant physiological response

α_{1A} Arterial vasoconstriction
    Vascular smooth muscle contraction
    Promotes cardiac hypertrophy
α_{1B} Promotes cardiac hypertrophy
α_{1D} Arterial vasoconstriction
α_{2A} Reduces sympathetic neurotransmission (including central sympathetic outflow)
Arterial vasoconstriction
α_{2B} Vasoconstriction
α_{2C} Modulates dopamine neurotransmission
    Inhibits hormone release from adrenal medulla
B_1 Heart (SA and AV nodes and His-Purkinje systems) increased automaticity, conduction velocity and contractility
B_2 Dilation of vasculature: arterioles and arteries
    Relaxation of bronchial smooth muscle
    Relaxation of pregnant uterine smooth muscle
B_3 Relaxation of bladder detrusor muscle
Source: Brunton LL, Chabner B, Knollman B. Goodman & Gilman's The pharmacological basic of therapeutics, 13th ed. McGraw-Hill, New York, 2017.

catecholamines. The main group is the β1-selective blockers that are frequently referred to as cardioselective blockers because these agents block β1-adrenoceptors on the heart. At high doses, however, β1-adrenoceptor selectivity diminishes, and the adverse effects of β2-adrenoceptor blockade then need to be considered. Drugs that block both types of adrenoceptors, β1- and β2-, are referred to as non-selective β-adrenoceptor antagonists. The use of all these drugs is contraindicated in people with asthma because of inhibition of bronchodilation mediated by β2-adrenoceptors.

KEY POINTS

The heart

- The heart comprises four chambers, two upper atria and two lower ventricles, which are supplied with blood and nutrients by the right and left coronary arteries.

- The myocardium or cardiac muscle tissue is comprised of sarcomeres, the basic contractile unit of the heart.

- Postganglionic fibres of the sympathetic nervous system release NA and innervate the SA node, atria and ventricles. Action of NA on β1 receptors located in both nodes and in atrial and ventricular muscles increases HR, **automaticity**, conduction velocity and force of contraction.

- Vagal nerve fibres of the parasympathetic nervous system, which release acetylcholine, are found primarily in the SA and AV nodes and atrial muscle. Acetylcholine acts on M_2 receptors of the SA node to decrease HR, on the AV node to decrease conduction velocity, and, to a limited extent, on the M_2 receptors on cardiac myocytes to reduce cardiac contractility.

- The cardiac conduction system comprises the SA and AV nodes, internodal pathways, the bundle of His, right and left bundle branches, and the Purkinje fibres.

- Cardiac output is a function of stroke volume and heart rate: $CO = SV \times HR$.

- Factors regulating stroke volume include the degree of stretch of heart fibres before contraction (preload), the force of contraction of the ventricles, and the pressure that must be overcome before the ventricles can eject the blood (afterload).

- The Frank-Starling law of the heart defines the relationship between the force of ejection and the length of cardiac muscle fibres.

- During pregnancy there are profound cardiovascular changes in the maternal body from as early as eight weeks. These include increased cardiac output, increased maternal blood volume, increased extracellular and plasma volume. Additionally, arterial under-filling, mediated through the effect of placental hormones and the RAA system are important in facilitating vasodilation and more be more important in the second half of pregnancy. These all play critical roles in circulation blood volume, blood pressure and uteroplacental perfusion which are disturbed in women experiencing hypertensive disorders of pregnancy. These are impacted in women with complex conditions such as preeclampsia and other pregnancy states, for example, twin pregnancy.

- Arterioles and capillaries are the main resistance vessels and regulate afterload. Venules and veins are capacitance vessels contributing to preload.

- Endothelial cells control vascular smooth muscle tone and play an active role in haemostasis and thrombosis.

- A rise in free calcium ion concentration is considered the primary event in increasing smooth muscle tone and causing vasoconstriction.

- The sympathetic nervous system (in conjugation with parasympathetic nervous system) is responsible for major physiological controls in the body, including blood pressure.

- The catecholamine noradrenaline acts as the neurotransmitter between sympathetic postganglionic nerves and effector organs. It is also released from modified postganglionic neurons in the adrenal medulla into the bloodstream (hormone) and from certain neurons.

- There are two major subtypes of adrenoceptors – alpha (α) and beta (β) – and they are stimulated by noradrenaline and adrenaline.

- Abrupt cessation of β-blockers can cause a rebound phenomenon. When stopping treatment, reduce dose gradually.

15.2 Hypertension in pregnancy

Hypertension is defined as an elevated systolic blood pressure, diastolic blood pressure, or both. In clinical practice, elevated systolic blood pressure is a greater predictor of cardiovascular risk than elevated diastolic pressure. However, as per SOMANZ Guidelines for the management of hypertensive disorders of pregnancy (see Online resources SOMANZ 2023; Lowe et al 2015), specific complexities that may develop in relation to pregnancy make accurate monitoring of both systolic and diastolic blood pressure highly relevant. Worldwide definitions of hypertension vary, and a suggested classification has been developed following a review of systems in the United States and Europe (Gabb et al 2016) (Table 15.2).

This classification also stratifies individuals based on blood pressure, the presence of risk factors and the degree of target-organ damage secondary to hypertension. The major risk factors in hypertensive patients include

TABLE 15.2 Review of systems in the United States and Europe

CATEGORY	SYSTOLIC BP (mmHg)	DIASTOLIC BP (mmHg)
Optimal	< 120	< 80
Normal	120–129	80–84
High–normal	130–139	85–89
Grade 1 (mild hypertension)	140–159	90–99
Grade 2 (moderate hypertension)	160–179	100–109
Grade 3 (severe hypertension)	≥ 180	≥ 110
Isolated systolic hypertension	≥ 140	< 90
Gestational hypertension > 20 w	≥ 140	≥ 90
Severe hypertension	≥ 160	≥ 110

Source: Adapted with permission from the National Heart Foundation of Australia. Guideline for the diagnosis and management of hypertension in adults 2016. © 2016 National Heart Foundation of Australia.

cigarette smoking, diabetes mellitus, raised total or LDL cholesterol or reduced HDL cholesterol, age (> 55 years male, > 65 years female), family history of heart disease, male gender (increased risk at any age compared with females), obesity, excessive alcohol intake and a sedentary lifestyle. Psychosocial risk factors include depression, social isolation and lack of quality support. Those populations most at risk include people of Aboriginal, Torres Strait Islander, Māori or Pacific Islander origin and those in lower socioeconomic groups. The target-organ damage or cardiovascular disease in hypertensive patients includes stroke or transient ischaemic attacks, kidney disease, retinopathy and various cardiac diseases such as angina, **heart failure**, left ventricular hypertrophy and prior MI.

Gestational hypertension, also known as pregnancy-induced hypertension (PIH), is a medical condition that develops after the 20th week of pregnancy and usually resolves after delivery. It is important to differentiate gestational hypertension from chronic hypertension that existed before pregnancy or before the 20th week of gestation. It is diagnosed when a pregnant woman, who previously had normal blood pressure, develops elevated blood pressure as a reading of 140/90 mm Hg or higher on two separate occasions, at least 6 hours apart. Often, gestational hypertension has no symptoms, and it is usually detected during routine prenatal checks. In some cases, gestational hypertension may present with further organ complications include symptoms of headaches, visual disturbances, abdominal pain, presence of protein in the urine and abnormal liver function, and blood coagulation complications, which have been discussed in Chapter 16.

Preeclampsia is a multifaceted multisystem disorder, characterised by the abrupt onset of hypertension (occurring after 20 weeks of gestation) and the presence of at least one additional related complication, such as proteinuria, maternal organ dysfunction, or uteroplacental dysfunction. Women who have experienced a hypertensive disorder of pregnancy, such as gestational hypertension or preeclampsia, may face long-term cardiovascular risks. Research suggests that these women have an increased likelihood of developing cardiovascular diseases, such as coronary artery disease and ischaemic stroke, later in life compared to those with normotensive pregnancies (Rayes et al 2023).

Drug therapy for hypertension in pregnancy

Non-pharmacological measures are the first step for managing hypertension in the non-pregnant person. However, for gestational hypertension or essential hypertension diagnosed for the first time during pregnancy, the first step of management is using pharmacological agents that mainly dilate the blood vessels (vasodilators including centrally acting and **calcium channel blockers**) or block the adrenergic agents (beta blockers) (Table 15.3). In the case of severe hypertension, the management is outlined in Table 15.4.

When instituting drug therapy, the lowest dose of the chosen drug is used, adding a second drug from a different drug class if necessary. The overriding goal of drug therapy is to lower the blood pressure, with minimal adverse effects. Figure 15.6 summarises the physiological factors controlling blood pressure (the sympathetic nervous system

TABLE 15.3 Antihypertensive medications in pregnancy

DRUG	DOSAGE	ACT	CONTRAINDICATIONS	PRACTICE POINTS
Methyldopa	250 mg–750 mg every 8 hours	Central	Depression	Slow onset of action over 24 hours Dry mouth, sedation, depression, blurred vision Withdrawal effect: rebound hypertension
Labetalol	100 mg–400 mg every 8 hours	Beta blocker with mild alpha vasodilator effect	Asthma, chronic airways limitation	Bradycardia, bronchospasm, headache, nausea, scalp tingling which usually resolves within 24 hours
Nifedipine	30 mg or 60 mg slow release every 12 hours	Calcium channel antagonist	Aortic stenosis	Severe headache in first 24 hours, flushing, tachycardia, peripheral oedema, constipation

TABLE 15.4 Medications for acute blood pressure lowering for severe hypertension

DRUG	FORMULATIONS	DOSE AND ADMINISTRATION	ONSET OF ACTION	ADVERSE REACTIONS
Nifedipine	10 mg & 20 mg immediate release tablet or capsule	10 mg or 20 mg orally Repeat after 30 minutes if BP not below threshold (max. 40 mg)	30–45 minutes	Headache Flushing
Labetalol	200 mg tablet 5 mg/mL IV vial	200 mg orally Repeat after 30 minutes if BP not below threshold, maximum 400 mg If BP not below threshold after 30 minutes, give 20 mg IV bolus slowly over 2 minutes Repeat doses of 40–80 mg every 10 minutes until BP controlled (max. 4 doses). Consider infusion after 2 bolus doses	Maximal effect usually occurs within 5 minutes after each dose	Bradycardia Hypotension Fetal bradycardia
Hydralazine	20 mg/mL IV powder vial	If BP not below threshold following administration of nifedipine, give 5 mg IV bolus over 5 minutes Repeat every 20 minutes until BP controlled (max. 30 mg)	20 minutes	Flushing Headache Nausea Hypotension Tachycardia

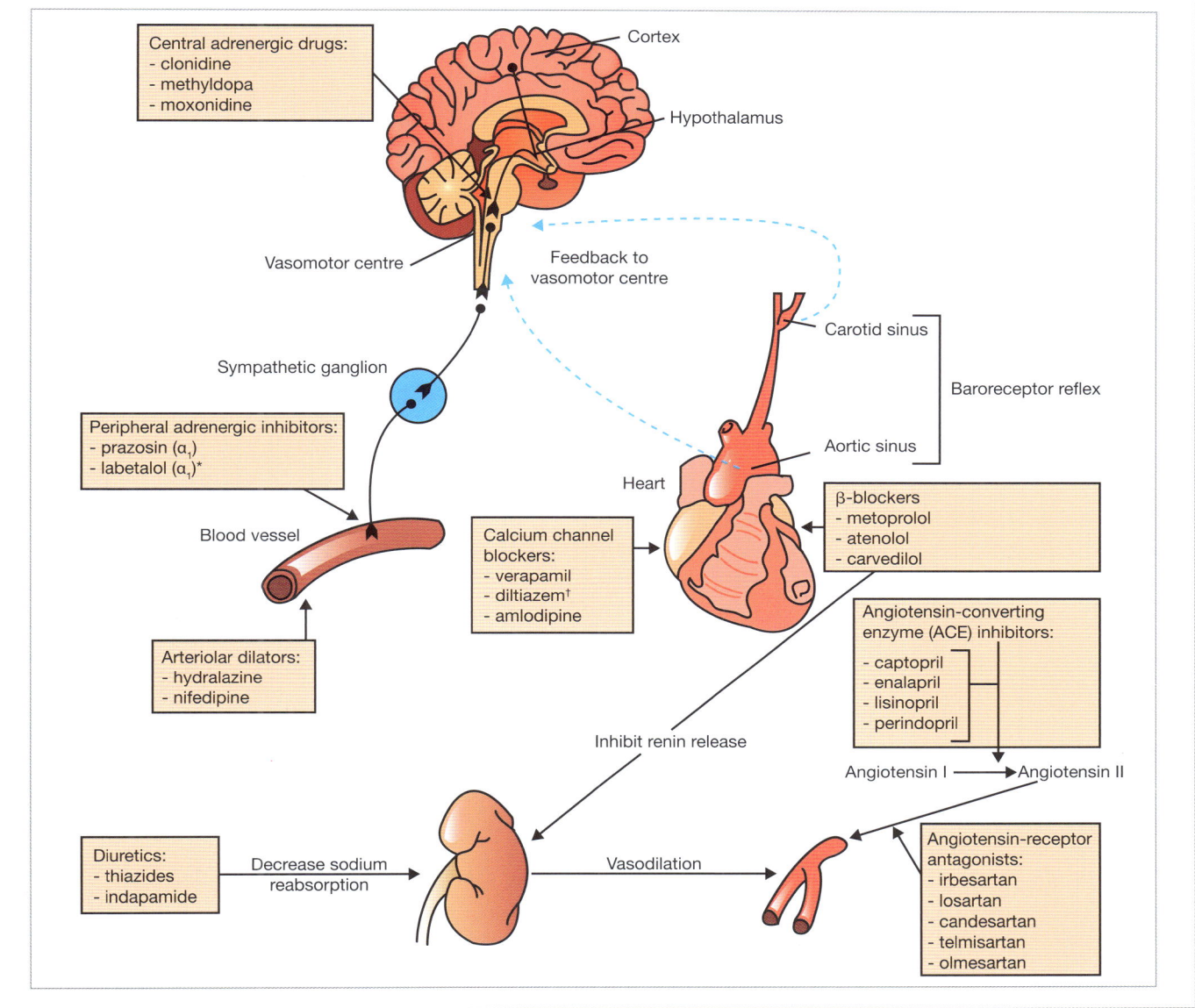

Physiological control of blood pressure and sites of action of some currently used oral antihypertensive drugs

Central adrenergic drugs:
- clonidine
- methyldopa
- moxonidine

Cortex

Hypothalamus

Vasomotor centre

Feedback to vasomotor centre

Carotid sinus

Baroreceptor reflex

Sympathetic ganglion

Aortic sinus

Heart

Peripheral adrenergic inhibitors:
- prazosin (α_1)
- labetalol (α_1)*

β-blockers
- metoprolol
- atenolol
- carvedilol

Blood vessel

Calcium channel blockers:
- verapamil
- diltiazem†
- amlodipine

Angiotensin-converting enzyme (ACE) inhibitors:
- captopril
- enalapril
- lisinopril
- perindopril

Arteriolar dilators:
- hydralazine
- nifedipine

Inhibit renin release

Angiotensin I ⟶ Angiotensin II

Diuretics:
- thiazides
- indapamide

Decrease sodium reabsorption

Vasodilation

Angiotensin-receptor antagonists:
- irbesartan
- losartan
- candesartan
- telmisartan
- olmesartan

FIGURE 15.6 * Labetalol acts on both α1- and β1- adrenoceptors. † Diltiazem acts on both the heart and arteriolar vascular smooth muscle.

and the RAAS) and indicates the sites of action of currently used oral antihypertensive drugs. For women with essential hypertension, review of antihypertensive drugs before conception is important since diuretics and drugs that act through the RAAS system are contraindicated in pregnancy.

This section focuses on antihypertensive drugs that are used in pregnancy. In pregnancy, first-line monotherapy regimens include:
- calcium channel blockers such as nifedipine (DM 15-1)

- β-adrenoceptor antagonists (beta blockers) such as labetalol
- centrally acting vasodilators such as methyldopa (DM 15-3).

Calcium channel blockers

Calcium channel blockers are medications that are effective in treating hypertension, including in pregnant women. These drugs work by inhibiting the influx of calcium ions into vascular smooth muscle and cardiac muscle cells, leading to vasodilation and a reduction in blood pressure.

DRUGS AT A GLANCE
Drugs affecting vascular smooth muscle

PHARMACOLOGICAL GROUP AND EFFECT	KEY EXAMPLES	CLINICAL USE
Antihypertensives *Calcium channel blockers* • Block inward movement of calcium through cell membranes of cardiac and smooth muscle cells • ↓ force of myocardial contraction • Dilate coronary arteries, which improves oxygen delivery to myocardium • Dihydropyridines are arteriolar vasodilators, which results in reduction in peripheral vascular resistance and blood pressure	Amlodipine	• Hypertension
	Clevidipine	• Hypertension (absence of oral treatment)
	Diltiazem	• Angina • Hypertension (controlled release)
	Felodipine	• Hypertension
	Lercanidipine	• Hypertension
	Nifedipine* (DM 15-1)	• Angina • Hypertension
Potassium channel activators • Relax vascular smooth muscle by acting on ATP-sensitive potassium channels • Antagonise action of ATP, which prevents closure of potassium channels • Cause hyperpolarisation and relaxation of vascular smooth muscle	Nimodipine	• Prevention/treatment neurological issues following aneurysmal subarachnoid haemorrhage
	Verapamil	• Angina • Atrial fibrillation/flutter • Hypertension • Supraventricular tachycardia (SVT)
Vasodilators • Direct arteriolar vasodilator (hydralazine) • Direct arteriolar/venous vasodilator (sodium nitroprusside)	Diazoxide	• Hypertensive emergency
	Minoxidil	• Severe refractory hypertension
	Hydralazine*	• Hypertensive emergency
Centrally acting antihypertensives • α₂ adrenoceptor agonist • ↓ sympathetic tone • ↓ blood pressure	Sodium nitroprusside	• Hypertensive emergency • Controlled hypotension during surgery • Acute heart failure
	Clonidine	• Hypertension
	Methyldopa*	• Hypertension

*Drugs highlighted in bold are used in pregnancy.

DRUG MONOGRAPH 15.1
Nifedipine

Nifedipine is a **calcium channel blocker** that blocks the inward movement of calcium through the slow channels of the cell membranes of cardiac and smooth muscle cells. Nifedipine has minimal effect on cardiac tissue at therapeutic doses. It acts principally on vascular smooth muscle, reducing peripheral vascular resistance. This results in widespread reduction in resistance to blood flow through the body (determined by the tone of the vascular musculature and the diameter of the blood vessels) and blood pressure. The haemodynamic change reduces afterload, which also decreases oxygen demand of the heart. In some circumstances, the reflex sympathetic response to vasodilation results in tachycardia, which contributes to the side effect profile of this class of drugs.

Pharmacokinetics and dosage and administration
See Table 15.5 for the pharmacokinetics of nifedipine. It is metabolised by CYP3A4 and has no known active metabolite.

Drug interactions
The common involvement of CYP3A4 leads to extensive drug interactions that vary for each of the other calcium channel-blocking drugs. Relevant drug information sources should always be consulted. Examples include:
- *β-adrenoceptor antagonists:* An increased risk of bradycardia occurs with co-administration with diltiazem, and monitoring of cardiac function is necessary. The combination with verapamil is not recommended because of the risk of heart block.
- *Carbamazepine and ciclosporin:* Diltiazem and verapamil increase plasma concentrations of carbamazepine and ciclosporin. Monitor such combinations closely, as dosage adjustments may be necessary.
- *Digoxin:* Increased plasma concentration of digoxin has been reported with co-administration of verapamil or diltiazem. Monitor digoxin plasma concentration closely whenever a calcium channel-blocking agent is started or discontinued or

DRUG MONOGRAPH 15.1
Nifedipine—cont'd

when dosage is changed. Monitor for prolonged AV conduction, bradycardia, or AV blocks, especially during the initial week of therapy, as digoxin dose may need to be changed.

- *Inhibitors of CYP3A4 (e.g. erythromycin, itraconazole, grapefruit juice):* May decrease metabolism of the calcium channel blockers, increasing the potential for adverse effects. Monitor and adjust dose if necessary.

Adverse reactions

Common adverse reactions are shown in Figure 15.7. Gingival hyperplasia is a rare adverse effect reported with amlodipine, diltiazem, felodipine, verapamil and, most often, nifedipine. It starts as an inflammation of the gums, usually in the first 9 months of therapy. When the drug is discontinued, this effect usually improves within 1–4 weeks. Good dental hygiene, along with professional teeth cleaning, is necessary to reduce the potential for this adverse effect.

TABLE 15.5 Pharmacokinetics and dosages of nifedipine

DRUG/INDICATION	TIME TO PEAK CONCENTRATION (h)	DURATION OF ACTION (h)	METABOLISM	USUAL ADULT ORAL DAILY DOSE
Nifedipine	0.5–1	4–8	Hepatic	◆10–20 mg twice daily to a max of 20–40 mg twice daily
Controlled release			Hepatic	20–30 mg once daily to a max of 90 mg daily (angina) or 120 mg daily (hypertension)

Source: Dosage information: Australian Medicines Handbook 2021, pp 264–268. Verify adult dose range using up-to-date drug/product information sources and pregnancy clinical guidelines.

WARNING AND CONTRAINDICATIONS

Calcium channel blockers should be used with caution in patients with severe bradycardia, congestive heart failure (caution with felodipine, nifedipine and nimodipine, as they have a slight negative **inotropic effect**), hypotension, acute MI, or liver or kidney impairment. Avoid use in patients with hypersensitivity to calcium channel blockers, cardiac shock, severe bradycardia, or congestive heart failure. (Use extreme caution with diltiazem and verapamil.) The use of clevidipine is contraindicated in severe aortic stenosis.

β-adrenoceptor antagonists

Beta-adrenoceptor antagonists, commonly known as beta blockers, are a class of medications widely used in the treatment of hypertension and other cardiovascular conditions during pregnancy. These drugs work by blocking the effects of catecholamines, such as adrenaline and noradrenaline, on beta-adrenergic receptors (Table 15.6).

Non-selective α₁- and β-adrenoceptor antagonists

Labetalol acts on both α1- and β-adrenoceptors and competitively antagonises the action of catecholamines. It is a complex drug that selectively blocks α1-, β1- and β2-adrenoceptors but also partially stimulates β2-adrenoceptors and inhibits the neuronal uptake of noradrenaline. Blockade of α1-adrenoceptors leads to a fall in peripheral vascular resistance, while blockade of β1-adrenoceptors prevents the reflex sympathetic stimulation of the heart. The drug is indicated for treating hypertension.

Mechanism of action

β-adrenoceptor antagonists competitively block β-adrenoceptor sites located on the heart, smooth muscle of the bronchi and blood vessels, kidney, pancreas, uterus, brain and liver. Cardiac muscle contains principally β1-adrenoceptors, while smooth muscle sites contain primarily β2-adrenoceptors.

Common adverse effects of calcium channel blockers

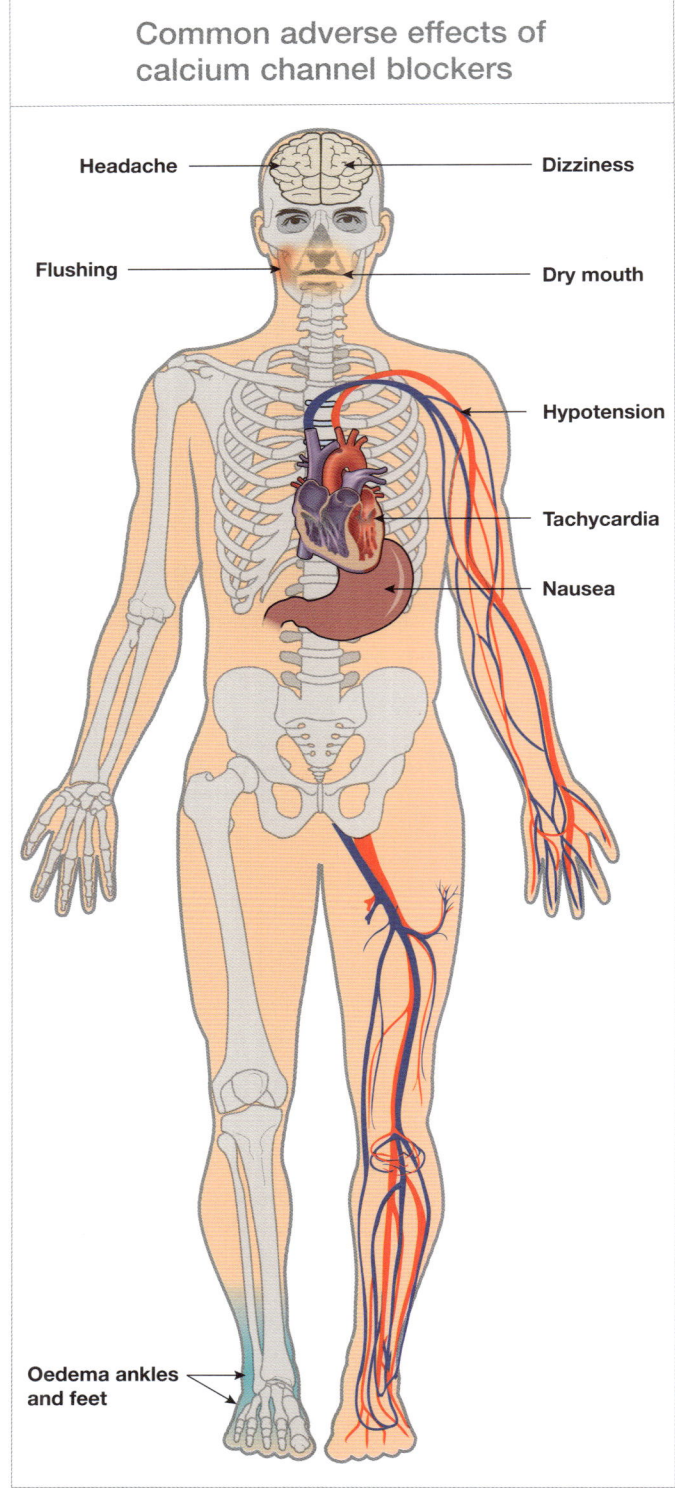

Headache — Dizziness

Flushing — Dry mouth

Hypotension

Tachycardia

Nausea

Oedema ankles and feet

FIGURE 15.7 Adverse effects vary between the drugs depending on the degree of vasodilation, which is greatest with the dihydropyridines such as nifedipine.

TABLE 15.6 Classification of β-adrenoceptor antagonists

TYPE	DRUGS
Selective β1-adrenoceptor antagonists	Atenolol, betaxolol,[a] bisoprolol, metoprolol, nebivolol[b]
Non-selective β1- and β2-adrenoceptor antagonists	Carvedilol,[c] labetalol, propranolol, sotalol, timolol[a]
Non-selective β1- and β2-adrenoceptor antagonists with ISA activity	Oxprenolol, pindolol

[a] Available as eyedrops only.
[b] Highly selective antagonist at β_1-adrenoceptors, and also causes vasodilation through release of nitric oxide.
[c] Also an α_1 antagonist.

Cardiovascular effects

Pharmacologically, blockade of β1-adrenoceptors on the heart decreases rate, conduction velocity, myocardial contractility and cardiac output (Fig 15.8).

Their antihypertensive actions result from decreased cardiac output (without a reflex increase in peripheral vascular resistance), diminished sympathetic outflow from the vasomotor centre in the brain to the peripheral blood vessels, and reduced renin release by the kidney.

Central nervous system effects

Adverse effects of β-blockers include fatigue, insomnia, nightmares and depression. Although many studies have investigated an association between lipophilicity and CNS effects, no clear correlation has been established. Studies have also identified that β-blockers decrease melatonin release via inhibition of central β1-adrenoceptors. Lower nocturnal melatonin concentration may contribute to the sleep disturbances.

Metabolic effects

Catecholamines are involved in the regulation of lipid and carbohydrate metabolism and, in response to hypoglycaemia, promote glycogen breakdown and mobilisation of glucose. Hence, blockade of β-adrenoceptors prevents an adequate response to hypoglycaemia in people with insulin-dependent diabetes and may also mask the symptoms.

Non-selective β-blockers raise plasma triglyceride concentration and lower high-density lipoprotein concentration, raising concerns that this may be undesirable in people with hypertension.

Pharmacokinetics

For the pharmacokinetics and usual adult dose range of β-blockers, see Table 15.7. These drugs are either metabolised in the liver or excreted as unchanged drug

Pharmacological effects of β-adrenoceptor antagonists

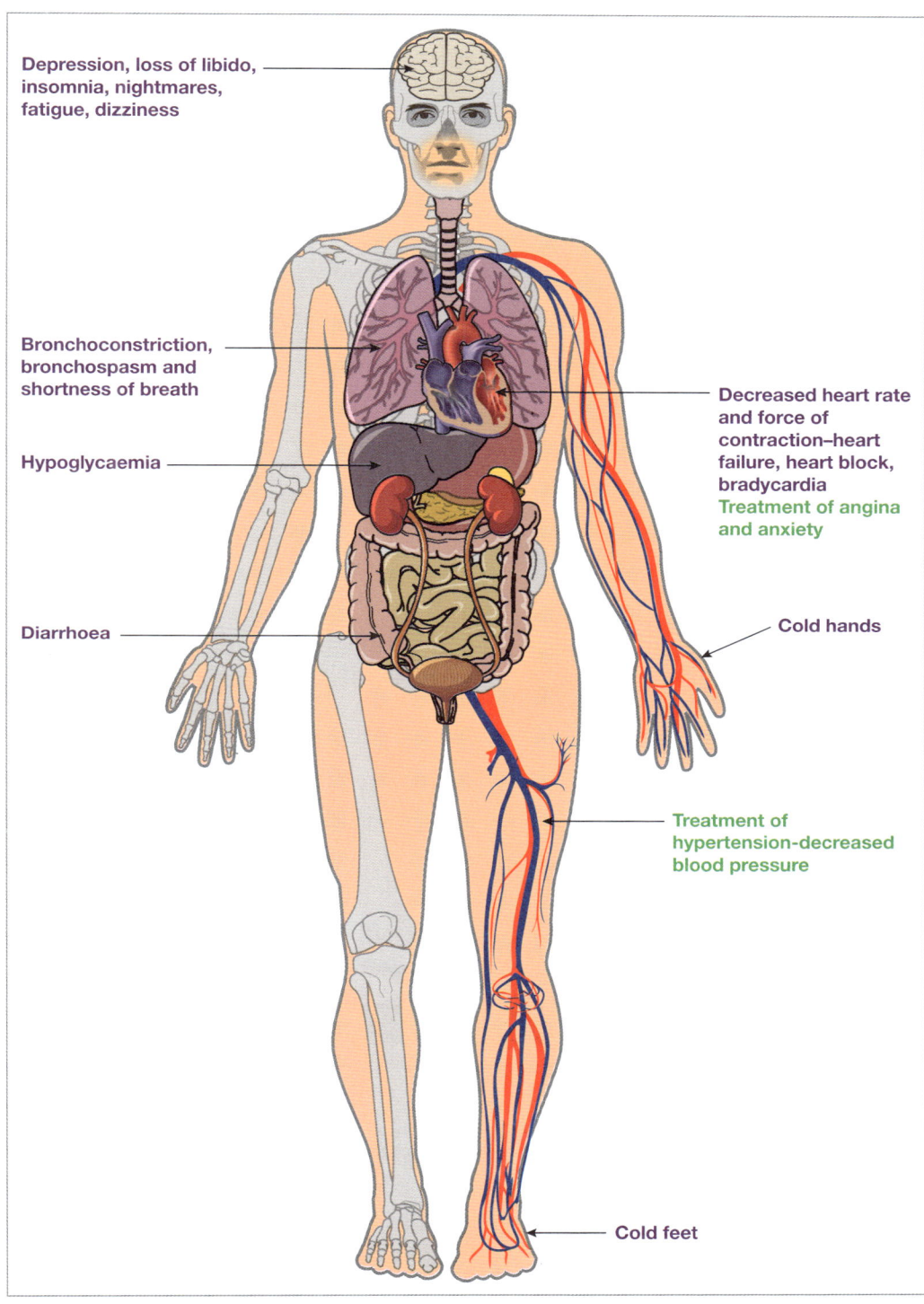

FIGURE 15.8

TABLE 15.7 Pharmacokinetics and adult dose range of β-adrenoceptor antagonists[a]

DRUG	ORAL BIOAVAILABILITY (%)	HALF-LIFE (h)	ELIMINATION	ADULT DOSE RANGE
Atenolol	~50	7–9	Renal (85–100%)	25–100 mg/day
Betaxolol	Ophthalmic preparation	14–22	Hepatic/renal (> 80%)	Eyedrops (5 mg/mL)
Bisoprolol	~88	10–12	Hepatic (50%) / renal (50%)	1.25–10 mg/day
Carvedilol	~30	6–10	Hepatic (> 75%)	6.25–50 mg/day
Labetalol	~33	6–8	Hepatic (95%)	200–800 mg/day
Metoprolol	~50	3–5	Hepatic (90%)	50–300 mg/day
Nebivolol	13% (EM)[b] and ~100% (PM)[b]	10 (EM)[b] and 35 (PM)[b]	Hepatic (99%)	1.25–10 mg/day
Pindolol	~75	3–4	Hepatic (50%) / renal (50%)	10–30 mg/day
Propranolol	~25	3–6	Hepatic (> 99%)	40–320 mg/day
Sotalol	~100	7–18	Renal (90%)	80–320 mg/day
Timolol	Ophthalmic preparation	5–6	Hepatic (85%)	Eyedrops

[a] Consult approved product information for individual drugs and doses for specific indications – for example, heart failure.
[b] CYP2D6 extensive metaboliser (EM) and poor metaboliser (PM) phenotypes.

by the kidneys. This allows the use of different agents in preexisting conditions of hepatic or renal impairment; for example, a drug such as metoprolol is metabolised by the liver, which is more suitable for use in those with renal impairment, whereas atenolol is more suitable in a person with hepatic disease because it is predominantly cleared by the kidneys.

Drug interactions and adverse reactions

See DI 15.1 for the drug interactions of β-blockers. Common adverse effects of β-blockers include insomnia, nightmares, depression, nausea, diarrhoea, dizziness, fatigue, hypotension, heart failure, heart block, bradycardia, cold hands and feet, bronchospasm, and shortness of breath. Use β-blockers with caution in

DRUG INTERACTIONS 15.1

β-adrenoceptor antagonists

DRUG	POSSIBLE EFFECTS AND MANAGEMENT
Adrenaline	Severe hypertension and bradycardia may occur with the use of non-selective beta antagonists. Use with extreme caution and monitor closely.
Antidiabetic agents, oral hypoglycaemic agents, insulin	May mask symptoms of hypoglycaemia such as increased heart rate and lowered blood pressure, and may prolong hypoglycaemic episodes, making monitoring difficult. Monitoring of blood glucose levels and dosage adjustments of the hypoglycaemic agent may be necessary.
Digoxin	May have an additive effect, increasing atrioventricular conduction time. Monitor heart rate and use with caution.
Calcium channel blockers (diltiazem and verapamil)	Enhanced cardiac-depressant effects, further decreasing rate, contractility, and conduction.
Clonidine	Combination may produce severe adverse reactions. Each drug is associated with withdrawal symptoms such as rebound hypertension. Avoid combination.
MAO inhibitors	Combination may result in hypotension and bradycardia. Use with caution and monitor closely.
Non–steroidal anti-inflammatory drugs	Antihypertensive effect of β-blockers may be reduced. Monitor blood pressure and avoid concurrent use.

patients with liver or renal function impairment, heart failure, diabetes, hyperlipidaemia, peripheral vascular disease, hyperthyroidism, myasthenia gravis or phaeochromocytoma. β-blockers are contraindicated in people with drug hypersensitivity, cardiogenic shock, heart block, bradycardia, severe hypotension, and asthma and chronic obstructive airways disease.

Withdrawal of a β-blocking drug

Abrupt cessation of β-blockers can cause a rebound phenomenon that exacerbates hypertension, angina, or ventricular dysrhythmias, and may precipitate a myocardial infarction. It is recommended that the dose of a β-blocking drug be halved every 2–3 days, reducing the dose over 8–14 days. The person should be advised to avoid vigorous physical exercise or activity during this time to decrease the risk of a myocardial infarction or cardiac dysrhythmia. If withdrawal signs occur (angina or chest pain, sweating, rebound hypertension, **dysrhythmias**, tremors, tachycardia, or respiratory distress), these may be controlled by temporary reinstitution of the drug.

Direct-acting vasodilators

Direct-acting **vasodilators** act directly on the smooth muscle cells of blood vessels to cause dilation, thereby lowering blood pressure and improving blood flow. There are different medications that directly dilate blood vessels, and hydralazine (DM 15.2) has been used in pregnancy as a potent vasodilator.

Centrally acting adrenergic inhibitors

The **centrally acting adrenergic inhibitors** clonidine, methyldopa and moxonidine are effective antihypertensive drugs. Methyldopa is considered an appropriate first-line agent in pregnancy due to its safety profile (DM 15.3).

DRUG MONOGRAPH 15.2
Hydralazine

Hydralazine hydrochloride produces its hypotensive effects by direct relaxation of vascular smooth muscle, particularly the arterioles, with a lesser effect on veins, leading to reduction in peripheral resistance. Consequently, renal blood flow is increased, providing an advantage in situations of renal failure. Hydralazine also maintains cerebral blood flow but causes sodium and water retention. As blood pressure falls the baroreceptor reflex is stimulated, causing an increase in heart rate and cardiac output. Unfortunately, this response limits the antihypertensive effects of the drug. Hydralazine also increases plasma renin activity. It is used in pregnancy and during labour to treat hypertensive emergencies due to its short onset of action.

Pharmacokinetics and dosage and administration

An oral dose of hydralazine has an onset of action of 45 minutes, and with IV administration the onset is 10–20 minutes. The peak effect is within 1 hour (orally) or 15–30 minutes (IV). The plasma half-life is 3–7 hours and duration of action is 3–8 hours. It is metabolised principally by acetylation in the liver, with the metabolites excreted by the kidneys.
Identification of a 'slow-acetylator' phenotype in both Caucasians (about 50%) and Asians (about 20%), which results in significant increases in the plasma concentration of the drug and hence the risk of toxicity.

Drug interactions

Concurrent drug administration with MAO inhibitors or other antihypertensives may result in severe hypotension.

Adverse reactions

Adverse reactions include diarrhoea, nausea, vomiting, tachycardia, anorexia, headache, facial flushing, stuffy nose, oedema, angina, rash, peripheral neuritis, and a systemic lupus erythematosus (SLE)-like syndrome. The SLE-like syndrome may include myalgia, arthralgia, arthritis, weakness, fever, and skin changes. Use with caution in women with angina, cerebral artery disease, and renal or hepatic impairment. The drug is contraindicated in people with hydralazine hypersensitivity, aortic dissection, severe tachycardia, and heart failure, and SLE.

DRUG MONOGRAPH 15.3
Methyldopa

Methyldopa is often used to treat hypertension in pregnant women, but in non-gestational hypertension its usefulness is limited by CNS and hepatic adverse effects. Although the exact hypotensive mechanism of methyldopa is unknown, the theory is that a metabolite of methyldopa (α-methylnoradrenaline) stimulates the central α2 adrenergic receptors, resulting in a reduction in sympathetic outflow to the heart, kidneys, and peripheral vasculature.

Pharmacokinetics, dosage and administration

The peak effect of methyldopa occurs in 4–6 hours after a single dose or in 48–72 hours with multiple dosing. The duration of action is 12–24 hours (after a single oral dose), 1–2 days (after multiple oral doses) or 10–16 hours (after IV administration).

Continued

DRUG MONOGRAPH 15.3
Methyldopa—cont'd

Methyldopa is metabolised to α-methylnoradrenaline within adrenergic nerve endings and in the liver to a sulfate conjugate (30–60%). Excretion is primarily by the kidneys.

Drug interactions

Methyldopa is subject to a number of drug interactions, including:
- *Iron* – Ferrous sulfate or gluconate may reduce bioavailability, interfering with blood pressure control.
- *Tricyclic antidepressants* – May reduce the antihypertensive effect of methyldopa, and an alternative antihypertensive should be considered.

Adverse reactions

Adverse reactions include drowsiness, dry mouth, headache, oedema of the feet and legs, fever, postural hypotension, impotency, insomnia, depression, anxiety, and nightmares. Use with caution in patients with depression (may be worsened) or renal dysfunction. Avoid use of methyldopa in patients with methyldopa hypersensitivity, hepatitis, cirrhosis, haemolytic anaemia or phaeochromocytoma.

KEY POINTS

Hypertension in pregnancy

For safety and effectiveness of antihypertensive drugs in pregnancy and lactation, the following considerations are important:

- The impact of hypertension on maternal health is a key consideration. Untreated or poorly controlled hypertension can lead to serious complications, such as preeclampsia or eclampsia. Antihypertensive therapy may be necessary to prevent these complications.

- The potential effects of hypertension during pregnancy on fetal development and neonatal outcomes must be considered. Certain medications, including ACE inhibitors, ARBs, and diuretics, may pose significant risks to fetal development. The choice of antihypertensive should consider their safety profile for the developing fetus as well as other effects on placental function and fetal growth.

- Different classes of antihypertensive drugs have varying safety profiles during pregnancy and lactation. For example, ACE inhibitors and angiotensin II-receptor blockers (ARBs) are generally contraindicated during pregnancy due to potential fetal harm.

- Regular monitoring of blood pressure and potential side effects is crucial during pregnancy and lactation. Adjustments to the medication regimen may be necessary based on maternal response.

- Antihypertensive therapy should be individualised.

- Regular monitoring of blood pressure and assessment of the mother and fetus during pregnancy, labour, birth, and postnatally are important.

- It is important to monitor the mother for signs and symptoms of preeclampsia and eclampsia, both during pregnancy and postnatally.

- There will be adjustments in the dosage of antihypertensive medications postnatally, changing the medications if required, and review and monitoring postnatally.

- The mother may switch to her pre-pregnancy medications after the birth of the baby in consultation with the treating physician.

- Education of the mother about the signs and symptoms of hypertension and hypotension postnatally is important, as well as education about the medications during the postnatal period.

- For lactating mothers, consideration of the transfer of antihypertensive drugs into breast milk is essential. The potential impact on the nursing infant should be weighed against the benefits of breastfeeding. See Chapter 10.

REVIEW EXERCISES

1 Kate, who had gestational hypertension, was discharged with thrice-daily (TDS) labetalol 200 mg following the birth of her baby. When last out shopping, she fainted in the street and was found to be hypotensive. Unfortunately, the postpartum blood pressure (BP) monitoring for Kate during her stay in the hospital was hit and miss, not providing an accurate reading of her postnatal BP. Discuss the physiological/pharmacological factors that could have contributed to her hypotensive episode.

2 Loan, with essential hypertension, had a change in her drug regimen to an ACE inhibitor and a diuretic following the birth of her daughter, like her pre-pregnancy routine. Discuss the impact of regular ibuprofen post-CS on her renal hemodynamics, considering her use of an ACE inhibitor and a diuretic. What education is essential for Loan's midwife to provide for Loan regarding medication management, medication interactions, and other potential impact of treatment given the change to her drug regime postnatally?

REFERENCES

Australian Medicines Handbook. Adelaide: Australian Medicines Handbook Pty Ltd 2021. 2006;129(Suppl 1): 169S–173S.

Gabb GM, Mangoni A, Anderson CS, et al. Guideline for the diagnosis and management of hypertension in adults 2016. Med J Aust. 2016:205(2);85-89. doi:10.5694/mja16.00526

Lowe SA, Bowyer L, Lust K, et al. SOMANZ guidelines for the management of hypertensive disorders of pregnancy 2014. Aust N Z J Obstet Gynaecol. 2015 Oct;55(5):e1-29. doi:10.1111/ajo.12399. Epub 2015 Sep 28. PMID: 26412014.

Rayes B, Ardissino M, Slob EAW, et al. Association of Hypertensive Disorders of Pregnancy With Future Cardiovascular Disease. JAMA Netw Open. 2023;6(2):e230034. doi:10.1001/jamanetworkopen.2023.0034

Salerno E. Pharmacology for health professionals. St Louis: Mosby 1999.

Soma-Pillay P, Nelson-Piercy C, Tolppanen H, et al. Physiological changes in pregnancy. Cardiovasc J Afr. 2016 Mar-Apr;27(2):89-94. doi: 10.5830/CVJA-2016-021. PMID: 27213856; PMCID: PMC4928162.

ONLINE RESOURCES

American Heart Association: https://www.heart.org/ (accessed 28 February 2022)

Cardiac Society of Australia and New Zealand: https://www.csanz.edu.au/ (accessed 28 February 2022)

European Society of Cardiology: https://www.escardio.org/ (accessed 28 February 2022)

National Heart Foundation of Australia – Guideline for the diagnosis and management of hypertension in adults 2016: https://www.heartfoundation.org.au (accessed 28 February 2022)

Safer Care Victoria – Hypertension in pregnancy 2018: https://www.safercare.vic.gov.au/best-practice-improvement/clinical-guidance/maternity/hypertension-in-pregnancy (accessed 16 January 2024)

Society of Obstetric Medicine Australia and New Zealand, Hypertension in pregnancy guideline, Sydney; 2023: https://www.somanz.org/content/uploads/2023/06/SOMANZ_Hypertension_in_Pregnancy_Guideline_2023_Updated_30.6.23.pdf (accessed 19 January 2024)

South Australia Perinatal Practice Guideline – Hypertensive disorders in pregnancy 2024: https://www.sahealth.sa.gov.au/wps/wcm/connect/aa782c004ee49dd483df8fd150ce4f37/Hypertensive+Disorders+in+Pregnancy_PPG_V5_2.pdf?MOD=AJPERES&CACHEID=ROOTWORKSPACE-aa782c004ee49dd483df8fd150ce4f37-ocQEdJI (accessed 16 January 2024)

CHAPTER 16

BLOOD AND BLOOD CLOTTING

Kirsten Small, Maryam Bazargan

Key Abbreviations

ADP	adenosine diphosphate
aPTT	activated partial thromboplastin time
HELLP	haemolysis, elevated liver enzymes, low platelets
HIT	heparin-induced thrombocytopaenia
INR	international normalised ratio
ITP	idiopathic thrombocytopaenic purpura
LMWHs	low-molecular-weight heparins
PT	prothrombin time
RBC	red blood cells
WBC	white blood cells

Key Terms

anaemia 309
anticoagulant drugs 315
antifibrinolytic drugs 321
antiplatelet agents 321
embolus 312
erythropoietin 307
ferritin 309

haematinics 309
haemostasis 312
haemostatic drugs 321
low-molecular-weight heparins 316
thrombocytopaenia 315
thrombus 312
transferrin 309

Chapter Focus

Blood is crucial for the maintenance of homeostasis, and disturbances of the haemopoietic or coagulation systems may manifest in illnesses such as anaemia or thromboembolic disease. Anaemia is common in pregnancy and the postpartum period. This chapter reviews the haematinic agents used in the treatment of anaemia.

Deep vein thrombosis and pulmonary embolism are less common but can complicate otherwise normal pregnancies. Thromboembolic disorders remain high on the list of causes of maternal mortality in high income countries. Preventing or managing the formation of thrombi or acute thromboembolic disorders involves the use of anticoagulant, thrombolytic, and antiplatelet agents. Specific haemostatic and antifibrinolytic drugs that hasten clot formation and reduce excessive bleeding after birth are increasingly used in maternity care. Drugs modifying coagulation pathways are potent, effective medications requiring a thorough knowledge of their pharmacology for safe administration and usage.

Key Drug Groups

Haematinic agents:
- folic acid, iron, vitamin B12

Anticoagulants:
- Antithrombin III-dependent: fondaparinux

Heparins:
- enoxaparin (DM 16.1), heparin

Vitamin K antagonists:
- warfarin (DM 16.2)

Antiplatelet drugs:
- aspirin

Haemostatic and antifibrinolytic drugs:
- protamine, tranexamic acid, vitamin K

Learning Outcomes

- Describe physiological changes occurring in pregnancy and the postnatal period impacting on blood and blood clotting and their clinical consequences.
- Discuss the use of haematinics for the treatment of anaemia and deficiency, including the formulations available, appropriate doses, adverse effects, and warnings.
- Describe the indications for anticoagulation in pregnancy and the postnatal period, the pharmacological options and the pros and cons of each.
- Outline the use of procoagulants in the prevention and management of peripartum haemorrhage and overdose with heparins and warfarin.

CRITICAL THINKING SCENARIO

Phillipa, who is 29 years old, has been admitted to her local hospital for an elective caesarean section for placenta praevia. She is known to have beta-thalassaemia minor. Her perioperative blood loss was estimated as 1.5 litres. Following surgery, she returns to the ward at 11 am. After being assessed at 5 pm to ensure her blood loss remains minimal, she is started on enoxaparin 40 mg subcutaneously once daily, to be continued for the duration of her hospital admission. Her haemoglobin concentration preoperatively was 120 g/dL and falls to 80 g/dL on day 1 postoperatively. Her obstetrician charts ferrous sulphate 325 mg daily combined with vitamin C 500 mg and asks her to continue using enoxaparin after discharge until she is fully mobile.

1   Discuss approaches to optimising haemoglobin levels in a woman with beta-thalassaemia during pregnancy and lactation. Describe the role of folate supplementation in preventing and treating anaemia.

2   Discuss the mechanism of action of enoxaparin.

3   Explain why Phillipa was commenced on enoxaparin 6 hours postoperatively, and why she should remain on the drug until fully mobile.

4   Outline the benefits and side effects of oral iron supplementation for Phillipa. Why is the addition of vitamin C useful? Is there any reason to be cautious about the use of iron in women with thalassaemia?

Introduction

The haemopoietic system comprises the blood and bone marrow (site of production of blood cells), complemented by the liver (storage of vitamin B12 for erythrocyte production), spleen (removal of expired blood cells and storage of platelets), and kidneys (erythropoietin production). Blood is a major transport medium, carrying drugs and nutrients absorbed from the gastrointestinal tract, oxygen from the lungs and hormones, electrolytes and so on to cells throughout the entire body. In addition, blood transports metabolic products from cells to the liver, kidneys, and lungs for excretion. Blood further helps to regulate body temperature in concert with changes in the vascular system modifying blood flow through the skin. Buffering is also an important function of blood, helping maintain the pH of human blood between 7.35–7.45. In addition to its transportation and regulatory roles, blood is integral to the process of coagulation and aids in immunity by producing antibodies.

16.1 Blood composition

Blood is composed of two components: cells and plasma. The blood volume of an adult is proportional to body size and is typically 4–6 L, of which approximately 55% is plasma. There are principally three types of blood cells: red blood cells (RBC), or erythrocytes, that transport oxygen and carbon dioxide; white blood cells (WBC), or leucocytes, that aid in the defence of the body against bacteria and infections; and platelets, or thrombocytes,

that are necessary for blood coagulation. Plasma is about 92% water and 8% plasma proteins (e.g. albumin, globulins, and fibrinogen). Plasma proteins play important roles in maintaining the osmotic pressure of blood, transporting some steroid hormones, and in binding numerous drugs (see Chapter 4). The globulins include the immunoglobulins, also called antibodies, which are important in the body's defence against viruses and bacteria. Fibrinogen is essential for blood clotting and is converted to fibrin by thrombin in the presence of calcium ions. In addition to proteins, plasma may contain thousands of other substances such as glucose, electrolytes, vitamins, hormones, and products of metabolism.

Blood cell production

During fetal development, many tissues (e.g. the liver, spleen, and thymus gland) participate in haemopoiesis, or blood cell production. After birth, haemopoiesis occurs only in the red bone marrow and, in adulthood, principally in the bone marrow of the vertebrae, sternum, ribs, and ilia. Differentiation and proliferation of precursor cells into the various types of blood cells is regulated by haemopoietic growth factors such as **erythropoietin** (EPO), thrombopoietin, and cytokines.

Renal secretion of EPO, a hormone regulating the production of RBCs in bone marrow, is stimulated by hypoxia and/or blood loss. With maximal bone marrow stimulation, RBC production can be increased seven-fold. Thrombopoietin, another hormone, is produced by the liver and substantially increases platelet production,

A simplified diagram of blood cell production (haemopoiesis) and the involvement of growth factors

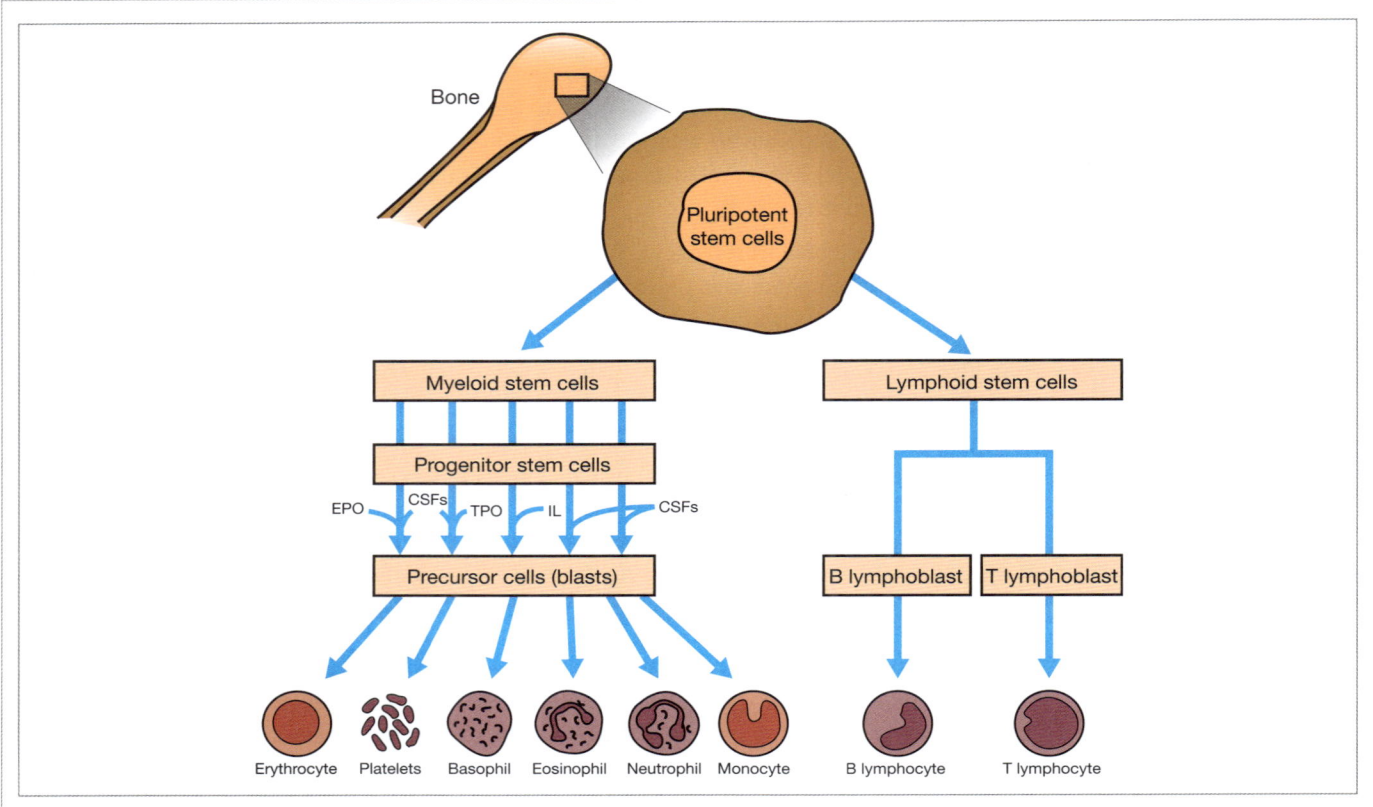

FIGURE 16.1 Cells originating from myeloid stem cells are produced in the bone marrow. Lymphoid stem cells arise in bone marrow, but development of lymphocytes is completed in lymphatic tissue. CSFs = colony-stimulating factors; EPO = erythropoietin; IL = interleukin; TPO = thrombopoietin.

while colony-stimulating factors and interleukins stimulate formation of leucocytes. A simplified diagram of blood cell differentiation is shown in Figure 16.1.

Red blood cells (erythrocytes)

Red blood cells, or erythrocytes, are small, non-nucleated, biconcave disc-shaped cells making up a large portion of the total blood volume. Without a nucleus, RBCs have negligible synthetic capacity and hence their life span is short (about 120 days). Expired cells are removed from the circulation and destroyed by phagocytes resident in the liver and spleen. A healthy adult female has $3.8–5.8 \times 10^{12}$ cells/L of blood. It is estimated that more than 100 million RBCs are produced/minute during adulthood, and production (erythropoiesis) and destruction of these cells is balanced to maintain a relatively constant level of RBCs.

Within the cytosol of RBCs are millions of haemoglobin molecules, the main function of which is the transport of oxygen. Each haemoglobin molecule consists of a protein called globin, composed of four polypeptide chains, four non-protein haem pigment molecules, and four iron atoms. Each polypeptide chain is associated with one haem and one iron ion (Fe^{2+}). Thus, one haemoglobin molecule combines in total with four oxygen molecules. Oxygen is transported from the lungs to the tissues, where it is released from haemoglobin and diffuses through the interstitial fluid into the cells. Haemoglobin can also combine with carbon dioxide carried from cells to the lungs for excretion. Haemoglobin is involved in blood pressure regulation by transporting the vasodilator nitric oxide, produced by endothelial cells lining blood vessels.

White blood cells (leucocytes)

White blood cells, or leucocytes, contain nuclei and are produced primarily in the bone marrow. They are classified according to the presence or absence of granules in the cell cytoplasm (Fig 16.1). The three types of granular leucocytes are neutrophils, eosinophils, and basophils. Aged cells that have different-shaped nuclear lobes and an increased number of nuclei (>2, >3, or >5) are referred to as polymorphonuclear leucocytes, or polymorphs. The other two types of leucocytes are lymphocytes and monocytes. These are produced mainly in lymph tissues and the spleen, thymus, tonsils, and various other lymphoid tissues, in the bone marrow, gastrointestinal tract, and elsewhere.

Platelets

Platelets, or thrombocytes, are small, disc-shaped, non-nucleated colourless cell fragments that split off from the megakaryocytes produced by the bone marrow (Fig 16.1). They have a short life span of about 5–8 days. Time-expired platelets are engulfed by resident macrophages in the spleen and liver. Platelets are essential for coagulation. A low concentration of platelets is known as **thrombocytopenia**.

KEY POINTS

Haemopoietic system

- The haemopoietic system comprises the blood and bone marrow, the liver, the spleen, and the kidneys.

- Blood transports drugs and nutrients absorbed from the gastrointestinal tract; oxygen from the lungs; and hormones, electrolytes, and other substances to cells throughout the entire body.

- Blood is composed principally of plasma and three types of blood cells: red blood cells, or erythrocytes; white blood cells, or leucocytes; and platelets, or thrombocytes.

16.2 Physiological changes in the haemopoietic system in pregnancy and the puerperium

Both blood volume and red cell mass increase progressively during pregnancy. At term, the average blood volume has increased by 30–45%, about 1.5 L. The increase in blood volume is proportionally greater than the increase in red cell mass, resulting in haemodilution. Red cell concentration and haemoglobin concentration fall. Mean cell volume increases slightly, reflecting a larger population of young red blood cells in the maternal circulation. The reduction in red cell concentration during pregnancy reduces blood viscosity and is believed to improve placental perfusion. Inadequate haemodilution, with the persistence of relatively high haemoglobin concentration, is associated with poor pregnancy outcomes (Dewey et al 2017).

Increasing red cell mass in pregnancy increases demand for iron, folic acid, and vitamin B12. In addition, fetal red blood cell production and other metabolic processes also make use of these **haematinics**. In the first few hours after birth, vaginal blood loss of up to 500 mL is common and begins the process of returning the expanded blood volume back to its pre-pregnancy level.

Anaemia

Anaemia is reduced oxygen-carrying capacity of the blood, and it often manifests as fatigue. Anaemias are classified based on the size and number of RBCs and haemoglobin concentration. Haemoglobin contains four haem moieties, each having one iron atom to which one oxygen molecule binds reversibly. In general, iron is obtained through a meat-containing diet, though non-haem sources of iron (such as legumes, green leafy vegetables, nuts, and grains) also contribute. Iron is absorbed from the duodenum and upper jejunum and carried in plasma bound to **transferrin**. On average, plasma contains approximately 4 mg iron; the daily turnover is about 30 mg (Fig 16.2). Iron as **ferritin** is stored in all cells. Most iron is stored in erythrocytes, with the next highest concentrations occurring in liver and bone marrow (stored as ferritin and haemosiderin) and in muscle, with small amounts in the spleen and bound in enzymes. Iron concentration is tightly controlled by the absorptive process, as the body has virtually no mechanism for excreting iron.

Anaemia in pregnancy

Physiological haemodilution in pregnancy means diagnostic criteria for anaemia are different to those for the non-pregnant population. The WHO defines anaemia as a haemoglobin concentration of less than 110 g/dL in the first and third trimester, and less than 105 g/dL in the second trimester (WHO 2016). Anaemia in pregnancy is common, with rates of around 10–15% in high income countries (Kangalgil et al 2021; Tang et al 2018). Screening all women for anaemia by measuring haemoglobin at their first antenatal assessment and again at 28 weeks of gestation is advised, with consideration for also testing ferritin levels in areas where the prevalence of iron deficiency anaemia is high (Department of Health 2019).

There are many causes of anaemia in pregnancy. Some are benign and self-limiting, like physiological haemodilution of pregnancy. Others have potentially serious consequences for the woman and her fetus, like haemoglobinopathies. Once a low haemoglobin concentration has been confirmed, further diagnostic evaluation is required to establish the underlying cause. This should include assessment of serum ferritin and total iron binding saturation, vitamin B12, red cell folate levels. Women from Asia, Africa, and Mediterranean

Distribution and turnover of iron in the body

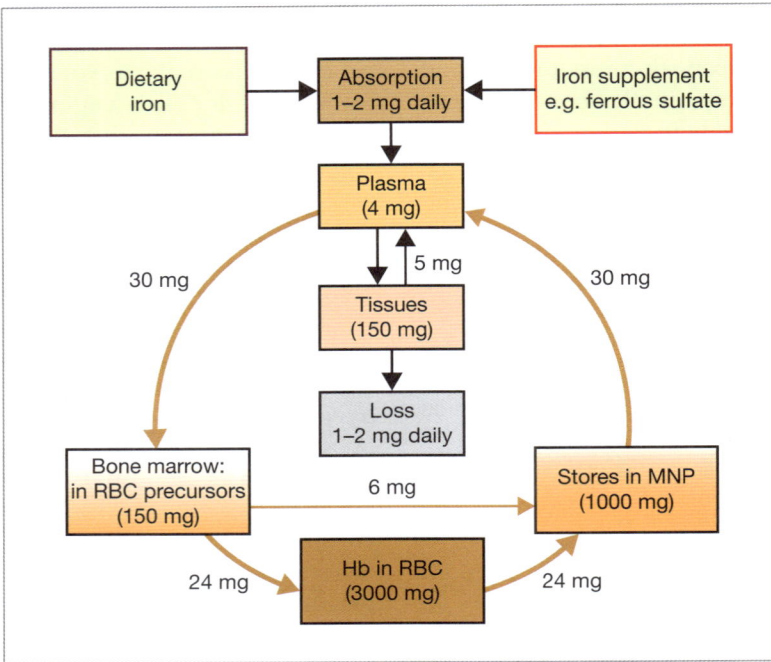

FIGURE 16.2 The quantities by the arrows indicate the usual amounts transferred each day. The transfer of 6 mg from red cell precursors to phagocytes represents aborted cells that fail to develop into functional red blood cells. Hb, haemoglobin; MNP, mononuclear phagocytes (mainly in liver, spleen, and bone marrow); RBC, red blood cells.

Source: Rang et al 2016, Chapter 25, Figure 25.1; used with permission.

regions should be offered haemoglobin electrophoresis testing for haemoglobinopathies, particularly if there is microcytosis or failure to respond to iron therapy.

Anaemia causes symptoms of fatigue and dyspnoea on exertion. Significant anaemia in later pregnancy reduces women's ability to compensate for increased postpartum blood loss. Identifying and treating anaemia during pregnancy reduces the symptom burden and can reduce the use of blood transfusion (Abdulrehman et al 2019). Reduced oxygen-carrying capacity can impact fetal growth and development, with further fetal consequences depending on the specific cause of the anaemia (Dewey et al 2017).

Iron deficiency and iron deficiency anaemia

Iron deficiency anaemia is characterised by small RBCs with reduced haemoglobin concentration but is not the only anaemia with this pattern. It is therefore important to assess iron status to confirm the diagnosis. Iron deficiency has other pathophysiological consequences than just anaemia. Iron is also an essential component of myoglobin, enzymes with a haem moiety (e.g. cytochromes and peroxidases) and metallo-flavoproteins

such as xanthine oxidase, which is involved in purine metabolism.

Iron deficiency and pregnancy

Pregnancy requires an estimated 1 g of additional iron to meet the requirements of the placenta, the fetus, and to ensure an appropriate increase in red cell mass during pregnancy. Common causes of iron deficiency include blood loss, increased iron requirements, malabsorption, or low dietary intake. Iron deficiency without anaemia is common in pregnancy, with prevalence rates ranging from 27–77% (Sharma et al 2021; Tang et al 2018). Specific pregnancy reference ranges for serum ferritin should be used. It is important to bear in mind that these have been determined by consensus, with little research having been conducted to determine threshold levels that reliably distinguish low iron stores leading to fetal iron insufficiency (Daru et al 2017). There is no current recommendation to screen serum ferritin routinely in pregnancy. It is important the fetus lays down adequate iron stores to ensure normal neurological development in the early months of life. Optimal (or delayed) cord clamping supports this (Qian et al 2019; McDonald et al 2013). Breast milk is lower in iron than artificial milk formulas. A breastfed neonate starting life with adequate iron stores has sufficient iron to support growth and increased red cell mass for 4–6 months, when additional dietary sources of iron are typically introduced.

Fetal iron loading is physiologically favoured, sometimes at the expense of maternal iron stores. In addition, the fetus prioritises red cell iron over tissue iron, so the development of anaemia is a late sign and brain function is likely already impacted. While adequate circulating maternal iron is important, it may not be enough to ensure adequate fetal iron stores in some situations. This is more likely when the woman smokes, has gestational diabetes or gestational hypertension, or in multiple pregnancy (Georgieff 2020).

Iron supplementation

Once iron deficiency anaemia has been diagnosed, iron supplementation along with dietary advice to optimise iron absorption is advised. Iron is administered orally as first-line therapy but can also be given parenterally if required. Iron dosage is expressed in terms of elemental iron:

- 1 mg elemental iron = ~3 mg ferrous sulphate (dried)
- 1 mg elemental iron = ~5 mg ferrous sulphate (as liquid)
- 1 mg elemental iron = ~3 mg ferrous fumarate.

The recommended dose of oral iron for treatment of iron deficiency during pregnancy is 40–80 mg of elemental iron. Iron is also available in combination with folic acid for preventing and treating folate deficiency, and with vitamin C to enhance absorption.

Adverse reactions with oral iron are gastrointestinal disturbances (e.g. abdominal pain, nausea, vomiting, diarrhoea, constipation, and black-coloured faeces). Symptoms relate to the dose of iron and can be minimised by taking supplements on an empty stomach and delaying food intake for 30 minutes. Alternate day dosing can also minimise gastrointestinal side effects while providing similar benefits. Oral iron supplementation has been associated with an increased risk of glucose intolerance (Zhang Rawal 2017).

Parenteral iron administration avoids gastrointestinal side effects. Intravenous options include iron sucrose, iron polymaltose, and ferric carboxymaltose. All appear equally effective in improving haemoglobin concentration, iron status, and symptoms (Qassim 2017). There is little evidence to suggest improvements in perinatal outcomes. Iron dextran can be administered intramuscularly. Although a rare occurrence, there is a risk of an anaphylactoid reaction with parenteral iron preparations. Extravasation of iron can result in potentially permanent skin staining (Crowley et al 2019). Women should be counselled regarding this possibility and care taken to avoid extravascular iron leakage.

As acute iron toxicity can be serious or even fatal in small children, iron formulations should be kept well out of reach and preferably locked away. To prevent an excessive intake of iron, oral and parenteral formulations of iron should not be used together. In cases of chronic iron overload, the iron chelators deferasirox, deferiprone, or desferrioxamine are administered. These drugs form complexes with the iron, and the complexes are then excreted in faeces or urine.

Following the initiation of iron therapy, regardless of the route, it is important to check for an appropriate response to therapy and to investigate further if symptoms and haemoglobin levels do not improve.

Folic acid and vitamin B12

In general, folic acid deficiency occurs through poor diet, while vitamin B12 deficiency arises from poor gut absorption (e.g. in Crohn's disease). Folic acid and vitamin B12 are both obtained through the diet and are necessary in DNA synthesis. Dietary folic acid is reduced to tetrahydrofolate (FH4). Vitamin B12 is required for conversion of methyl-FH4 to FH4. Hence, a deficiency of either nutrient results in defective DNA synthesis. Red blood cell replacement requires rapid DNA synthesis to support cell division and is reduced by deficiency of folate and/or vitamin B12.

Folic acid in pregnancy

Folic acid plays an important role in the development of the fetal nervous system and other body organs. Supplementation around the time of conception and in the first trimester reduces the occurrence of neural tube defects (such as anencephaly and spina bifida) (Moussa et al 2016). A dose of 0.5 mg (Australia) or 0.8 mg (New Zealand) daily is recommended for all women, and 5 mg for women at higher risk for neural tube defects. Australia and New Zealand fortify cereal grain products with additional folic acid as a public health measure to prevent neural tube defects. While folate deficiency (with or without anaemia) can complicate pregnancy, fortified foods have reduced this rate (Rogers et al 2018).

Vitamin B12 in pregnancy

Like folic acid, vitamin B12 plays important roles in nervous system development and growth (Finkelstein et al 2015). Fetal vitamin B12 status reflects maternal levels and there are active transport mechanisms to support the movement of vitamin B12 across the placenta. Vitamin B12 deficiency in pregnancy is uncommon in high income countries and is associated with higher rates of pregnancy loss; fetal growth restriction and small for gestational age babies; and alterations in maternal blood glucose levels (Saravanan et al 2021).

Treating folic acid and/or vitamin B12 deficiency

Vitamin B12 deficiency should be excluded before prescribing folic acid for treatment of deficiency. Without adequate vitamin B12, folic acid will not be converted to the active FH4 form. In addition, check for other medications, as some drugs (e.g. antiepileptics and dihydrofolate reductase inhibitors such as methotrexate and trimethoprim) cause folic acid deficiency. Except in special circumstances, folic acid is administered orally. Adverse reactions with folic acid are rare.

Vitamin B12 supplements are available as hydroxocobalamin and cyanocobalamin. Long-term use of metformin has been associated with vitamin B12 deficiency (Infante et al 2021). Hydroxocobalamin is administered intramuscularly, while cyanocobalamin is available as both an oral and an injectable (IM) formulation. In cases of malabsorption, oral formulations are inappropriate and vitamin B12 injections will be required. Adverse reactions are rare.

See Clinical Focus Box 16.1 for further information about the clinical uses of iron, folic acid, and vitamin B12 in pregnancy.

CLINICAL FOCUS BOX 16.1

Clinical uses of iron, folic acid, and vitamin B12

Iron

- Prevention/treatment of iron deficiency anaemia

Folic acid

- Folate-deficiency anaemia
- Prevention of neural tube defect in fetuses
- Prevention/treatment of methotrexate-induced toxicity

Vitamin B12

- Prevention/treatment of vitamin B12 deficiency

KEY POINTS

Haematinics

- A reduced oxygen-carrying capacity of the blood is referred to as anaemia.
- Different types of anaemia are classified based on the size and number of functional RBCs and the haemoglobin concentration.
- Iron concentration is tightly controlled by the absorptive process, as the body has virtually no mechanism for excreting iron.
- Haematinics commonly used to treat anaemia include iron, folic acid, and vitamin B12.
- Iron is carried in plasma bound to transferrin and stored in cells as ferritin.
- Folic acid is used to treat folate-deficiency anaemia, to prevent neural tube defects in the developing fetus, and to prevent toxicity from methotrexate.
- Vitamin B12 is available as hydroxocobalamin and cyanocobalamin for oral or intramuscular administration.

16.3 Blood clotting

Blood clotting protects against excessive haemorrhage but must be balanced against the risk of **thrombus** formation (an aggregation of platelets, fibrin, clotting factors, and cellular blood elements) that can obstruct blood flow and cause ischaemia. Risk factors for venous thrombosis include inherited thrombophilia disorders, prolonged immobilisation, operative procedures, dehydration, current or recent pregnancy, and use of the oral contraceptive pill.

An **embolus**, a mass of undissolved matter broken off from a thrombus, can travel in the vascular system and lodge, causing ischaemia, infarction, and death. In contrast, a defect in the blood coagulation cascade can lead to excessive bleeding or haemorrhage.

The haemostatic mechanism

Haemostasis is a process that spontaneously stops bleeding from damaged blood vessels, and is achieved by three sequential steps:

Step 1 Vasoconstriction. This response instantly slows blood flow from and through the ruptured vessel.

Step 2 Platelet plug formation. Blood vessel injury exposes collagen in the underlying connective tissue. Platelets become activated and adhere to the exposed collagen. A dense aggregate known as a platelet plug is formed. This attachment triggers the release of adenosine diphosphate (ADP) and thromboxane A2, leading to further activation of nearby platelets and vasoconstriction through the action of thromboxane A2. Because this plug is relatively unstable, it can stop bleeding quickly, provided damage to the vessel is tiny.

Step 3 Blood coagulation. For long-term effectiveness the platelet plug must be reinforced with fibrin. This involves a series of chemical coagulation or clotting reactions. Blood coagulation ultimately results in the formation of a stable fibrin clot, a meshwork of fibrin threads that entraps platelets, blood cells, and plasma. The chemical events in blood coagulation involve two distinct pathways: the intrinsic pathway and the extrinsic pathway. See Figure 16.3 for an illustration of these two pathways and the sites of action of anticoagulant medications.

KEY POINTS

Blood coagulation

- Haemostasis stops bleeding from damaged blood vessels and is achieved by three sequential steps: (1) vasoconstriction, (2) platelet activation and adhesion, and (3) activation of coagulation and fibrin formation.
- Venous thrombosis occurs in areas where blood flow is reduced or stasis occurs.
- Blood coagulation involves two distinct pathways: the intrinsic pathway and the extrinsic pathway.

Coagulation cascade for the intrinsic and extrinsic pathways

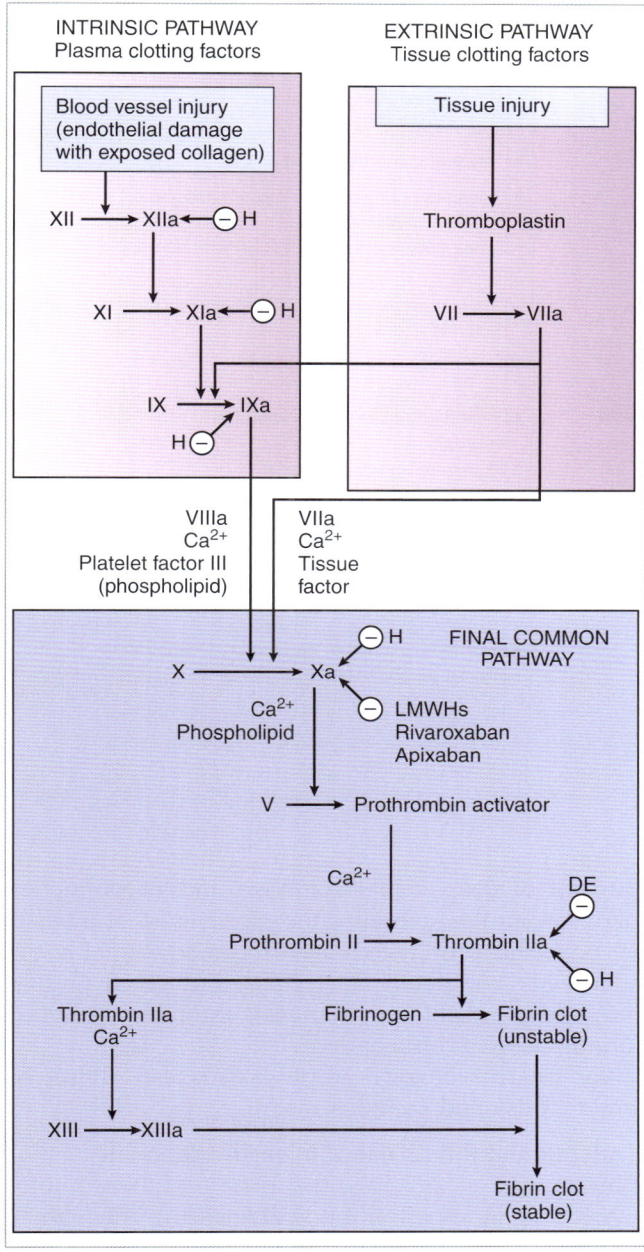

FIGURE 16.3 Final pathway (activation of factor X) is common to both the intrinsic and extrinsic pathways. Sites of action of anticoagulant drugs denoted; H = heparin; LMWHs = low-molecular-weight heparins; DE = dabigatran etexilate; $\ominus$ = inhibition

16.4 Physiological changes in the coagulation system in pregnancy and the puerperium

Pregnancy is a hypercoagulable state. Increased hepatic production of clotting factors is stimulated by the hormonal environment of pregnancy. Consequently, the levels of clotting factors, such as fibrinogen and prothrombin, increase (Thornton 2010). Platelet concentration falls, and further reductions can occur with conditions such as preeclampsia. Fibrinolytic activity is reduced in pregnancy but promptly returns to pre-pregnancy levels in the first hour after birth.

Thromboembolic disorders and pregnancy

Deep vein thrombosis and the associated risk of pulmonary embolism are more common during pregnancy and the early postpartum period than for non-pregnant women due to the hypercoagulability of pregnancy. This risk is further compounded by major surgery (e.g. caesarean section), dehydration (e.g. secondary to hyperemesis gravidarum), immobilisation (e.g. long-haul flights), smoking, high body mass index, and preexisting thrombophilias such as factor V Leiden. A previous history of venous thromboembolism is associated with an approximately 10% risk of recurrence during pregnancy (Thornton 2010).

Screening, and repeated re-screening, for risk of venous thromboembolism is recommended during pregnancy and the postnatal period. A variety of risk scoring tools exist. Few have been validated to confirm their accuracy or ability to reduce the incidence of venous thromboembolism while avoiding bleeding complications (Raia-Barjat et al 2022).

Placental function disorders and thrombophilias

Thrombophilias are conditions that result in a procoagulant state. They include the autoimmune condition antiphospholipid syndrome, and the genetic conditions Factor V Leiden, Protein C or S deficiency (or dysfunction), antithrombin deficiency, and G20210A prothrombin gene mutation. Thrombophilias have been associated with higher risk for preeclampsia, placental abruption, fetal growth restriction, and recurrent and late miscarriage, presumed to be mediated by placental damage due to microthrombi in the placental bed.

DRUGS AT A GLANCE
Drugs affecting thrombosis and haemostasis

PHARMACOLOGICAL GROUP AND EFFECT	KEY EXAMPLES	CLINICAL USE IN MIDWIFERY
Heparins Inactivate factor IIa (thrombin) and factor Xa by binding to antithrombin III action of antithrombin III on factor Xa (LMWHs) ↓ binding to thrombin (LMWHs)	Enoxaparin (LMWH)	• Prevention of VTE • Prevention of placenta mediated disorders in women with recurrent pregnancy loss • Treatment of VTE
	Heparin	• Prevention and treatment of VTE
Vitamin K antagonist Inhibits VKORC1, which inhibits synthesis vitamin K–dependent clotting factors (II, VII, IX, and X)	Warfarin	• Prevention of thromboembolism associated with prosthetic heart valves • Prevention/treatment of VTE in women unable to use heparins
Antithrombin-III-dependent anticoagulant Binds ATIII potentiating neutralisation of factor Xa by antithrombin which inhibits thrombin formation and thrombus development	Fondaparinux	• Prevention/treatment of VTE in women unable to use heparins and warfarin
Antifibrinolytics Competitive inhibitor of plasminogen activation	Tranexamic acid	• Reduction of bleeding related to • surgery • postpartum haemorrhage
Antiplatelet drugs Inhibitor of COX-1 ↓ thromboxane A_2 synthesis and platelet aggregation Inhibits phosphodiesterase activity ↑ platelet cAMP	Aspirin	• Prevention of preeclampsia, fetal growth restriction, preterm birth in women at risk
Heparin antagonist Forms complex with heparin Dissociates the heparin-AT III complex reducing the anticoagulant effect of heparin	Protamine	• Overdose with either heparin or enoxaparin • Risk of severe haemorrhage

LMWH = low-molecular-weight heparins; VTE = venous thromboembolism

Homozygous states of the genetic conditions, the combination of more than one condition, or when one is combined with a family history of venous thromboembolism are associated with higher risk for venous thromboembolism (Ormesher et al 2017). Women with a history of recurrent miscarriage who have antiphospholipid antibodies (such as anticardiolipin or beta-2 glycoprotein 1 antibodies) are at high risk of placental mediated disorders and this risk can be reduced by using low-dose aspirin and low-molecular weight heparin (Hamulyák et al 2020). The association between placental mediated disorders and other thrombophilias is less clear and current evidence of benefit from thromboprophylaxis is limited. Routine screening for thrombophilias is therefore not currently advised (Ormesher et al 2017).

Anticoagulation and pregnancy

Anticoagulation is recommended during pregnancy and the postpartum period for women at increased risk for venous thromboembolism; for the prevention of pregnancy loss and other complications for women with antiphospholipid antibody syndrome; and for the treatment of deep vein thrombosis and/or pulmonary embolism. Studies examining the effectiveness of antenatal and postnatal prophylaxis have been low quality and undersized (Middleton et al 2021), but given findings from non-pregnant populations, thromboprophylaxis continues to be recommended.

Non-pharmacological prophylaxis is also advised for women at risk and includes:

- attention to fluid balance to ensure adequate hydration
- encouraging mobilisation, and ensuring adequate analgesia is available to achieve this if required
- well-fitting antiembolism stockings
- pneumatic devices that produce intermittent compression of the feet or calves. These are advised when mobilisation is not possible.

Drug selection for anticoagulation in pregnancy should focus on drugs that:

- are highly effective
- have a half-life permitting once or twice daily dosing, but not so long that the procoagulant effect persists long after cessation

- minimise the risk of bleeding and other adverse effects
- cross the placental barrier in minimal concentrations and thereby minimise fetal risks
- where transplacental transfer does occur, are not teratogenic
- are readily reversible, so that when labour begins or surgery is indicated, the risk of heavy bleeding can be reduced
- are cost effective
- can be administered by a route that is acceptable to the user.

Research for new anticoagulant agents rarely includes pregnant and lactating women. Consequently, most agents advised for use in pregnancy and lactation are older medications with parenteral routes of administration.

Bleeding disorders and pregnancy

Heavy bleeding can complicate birth. Some bleeding disorders predate pregnancy and increase the chance of bleeding during pregnancy, labour, and the early postnatal period. Pregnancy complications, for example preeclampsia, may dysregulate the coagulation system and favour bleeding. Management of bleeding disorders in pregnancy should involve consultation with a haematologist. Ongoing bleeding that fails to respond to usual treatment should prompt consideration of a bleeding disorder.

Thrombocytopaenia in pregnancy

The most common cause of **thrombocytopaenia** in pregnancy is gestational thrombocytopaenia. This benign condition is seen in the third trimester, with platelet counts typically in the $90–150 \times 10^9$ /L range. There is no associated risk of haemorrhage and no contraindication to the use of epidural analgesia or spinal anaesthesia.

Gestational thrombocytopaenia must be distinguished from idiopathic thrombocytopaenic purpura (ITP) and other causes of thrombocytopaenia (e.g. HELLP syndrome). ITP predates pregnancy but may be diagnosed for the first time in pregnancy. Antiplatelet antibodies increase the rate of removal of platelets from the circulation. Antiplatelet antibodies may cross the placenta, so the fetus can also be at risk for bleeding. It is therefore advised that fetal spiral electrodes not be used for cardiotocograph monitoring, and vacuum extraction and complicated forceps assisted birth be avoided (Lefkou et al 2018). Haemostasis remains normal for most people with ITP. When bleeding does occur and platelets levels are very low, treatment with corticosteroids and/or intravenous gammaglobulin can be used (Thornton 2010).

Inherited coagulopathies and pregnancy

Von Willebrand disease, haemophilia A and B, factor XI and other clotting factor deficiencies, and congenital platelet disorders increase the risk of bleeding and can complicate pregnancy. Von Willebrand disease, due to deficient or defective von Willebrand factor, affects 1–3% of the population and is the most common inherited coagulopathy to complicate pregnancy (Hermans et al 2018). In women, von Willebrand disease often presents as menorrhagia and may also be diagnosed after severe epistaxis (nasal bleeding), marked bruising, or heavy bleeding after dental extraction. In the most common form of von Willebrand disease (type I), von Willebrand factor levels rise during pregnancy, so antenatal complications are rare. These levels drop after birth, so postpartum blood loss can be a concern. When von Willebrand factor activity levels are low, desmopressin can be used to increase the levels (Lefkou et al 2018). Tranexamic acid is useful in both preventing and treating haemorrhage in women with von Willebrand disease.

Haemorrhage and disseminated intravascular coagulopathy

Widespread activation of clotting pathways consumes clotting factors and platelets, ultimately leading to a tendency for bleeding. This is known as disseminated intravascular coagulopathy (DIC). In pregnancy, amniotic fluid embolism, abruption, preeclampsia, and sepsis can trigger DIC. Management in pregnancy includes identifying and treating the cause, and replacement of the consumed factors and platelets with blood products (Lefkou Hunt 2018).

> **KEY POINTS**
>
> **Physiological changes in the coagulation system in pregnancy and the puerperium**
>
> - Pregnancy is a procoagulant state, and thromboembolic disorders are more common.
> - Thrombophilias increase the incidence of placental dysfunction and this is thought to be mediated by the formation of microthombi in the placental vasculature. Anticoagulants and antiplatelet agents are used to reduce this risk.
> - Gestational thrombocytopenia and von Willebrand's disease are the most common bleeding disorders in pregnancy.

Drugs capable of modifying thrombosis and haemostasis include:

- anticoagulant drugs
- antiplatelet agents
- haemostatic and antifibrinolytic drugs.

16.5 Anticoagulant drugs

Anticoagulant drugs (Fig 16.4) are commonly used as prophylaxis during pregnancy and the postnatal period

Sites of action of drugs interacting with the coagulation cascade and the fibrinolytic and platelet activation pathways

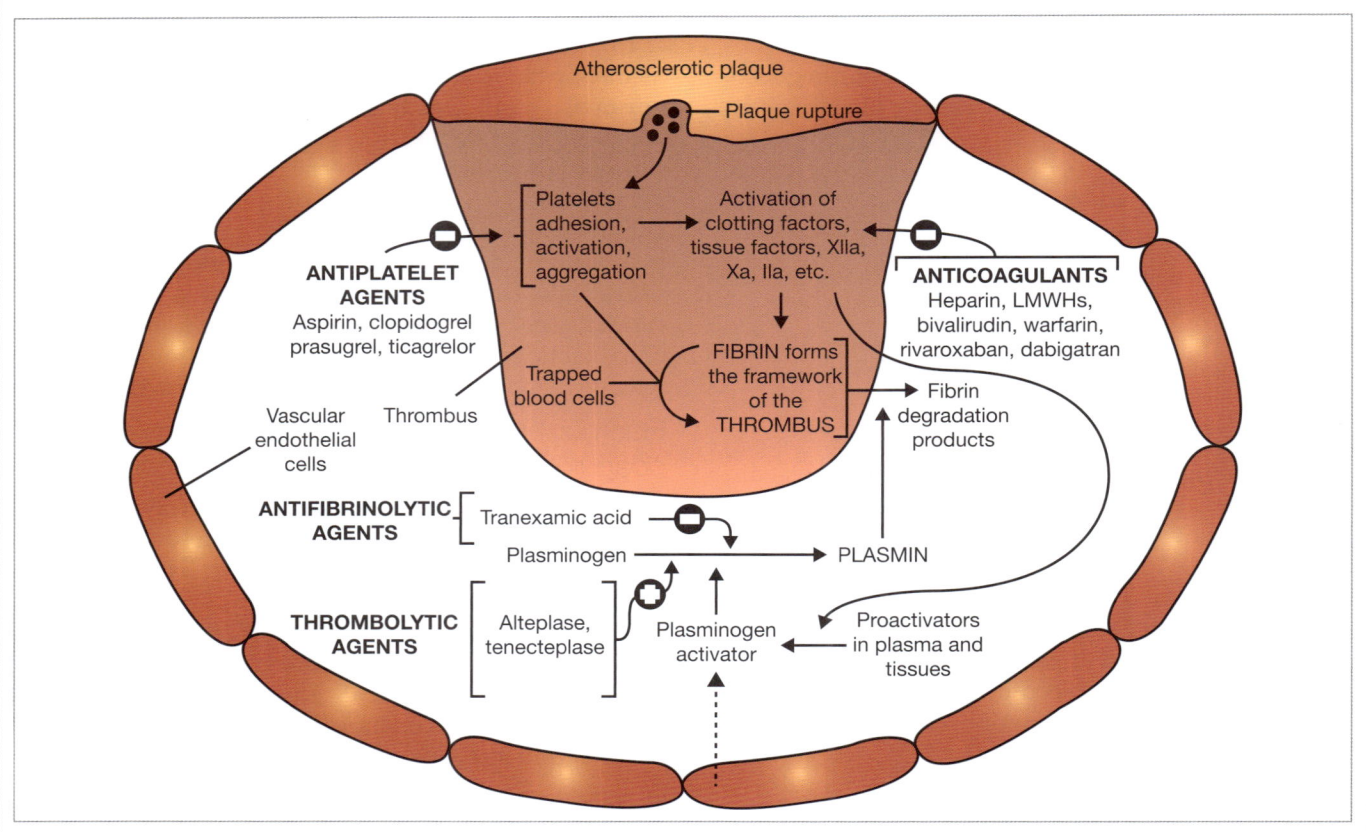

FIGURE 16.4

Source: Adapted from Rang et al 2012, Figure 24.10; reproduced with permission.

for women with risk factors for thromboembolism. They act by preventing fibrin deposits and extension of a thrombus, and therefore avoid complications of thromboembolism. Anticoagulant drugs have no direct effect on existing clots or on ischaemic tissue. Although long-term anticoagulant therapy remains controversial, there is evidence that anticoagulant therapy reduces the incidence of thrombosis.

Anticoagulant drugs used in maternity practice include:

- heparin and the **low-molecular-weight heparins** (LMWHs) including enoxaparin (DM 16.1)
- the vitamin K antagonist warfarin (DM 16.2)
- the antithrombin III-dependent anticoagulant fondaparinux.

Heparin and LMWHs are the drugs of first choice if a rapid anticoagulant effect is required because their onset is immediate if administered intravenously. They are considered the safest options in pregnancy. Warfarin is a teratogen and should be used with caution in pregnancy but has the convenience of oral administration. Fondaparinux is occasionally used in pregnancy when heparins and warfarin are contraindicated.

Low-molecular-weight heparins

Currently, there are three LMWHs on the market – dalteparin, enoxaparin, and nadroparin – and one heparinoid, danaparoid. The LMWHs are fragments approximately one-third the size of standard heparin and are prepared by enzymatic or chemical cleavage of unfractionated heparin. This difference in molecular weight produces an anticoagulant with properties considerably different from those of heparin. The LMWHs are administered subcutaneously. They are considered safer and require less monitoring than standard heparin (CFB 16.2).

DRUG MONOGRAPH 16.1
Enoxaparin

Enoxaparin is a LMWH produced by partial depolymerisation of unfractionated heparin. It is indicated for preventing and treating venous thromboembolism (VTE) (e.g. during pregnancy or after caesarean section).

Mechanism of action

The LMWHs, including enoxaparin, bind to and accelerate the action of antithrombin III (Fig 16.3). Binding potentiates inactivation of factor Xa and factor IIa (thrombin), ultimately resulting in decreased thrombin formation and hence preventing fibrin clot formation. Enoxaparin has a four-fold greater effect on factor Xa than on factor IIa.

Pharmacokinetics

Following subcutaneous administration, the bioavailability of enoxaparin is 91% and the volume of distribution is small (5–9 L) due to confinement to the vascular space. It has limited oral bioavailability, therefore even if present in breast milk, neonatal exposure is minimal. Enoxaparin undergoes desulfation and depolymerisation in the liver, producing smaller fragments with decreased biological activity. Both the parent drug and the smaller fragments are renally excreted. The elimination half-life is 3–5 hours.

Drug interactions

Drug interactions with the LMWHs include any drugs that potentially affect the clotting process, and current drug information sources should be consulted. In addition, heparins can cause hyperkalaemia, and combinations that increase this risk should be avoided or the plasma potassium concentration should be monitored.

Adverse reactions

Adverse reactions commonly include:
* bleeding, bruising
* injection site reactions, e.g. pain and rarely, skin necrosis
* hyperkalaemia.

Warnings and contraindications

Refer to the section on heparins in the text.

Dosage and administration

Enoxaparin is administered subcutaneously, and the dosage varies depending on the situation. For example, for postoperative prophylaxis 20–40 mg is administered once daily for 7–10 days or until mobile.

CLINICAL FOCUS BOX 16.2

Clinical uses of low-molecular-weight heparins

* Prevention of VTE for women at high risk during pregnancy
* Prevention of VTE for women at high risk postpartum
* Treatment of DVT and pulmonary embolus
* Prevention of pregnancy loss and other placenta mediated disorders for women with recurrent pregnancy loss, along with aspirin

Mechanism of action

Both types of heparin inactivate factor Xa. Unfractionated heparin also inactivates thrombin (IIa) by binding, at the same time, to both antithrombin III and thrombin. In contrast, LMWHs increase the action of antithrombin III on factor Xa but, because of their small size, LMWHs cannot bind antithrombin III and thrombin at the same time. Hence, they have an enhanced capacity to inhibit factor Xa, which contributes to their improved antithrombotic effect. See Table 16.1 for a comparison of unfractionated heparin and LMWHs.

Pharmacokinetics

Compared to standard heparin, LMWHs have a lower affinity for endothelial cells, macrophages, and plasma proteins; increased bioavailability; and a more predictable clearance that is independent of dose. Hepatic clearance plays a minor role and elimination is principally via the kidneys, hence their biological half-life is prolonged in renal failure. For LMWHs, consider dose reduction in severe renal impairment. LMWHs have a longer half-life than heparin (2–4 times greater) when given subcutaneously and their anticoagulant effect also lasts longer.

Unfractionated and LMWHs are large molecules and there is little transplacental transfer or entry into breast milk. They are therefore considered safe to use during pregnancy and lactation.

Drug interactions and adverse reactions

Drug interactions with the heparins include any drugs that affect the clotting process, and current drug information sources should be consulted. In addition, the heparins can cause hyperkalaemia, and combinations that increase this risk should be avoided or plasma potassium concentration monitored.

Bleeding is a well-known complication of heparin therapy, and the LMWHs have a similar risk. Common

TABLE 16.1 Comparison of regular heparin and low-molecular-weight heparins

PROPERTY	REGULAR HEPARIN	LOW-MOLECULAR-WEIGHT HEPARIN
Molecular weight range	3,000–30,000	1,000–10,000
Average molecular weight	12,000–15,000	4,000–6,000
Mechanism of action	Inactivates factor Xa and IIa (thrombin)	Inactivates factor Xa
aPTT monitoring required	Yes	No
Inhibition of platelet function	++++ (high)	++ (medium)
Route of administration	IV, SC	SC
Protein binding	++++ (high)	+ (low)
Vascular permeability increased	Yes	No
Reversal of effects	Protamine	Protamine (partially effective)

adverse reactions include local irritation such as erythema, haematoma, urticaria, and pain at the injection site.

Some people develop an immunological response to heparins, known as heparin-induced thrombocytopaenia (HIT). Binding of the resultant antibodies leads to platelet activation and aggregation, causing widespread thrombosis and thrombocytopaenia. The incidence of HIT is less with LMWH than with unfractionated heparin and data on osteoporosis also indicate a decreased incidence. Danaparoid may be used as an alternative to heparin or LMWH in people with HIT, as cross-reactivity occurs in fewer than 10% of people.

Warnings and contraindications

Use LHWH with caution in women undergoing any procedure that increases the potential of bleeding, including induction of labour. Avoid use in people with LMWH or heparin hypersensitivity, bleeding disorders, severe hypertension, stroke, thrombocytopenia, severe liver or kidney disease, endocarditis, or retinopathy. People with renal impairment have a higher risk of bleeding with LMWHs because they are eliminated by renal excretion. (See 16.7 Haemostatic and Antifibrinolytic Drugs for a discussion of the role of protamine in reversing heparin-induced bleeding.)

Vitamin K antagonists – Warfarin

These drugs were discovered following an outbreak of a haemorrhagic disorder in cattle eating spoiled sweet clover in 1929, when the active constituent was identified as bis-hydroxycoumarin. Synthesised analogues, including warfarin (the name comes from the **W**isconsin **A**lumni **R**esearch **F**oundation, and **arin** from coumarin), were originally thought to be too toxic and were used as rodenticides. Following the survival of a man in 1951 after repeated suicide attempts using high doses of the rat poison, warfarin was introduced as an anticoagulant for humans in 1959 (DM 16.2). Table 16.2 provides a

---

DRUG MONOGRAPH 16.2

Warfarin

Warfarin interferes with hepatic synthesis of the vitamin K–dependent clotting factors (II, VII, IX and X, and various other anticoagulant proteins) leading to the production of non-functional coagulation factors (Fig 16.4). Factor VII is depleted quickly. The sequential depletion of factors IX, X and II follows. Warfarin does not affect established clots but prevents further extension of formed clots, diminishing the potential for secondary thromboembolic complications. The main advantage of warfarin is that it is effective orally and can be given once daily after the maintenance dose has been established.

Indications

Warfarin is indicated for the prophylaxis and treatment of DVT and pulmonary thromboembolism. It is also used for the prophylaxis of thromboembolism in people with prosthetic heart valves.

Pharmacokinetics

Warfarin is well absorbed from the gastrointestinal tract and has a systemic bioavailability of more than 95%. Peak plasma concentration occurs in 3–9 hours and its duration of action is 2–5 days. Warfarin is highly protein-bound (99%), and plasma half-life varies from 25–60 hours, with an average of 40 hours. Warfarin crosses the placenta, and fetal plasma concentration is similar to that of the maternal circulation.

DRUG MONOGRAPH 16.2
Warfarin—cont'd

Warfarin is metabolised in the liver by CYP enzymes including CYPIA2, CYP2C9, and CYP3A4. Genetic variability in the expression of the specific enzymes responsible for warfarin metabolism (especially CYP2C9) accounts for the large variability observed in warfarin dose requirements. Reduced metabolism of warfarin, and thus increased warfarin plasma concentration, is more prevalent in European, African, and Asian populations.

Drug interactions

Current drug information resources should always be consulted. Numerous drugs, including antimicrobials, cardiovascular drugs, analgesics, anti-inflammatory drugs, immuno-modulators, gastrointestinal drugs, antineoplastics and central nervous system drugs, and St John's wort interact with warfarin. Certain foods (such as grapefruit) can also interact with warfarin. The international normalised ratio (or INR) should be monitored frequently when instituting, ceasing, or altering other drug therapy.

Adverse reactions

Adverse reactions include:
- bleeding (common)
- rarely, alopecia, anorexia, abdominal cramps or distress, leucopenia, nausea, vomiting, diarrhoea, purple toes syndrome, and kidney damage.

Warnings and contraindications

- Avoid use in the elderly.
- Contraindicated in people with liver disease.
- Avoid use in pregnancy, particularly during the first trimester. The risk of abortion and teratogenicity is high, and fetal abnormalities and facial anomalies have been reported if warfarin is administered during weeks 6–12 of pregnancy. Administration during the second and third trimesters is associated with central nervous system abnormalities. Women with prosthetic heart valves have a high risk for valve-related thrombotic events and are typically managed on warfarin. Changing to a LMWH eliminates fetal risk but is associated with a higher rate of valve complications than continuation of warfarin. Individualised decision making in consultation with the woman's cardiologist should take place when planning pregnancy, or early in the first trimester when pregnancy was unplanned. If warfarin is continued, consideration should also be given to switching to LMWH in late pregnancy to take advantage of the shorter half-life in the lead-up to labour, to avoid peripartum bleeding risks.
- Avoid use in people with known anticoagulant drug hypersensitivity; any medical or surgical condition associated with bleeding (aneurysm, cerebrovascular bleeding, surgery, and severe trauma); blood disorders; severe uncontrolled hypertension; pericarditis; severe diabetes; ulcers; visceral cancer; vitamin C or vitamin K deficiencies; endocarditis; or severe liver or kidney impairment.
- Brands of warfarin should not be interchanged due to a lack of bioequivalence data.

Dosage and administration

Warfarin should be taken at the same time each day, and the usual dose is 5 mg daily for 2 days and then adjusted according to the INR. The maintenance dose is in the range 1–10 mg daily. The INR range varies with specific indications, and local guidelines should be consulted. Several algorithms are available to aid with warfarin dosing and can be accessed at the International Warfarin Pharmacogenetics Consortium website (https://www.pharmgkb.org/page/iwpc) and www.warfarindosing.org.

TABLE 16.2 Anticoagulant drugs: Comparison of heparin and warfarin

	HEPARIN	WARFARIN
Onset of action	Immediate	Slow (24–48 hours)
Route of administration	Parenteral	Oral
Duration of action	Short (< 4 hours)	Long (2–5 days)
Laboratory test for dosage control	Activated partial thromboplastin time (aPTT)	Prothrombin time (PT)
Antidote	Protamine	Vitamin K, whole blood or plasma
Pregnancy	Heparin and LMWH used. LMWH not recommended in pregnant women with prosthetic heart valves due to evidence of inadequate anticoagulation	Generally contraindicated (may be used in second trimester if indicated)
Lactation	Safe to use	Safe to use

Site of action of warfarin and the role of vitamin K

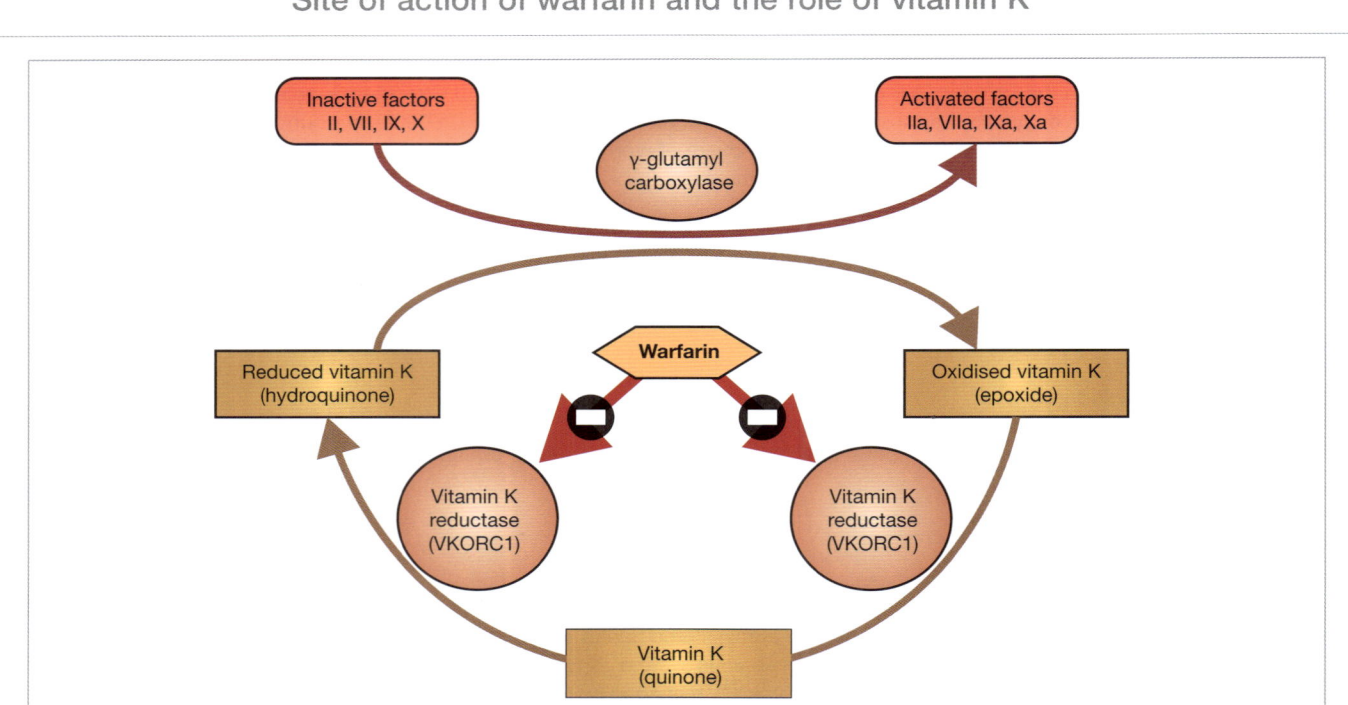

FIGURE 16.5 The oxidation of the reduced form of vitamin K (the hydroxyquinone) forming oxidised vitamin K (the epoxide) is coupled to the carboxylation of the inactive factors II, VII, IX, and X. The vitamin K reductase complex 1 (VKORC1) then regenerates the reduced form of vitamin K via initial formation of vitamin K quinone. Warfarin inhibits VKORC1 and, hence, both the regeneration of reduced vitamin K and formation of the activated clotting factors.

comparison of heparin and warfarin. Figure 16.5 illustrates the site of action of warfarin and the importance of the role of vitamin K. (See also 16.7 Haemostatic and Antifibrinolytic Drugs.)

Fondaparinux: Antithrombin-III-dependent anticoagulant

Fondaparinux is a synthetic antithrombin-III-dependent anticoagulant. It binds AT III, potentiating the neutralisation of factor Xa by antithrombin, inhibiting both thrombin formation and thrombus development. It does not inhibit thrombin (activated factor IIa) and has no antiplatelet activity. Fondaparinux is as effective and as safe as the LMWHs. It is used to prevent VTE in high-risk surgery such as hip fracture or replacement. Administered subcutaneously, the long half-life of 17 hours permits once-daily administration. As with the heparins, this drug is contraindicated in co-existing bleeding disorders and in cases of renal impairment. The latter is important because fondaparinux is excreted unchanged in urine.

When both warfarin and a heparin are contraindicated, fondaparinux direct factor Xa inhibitor may be considered for use in pregnancy or the postpartum period. While

fondaparinux has not been widely used in this population, there is some data to support that it is effective, well tolerated, and safe during pregnancy and lactation (Dempfle et al 2021).

KEY POINTS

Anticoagulants

- Heparin produces its anticoagulant effect by combining with antithrombin III to form a complex that acts at multiple sites in the normal coagulation system, inactivating factors IXa, Xa, XIa and XIIa. Inactivation of factor Xa of the intrinsic and extrinsic pathways prevents the conversion of prothrombin to thrombin, thereby inhibiting the formation of fibrin from fibrinogen.

- The LMWHs are fragments of standard heparin prepared by enzymatic or chemical cleavage. They inactivate factor Xa more potently than factor IIa.

- LMWHs are considered safer, easier to administer and require less monitoring than standard heparin. Bleeding is a well-known complication of heparin therapy, and the LMWHs have a similar risk.

- Warfarin is an orally administered anticoagulant and is indicated for women with mechanical heart valves.

- Many drugs interact with warfarin, and the INR should be monitored frequently when instituting, ceasing, or altering other drug therapy.

- The synthetic antithrombin-III-dependent anticoagulant is fondaparinux, which binds AT III, potentiating the neutralisation of factor Xa by antithrombin and inhibiting both thrombin formation and thrombus development.

16.6 Antiplatelet agents

Aspirin

Platelet dysfunction has been considered as a potential cause for placenta mediated disorders, including preeclampsia, fetal growth restriction, and preterm birth. Platelets adhere to a thrombogenic surface and are activated by mediators such as platelet activating factor, thromboxane A_2 (which binds to Tx receptors), ADP (which binds to $P2Y_{12}$ and $P2Y_1$ receptors) and thrombin, resulting in platelet aggregation. Platelet microthrombi occurring in the placental microvasculature can lead to areas of infarction and malfunction.

Our knowledge of the role of platelets in thromboembolic disease and our understanding of the pharmacology of aspirin has led to considerable development of drugs with antiplatelet activity. Only aspirin has a history of use in pregnancy, and it continues to be used in low dose for the prevention of preeclampsia, fetal growth restriction, preterm labour, and recurrent pregnancy loss.

Mechanism of action

Aspirin causes a long-lasting functional deficit in platelets by irreversibly inhibiting the cyclooxygenase enzyme COX-1 necessary for thromboxane A_2 synthesis. Thromboxane A_2 promotes platelet aggregation and vasoconstriction, and thus aspirin suppresses these actions. Platelets lack the metabolic capacity to synthesise new COX-1, so the deficit induced by aspirin lasts 8–10 days until new platelets are synthesised. This effect on platelet function explains both the effectiveness of aspirin as an **antiplatelet agent** and its prolonged action.

Studies have established the effectiveness of aspirin therapy for reducing the risk of developing preterm preeclampsia, or fetal growth restriction, when commenced prior to 16 weeks of gestation in women at risk (Ghazanfarpour et al 2020). Lower rates of preterm birth have also been found with aspirin use, regardless of the gestational age at commencement. Low-dose aspirin (75–150 mg/day) is advised for these indications in pregnancy with no increased risk for abruption and antepartum haemorrhage at these doses.

Pharmacokinetics

Aspirin is rapidly absorbed from the stomach after oral administration, reaching peak levels at 2 hours (Shanmugalingam et al 2019). Aspirin is metabolised in the liver to salicylic acid and other metabolites then renally excreted. At higher doses, salicylic acid contributes to the anti-inflammatory and analgesic effects of aspirin. While the half-life is short at 2.5 hours, the non-reversible impact of aspirin on COX-1 produces long-lasting clinical effects.

Adverse effects

Low-dose aspirin is generally well tolerated. Gastrointestinal side effects such as dyspepsia and abdominal pain can occur, even with low doses. Long-term aspirin use has been associated with bleeding and gastric ulceration. At large doses, the metabolites of aspirin are hepatotoxic. Aspirin allergy can complicate the management of asthma for people sensitive to it.

KEY POINTS

Antiplatelet drugs

- Platelets play a critical role in thrombosis.

- Platelets adhere to a thrombogenic surface and are activated by mediators such as platelet activating factor, thromboxane A_2, ADP, and thrombin, resulting in platelet aggregation.

- The antiplatelet drug used in pregnancy is aspirin, which binds irreversibly to platelet COX-1.

16.7 Haemostatic and antifibrinolytic drugs

Haemostatic and **antifibrinolytic** drugs are compounds used to control and prevent bleeding, including drug-induced over-anticoagulation. This group of drugs includes tranexamic acid, protamine, and vitamin K. These agents are used to control rapid blood loss.

Tranexamic acid

Tranexamic acid, an antifibrinolytic drug, is a competitive inhibitor of plasminogen activation. At high doses, it is a non-competitive inhibitor of plasmin. It is indicated for use in heavy menstrual bleeding and the prevention and management of postpartum haemorrhage. Research confirms administration of tranexamic acid during postpartum haemorrhage reduces the amount and duration of bleeding, the use of blood transfusion, and death (Bouthors et al 2022). Evidence for prophylactic use for either vaginal birth or caesarean section is less clear.

Tranexamic acid can be administered orally, intramuscularly, or intravenously. Doses of 1 gram administered intravenously are commonly used in the management of postpartum haemorrhage. No significant drug interactions have been reported. Adverse reactions include nausea, vomiting, diarrhoea, visual disturbances, thrombosis, hypotension, and thromboembolism. There is limited evidence regarding the use of tranexamic acid during breastfeeding, but it is minimally excreted into breast milk. Avoid use in people with tranexamic acid hypersensitivity, colour vision defects, haematuria, subarachnoid haemorrhage, a history of thrombosis, or renal impairment.

Protamine (reverses heparin's action)

Protamine, a protein-like substance derived from the sperm and mature testes of salmon and other fish, is a heparin antagonist and is used in over-anticoagulation. Protamine is a very weak anticoagulant alone, but when the sulphate form is given in conjunction with heparin, a complex is formed that dissociates the bond between heparin and AT III, thus reducing the anticoagulant action of heparin. Protamine is a basic protein (containing many free amino groups) and combines with heparin to form an inactive complex.

Protamine is indicated to treat an overdose of LMWH or standard heparin that leads to haemorrhage. Blood transfusions may also be necessary. It is administered intravenously and has an onset of action within 1 minute. Its duration of action is approximately 2 hours.

Adverse reactions include back pain, a feeling of warmth or tiredness, flushing, nausea, and vomiting. Less often reported are bradycardia, sudden hypotension, shock, dyspnoea (all related to the too-rapid administration of protamine), bleeding (caused by protamine overdose or a rebound of heparin activity), hypertension, and anaphylaxis.

Use protamine with caution in people who have been exposed to either protamine or protamine insulin in the past. Antibodies to protamine may have developed, which increases the risk of an allergic reaction. Avoid use in people with protamine hypersensitivity.

Protamine is administered by slow intravenous injection over 10 minutes. One milligram of protamine is necessary to neutralise around 100 units of standard heparin, if injected within 15 minutes of heparin administration. As heparin is cleared quite rapidly, a reduction in the dose of protamine is necessary if it is administered more than 15 minutes after the heparin dose. The standard dose of protamine (1 mg) will partially neutralise 1 mg of enoxaparin. Close monitoring with blood coagulation tests is required.

Vitamin K (reverses warfarin's action)

Vitamin K (phytomenadione) is essential to the hepatic synthesis of prothrombin (factor II) and factors VII, IX and X. Vitamin K may be given as an antidote for excessive anticoagulation with warfarin if cessation of warfarin therapy is not sufficient (Fig 16.4). Local guidelines should be followed when administered to reverse the anticoagulant effect of warfarin (Tran et al 2013). When vitamin K is given concurrently with warfarin, the anticoagulant effect is reduced.

A deficiency of vitamin K leads to hypoprothrombinaemia and haemorrhage. Vitamin K is also used to prevent and treat hypoprothrombinaemia. Prothrombin deficiency can occur because of inadequate absorption of vitamin K from the intestine or because of destruction of intestinal organisms, which might occur with antibiotic therapy. It is also seen in newborns, who are yet to establish intestinal organisms. Vitamin K is routinely offered to newborns to help prevent vitamin K deficiency bleeding. Although prothrombin levels may be normal at birth, they decline until about day 6–8, when the neonate is a risk for the classical form of vitamin K deficiency.

The onset of action for oral phytomenadione is 6–12 hours, and for the injectable form it is 1–2 hours. Vitamin K is metabolised in the liver and excreted via the kidneys and in the bile. Hence it is used with caution in people with biliary atresia, pancreatic insufficiency, or fat malabsorption syndromes. Adverse reactions include facial flushing, taste alterations, and redness or pain at the injection site.

KEY POINTS

Haemostatic and antifibrinolytic drugs

- The haemostatic and antifibrinolytic agents are used to control and prevent bleeding and reduce blood loss.
- This group of drugs includes tranexamic acid, protamine, and vitamin K.
- Tranexamic acid is an antifibrinolytic agent used in the management of postpartum haemorrhage.
- Protamine reverses the anticoagulant effects of the heparins.
- Vitamin K reverses the action of warfarin.

REVIEW EXERCISES

1 Benita, aged 26 years, has a prosthetic heart valve and is on warfarin therapy. She is planning pregnancy and has been advised to consider stopping warfarin and changing to heparin therapy. She asks you to explain what the pros and cons of this change are. Make a list of the key points you would discuss with her to answer her query.

2 Jocasta is 28 years old and 20 weeks pregnant. She has been diagnosed with iron deficiency anaemia and has been treated with iron 100 mg daily. However, her most recent haemoglobin, 3 weeks after commencing iron therapy, was unchanged from her previous test. Make a list of possible explanations for the lack of improvement.

REFERENCES

Abdulrehman J, Lausman A, Tang GH, et al. Development and implementation of a quality improvement toolkit, iron deficiency in pregnancy with maternal iron optimization (IRON MOM): a before-and-after study. PLoS Med. 2019, Aug;16(8): e1002867. doi.org/10.1371/journal.pmed.1002867

Bouthors A-S, Giliot S, Sentilhes L, et al. The role of tranexamic acid in the management of postpartum haemorrhage. Best Prac Res Clin Anaesthesiol. 2022;36:411-426. doi.org/10.1016/j.bpa.2022.08.004

Crowley CM, McMahon G, Desmond J, et al. Skin staining following intravenous iron infusion. BMJ Case Rep. CP 2019;12:e229113. doi.org/10.1136/bcr-2018-229113

Daru J, Allotey J, Pena-Rosas, JP, et al. Serum ferritin thresholds for the diagnosis of iron deficiency in pregnancy: a systematic review. Transfus Med. 2017 Jun;27(3):167-174. doi.org/10.1111/tme.12408

Dempfle C-E, Koscielny J, Lindhoff-Last E, et al. Fondaparinux pre-, peri-, and/or postpartum for the prophylaxis/treatment of venous thromboembolism (FondaPPP). Clin App Thromb Hemost. 2021;27:1-8. doi:10.1177/10760296211014575

Department of Health. 2019. Pregnancy Care Guidelines: Anaemia. https://www.health.gov.au/resources/pregnancy-care-guidelines/part-f-routine-maternal-health-tests/anaemia

Dewey KG, Oaks BM. U-shaped curve for risk associated with maternal hemoglobin, iron status or iron supplementation. Am J Clin Nutr. 2017;106:1694S-702S.

Finkelstein J, Layden A, Stover P. Vitamin B12 and perinatal health. Adv Nutr. 2015;6:552-563. doi:10.3945/an.115.008201

Georgieff, MK. Iron deficiency in pregnancy. Am J Obstet Gynecol. 2020, Oct;223(4):516-524. doi.org/10.1016/j.ajog.2020.03.006

Ghazanfarpour M, Sathyapalan T, Banach M, et al. Prophylactic aspirin for preventing preeclampsia and its complications: an overview of meta-analyses. Drug Discov Today. 2020;25(8):1487-1501. doi.org/10.1016/j.drudis.2020.05.011

Hamulyák EN, Scheres LJJ, Marijnen MC, et al. Aspirin or heparin or both for improving pregnancy outcomes in women with persistent antiphospholipid antibodies and recurrent pregnancy loss. Cochrane Database Syst Rev. 2020 May 2;5(5):CD012852. doi:10.1002/14651858.CD012852.pub2. (accessed 19 February 2023).

Hermans C, Kulkarni R. Women with bleeding disorders. Haemophilia. 2018;24(6):29-36. doi:10.1111/hae.13502

Infante M, Leoni M, Caprio M, et al. Long-term metformin therapy and vitamin B12 deficiency: an association to bear in mind. World J Diabetes. 2021;12(7):916-931. doi:10.4239/wjd.v12.i7.916

Lefkou E, Hunt, B. Bleeding disorders in pregnancy. Obs Gynaecol Reproductive Med. 2018;28(7):189-195. doi.org/10.1016/j.ogrm.2018.06.002

McDonald SJ, Middleton P, Dowswell T, et al. Effect of timing of umbilical cord clamping of term infants on maternal and neonatal outcomes. Cochrane Database Syst Rev. 2013 Jul 11;2013(7):CD004074. doi:10.1002/14651858. (accessed 10 February 2023).

Middleton P, Shepherd E, Gomersall JC. Venous thromboembolism prophylaxis for women at risk during pregnancy and the early postnatal period. Cochrane Database Syst Rev. 2021 Mar 29;3(3):CD001689. doi:10.1002/14651858.CD001689.pub4

Moussa H, Nasab S, Haida Z, et al. Folic acid supplementation: what is new? Fetal, obstetric, long-term benefits and risks. Future Science. 2016;2(2):FSO116. doi:10.4155/fsoa-2015-0015

Ormesher L, Simcox LE, Tower C, et al. 'To test or not to test', the arguments for and against thrombophilia testing in obstetrics. Obstet Med. 2017, Jun;10(2):61-66. doi.org/10.1177/1753495X17695696

Qian Y, Ying X, Wang P, et al. Early versus delayed umbilical cord clamping on maternal and neonatal outcomes. Arch Gynecol Obstet. 2019;300:531-543. doi.org/10.1007/s00404-019-05215-8

Raia-Barjat T, Edebiri O, Chauleur C. Venous thromboembolism risk score and pregnancy. Front Cardiovasc Med. 2022;9:863612. doi:10.3389/fcvm.2022.863612

Rang HP, Dale JM, Ritter JM, et al. Rang and Dale's pharmacology, 7th edn. Elsevier Ltd, 2012.

Rogers L, Cordero A, Pfeiffer C, et al. Global folate status in women of reproductive age: a systematic review with emphasis on methodological issues. Ann NY Acad Sci. 2018;1431:35-57. doi: 10.1111/nyas.13963

Shanmugalingam R, Wang X, Münch G, et al. A pharmacokinetic assessment of optimal dosing, preparation, and chronotherapy of aspirin in pregnancy. Am J Obstet Gynecol. 2019 Sep;221(3):255.e1-255.e9. doi.org/10.1016/j.ajog.2019.04.027

Sharma AJ, Ford ND, Bulkley JE, et al. Use of the electronic health record to assess prevalence of anemia and iron deficiency in pregnancy. J Nutr. 2021, Nov 2;151(11):3588-3595. doi.org/10.1093/jn/nxab254

Saravanan P, Sukumar N, Adaikalakoteswari A, et al. Association of maternal vitamin B12 and folate levels in early pregnancy with gestational diabetes: a prospective UK cohort study (PRiDE study). Diabetologia. 2021;64:2170-2182. doi.org/10.1007/s00125-021-05510-7

Tang G, Lausman A, Petrucci J, et al. Prevalence of iron deficiency in pregnancy: a single centre Canadian study. Blood. 2018;132(Supp1):4896-4896. doi.org/10.1182/blood-2018-99-116792

Tran HA, Chunilal SD, Harper PL, et al. An update of consensus guidelines for warfarin reversal. Med J Aust. 2013;198(4):198-199.

World Health Organization (2016). WHO recommendations on antenatal care for a positive pregnancy experience. Geneva: World Health Organization, 2016. https://apps.who.int/iris/rest/bitstreams/1064182/retrieve

Zhang C, Rawal S. Dietary iron intake, iron status and gestational diabetes. Am J Clin Nutr. 2017;106:1672S-1680S.

ONLINE RESOURCES

International Warfarin Pharmacogenetics Consortium: https://www.pharmgkb.org/page/iwpc

Melbourne Haematology, Anticoagulation (blood thinning) in pregnancy: http://www.melbournehaematology.com.au/fact-sheets/anticoagulation-blood-thinning-in-pregnancy.html

UpToDate, Use of anticoagulants during pregnancy and postpartum: https://www.uptodate.com/contents/use-of-anticoagulants-during-pregnancy-and-postpartum

CHAPTER 17

PREMATURE LABOUR AND BIRTH

Michelle Gray, Roslyn Donnellan Fernandez

Key Abbreviations

CTG	cardiotocograghy
fFN	fetal fibronectin
FHR	fetal heart rate
GBS	group B streptococcus
LFT	liver function test
LLETZ	large loop excision of the transformation zone
OA	occiput anterior
SABA	short-acting β2 agonist

Key Terms

cervical cerclage 328
cervical length 327
corticosteroid 329
hyaline membrane
  disease 333
pessaries 328
prematurity 326

premature birth 325
preterm 325
progesterone 328
premature rupture of
  membranes 326
tocolytic 329
uterotonic 329

Chapter Focus

This chapter focuses on prematurity and on the pharmacology relevant to the management of premature labour and birth. The content informs midwives' understanding of the pathophysiological causes that increase the risk of premature labour and birth. It provides an overview of diagnostic and screening assessments, and describes contemporary treatments available in Australia. A preliminary case study provides a contextual scenario to direct readers' learning.

Key Drug Groups

- Magnesium sulphate
- Calcium channel blockers
- B-adrenergic receptor agonists
- Cyclooxygenase inhibitors
- Oxytocin receptor antagonists:
  - atosiban
- Nitric oxide donors

Learning Outcomes

- Understand the pathophysiological causes that increase the risk for premature labour and birth for a woman and her baby.
- Identify the signs and symptoms of premature labour that suggest the potential risk of premature birth.
- Demonstrate an understanding of the screening and diagnostic assessments that cover contemporary treatments for premature labour and birth available in Australia and New Zealand.
- Understand the pharmacology relevant to the management of premature labour and birth for the woman and her baby.
- Describe the key drug groups used in treating a woman and her baby who experience premature labour and birth, including the midwife's role in medication management.

CRITICAL THINKING SCENARIO

Casey is 30 weeks pregnant and reporting uncomfortable lower back pain. She is G2P1 (Gravida 2, Parity 1). Casey is accompanied by her partner Melanie. This pregnancy and the couple's previous child (Max, 4 years old) were conceived through donor sperm provided by a friend. Casey has used vaginal progesterone pessaries during both pregnancies. The family lives off-grid, in a small regional town. Casey is concerned that she has a muscle strain from tending her vegetable garden. Even after a warm bath she cannot get comfortable and has not been able to sleep. They have dropped Max off with friends this morning before attending the local hospital.

1   What signs and symptoms could Casey present with, for you to suspect premature labour?

2   What assessments will you make to determine if she is in premature labour?

In your assessment you note the following:

BP 140/80, P92, T37.8C, R18

Abdominal palpation: Fundus = 31 cm, Lie longitudinal, Position OA, FHR heard. Fetal movements felt today. On palpation the uterus is non-tender to touch. Mild tightening can be palpated lasting 30–40 secs 2:10.

3   What characteristics might you observe on a CTG performed at 30 weeks?

4   What screening tests can be performed to determine if Casey is in premature labour?

5   What is the role of progesterone pessaries?

6   Who from the multi-disciplinary team will you involve in Casey's care and what other resources or standards will guide your practice?

7   If Casey is in labour, diagnosed by changes to her cervix, she will need to be moved to a tertiary hospital with a neonatal intensive care unit. Outline the treatment options, first-line pharmacological management, and the organisation of the transfer.

Introduction

The World Health Organization (WHO) estimates that globally, 13.4 million babies were born **preterm** in 2020, with approximately 900,000 premature infants dying in 2019 due to complications associated with preterm birth (Ohuma et al 2023). Preterm birth complications are the leading cause of death among children under 5 years of age and were responsible for approximately 900,000 deaths in 2019 (Perin et al 2022). The WHO suggests that three-quarters of these deaths could have been prevented.

The Australian Preterm Birth Prevention Alliance (see Online resources; APBPA) reports that 26,000 Australian babies are born preterm every year, and for babies of Aboriginal and Torres Strait Islander descent this rate is doubled. The Australian Institute of Health and Welfare's (AIHW) 2023 report indicates there has been little change in the proportion of preterm birth in Australia over the last decade; 8.3% (2011) and 8.2% (2021). In New Zealand, data for 2020 indicate a rate of preterm birth of 7.9%, with the rate varying by ethnic groupings from highest to lowest: Māori (9%); Pasifika (8.1%); Indian (8.8%); Asian (7.3%); and European (7.1%).

17.1 Prematurity definitions and causes

Premature labour

The physiology of labour is covered in Chapter 8. Premature onset of labour through stimulation of stretch receptors within the myometrium and/or the spontaneous rupture of membranes can initiate premature labour. Premature labour is defined as when regular contractions or tightenings result in the opening of the cervix after week 20 and before 37 completed weeks of pregnancy.

Premature birth

Premature birth is defined as an infant born alive prior to 37 completed weeks of gestation. The WHO (2023) also defines the sub-categories of premature birth based on gestational age as:

- Extremely preterm (< 28 weeks)
- Very preterm (28 to < 32 weeks)
- Moderate to late preterm (32–37 weeks).

Risk factors for preterm birth include having a prior preterm birth, recurrent urinary tract infections, and being pregnant with multiples. Complications associated with babies who are born preterm include immature lungs, difficulty regulating body temperature, feeding difficulties and poor weight gain. Preterm babies usually require intensive nursery care, medication, and sometimes surgery. Currently there are few medicines in use for managing preterm labour or preventing spontaneous preterm birth from occurring (McDougall et al 2023).

Although the percentages in Box 17.1 represent a small portion of total births in Australia, Dodd et al (2009) reported **prematurity** accounts for almost 70% of the total perinatal mortality. Preterm babies are more likely to be admitted to a special care nursery or neonatal intensive care unit (72%) than babies born at term (10%) or post term (13%). More recently, Ohuma et al (2023) reported on national, regional, and worldwide estimates of preterm birth in 2020, with trends from 2010. In their international systematic review they found that there has been no measurable change in the preterm birth rates over the last decade.

There are several defining gestations that suggest maturity of certain body systems:

- *At 34 weeks*, defined as early preterm, a baby's lungs are immature.

- *After 28–32 weeks* a baby is very preterm; the skin is thin and thermoregulation is a challenge. The baby may have a good sucking reflex but will tire quickly and require supplement tube feeds at the breast.
- *Before 28 weeks* – whereas survival rates for babies born at 28 weeks can be between 80–90%, being born earlier than 28 weeks is considered extremely preterm, and the survival rate drops considerably for babies for each gestational week lost.
- *At 23 weeks* a baby with access to medical treatment in a well-resourced setting still has just a 45% chance of surviving (Rysavy et al 2021).

Causes of prematurity

The cause of premature labour is sometimes unknown – *idiopathic*, meaning we do not know the cause of premature birth. However, known causes can be linked to physical, emotional, psychological, or environmental triggers (Ohuma et al 2023).

There are many hypothesised emotional and psychological causes of premature labour. For example, a distressing emotional incident such as the death of someone close; environmental triggers such as earthquakes and flooding; or witnessing a life-threatening event such as war have all been hypothesised as the cause of preterm birth. Flooding has been reported to cause an increase in hypertension and low birth weights in babies; however, there is no correlation with an increase in premature births (Partash et al 2022).

Seismic activity has been found to affect birth gestation for mothers who feel the quake (Glynn et al 2001). More recently, Amarpoor et al (2023) also found an increase in preterm birth outcomes among mothers who experienced earthquake when compared before and after the Varzaghan earthquake. However, other studies have suggested pregnant women who experienced the New Zealand earthquakes in 2011 were only affected if they were in their first or third trimester (Kutinova Menclova et al 2020).

Infection

Infection is one of the main causes of premature labour and birth. Infection is covered in detail in Chapter 12. Chorioamnionitis, bacterial vaginosis, group B streptococcus (GBS), and urinary infections are all well-documented causes of premature labour (Morgan et al 2023). Consequently, widespread use of antibiotics in these scenarios is common. While antibiotic use in cases of **premature rupture of membranes** has led to prolonging the pregnancy, evidence suggests that in the case of preterm labour with intact membranes prophylactic use of antibiotics does not improve the overall outcomes for neonates (Flenady et al 2013). The review by Flenady et al (2013) suggested potential short- and long-term detrimental consequences on children exposed to antibiotics prophylactically in scenarios of

---

BOX 17.1 Australia's mothers and babies: Preterm birth statistics (AIHW 2023)

- The proportion of babies born between 20 and 36 weeks remained steady between 2011 (8.3%) and 2021 (8.2%) with a peak of 8.7% reached most recently in 2018.
- The proportion born between 37 and 39 weeks increased (e.g. babies born at 38 weeks increased from 19% in 2011 to 23% in 2021).
- The proportion born from 40 weeks onwards decreased (e.g. babies born at 40 weeks decreased from 25% in 2011 to 20% in 2021).
- Almost 1 in 10 babies (8.2%) were born preterm and of these the majority were born between 32 and 36 completed weeks.
- Babies born to mothers who smoked at any point during pregnancy were more likely to be born preterm (13%) than babies born to mothers who had not smoked (7.6%).
- Most singleton babies were born at term (93%), while twins and babies of other multiple births were more likely to be born preterm (57% for twins and 100% for other multiples).

Source: AIHW 2023, Australia's mothers and babies: https://www.aihw.gov.au/reports/mothers-babies/australias-mothers-babies/contents/baby-outcomes/gestational-age

preterm labour. However, vaginal bacterial infections, specifically vaginal dysbiosis caused by four microbial species – *ureaplasma urealyticum, streptococcus agalactiae, candida albicans and gardnerella vaginalis* – have been found to cause premature labour. A reduction or absence of lactobacilli and presence of pathogenic microbial species was found in all women in a study conducted by Arena and Dacco (2021). Of the total cohort admitted to the hospital for premature labour, 81.63% (n=200) responded to the tocolytic treatment with arrest of the contractions and could be eventually discharged, while 18.36% of women (n=45) did not respond to the treatment and delivered prematurely (before 37 completed weeks).

Physical causes

Physical causes of premature labour or birth include maternal age, depression (Yonkers et al 2014), injury from a fall, motor vehicle accident, or previous premature birth (Dodd et al 2013) and multiple births (see Online resources; APBPA 2023). Previous pregnancy loss at 16–24 weeks or previous preterm birth at less than 34 weeks is also a risk factor for subsequent further premature labour.

Other physical causes include placental abruption – where the placenta separates from the uterus during pregnancy, and/or cervical weakness that may have resulted from previous surgery (two or more LLETZ, previous cone biopsy, previous LLETZ of more than 10 mm depth, uterine anomaly [Liu et al 2023; Miyakoshi et al 2021]).

Lifestyle factors

Many lifestyle habits and addictions such as alcohol intake, drug use (prescription and illicit), and smoking have been linked to an increase in the incidence of premature labour and birth. Babies are more likely to be born premature if their mothers smoked (13%) compared to mothers who do not smoke (8%) (see Online resources; APBPA 2023). See Chapter 21 for further information regarding drugs of addiction and substance dependence during pregnancy.

Women should be cautioned to avoid ingesting all foreign substances and avoid non-essential treatments during pregnancy. For instance, some essential oils are known to be abortigenic and/or cause bleeding during pregnancy (Dotsoky et al 2021). Prematurity has been linked to antepartum haemorrhage. Furthermore, acupressure applied too early or indirectly can cause uterine activity. Thus, women should be cautioned that complementary or alternative therapies are not without risk (Steel et al 2015).

Premature rupture of membranes

Flenady et al (2013) determined that prophylactic use of antibiotics in preterm labour with intact membranes did not improve the overall outcomes for the neonates. Plus, their review suggested potential short- and long-term detrimental consequences on children exposed to antibiotics prophylactically.

However, in preterm premature ruptured membranes between 24–31 weeks third-generation cephalosporins have been found to improve neonatal outcomes when compared to amoxicillin (Lorthe et al 2022).

Continuity of care provided by a known midwife or group of midwives has proven to reduce the incidence of premature labour. A Cochrane Review in 2016 reviewed 15 trials involving 17,674 women and reported that women have a 24% lower risk of premature labour when cared for by a midwife in a continuity of care model (Sandall et al 2016).

17.2 Diagnosis of premature labour

Signs and symptoms of premature labour

Signs and symptoms of premature labour can be vague and nondescript; low back pain, a dull ache, or just a feeling of pressure may be all the woman reports. A cardiotocograph (CTG) is not advised before 28 weeks and mild tightening would not be detectable by tocography. Therefore, the midwife needs to have acute observation skills and be vigilant in detecting even mild tightening on palpation of the abdomen to detect any uterine activity.

A thorough history should be taken from the woman and her birth support persons to determine any risk factors and the time scale of events. Non-invasive physical assessments should be performed to assist with planning the management of the pregnant woman. Medical and obstetric details, including physiological and psychosocial history, need to be documented to capture a comprehensive picture of possible causes.

A transvaginal ultrasound scan of the cervix in the mid-trimester

Best practice recommendations advocate for the **cervical length** to be measured routinely at the morphology scan and any other scan completed between 16–24 weeks gestation. Using an abdominal scanner, a cervical length a minimum of 35 mm is considered adequate (APBPA n.d.). A short cervix measured during the mid-trimester has been found to be a strong indicator of premature labour. If a transvaginal ultrasound determines the cervical length is shorter than 25 mm, regular transvaginal cervical length (VCL) monitoring (2–3 times weekly from 13 weeks until 22 weeks) is considered necessary surveillance for women at risk of premature labour. If cervical length is confirmed to be

25 mm or less, at $\leq$ 24 weeks, vaginal **progesterone pessaries** are recommended as a prophylaxis to prevent preterm labour and birth (Kabiri et al 2023). In cases where the cervical length is measured by transvaginal scan at less than 10 mm between 16–24 weeks, a **cervical cerclage**, and/or nightly progesterone pessary is recommended (APBPA, n.d.). Cervical cerclage at 13–14 weeks has been suggested for those who have had more than two previous affected pregnancies.

Assessments that assist in diagnosis

When a woman presents with suspected premature labour, initial physical assessment by the midwife involves observation of temperature, pulse, respirations, and blood pressure to establish if there are any signs of infection. These vital signs should be monitored every 30 minutes until the woman's contractions cease. Maternal hypotension should be resolved with intravenous fluids in the first instance.

Establishing micturition and bowel action can be informative as a urine infection and diarrhoea can both have a stimulating effect on uterine activity. Physical assessments should be non-invasive to avoid touching the cervix and stimulating further hormone release. An intravenous cannula would provide access for the administration of medication and the mother's consent for the insertion and baseline measurements of electrolytes, urea, and creatinine and liver function test (LFT) levels should be requested.

The history taking will determine if there has been any vaginal secretion loss, such as blood, liquor, or mucus. In this case the woman will be asked to wear a sanitary towel to collect any vaginal loss for visualisation and assessment of odour. Blood loss can be assessed for colour. Dark brown blood is a sign of an old bleed and is of less concern. Bright red blood is fresh active bleeding, and the source needs to be determined as soon as possible by viewing the cervix and cervical os. Liquor can vary in colour and smell. Normal, healthy liquor is clear or straw coloured and non-offensive in odour. Liquor that is pinkish or red means that there is uterine or placental bleeding. Liquor can be greenish to brown if the fetus has passed meconium in utero. Finally, liquor that has a pungent smell usually indicates a sign of infection. Any of these signs suggests a need for consultation and referral to an obstetrician for further investigation and internal examination of the cervix and cervical os-uteri. After the rationale for the procedure has been explained, consent, including affirmation of the woman's understanding of treatment options, should be gained before proceeding.

Premature rupture of membranes

- Visualisation of the cervix will require a speculum and a good light source.

- The speculum should be lubricated with water rather than lubricant before being placed into the vagina. The use of water instead of lubricant avoids any contamination of vaginal swabs or testing for rupture of membranes.
- Nitrazine paper can be used to confirm alkalinity of any vaginal secretions. Liquor wiped onto a glass slide will also create a fern pattern.
- The biochemical test for placenta alpha macroglobulin-1 (PAMG-1) is a reliable test for confirming prolonged rupture of membranes (PROM); alternatively testing for presence of **fetal fibronectin (fFn)** may be undertaken (Brown et al 2020) (CFB 17.1).

CLINICAL FOCUS BOX 17.1

Assessments to assist decision making about imminent birth

The cervicovaginal fetal fibronectin and Actim Partus tests are useful for determining a plan of care with the woman and the transfer team. The fFn and Actim Partus test should be used on intact membranes, no vaginal bleeding, no sexual intercourse or vaginal examination in the past 24 hours and a cervix less than 3 cm.

'Fetal fibronectin is an extra cellular matrix glycoprotein localized at the maternal membrane' (p881). In healthy pregnancies fFn is found in very low levels in the cervicovaginal secretions. Levels greater than or equal to 50 mg/ml at or after 22 weeks of pregnancy are associated with an increased risk of spontaneous premature birth, (Berghella et al 2019).

The absence of fFN in the cervical secretions is a very useful negative predictor of imminent birth (negative predictive value for birth within 7 days, 97–98%).

'The Actim Partus test examines levels of phosphorylated insulin-like growth factor binding protein-1 (phIGFBP-1) synthesised by maternal decidual cells' (Berghella et al 2019).

Biochemical tests such as fFN are used to screen pregnant women who are within 26 weeks and 34 weeks of gestation and are having symptoms of premature labour. The test may be beneficial in predicting the risk of premature birth.

The tests should be used only on those who:

- have intact amniotic membranes
- have a cervix that has not dilated more than 3 cm
- do not have more than slight vaginal bleeding
- do not have cervical cerclage
- have not had sexual intercourse or a pelvic examination in the past 24 hours.

The tests are not recommended for screening asymptomatic women even if they are considered to be at high risk for premature labour and birth.

Transfer of the mother and fetus in utero

Preterm birth is responsible for increased morbidity and mortality. The outcome is determined by the location of the mother at the time of birth. Imminent birth requires services to come to the mother; however, when and where possible the mother should be transported to the highest tertiary services accessible in the time available. However, the actual time of birth is often difficult to predict. Amnio-indicators can assist in determining time scales.

Transfer requires resources to support the safe journey of the mother, and planning should anticipate for all eventualities. Birth en route would require a heat source and oxygen for management of the preterm infant. Prior to transportation, the best possible outcome for the infant is achieved through the administration of steroids (McGoldrick et al 2020).

Cervicovaginal fFN and Actim Partus tests are useful for determining a plan of care with the woman and the transfer team. Clinical Focus Box 17.1 identifies in which circumstances these tests are useful.

KEY POINTS

Diagnosis of premature labour

- Many pregnant women experience symptoms that suggest preterm labour. These may include uterine contractions, lower back pain or pelvic pressure, or cramping.

- Changes in vaginal discharge, cervical softening, cervical effacement, and dilation.

- Not all symptomatic women will actually have a preterm birth (Pincombe et al 2023).

17.3 Medications in the management of preterm labour and premature birth

The following medications are used in the management of preterm labour to prevent or manage premature birth.

Antibiotic therapy

Treatment of infection during pregnancy is often aggressive to prevent premature labour and birth. This is covered in Chapter 12. A broad-spectrum intravenous antibiotic is usually commenced (group B Streptococcus antibiotic prophylaxis) while specific cultures are grown from blood, urine, and vaginal swab specimens.

Corticosteroids

Betamethasone 11.4 mg given 24 hours apart between 23 and 33 weeks has been shown to reduce the incidence of respiratory distress syndrome, intraventricular haemorrhage, and neonatal mortality. Tocolysis, an obstetrical procedure carried out with the use of medications for the purpose of delaying the birth of a baby in women presenting with preterm contractions is used to inhibit labour to allow time for the **corticosteroid** to be administered 24 hours apart.

Uterotonics and tocolytics

Tocolytics are administered with the aim of inhibiting or reducing uterine activity. Tocolytic medications act by relaxing the uterine muscles, delaying birth, and allowing more time for the baby to mature, including time for administration of pre-birth medications. In the premature pregnancy under 34 weeks tocolytics can be used to avert labour progress until the administration of corticosteroids to the mother, and sufficient time for the increase of surfactant in the fetal lungs to prevent respiratory distress syndrome, intraventricular haemorrhage, and neonatal mortality. McGoldrick et al (2020) advocate that tocolytics alone do not improve outcomes but are useful for gaining time to deliver corticosteroid therapy and transfer to an appropriate unit with neonatal services.

Most uterine medications have not been approved by the FDA as there is insufficient evidence to endorse their effectiveness (Fauche-Camargo 2022). However, this only applies below 34 weeks gestation.

Prior to commencing **uterotonics** or tocolytics it is important to ascertain maternal and fetal wellbeing to confirm that delaying birth will not be detrimental to the mother or infant. In the case of placental abruption, antepartum haemorrhage, intrauterine growth restriction, or prolonged rupture of membranes, birth may be the best outcome.

Calcium channel blockers

Calcium channel blockers are used as the first-line tocolytic as they relax smooth muscle by directly blocking absorption of calcium by the myometrial cells and preventing calcium release from the sarcoplasmic reticulum (Fig 17.1) Calcium is necessary for myosin light-chain kinase (MLCK). If calcium channels are blocked, muscle contraction is reduced/ceased due to a lack of calcium ions in the myometrium cells. No calcium=no MLCK.

Contractant and relaxant pathways of a myometrial cell

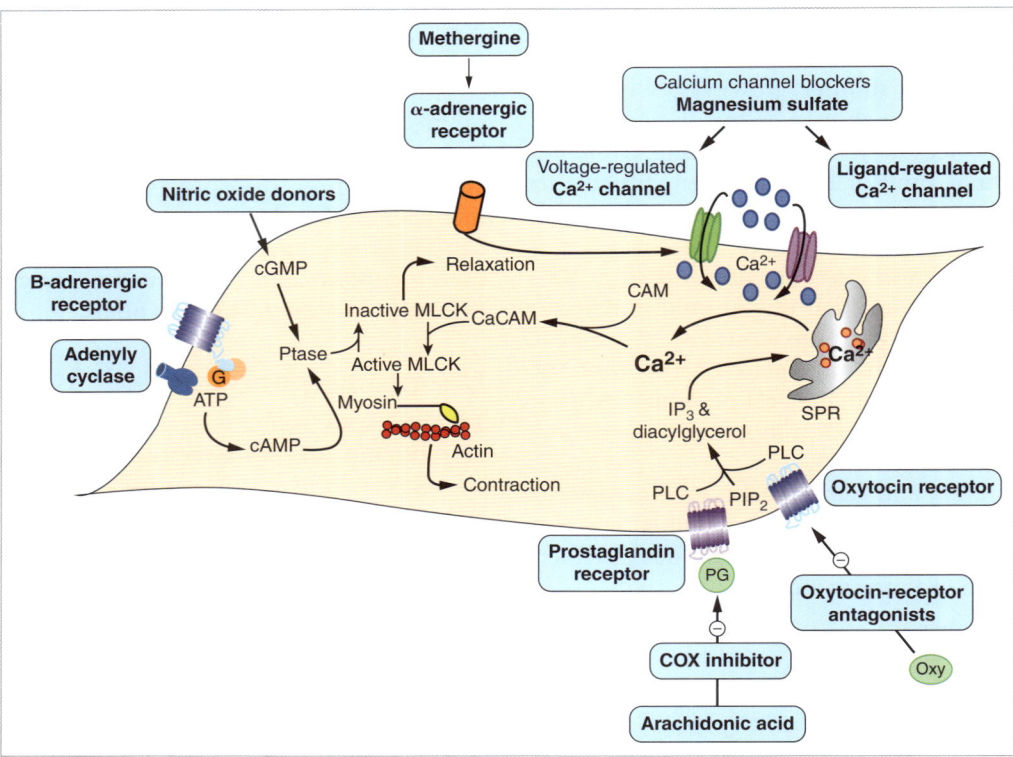

FIGURE 17.1 CaCAM, calcium–calmodulin complex; CAM, calmodulin; IP3, inositol triphosphate; MLCK, myosin light-chain kinase; Oxy, oxytocin; Pg, prostaglandin; PIP2, phosphatidylinositol 4,5-biphosphate; PLC, phospholipase C; Ptase, phosphate kinase; SPR, sarcoplasmic reticulum.

Source: Fouche-Camargo, JS. Uterotonics and tocolytics. In: Clinical pharmacology during pregnancy (pp. 323-338). Academic Press 2022.

DRUG MONOGRAPH 17.1
Nifedipine/Adalat

Unless contraindicated, the first-line tocolytic to be used should be nifedipine immediate release (IR) (Flenady et al 2014; Songthamwat et al 2018). Oral nifedipine has been reported as an effective calcium channel blocker with the least complications (Hanley et al 2019).

The National Institute of Clinical Excellence (NICE) guidelines recommend an oral dose of 20 mg initially followed by doses of 10–20 mg, 3–4 times daily, dependent on uterine activity. Immediate release only should be used as adverse effects have been reported from the sustained release or sublingual forms of medication (Rath et al 2018).

Tocolysis should not be commenced when the best outcome would be birth.

Contraindications to the use of nifedipine include antepartum haemorrhage, preeclampsia, chorioamnionitis, fetal distress, hypotension, cardiac disease including cardiac conduction defects and left ventricular failure. Caution should be taken with simultaneous administration of magnesium sulphate (MgSO4) and concomitant use of betamimetics such as salbutamol.

Dosage

The initial and second dose of 20 mg of nifedipine IR should be chewed to increase the rate of absorption. After 30 minutes, if the contractions persist, the woman should be administered a further 20 mg nifedipine IR orally. The full tocolytic effect may not be seen for 30–60 minutes and therefore other alternative/additional tocolytic treatments are contraindicated in the first 2 hours after consuming nifedipine IR.

After 3 hours, if the contractions continue the administration of nifedipine should continue: nifedipine IR 20 mg every 3–8 hours until contractions cease or birth occurs. A maintenance dose of 20 mg, three times per day for 48–72 hours may be given when indicated. The maximum recommended dose is 160 mg/24 hours.

If contractions continue after 2 hours, a second-line tocolytic should be considered by the treating obstetrician consultant.

DRUG MONOGRAPH 17.2
Magnesium sulphate

Historically, magnesium was used in the 1960s due to its ability to reduce contractibility (Kumar et al 1963). Magnesium decreases calcium concentrations in the cellular structures and thus prevents contractibility. Magnesium is still used as a tocolytic in the USA; however, elsewhere magnesium sulphate has also been found to be beneficial for gestations less than 32 weeks in providing neurological protection for a maximum of 48 hours. Magnesium sulphate (MgSO4) administration to the woman in preterm labour has been linked with the prevention of cerebral palsy (CP) since 1995 (Doyle et al 2009; Chollat et al 2018).

Cerebral palsy is a motor and/or postural dysfunction which is not progressive and may be associated with cognitive impairment. CP has a prevalence of 2:1000 live births and the principal obstetric risk factors for CP are preterm birth (before 34 weeks) and low birth weight. A Cochrane meta-analysis review in 2009 concluded that antenatal MgSO4 therapy given to women at risk of preterm birth substantially reduced the risk of CP in their child (RR.68 CI .54–.87, five trials, 6145 infants) (Doyle et al 2009).

Australian perinatal practice guidelines advocate that MgSO4 is given to all women in preterm labour where birth is anticipated before 30 weeks (Skubisz et al 2024).

Administration of MgSO4

Magnesium sulphate is administered within 4 hours of the impending birth: 4 g over a 20-minute period, continued at 1 g/hour for 4 hours then the infusion is ceased. Magnesium sulphate therapy needs vigilance, hence close supervision requires the infusion to be administered through an infusion pump. If the birth occurs before the 4-hour mark, discontinue the infusion at the time of birth. Urgent delivery for fetal or maternal indications should not be delayed to achieve MgSO4 administration. Monitoring requires assessment of vital signs and observation for side effects and magnesium toxicity. Magnesium sulphate administration can cause flushing, nausea, headache, generalised muscle weakness and diplopia. Signs of toxicity are absent deep tendon reflexes, respiratory depression, pulmonary oedema, cardiac arrythmias and cardiopulmonary arrest. The antidote for these signs of toxicity is calcium gluconate (Chakraborty et al 2022).

Second-line tocolytics – Cydooxygenase inhibitors

'Cydooxygenase (COX) inhibitors prevent the conversion of arachidonic acid to prostaglandin' (Fouche-Camargo 2022). Prostaglandins stimulate myometrial gap junction formation and increase the intracellular calcium levels, COX inhibitors halt progesterone formation and thus prevent labour (Fouche-Camargo 2022).

DRUG MONOGRAPH 17.3
Salbutamol

Salbutamol, the β_2-adrenoceptor agonist, causes smooth muscle relaxation and dilation of the airways. Short-acting beta-2 agonists (SABAs), such as salbutamol and terbutaline, have a rapid onset of action (15 minutes) and their effects last for up to 4 hours. SABAs may be used as a second-line tocolytic, in the absence of contraindications.

Caution

Salbutamol must not be used in addition to nifedipine IR, as the two drugs have potentially synergistic actions. Salbutamol should be used with care, as it is associated with maternal tachycardia, hypotension, tremor, pulmonary oedema, hyperglycaemia, and hypokalaemia, and is contraindicated in the presence of:
- maternal or fetal cardiac disease
- insulin-dependent diabetes
- thyroid disease.

An IV infusion pump must be prepared for administration of the salbutamol infusion. An infusion of 5 mg (5 mL ampoule Ventolin Obstetric Injection) in 100 mL of normal saline (50 microg /mL solution) is commenced at 12 mL/hour (10 microg/minute) and increased by 4 mL/hour (3.3 microg/minute) every 30 minutes until:
- contractions cease
- maternal pulse rate reaches 120 beats/minute, or
- the infusion rate reaches a maximum of 36 mL/hour (30 microg/minute).

Continued

DRUG MONOGRAPH 17.3
Salbutamol—cont'd

Contraindications to salbutamol infusion
- Maternal or fetal cardiac disease
- Thyroid disease
- Insulin-dependent diabetes

Precautions
- Baseline electrolytes, urea and creatinine before commencement of infusion; repeat as necessary if abnormal
- Baseline maternal blood sugar level; repeat 4-hourly if abnormal
- Cardiovascular examination including auscultation of lung bases once in the first 24 hours of therapy
- No additional intravenous fluids to avoid fluid overload
- Half-hourly maternal pulse, BP and respiratory rate until the maintenance dose is reached
- Reduce the infusion if maternal pulse is > 120 bpm
- CEASE the infusion and request medical review immediately if there is chest pain, dyspnoea or the respiratory rate is > 30/min
- Baseline electronic fetal heart rate monitoring
- Do not exceed 48 hours of salbutamol therapy. Only in exceptional circumstances should the treatment be continued for more than 24 hours.

DRUG MONOGRAPH 17.4
Indomethacin

Indomethacin is a non-steroidal anti-inflammatory drug (NSAID), cyclooxygenase inhibitor (Munjal & Allam 2023). Indomethacin is a second-line drug in the treatment of premature labour and is used when there are contraindications to other tocolytics. Indomethacin is often used in association with the insertion of a cervical suture at pre-viable gestations, prior to 32 weeks gestation.

Dosage
Indomethacin is administered orally or rectally. Oral administrations are rapidly absorbed into the plasma and circulated around the body – protein-bound. In Australia the initial dose is administered as a 100 mg rectal suppository followed by a 25 mg oral dose every 4 hours for 48 hours. If regular uterine contractions persist 1–2 hours after the initial 100 mg suppository, an additional 100 mg suppository is administered before beginning oral therapy. Indomethacin is eliminated via the liver and kidneys and the half-life is approximately 4.5 hours. Administration should be ceased if birth becomes imminent.

Contraindication
Peptic ulceration

Side effects
Prolonged use of indomethacin has the potential to cause narrowing or occlusion of the fetal ductus arteriosus, reduction in fetal renal function, fetal pulmonary hypertension and/or reduced renal function. However, evidence-based practice does not advocate for prolonged use for greater than 48 hours, or at gestations greater than 34 weeks. Therefore, these potential side effects do not contraindicate the use of indomethacin if first-line options cannot be administered due to unavailability, contraindications, or in the case of the need for transportation and the inability to monitor the mother in transit.

DRUG MONOGRAPH 17.5
Nitric oxide donors/Nitroglycerine/Glyceryl Trinitrate (GTN)

Nitric oxide (NO) acts as a second messenger to increase Ca+2 uptake.
Nitric oxide (NO) promotes uterine quiescence in pregnancy, by causing vasodilation and relaxation of smooth muscles by increasing guanosine monophosphate (cGMP) which inactivates MLCK leading to relaxation of smooth muscle (Fouche-Camargo 2022).
In the event of acute situations such as inversion prolapse of the uterus, relief of head entrapment after breech birth, or planned procedures such as external cephalic version or caesarean section, nitroglycerin (NG) can be administered intravenously to facilitate immediate management in the relaxation of the cervix and uterine activity.
GTN patches provide continuous plasma nitrate concentration up to 24 hours. Peak action occurs 1–2 hours after application.

DRUG MONOGRAPH 17.5
Nitric oxide donors/Nitroglycerine/Glyceryl Trinitrate (GTN)—cont'd

Dosage

NG 100–200 mcg IV. The half-life of NG is very short: 1–4 minutes.

GTN 5–10 mg (1 to 2 patches) applied to the abdominal skin – transdermal GTN patch and the patch repeated one hour later if the contractions persist (maximum dose 20 mg in 24 hours).

Side effects

- Headache
- Facial flushing
- Hypotension and tachycardia
- Uterine atony

Atosiban (Tractocile)

Atosiban is an oxytocin receptor antagonist that inhibits oxytocin from binding to receptors in the myometrium and decidua (Fig 17.2). Atosiban has fewer side effects than other tocolytics but is more expensive than adrenergic agents.

Progesterone

Progesterone enhances the acquiescence of the uterus to keep the muscle fibres relaxed and reduce myometrial activity. Vaginal progesterone pessaries have been found to be effective in reducing the incidence of premature birth in pregnancies with a short cervix detected on the anomaly scan, and in women who have had a previous premature birth. Natural vaginal progesterone 200 mg pessaries used each night from 16–36 weeks gestation for women who are less than 5 cm dilated have been found to be the most effective in postponing birth for all cases in which there is a history of spontaneous preterm birth (with or without preterm pre-labour rupture of membranes) (APBPA n.d.). Long-term studies following infants up to 4 years of age have found no long-term impact of the use of progesterone pessaries (Northen et al 2007).

CLINICAL FOCUS BOX 17.2

Midwifery care of the mother receiving tocolytic therapies

The side effects of tocolytics are numerous and can exacerbate the woman's anxiety. Palpations caused by tachycardia, flushing from vasodilation, nervousness, dizziness and breathlessness all add to her sense of 'impending doom' and panic. The midwife needs to offer the woman reassurance that these are side effects of the medication.

Premature uterine activity will cause significant stress and anxiety in the pregnant woman as she fears for the wellbeing of her unborn child. The multi-disciplinary team each play a role in being conscious of the language they use when conversing with the mother directly, or with the team in her presence. Providing clear, honest information and being truthful about the anticipated outcome and care the infant will require after birth enables the parents to understand and prepare themselves for uncertain eventualities (Bry et al 2019).

While advances in science and technology have significantly seen improvement in survival rates of premature infants in the last few decades, gestational impacts on fetal anatomical and physiological development and survival prior to 24 weeks often incurs disability and morbidity, including complications such as **hyaline membrane disease** that can require extended treatment during the early years of the infant's life.

Neonates born prematurely (before 37 completed weeks) need intensive medical attention and are often admitted into the special care nursery (SCN). The SCN combines advanced technology and trained healthcare professionals to provide specialised care for the tiniest of neonates. The SCN may also have intermediate or continuing care areas for neonates who are not as sick but do need specialised nursing care. Some hospitals do not have the personnel or a SCN and neonates must be transferred to another hospital. Specialist treatments, medications, and newborn intensive care therapies are outside the scope of this book.

17.4 Complementary and alternative therapies

A thorough history must be taken from women experiencing premature labour to rule out any potential cause of uterine tightening. For instance, while Bowman et al (2021) have reported that there is no credible evidence to support raspberry leaf as a uterine stimulant they did find that 'laboratory studies have identified that raspberry leaf contains several active constituents' (p 8) which cause both relaxation and stimulation of the smooth muscle. Thus, caution should be urged to women at risk of premature labour, to avoid complementary therapies without the supervision of qualified practitioners.

Dietary supplementation

Calcium supplementation has been reported to have the potential to reduce premature birth. In a Cochrane review a random placebo-controlled study found that of 524 healthy primigravid women with a low calcium RDI, a supplementation of 2 g daily reduced the risk of premature birth by 49% compared with placebo (Villar et al 2006).

CONCLUSION

Choice of tocolytic will depend on location and available options. It is important to provide treatment based on the best available evidence which should be guided by contemporary protocols. The selection of the treatment must occur in collaboration and with the consent of the mother so she is aware of the side effects and associated risks to her baby. While the choice of medication falls in the parameters of the obstetric team, maternal observation, assessment, and collaborative multi-disciplinary management of the woman in preterm labour is within the scope of the midwife.

REVIEW QUESTIONS

Casey's contractions are palpated at three every 10 minutes and an intravenous infusion of salbutamol is recommended.

1 What considerations need to be made before the infusion is commenced?

2 What information needs to be provided to Casey to enable her to make an informed choice?

3 What observations will you as the midwife need to make to monitor the effects of the tocolytic therapy?

4 What are the adverse side effects experienced by women receiving tocolytic therapy?

5 What action would the midwife take to resolve or support the woman?

6 What actions/preparations should be made in case the tocolytics are ineffective?

REFERENCES

Australian Institute of Health and Welfare. Australia's mothers and babies (2023). https://www.aihw.gov.au/reports/mothers-babies/australias-mothers-babies/contents/baby-outcomes/gestational-age (accessed 22 January 2024)

Amarpoor Mesrkanlou H, Ghaemmaghami Hezaveh S, Tahmasebi S, et al. The effect of an earthquake experienced during pregnancy on maternal health and birth outcomes. Disaster Med Public Health Prep. 2022 Jun;17:e157. doi: 10.1017/dmp.2022.132

Arena B, Daccò MD. Evaluation of vaginal microbiota in women admitted to the hospital for premature labour. Acta Biomed. 2021;92(5):e2021292. doi.org/10.23750/abm.v92i5.9925

Australian Preterm Birth Prevention Alliance. Midwifery continuity of care. https://www.pretermalliance.com.au/Alliance-News/Latest-News/Midwifery-Continuity-of-Care (accessed 12 December 2023)

Berghella V, Saccone G. Fetal fibronectin testing for reducing the risk of preterm birth. Cochrane Database Syst Rev. 2019 Jul;7(7):CD006843. doi: 10.1002/14651858.CD006843.pub3 (accessed 18 June 2024)

Bowman R, Taylor J, Muggleton S, et al. Biophysical effects, safety and efficacy of raspberry leaf use in pregnancy: a systematic integrative review. BMC Complement Med Ther. 2021;21:56. doi: 10.1186/s12906-021-03230-4

Brown SR. Placental alpha macroglobulin-1 (PartoSure) immunoassay to assess the risk of spontaneous preterm birth. Am Fam Physician. 2020 Sep 1;102(5):269-270. PMID: 32866362

Bry A, Wigert H. Psychosocial support for parents of extremely preterm infants in neonatal intensive care: a qualitative interview study. BMC Psychol. 2019;7:76. doi.org/10.1186/s40359-019-0354-4

Chakraborty A, Can AS. Calcium gluconate. [Updated 2022 Jun 4]. In: Treasure Island (FL): StatPearls Publishing; 2024 Jan. https://www.ncbi.nlm.nih.gov/books/NBK557463/

Chollat C, Marret S. Magnesium sulfate and fetal neuroprotection: overview of clinical evidence. Neural Regen Res. 2018;13(12):2044-2049. doi.org/10.4103/1673-5374.241441

Dodd JM, Crowther CA, McPhee AJ, et al. Progesterone after previous preterm birth for prevention of neonatal respiratory distress syndrome (PROGRESS): a randomised controlled trial. BMC Pregnancy Childbirth. 2009;9:6. PubMed PMID: 19239712. Pubmed Central PMCID: 2653463. http://www.ncbi.nlm.nih.gov/pubmed/19239712

Dotsoky NS, Setzer WN. Maternal reproductive toxicity of some essential oils and their constituents. Int J Mol Sci. 2021 Feb 27;22(5):2380. doi: 10.3390/ijms22052380. PMID: 33673548; PMCID: PMC7956842

Doyle LW, Crowther CA, Middleton P, et al. Antenatal magnesium sulphate and neurological outcomes in preterm infants: a systematic review. Obstet Gynaecol. 2009;113(6):1327-1333. doi: 10.1097/AOG.0b013e3181a60495

Fauche-Camargo, JS. Uterotonics and tocolytics (Ch 18) In: Clinical pharmacology during pregnancy, 2nd edn. Mattison D, Halbert LA (eds). Academic Press, Elsevier, UK and US.

Flenady V, Hawley G, Stock OM, et al. Prophylactic antibiotics for inhibiting preterm labour with intact membranes. Cochrane Database Syst Rev. 2013;(12):CD000246. doi: 10.1002/14651858.CD000246.pub2

Flenady V, Wojcieszek AM, Papatsonis DNM, et al. Calcium channel blockers for inhibiting preterm labour and birth. Cochrane Database Syst Rev. 2014;(6):CD002255. doi: 10.1002/14651858.CD002255.pub2

Glynn LM, Wadhwa PD, Dunkel-Schetter C, et al. When stress happens matters: effects of earthquake timing on stress responsivity in pregnancy. Am J Obstet Gynecol. 2001;184:637-642. doi: 10.1067/mob.2001.111066

Government of South Australia, Department for Health and Wellbeing. South Australian perinatal practice guideline: magnesium sulphate for neuroprotection of the fetus in women at risk of preterm birth. https://www.sahealth.sa.gov.au/wps/wcm/connect/86f3f2804ee4f45294189dd150ce4f37/magnesium-sulphate-neuroprotection-preterm-wchn-ppg-19062012.pdf?mod=ajperes

Government of Western Australia, North Metropolitan Health Service, Women and Newborn Health Service. King Edward Memorial Hospital clinical practice guideline; magnesium sulphate for neuroprotection of the fetus [Reviewed September 2016]. https://www.kemh.health.wa.gov.au/~/media/HSPs/NMHS/Hospitals/WNHS/Documents/Clinical-guidelines/Obs-Gyn-Guidelines/Preterm-Labour-Magnesium-Sulphate-for-Neuroprotection-of-the-Fetus.pdf?thn=0

Hanley M, Sayes L, Reiff ES, et al. Tocolysis: a review of the literature. Obstet Gynaecol Surv. 2019;74:50-55 doi: 10.1097/OGX.0000000000000635

Kabiri D, Raif Nesher D, Luxenbourg D, et al. The role of vaginal progesterone for preterm birth prevention in women with threatened labor and shortened cervix diagnosed after 24 weeks of pregnancy. Int J Gynecol Obstet. 2023;161:423-431. doi: 10.1002/ijgo.14465

Kumar D, Zourlas P, Barnes A. In vitro and in vivo effects of magnesium sulfate on human uterine contractility. Am J Obstet Gynaecol. 1963;86:1036-1040.

Kutinova Menclova A, Stillman S. Maternal stress and birth outcomes: evidence from an unexpected earthquake swarm. Health Econ. 2020 Dec;29(12):1705-1720. https://doi.org/10.1002/hec.4162

Liu R, Liu C, Ding X. Association between loop electrosurgical excision procedure and adverse pregnancy outcomes: a meta-analysis. J Matern Fetal Neonatal Med. 2023 Dec;36(1):2183769. doi: 10.1080/14767058.2023.2183769

Lorthe E, Letouzey M, Torchin et al. Antibiotic prophylaxis in preterm premature rupture of membranes at 24–31 weeks' gestation: perinatal and 2-year outcomes in the EPIPAGE-2 cohort. BJOG. 2022 Aug;129(9)1560-1573. https://doi.org/10.1111/1471-0528.17081

McDougall ARA, Hastie R, Goldstein M, et al. New medicines for spontaneous preterm birth prevention and preterm labour management: landscape analysis of the medicine development pipeline. BMC Pregnancy Childbirth. 2023 Jul 18;23(1):525. doi: 10.1186/s12884-023-05842-9. PMID: 37464260; PMCID: PMC10354994

McGoldrick E, Stewart F, Parker R, et al. Antenatal corticosteroids for accelerating fetal lung maturation for women at risk of preterm birth. Cochrane Database Syst Rev. 2020 Dec;12(12):CD004454. doi: 10.1002/14651858.CD004454.pub4

Miyakoshi K, Itakura A, Abe T, et al. Risk of preterm birth after the excisional surgery for cervical lesions: a propensity-score matching study in Japan. J Matern Fetal Neonatal Med. 2021 Mar;34(6):845-851. doi: 10.1080/14767058.2019.1619687. Epub 2019 May 30. PMID: 31092078

Morgan JA, Zafar N, Cooper DB. Group B streptococcus and pregnancy. [Updated 2023 Jul 24]. In: StatPearls [Internet]. Treasure Island (FL): StatPearls Publishing; 2023 Jan. https://www.ncbi.nlm.nih.gov/books/NBK482443/ (accessed 22 January 2024)

Munjal A, Allam AE. Indomethacin. [Updated 2023 Jan 31]. In: StatPearls [Internet]. Treasure Island (FL): StatPearls Publishing; 2024 Jan. https://www.ncbi.nlm.nih.gov/books/NBK555936/

Northen AT, Norman GS, Anderson K, et al. Follow-up of children exposed in utero to 17 alpha-hydroxyprogesterone caproate compared with placebo. Obstet Gynecol. 2007 Oct;110(4):865-872. doi: 10.1097/01.AOG.0000281348.51499.bc. PubMed PMID:17906021

Ohuma E, Moller A-B, Bradley E, et al. National, regional, and worldwide estimates of preterm birth in 2020, with trends from 2010: a systematic analysis. Lancet. 2023;402(10409):1261-1271. doi: 10.1016/S0140-6736(23)00878-4

Partash N, Naghipour B, Rahmani SH, et al. The impact of flood on pregnancy outcomes: a review article. Taiwan J Obstet Gynecol. 2022 Jan;61(1):10-14. doi.org/10.1016/j.tjog.2021.11.005

Perin J, Mulick A, Yeung D, et al. Global, regional, and national causes of under-5 mortality in 2000-19: an updated systematic analysis with implications for the Sustainable Development Goals. Lancet Child Adolesc Health. 2022;6(2):106-115.

Pincombe J, Pairman S, Tracy SK, et al (eds). Midwifery: preparation for practice, 4th edn. 2023: Elsevier, Australia.

Rath W, Kehl S. Acute tocolysis – a critical analysis of evidence-based data. Geburtshilfe Frauenheilkd. 2018 Dec;78:1245-1255. doi: 10.1055/a-0717-5329

Rysavy MA, Mehler K, Oberthür A, et al. An immature science: intensive care for infants born at ≤23 weeks of gestation. J Pediatr. 2021 Jun;233:16-25.e1. doi: 10.1016/j.jpeds.2021.03.006. Epub 2021 Mar 7 (accessed 22 January 2024)

Sandall J, Soltani H, Gates S, et al. Midwife-led continuity models versus other models of care for childbearing women. Cochrane Database Syst Rev. 2016 Apr;4(4):CD004667. doi: 10.1002/14651858.CD004667.pub5 (accessed 06 August 2023)

Skubisz M, Smith R, Earl A, et al. Preterm labour and birth PPG033 [Internet]. South Australian Perinatal Practice Guideline. SA Health, Government of South Australia. 2024 [updated 7 May 2024, version 8]. Available from: http://www.sahealth.sa.gov.au/perinatal

Songthamwat S, Na Nan C, Songthamwat M. Effectiveness of nifedipine in threatened preterm labor: a randomized trial. Int J Womens Health. 2018 Jun 15;10:317-323. doi: 10.2147/IJWH.S159062. PMID: 29942162; PMCID: PMC6007202

Steel A, Adams J, Sibbritt D, et al. The outcomes of complementary and alternative medicine use among pregnant and birthing women: current trends and future directions. Women's Health. 2015;11(3):309-323. doi: 10.2217/WHE.14.84

Villar J, Abdel-Aleem H, Merialdi M, et al. World Health Organization randomised controlled trial and calcium supplementation among low calcium intake pregnant women. American Journal Obstetrics and Gynaecology. 2006 Mar;194(3); 639-649. doi: 10.1016/j.ajog.2006.01.068

World Health Organization. Born too soon, a decade of action on preterm birth. Global report, 9 May 2023. https://apps.who.int/iris/rest/bitstreams/1501073/retrieve

World Health Organization. Preterm birth. Fact sheet, 10 May 2023. https://www.who.int/news-room/fact-sheets/detail/preterm-birth

ONLINE RESOURCES

Australian Preterm Birth Prevention Alliance. Midwifery continuity of care: https://www.pretermalliance.com.au/Alliance-News/Latest-News/Midwifery-Continuity-of-Care

Lancet. Small Vulnerable Newborn Series, 2020: https://www.thelancet.com/journals/lancet/article/PIIS0140-6736(20)31906-1/fulltext

World Health Organization. Born too soon: global action report on preterm birth. 2012: https://www.who.int/publications/i/item/9789241503433

World Health Organization. Preterm birth. Fact sheet, 10 May 2023: https://www.who.int/news-room/fact-sheets/detail/preterm-birth

World Health Organization. Protect the promise: 2022 progress report on the Every Woman Every Child Global Strategy for Women's, Children's and Adolescents' Health (2016–2030). WHO and United Nations Children's Fund, 2022: https://www.who.int/publications/i/item/9789240060104

Born too soon: decade of action on preterm birth. Geneva: World Health Organization; 2023. Licence: CC BY-NC-SA 3.0 IGO. (https://creativecommons.org/licenses/by-nc-sa/3.0/igo/) https://data.unicef.org/resources/born-too-soon-decade-of-action-on-preterm-birth/

CHAPTER 18

ASTHMA

Kirsten Small, Michelle Gray

Key Abbreviations

cAMP	cyclic 3,5-adenosine monophosphate
DPI	dry powder inhaler
GMP	guanosine monophosphate
ICS	inhaled corticosteroids
IgE	immunoglobulin E
LABAs	long-acting β_2-agonists
LAMAs	long-acting muscarinic antagonists
MDI	metered-dose inhaler
$PaCO_2$	partial pressure of carbon dioxide in arterial blood
PaO_2	partial pressure of oxygen in arterial blood
PGs	prostaglandins
pMDI	pressurised metered-dose inhaler
SABAs	short-acting β_2-agonists
SAMAs	short-acting muscarinic antagonists

Key Terms

β_2-adrenoceptor agonists 348
aerosol 344
anticholinergics 352
asthma 339
bronchoconstriction 340
bronchodilator 348
controller 348
corticosteroids 352
hypercapnia 338
hypoxia (hypoxaemia) 338
immunomodulating drugs 340
leukotriene-receptor antagonists 354
long-acting β_2-agonists 348
long-acting muscarinic antagonists 352
mast-cell stabilisers 347
muscarinic receptors 339
nebuliser 345
pressurised metered-dose inhaler 345
preventer 352
puffer 345
reliever 348
respiration 338
short-acting β_2-agonists 348
short-acting muscarinic antagonists 352
spacer 345
xanthine derivatives 350

Chapter Focus

The respiratory system maintains the exchange of oxygen and carbon dioxide between the lungs and cells, and regulates the pH of body fluids. This chapter briefly reviews relevant respiratory system anatomy and physiology, and describes how drugs are administered by inhalation. The pathophysiology of asthma and the significance of asthma during pregnancy and the puerperium are outlined. Drugs used for asthma management during pregnancy are discussed: bronchodilators, symptom controllers and anti-inflammatory agents.

Australia and New Zealand have a high prevalence of respiratory tract diseases. Asthma exacerbation poses additional risks to the health of the mother during pregnancy and poorly managed asthma can have health impacts for the unborn child, including increased risk for developing asthma themselves. An underpinning knowledge of the structure, function, and pathophysiology of the respiratory tract is fundamental to understanding the drug groups used to treat asthma.

Key Drug Groups

1 Bronchodilator drugs:

β_2-adrenoceptor agonists
- Long-acting (LABAs; controllers): formoterol (eformoterol), salmeterol, indacaterol
- Short-acting (SABAs): **salbutamol, terbutaline** (DM 18.1)

Methylxanthines
- aminophylline, theophylline (DM 18.2)

Anticholinergics (muscarinic antagonists)
- Long-acting (LAMAs): tiotropium, aclidinium, umeclidinium, glycopyrronium bromide (glycopyrrolate)

- Short-acting (SAMAs): ipratropium bromide

2 Prophylactic antiasthma drugs (preventers):
- Inhaled (gluco)corticosteroids: beclometasone (DM 18.3), budesonide, fluticasone, ciclesonide

3 Other drug groups:
- Leukotriene-receptor antagonists (LTRAs): montelukast
- +monoclonal antibodies: omalizumab, mepolizumab

Learning outcomes

- Describe aspects of respiratory anatomy and physiology relevant to asthma.
- Describe the changes in the respiratory system during pregnancy.
- Discuss why and how drugs are administered via inhalation.
- Describe the principles of pharmacological management of asthma in pregnancy.
- Describe the mechanism of action, dose, frequency, adverse effects, and safety of medications used to manage asthma in pregnancy.

CRITICAL THINKING SCENARIO

Peter calls an ambulance for his partner, Jenny, who has a runny nose, dry cough, and rapid onset of breathing difficulties. Jenny is 22 years old and 13 weeks pregnant with the couple's first child. Jenny was diagnosed with chronic persistent asthma as a child. Her general practitioner usually helps Jenny with her asthma management. She has prescribed an asthma preventer puffer of low-dose inhaled fluticasone propionate, 50 micrograms pMDI via spacer, one puff taken twice daily. The paramedics note that Jenny has moderate work of breathing, tight wheeze on stethoscope auscultation of the chest, and tachycardia. She can speak in sentences. She is given six puffs of salbutamol 100 micrograms via spacer over 5 minutes, with some improvement in her symptoms. This dose is repeated during transit to the local hospital. Jenny states she has not been using her puffer as she has concerns about potential harm to her developing baby from the medications.

1   Why was Jenny originally prescribed low-dose fluticasone propionate and administered salbutamol by the paramedics?

2   What classes of drugs are these and what are their mechanisms of action? Are they appropriate for use in pregnancy?

3   Explain the roles of the pMDI and spacer.

4   What specific factors will be taken into consideration related to medication management when Jenny undergoes medical review for this exacerbation of her asthma and why?

Introduction: The respiratory system, asthma and its treatment

This chapter reviews the anatomy and physiology of the respiratory system as a basis for a discussion of pathophysiology and the pharmacological treatment of asthma. The respiratory system includes all structures involved in the movement and exchange of oxygen and carbon dioxide (Figs 18.1 and 18.2). Oxygen is supplied to the body through the process of **respiration**, a term loosely used to describe three distinct but interrelated processes: pulmonary ventilation (inspiration and expiration), gas transport, and cellular respiration.

The respiratory system also participates in warming, filtering, and moistening inspired air, in the senses of smell and taste, producing sounds (speech), assisting in the control of pH, in removal of foreign bodies and mucus, in immune system defence mechanisms, in inactivation of many biogenic amines and autacoids, and in temperature regulation.

18.1 Control of respiration

Respiration is normally under involuntary central and autonomic control. The basic rhythm for respiration is maintained via the medulla oblongata at 12–18 breaths per minute in adults. Regulation is achieved primarily through changes in concentrations of oxygen, carbon dioxide, and hydrogen ions in body fluids. An increase in carbon dioxide tension in the blood (**hypercapnia**) directly stimulates the inspiratory and expiratory centres, increasing the rate and depth of breathing. If arterial oxygen concentration falls below about 60% of normal (**hypoxaemia**), chemoreceptors are stimulated to increase alveolar ventilation.

Physiological adjustments in the respiratory system during pregnancy impact asthma symptoms and pulmonary lung function assessment (Conte et al 2018). Progesterone favours bronchodilation, while diaphragmatic elevation from the enlarged uterus reduces residual volume and functional residual capacity. Forced expiratory volume in 1 second (FEV1) and forced vital capacity – common markers of asthma control – remain unchanged by pregnancy. Arterial blood gases typically show higher arterial oxygen pressure (PaO_2), lower carbon dioxide pressure ($PaCO_2$), and a slight rise in pH. Pregnancy-specific reference ranges for blood gases should be used. Dyspnoea is common as pregnancy progresses, even in uncomplicated pregnancy. Suspect asthma if dyspnoea is associated with wheezing or cough.

Regulation of the glands and musculature of the respiratory tract

Autonomic innervation

Parasympathetic: The predominant innervation of human airways is by cholinergic nerves which, via the vagus nerve, synapse in ganglia located in the wall of the bronchi. Parasympathetic stimulation

Structures associated with the respiratory system

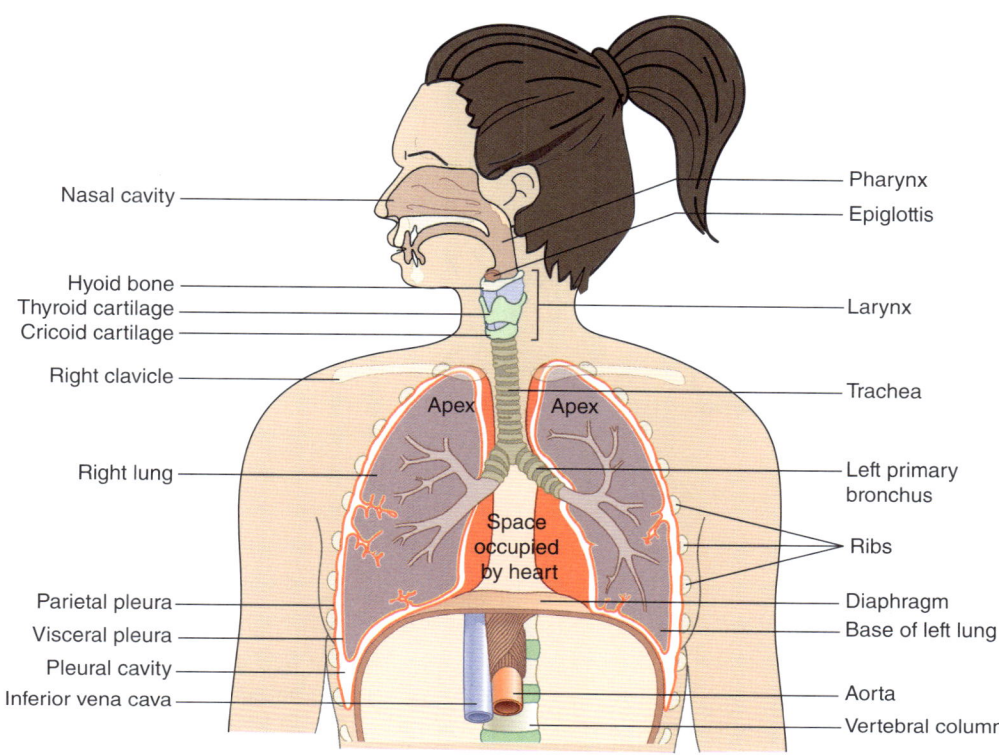

FIGURE 18.1

Source: Waugh & Grant 2014, Figure 10.1.

leads to activation of M_3 **muscarinic receptors** on smooth muscle and glandular tissue, leading to contraction (and thus bronchoconstriction) and secretion, respectively.

Sympathetic: There are no sympathetic nerves innervating the airways. However, there are many β2 receptors. When activated by circulating catecholamines – predominantly adrenaline (epinephrine) – bronchial smooth muscle relaxation occurs.

- Bronchial smooth muscle is innervated by the parasympathetic nervous system. The parasympathetic nervous system mediates bronchoconstriction via M_3 muscarinic receptors.

- β₂-adrenoceptors in bronchi are activated by circulating adrenaline, leading to bronchodilation.

18.2 Asthma – An overview

Asthma is a chronic inflammatory disease of the airways leading to obstruction of the passage of air into and out of the lungs. Asthma affects more than 300 million people worldwide. Just under 2.7 million (10.7%) Australians have asthma (ABS 2022), and 11% of Australians and 12% of adult New Zealanders report taking current asthma medication. The prevalence of asthma varies by socioeconomic area. In Australia, prevalence is highest for those living in the lowest socioeconomic areas compared with those living in the highest areas (males: 13% and 10%, respectively; females: 16% and 10%, respectively).

Tracheobronchial tree and bronchial smooth muscle

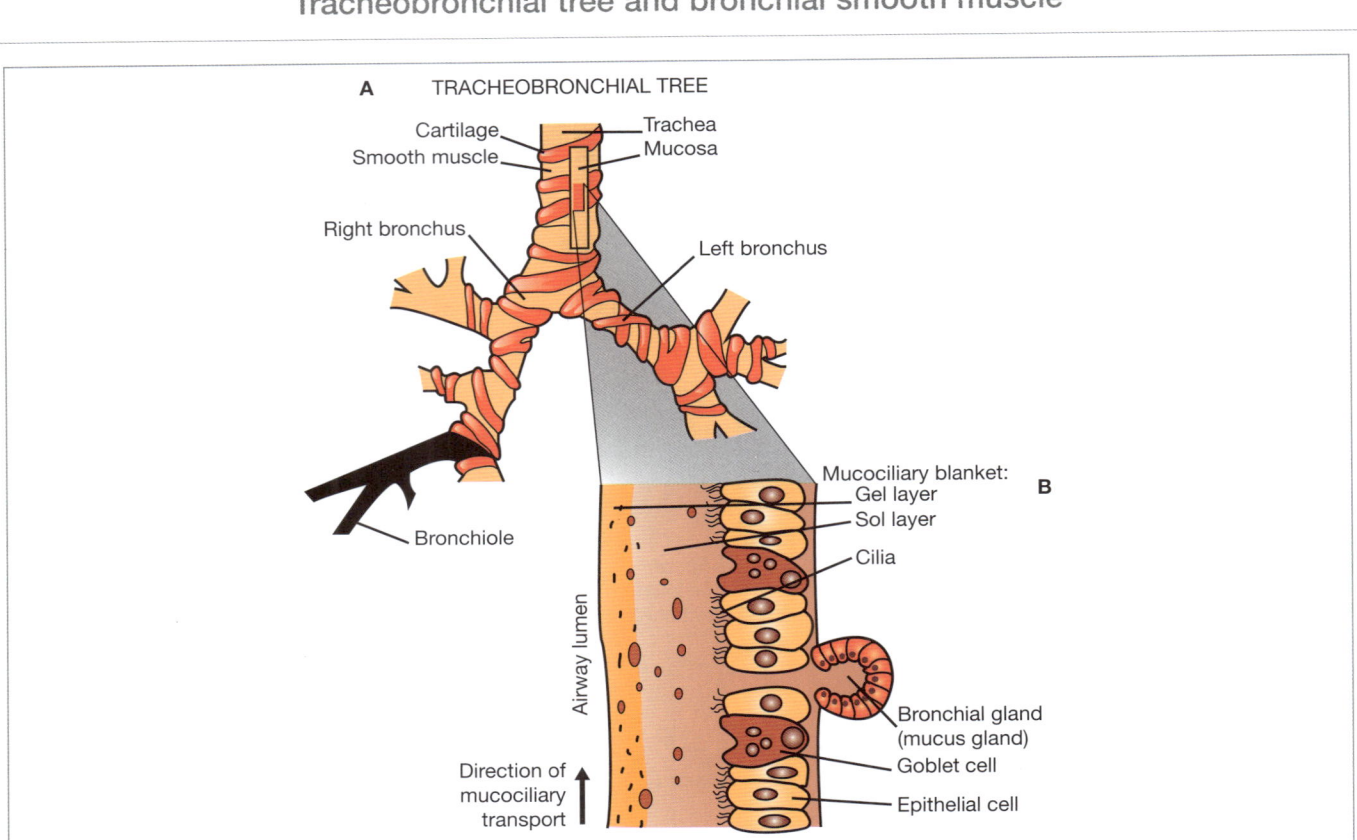

FIGURE 18.2 A Diagram of tracheobronchial tree; **B** Longitudinal section of the inner lining of an airway, magnified approximately ×200.

Source: Salerno 1999; used with permission.

Effective asthma management requires accurate diagnosis, achieving and maintaining good control, and regular monitoring and review. The rationales for use of drugs in asthma are to relieve and control symptoms, prevent acute asthma and deaths, and maintain best lung function and quality of life (Australian Medicines Handbook 2020; Ministry of Health 2018; NAC 2018; National Asthma Council Australia 2020).

By the early 20th century, asthma was being treated with adrenaline (epinephrine) injections, anticholinergics, and coffee (containing methylxanthines). Other β-agonists and corticosteroids were introduced in the 1950s, and long-acting β-agonists (LABAs) in the 1980s. Later treatments include long-acting muscarinic antagonists (LAMAs) and **immunomodulating drugs** (Global Initiative for Asthma 2016; Trivedi et al 2014) (Asthma Australia – see Online resources).

Pathophysiology of asthma

The hallmarks of asthma are reversible **bronchoconstriction**, chronic inflammation of the epithelium of the airways, and increased mucus secretion. There is airway hypersensitivity to a variety of stimuli, leading to episodes of wheezing, breathlessness, and coughing. Many physiological mediators are involved in the pathogenesis of an asthma attack, including leukotrienes, interleukins, histamine, prostaglandins (PGs), other cytokines and nitric oxide, as well as autonomic neurotransmitters (Page et al 2017). The term 'asthma' is now understood as an umbrella diagnosis for several diseases with distinct pathways (endotypes) and variable clinical presentations (phenotypes) (Kuruvilla et al 2019; Page et al 2017).

The early phase of an acute attack involves vasodilation and increased capillary permeability, with infiltration of bronchial mucosa by white blood cells. Numerous immune cell types are involved, particularly mast cells, eosinophils, macrophages, and Th2 and CD4$^+$ lymphocytes. Activation of these cells leads to release of dozens of pro-inflammatory mediators and cytokines, notably nuclear factor κB, interleukin-2, -4, -5, and -13, and tumour necrosis factor-α, as well as immunoglobulin E (IgE).

The inflammatory process involves vascular leakage, contraction of bronchial smooth muscle (bronchoconstriction), inflammatory cell infiltration, increased oedema and mucus production, impaired mucociliary function and, eventually, thickening of airway walls, airway hyper-reactivity and irreversible airways obstruction (Fig 18.3). The late-phase (chronic) response involves inflammation, proliferation of fibroblasts and fibrosis, oedema of the airway mucosa, necrosis of bronchial epithelial cells, and airway wall remodelling with increased collagen deposition. Expiration is particularly impaired, leading to air trapping, hypoxaemia, and raised partial pressure of CO_2.

The principal signs and symptoms are wheezing and cough, tachypnoea or dyspnoea (rapid or difficult breathing), chest tightness, tachycardia, fatigue, sweating, difficulty speaking in sentences, and anxiety. If bronchoconstriction is not reversed, status asthmaticus occurs, with respiratory acidosis and life-threatening respiratory failure.

Asthma in pregnancy

Asthma is the most common chronic condition complicating pregnancy, affecting between 8 and 13% of pregnant women (Murphy 2022). In most women, symptoms remain stable during pregnancy but exacerbations can occur for some. Risk factors for exacerbation during pregnancy are increased age, body weight, and parity; smoking; and moderate-to-severe asthma.

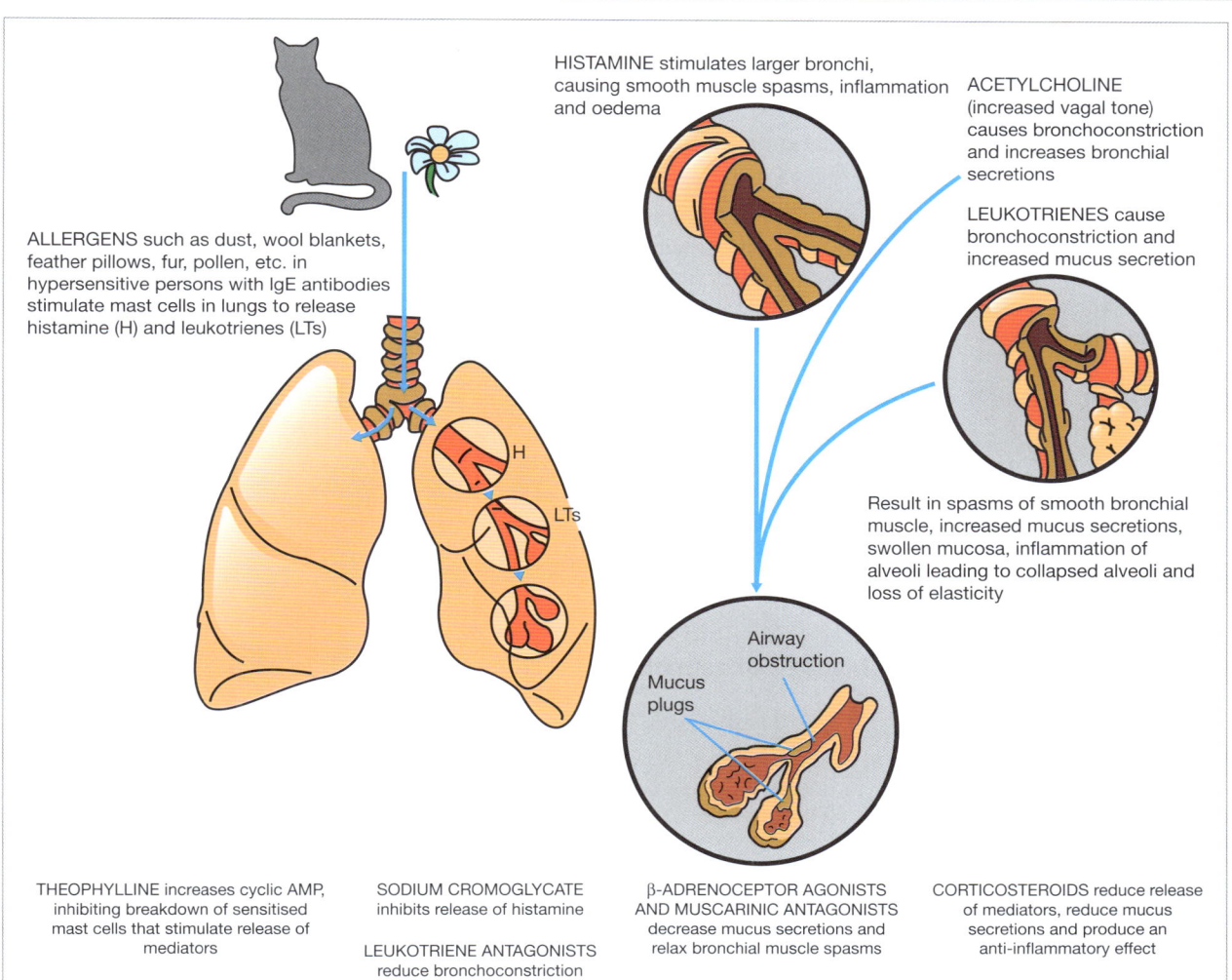

The airways and mediators in asthma, and effects of various antiasthma medications

HISTAMINE stimulates larger bronchi, causing smooth muscle spasms, inflammation and oedema

ACETYLCHOLINE (increased vagal tone) causes bronchoconstriction and increases bronchial secretions

LEUKOTRIENES cause bronchoconstriction and increased mucus secretion

ALLERGENS such as dust, wool blankets, feather pillows, fur, pollen, etc. in hypersensitive persons with IgE antibodies stimulate mast cells in lungs to release histamine (H) and leukotrienes (LTs)

H

LTs

Result in spasms of smooth bronchial muscle, increased mucus secretions, swollen mucosa, inflammation of alveoli leading to collapsed alveoli and loss of elasticity

Airway obstruction

Mucus plugs

THEOPHYLLINE increases cyclic AMP, inhibiting breakdown of sensitised mast cells that stimulate release of mediators

SODIUM CROMOGLYCATE inhibits release of histamine

LEUKOTRIENE ANTAGONISTS reduce bronchoconstriction

β-ADRENOCEPTOR AGONISTS AND MUSCARINIC ANTAGONISTS decrease mucus secretions and relax bronchial muscle spasms

CORTICOSTEROIDS reduce release of mediators, reduce mucus secretions and produce an anti-inflammatory effect

FIGURE 18.3 H = histamine; LTs = leukotrienes

Source: Adapted from Rang et al, 2003; used with permission.

Women with asthma are at risk for pregnancy complications, most of which can be mitigated by achieving good symptom control (Popa et al 2021). Higher rates of low birth weight and small-for-gestational-age fetuses, preterm birth, admission to the neonatal intensive care, and neonatal death have been reported. The risk is higher still for Australian Indigenous women (Clifton et al 2022). Women with asthma are more likely to develop gestational diabetes or hypertensive disorders during pregnancy and are more likely to require critical care after caesarean section (Murphy 2022).

The principles of asthma management in pregnancy are (Murphy 2022) (Fig 18.4):

- regular monitoring of symptoms and lung function
- medication use to achieve symptom control
- encouragement of proactive self-management, with a written action plan, and knowledge about inhaler technique
- multi-disciplinary management, involving the woman's general practitioner, respiratory physician, obstetrician, midwife, neonatologist, and others as required
- management of co-morbidities
- avoidance of triggers, support the achievement of smoking cessation, encourage vaccination against respiratory infections.

Initial or booster vaccinations for COVID-19 and seasonal influenza is considered safe and effective during pregnancy (see Chapter 11). Both vaccines are particularly recommended for women with asthma in order to prevent severe asthma exacerbations (Centre of Excellence in Treatable Traits 2023).

Pregnant women with asthma are advised to see their usual care provider and update their action plan to take their pregnancy into consideration. Inappropriate cessation of asthma medications is common in early pregnancy, and women can be advised of both the safety and importance of continuing effective therapy (Popa et al 2021). Acute exacerbations of asthma complicates labour in around 10% of women (Conte et al 2018).

Asthma and lactation

Inhaled antiasthma drugs are safe for lactating women and their babies. Spacing dose administration and breastfeeding times may be necessary when using oral corticosteroids. General advice is to take the dose immediately after feeding the baby.

Drugs used in asthma

Many types of drugs are used to interrupt the various pathophysiologic pathways in asthma. The main groups are:

- bronchodilators (β_2-receptor agonists, theophyllines, and anticholinergics)
- controller or preventer medications (long-acting β_2-receptor agonists [controllers], inhaled corticosteroids [ICS], leukotriene-receptor antagonists, 5-lipoxygenase inhibitors, and antibodies).

Figure 18.5 gives an overview of the mechanisms of action of asthma medications on inflammation and bronchial smooth muscle contraction. Aspects of their clinical use are summarised in Table 18.1.

There is a large degree of variability in the response to bronchodilators, ICS, and leukotriene modifiers, some of which is attributed to genetic variation. Choice of drugs depends on personal factors, aetiological factors,

---

Key features of asthma management in pregnancy

Key features of asthma management in pregnancy

Regular monitoring	Medication use	Self-management education	Multi-disciplinary team
• Symptoms • Lung function	• As for non-pregnant • Important for asthma control	• Inhaler technique • Written action plan • Knowledge • Adherence	• Co-morbidity management • Smoking cessation • Vaccinations

FIGURE 18.4

Source: Murphy VE. Asthma in pregnancy–management, maternal co-morbidities, and long-term health. Best Prac Res Clin Obstet Gynaecol. 2022 Dec;85(Pt A):45-56.

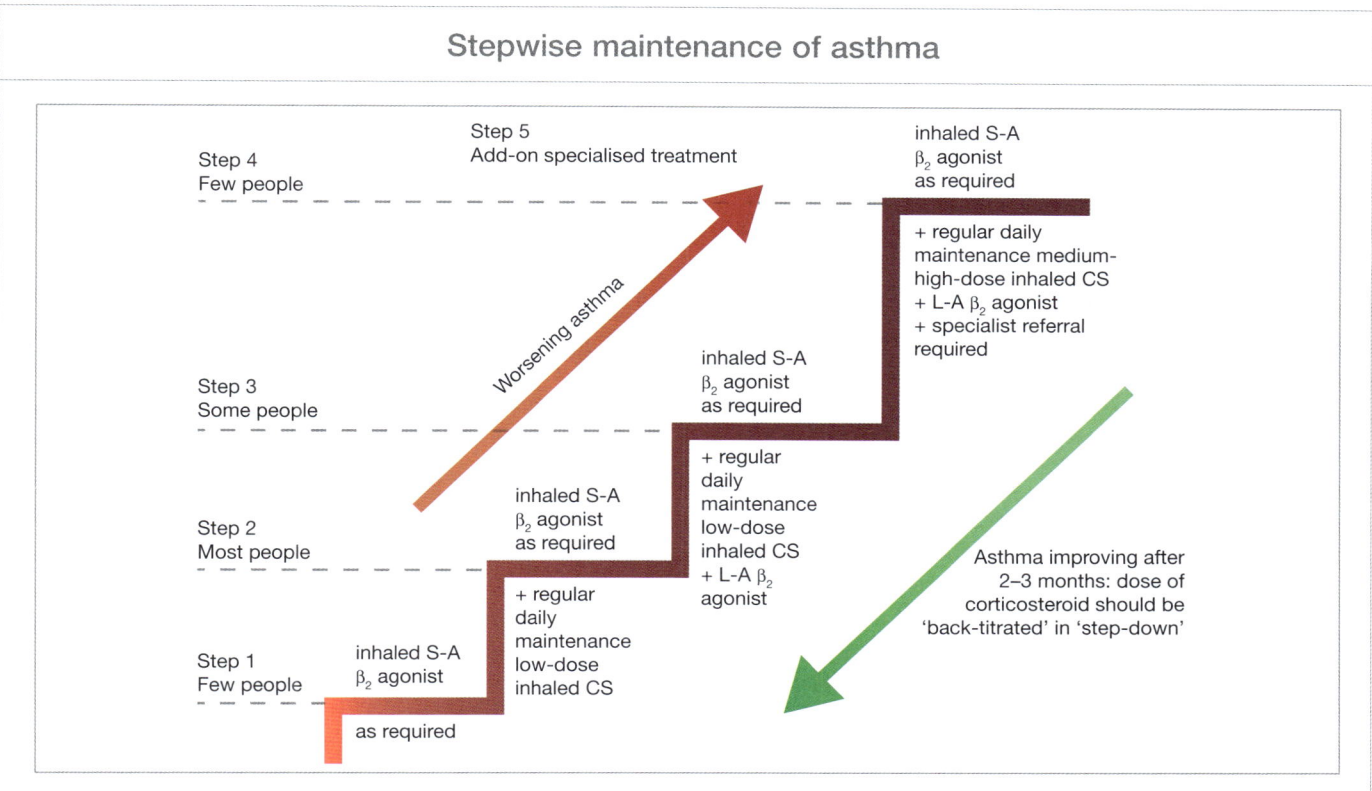

Stepwise maintenance of asthma

Step 5
Add-on specialised treatment

Step 4
Few people

inhaled S-A β₂ agonist as required

+ regular daily maintenance medium-high-dose inhaled CS
+ L-A β₂ agonist
+ specialist referral required

Step 3
Some people

inhaled S-A β₂ agonist as required

+ regular daily maintenance low-dose inhaled CS + L-A β₂ agonist

Worsening asthma

Asthma improving after 2–3 months: dose of corticosteroid should be 'back-titrated' in 'step-down'

Step 2
Most people

inhaled S-A β₂ agonist as required

+ regular daily maintenance low-dose inhaled CS

Step 1
Few people

inhaled S-A β₂ agonist

as required

FIGURE 18.5 CS = corticosteroid; L-A = long-acting; S-A = short-acting. Persistent: > 3–4 attacks/week; moderate: asthma not controlled by low-dose inhaled CS + β₂-agonist

Source: National Asthma Council Australia, 2020.

TABLE 18.1 Summary of drugs used in asthma

DRUG GROUP	EXAMPLE	FORMULATION/ ROUTE	ONSET (min)	DURATION (h) OR FREQUENCY (/d)	USAGE
Relievers					
SABAs	Salbutamol	DPI, pMDI, neb, PO, IV (IM, SC)	5–15	3–6 h; neb: 3–4/d	Reliever + ex-ind
	Terbutaline	DPI, SC	5–15	3–6 h	Reliever + ex-ind
LABAs (rapid)	Formoterol (eformoterol)	DPI	Fast 1–3	>12 h; admin 2/d	Reliever + controller in people on inhaled CSs
Anticholinergics (SAMAs)	Ipratropium	pMDI, neb	Short	6 h; admin 3–4/d	Adjunct in acute severe asthma
Anticholinergics (LAMAs)	Tiotropium	DPI	30	Long-acting up to 24 h	Maintenance in mod-severe asthma
Theophyllines	Aminophylline	Slow IV injection or infusion			Adjunct in severe persistent asthma
	Theophylline	CR tablets, syrup	1–2 hrs	CR admin 2/d; syrup 4/d	Adjunct in severe persistent asthma
Controllers					
LABAs	Salmeterol	DPI, pMDI	10–20	>12	Controller combined with inhaled CSs
Preventers		Beclometasone	pMDI	Admin 2/d	Maintenance in persistent asthma

Continued

TABLE 18.1 Summary of drugs used in asthma—cont'd

DRUG GROUP	EXAMPLE	FORMULATION/ ROUTE	ONSET (min)	DURATION (h) OR FREQUENCY (/d)	USAGE
Corticosteroids (ICS)	Budesonide	DPI, neb		Admin 2/d	Maintenance in persistent asthma
	Ciclesonide	pMDI		Admin 1/d	Maintenance in persistent asthma
	Fluticasone	DPI, pMDI, neb		Admin 2/d	Maintenance in persistent asthma

Admin = administer; CR = controlled-release; CSs = corticosteroids; d = day; DPI = dry powder inhaler; ex-ind = prevention of exercise-induced asthma; ICS = inhaled corticosteroids; IV = intravenous; LABA= long-acting β₂-agonist; LAMA = long-acting muscarinic antagonist; neb = nebuliser; PO = oral; pMDI = pressurised metered-dose inhaler; SAMA = short-acting muscarinic antagonist; SABA= short-acting β₂-agonist; SC = subcutaneous

Sources: Based on information in Australian Medicines Handbook, 2020; Respiratory Expert Group, 2020.

drug factors such as adverse drug reactions, and classified severity and frequency of asthma attacks.

The stepwise pharmacological treatment is discussed later in this chapter (Fig 18.5). Older classifications referred to asthma as mild, moderate, or severe:

Mild – intermittent attacks (fewer than 1–2 per week), or nocturnal asthma twice or less monthly. Peak expiratory flow (PEF) over 80% predicted (i.e. > 80% of the expected level), normal after bronchodilator use, PEF variability under 20%.

Moderate – attacks more than twice weekly, nocturnal asthma symptoms more than twice per month, and use of a bronchodilator β-agonist inhaler required nearly daily. PEF 60–80% predicted, normal after bronchodilator use, PEF variability 20–30%.

Severe – frequent and continuous asthmatic symptoms, including nocturnal asthma and having been hospitalised for asthma in the previous year.

Currently, the severity of asthma is assessed retrospectively, reviewing the level of treatment that has been required to control the symptoms and exacerbations. This is, once the person has been on a controller for several months and, if possible, step-down treatment has been undertaken to determine the minimum effective level of treatment.

According to the *Australian Asthma Handbook* (2021), good asthma control is having, in the previous 4 weeks:

- daytime symptoms fewer than 2 days a week
- need for a short-acting reliever fewer than 2 days a week (not including doses for preventing exercise-induced bronchoconstriction)
- no limitation of activity
- no symptoms during the night or on waking.

Further classification includes partial control or poor control.

The overall management of asthma is summarised after discussion of the groups of drugs commonly used in treatment and their methods of delivery.

KEY POINTS

The pathophysiology of asthma

- Asthma is a condition involving impaired autonomic control as well as inflammatory processes.

- The principal signs and symptoms of asthma include wheezing and cough, tachypnoea or dyspnoea (rapid or difficult breathing), chest tightness, tachycardia, fatigue, sweating, difficulty speaking sentences, and anxiety.

- The early phase of an acute attack involves vasodilation and increased capillary permeability, infiltration of immune cell types and the release of dozens of pro-inflammatory mediators and cytokines. Constriction of the airways can be produced by neuropeptides and cytokine mediators released during inflammatory responses.

- The late-phase (chronic) response involves inflammatory processes, proliferation of fibroblasts and fibrosis, oedema of the airway mucosa, necrosis of bronchial epithelial cells, and airway wall remodelling with increased collagen deposition.

- Asthma can complicate pregnancy and is largely managed with the same approaches as it is outside of pregnancy.

18.3 Considerations for drug delivery to the airways

While oral administration of medications is the most common route, drug delivery via the respiratory system is also useful. Inhalation of drugs can be applied in the treatment of respiratory illness, where the reduction in circulating drug levels in other parts of the body minimises (but does not eliminate) side effects.

Aerosols

An **aerosol** is a suspension of fine liquid or solid particles dispersed in a gas or in solution. Aerosol drugs are commonly delivered by inhalation but can also be administered to the skin (as topical sprays) or to body cavities (ear, nose). After inhalation, some particles are deposited in the respiratory tract. The remainder tends to be swallowed, depending on droplet size. Inhalation may be via steam, from a nasal spray, or with devices like metered-dose inhalers (MDI) (Fig 18.6A), spacers (Fig 18.6B), dry powder inhalers (DPI) (Fig 18.6C, D), face masks, and nebulisers (Fig 18.6E).

Aerosol therapy has many advantages:

- Drug administration is convenient.
- There is minimal irritation, contamination, or systemic adverse effects.
- Lower doses can be given than by systemic administration.
- The drug is delivered rapidly to the desired site of action.
- Inhaled aerosols can promote bronchodilation, pulmonary decongestion, loosening of secretions, topical application of corticosteroids and other drugs, and moistening of inspired air.

A disadvantage of aerosol therapy is the expertise required to use an inhaler correctly. If the person uses their inhaler poorly, they will have poor asthma control. Incorrect inhaler use is common. It is important that health professionals assist with education regarding correct usage of these devices (see Online resources – inhaler techniques). Information about the correct use of puffers and inhalers is provided in Clinical Focus Box 18.1.

Pressurised metered-dose inhalers

Pressurised metered-dose inhalers (pMDIs) are small hand-held 'puffers' containing multiple doses of the active drug, mixed with a dispersing agent and a propellant, in a canister (Fig 18.6A). The canister is shaken and then the trigger is depressed (while inhaling) to deliver an accurate dose of the aerosol.

Effective use of pMDIs requires good hand–breath coordination, which can be difficult for some. Breath-activated MDIs, spacers (Fig 18.6B), and face masks improve drug administration (CFB 18.1). Breath-activated MDIs release a mist of medicine when inhalation occurs.

CLINICAL FOCUS BOX 18.1

Puffers and spacers

Correct use of inhaler devices maximises drug delivery to the airways. With pMDI **puffers**, the technique is as follows:

1. Take the cap off the puffer's mouthpiece.
2. Hold the puffer upright and shake it well.
3. Breathe out slowly and gently without emptying the lungs.
4. Put the mouthpiece between the teeth and close the lips around it without biting.
5. Tilt the head back slightly and, while breathing in slowly, press down on the top of the aerosol canister and continue to breathe in deeply.
6. Take the puffer away from the mouth and hold the breath for as long as possible, then breathe out gently.
7. Click the cap back onto the puffer.
8. If the inhaler delivered a corticosteroid, rinse the mouth with water and spit out.

The technique for handling different styles of inhalers varies, but the inhaling drug–breath holding–exhaling method is similar. Cleaning techniques for devices should be checked from information supplied with the inhaler. The simplest way to determine when a puffer is running out of drug is to count and keep a record of the number of times it has been used.

People with poor hand–breath coordination sometimes find it easier to use a puffer with a **spacer** (Fig 18.6B). Spacers should be washed monthly (with dishwashing detergent) and air-dried.

Dry powder inhalers

DPIs are like breath-activated MDIs, except the drug is delivered as finely divided particles rather than in aerosol solution. Examples are the 'Accuhaler™', a compact device with a foil strip inside containing doses of finely powdered drug (Figs 18.6C, D), and the 'Turbuhaler', in which the drug is loaded as a capsule which is then broken when the base is rotated, releasing the active drug. Mouthpieces of inhalers need regular cleaning. Manufacturers' instructions for specific devices should be followed.

Nebulisers

Nebulisers ('pumps'; Fig 18.6E) use compressed air or oxygen (Fig 18.6F), or ultrasonic energy, to produce a fine aerosol mist from a solution of the drug. Nebulisers are useful for delivering large doses inhaled by mouth over long periods, especially in severe asthma attacks. The aerosol drug or solution may irritate facial skin and may contribute to the spread of bacteria. Nebulisers can be costly to purchase.

Inhaled drugs

Drugs administered by inhalation are generally intended for local effects only. However, the lung is an absorptive organ (think: oxygen), so it is also a route for drugs to enter the systemic circulation. As an example, inhaled bronchodilator $\beta2$-agonist aerosols produce systemic effects after pulmonary absorption. The drug stimulates $\beta3$ and $\beta1$-adrenoceptors, causing tremor and tachycardia, respectively. Absorption of drugs is generally rapid due to the highly vascular pulmonary

Devices for drug administration

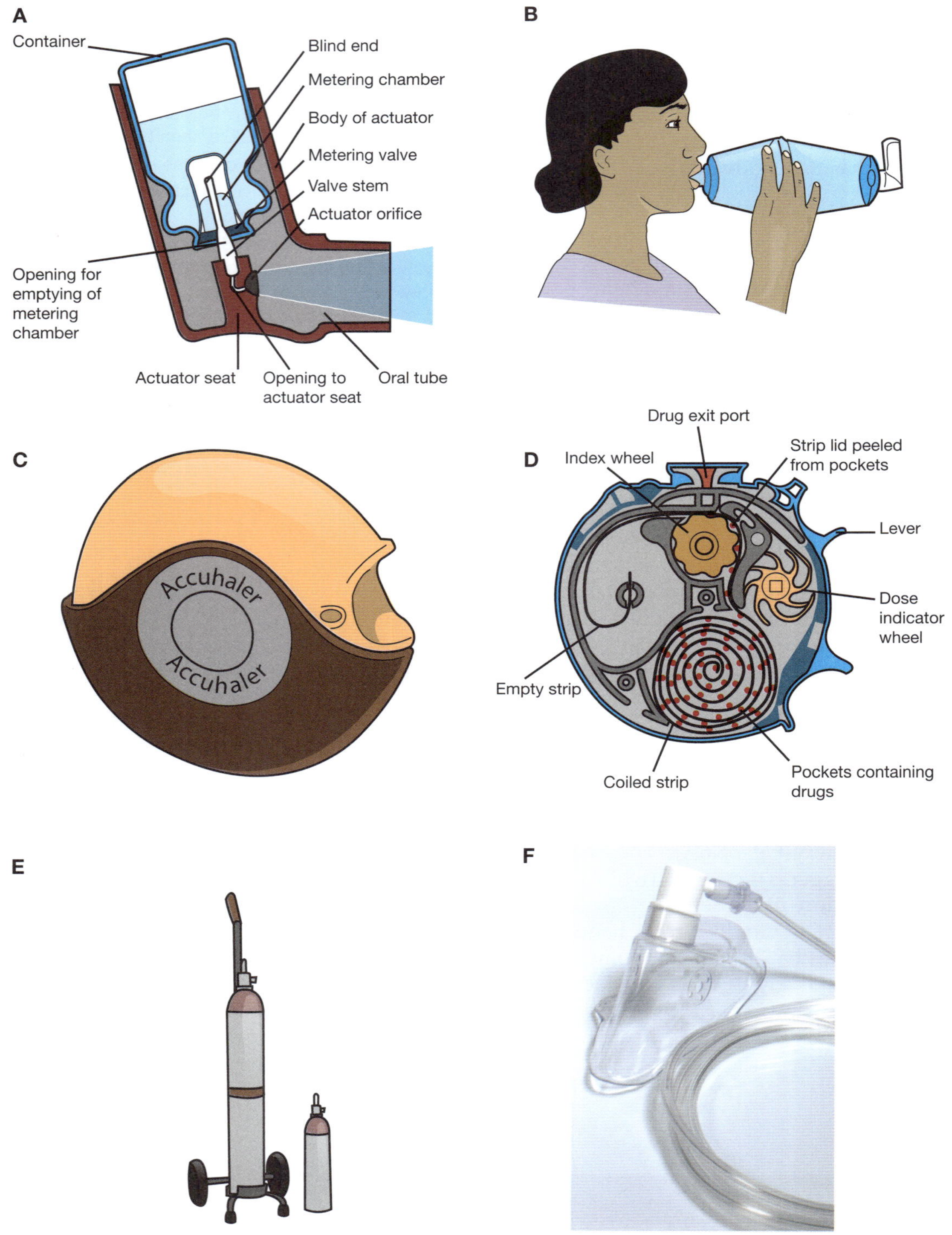

A

- Container
- Blind end
- Metering chamber
- Body of actuator
- Metering valve
- Valve stem
- Actuator orifice
- Opening for emptying of metering chamber
- Actuator seat
- Opening to actuator seat
- Oral tube

B

C

Accuhaler
Accuhaler

D

- Drug exit port
- Index wheel
- Strip lid peeled from pockets
- Lever
- Dose indicator wheel
- Empty strip
- Coiled strip
- Pockets containing drugs

E

F

FIGURE 18.6 A Pressurised metered-dose inhaler (pMDI, or 'puffer') shown in cross-section. **B** pMDI in combination with a large-volume spacer. **C** Accuhaler™. **D** Accuhaler; cross-section. **E** Gas cylinder on trolley. **F** Nebuliser bowl, tubing, and mask.

*Sources: **A**, **C** and **D**: courtesy GlaxoSmithKline, Australia; used with permission; **E**: Dreamstime/Podius; **F**: iStock/Hulldud30.*

DRUGS AT A GLANCE
Drugs used in the treatment of asthma

PHARMACOLOGICAL GROUP AND EFFECT	KEY EXAMPLES	CLINICAL USE
Relievers		
Bronchodilators		
Short-acting β₂-receptor agonists (SABAs) • Stimulate β₂-adrenoceptors in smooth muscle leading to muscle relaxation	Salbutamol and terbutaline	Acute relief of asthma symptoms Tocolysis
Methylxanthines • Proposed inhibition of phosphodiesterase (the enzyme that metabolises cAMP), leading to increased intracellular levels of cAMP, smooth muscle relaxation and bronchodilation. • Inhibit cyclic GMP (guanosine monophosphate) specific phosphodiesterase. • Competitive antagonism of adenosine at adenosine receptors	Theophylline, aminophylline	Acute relief of asthma symptoms (rarely used)
Short-acting muscarinic antagonists (SAMAs) • Block muscarinic M3 receptors on glands and smooth muscles to reduce secretions and relax smooth muscles of airways	Ipratropium bromide	Symptomatic treatment of asthma
Long-acting muscarinic antagonists (LAMAs) • Block muscarinic M3 receptors on glands and smooth muscles to reduce secretions and relax smooth muscles of airways (duration of action of over 24 hours)	Tiotropium, glycopyrronium bromide (glycopyrrolate), aclidinium, and umeclidinium	Maintenance treatment of asthma (with adjuncts; ICS, LAMA, LABA combinations)
Controller Medications		
Long-acting β₂-receptor agonists (LABAs) • Allosteric binding of agonists at the β₂ receptors leads to prolonged relaxation of bronchial smooth muscle	Salmeterol Formoterol (eformoterol) Indacaterol	Maintenance treatment of asthma (with inhaled corticosteroids)
Preventer Medications		
Corticosteroids • Inhibit gene transcription and the enzyme phospholipase A2, inhibiting the production of inflammatory mediators	Fluticasone, budesonide, beclometasone	Maintenance treatment of asthma
Monoclonal antibodies • Recombinant humanised monoclonal antibody, complexes with free IgE antigens to prevent their binding to mast cells • Target human interleukin-5 (IL-5) (inflammatory mediator) with high affinity and specificity	Omalizumab	Maintenance treatment of moderate-to-severe allergic asthma in people treated with inhaled corticosteroids and with raised serum IgE levels
	Mepolizumab	Severe refractory eosinophilic asthma
Leukotriene-receptor antagonists (LTRAs) • Block receptors for the cysteinyl leukotrienes (LTC4, LTD4 and LTE4), mediators of inflammation in both early and late phases of asthma; also inhibit other pro-inflammatory cytokines	Montelukast	Maintenance treatment of asthma
Oxygen • Reduces mortality in severe hypoxia		Acute severe asthma

capillary system and depends on the lipid solubility of the inhaled drug, the aerosol particle size, and pulmonary function.

Potential problems from aerosol administration include oral fungal infections after corticosteroid inhalation, or ocular effects if the aerosol mist reaches the eyes (e.g. in the case of ipratropium administration). A considerable proportion of an inhaled drug dose is swallowed, so it may produce systemic effects if not digested or metabolised rapidly.

When two or more inhalers are prescribed together, such as when a corticosteroid or **mast-cell stabiliser** puffer is prescribed along with a bronchodilator puffer, it is important that the *bronchodilator* is administered 5 minutes *before* the other drug to promote bronchodilation and maximise inhalation of the second aerosol.

KEY POINTS

Drug delivery to airways

■ An aerosol is a suspension of fine particles, liquid or solid, dispersed in gas to body cavities.

- Aerosol therapy is convenient and rapid, provides minimal systemic effects, allows for lower doses of drugs, promotes bronchodilation and decongestion, and enables topical administration of drugs such as corticosteroids to airways.
- Devices for drug administration by inhalation include nasal sprays, pMDIs, DPIs, and nebulisers.
- Systemic effects can occur with inhaled drugs.
- Teaching proper techniques for use and cleaning of a pMDI or other inhalation devices is important. Spacer units are suggested when hand–breath coordination is an issue.

18.4 Bronchodilator drugs

β-adrenoceptor agonists

Bronchodilator drugs are used to treat pulmonary diseases such as asthma, chronic bronchitis, and emphysema. Ephedrine, an alkaloid from the plant *Ephedra sinica*, was introduced from traditional Chinese medicine into Western medicine in 1923. Ephedrine is a sympathomimetic amine related structurally to adrenaline (a hormone from the adrenal medulla). It predominantly acts indirectly via release of noradrenaline from adrenergic nerve terminals. Thus, it has effects on both α- and β-adrenoceptors. Adrenaline, also a non-selective α- and β-adrenoceptor agonist, is still used clinically for asthma (and for anaphylactic reactions and cardiovascular effects) but has a short duration of action. Effects mediated by α-adrenoceptors (especially vasoconstriction and hypertension) and β1-adrenoceptors (cardiac stimulation) generate adverse reactions in the context of asthma therapy, so much research effort has gone into the development of specific β2-agonist bronchodilators to avoid such reactions (Matera et al 2020b).

Mechanism of action

Activation of β2-adrenoceptors in bronchial smooth muscle leads to increased formation of cyclic 3,5-adenosine monophosphate (cAMP), enhancement of calcium extrusion from the cell, and binding of intracellular calcium, which lowers the concentration of intracellular calcium and strongly relaxes bronchial smooth muscle (Fig 18.7). **β2-adrenoceptor agonists** are the most effective bronchodilators, acting as functional antagonists of airway smooth muscle contraction. Agonist actions on β2-adrenoceptors in the uterus cause relaxation of uterine smooth muscle (tocolysis), so the drugs have also been used to delay threatened preterm birth and during external cephalic version (see Chapter 17).

Administration

The optimal route of administration of β2-agonists is by inhalation. 'Puffers' and 'pumps' deliver low doses of drug directly to the airway smooth muscle and have rapid and relatively specific effects. Some inhaled drug is inevitably deposited in the oropharynx and swallowed where it may be absorbed into the systemic circulation and cause adverse reactions. In rare cases, propellants may induce cardiac dysrhythmias or allergic reactions. In emergencies, systemic administration may be required. Adrenaline, salbutamol, and terbutaline can be administered by injection. Salbutamol is also available in a syrup form, useful for children.

Adverse effects

While agonists with relatively specific actions on β2-adrenoceptors are available, they may in high doses also stimulate α- and β1-receptors, so adverse effects in the cardiovascular system (vasoconstriction, vasodilation and reflex tachycardia, pulmonary vasodilation), skeletal muscle (fine tremor), metabolism (ketoacidosis, mobilisation of triglycerides), and CNS (headaches, nausea, and anxiety) may occur. The reverse is also true: β1-adrenoceptor antagonists used in cardiovascular disease may have potentially life-threatening bronchoconstrictor (β2 antagonism) effects in people with asthma.

Non-selective β-agonists may downregulate receptors over time, leading to tolerance to the bronchodilator effects of these agents, which encourages overuse and exacerbates adverse effects arising from cardiac and vascular actions. In addition, people with particular polymorphisms of the β2-adrenoceptor appear to experience reduced lung function and increased asthma exacerbations.

Short-acting β2-agonists (relievers)

Short-acting β2-agonists (SABAs) are fast-acting bronchodilators, used as **relievers** in first-line treatment for acute relief of asthma symptoms. Salbutamol (also known as albuterol, and by its first trade-name Ventolin) and terbutaline are described in Drug Monograph 18.1. They are also used to prevent exercise-induced asthma and for their tocolytic effects during pregnancy. Over-dependence on β2-agonists (high dose use on more than 3 days per week) may indicate other aspects of asthma management, including preventive use of anti-inflammatory drugs and monitoring of FEV1 (forced expiratory volume in 1 second), are not optimal. Inhaled SABAs are safe in pregnancy and lactation.

Long-acting β2-agonists (controllers)

Long-acting β2-agonists (LABAs) commonly used include salmeterol and formoterol (eformoterol). Due to their allosteric actions at the β2 receptors and greater lipid solubilities they have prolonged actions, with half-lives in the range 6–12 hours (indacaterol up to 24 hours). They are administered once or twice daily by MDI or DPI. They are useful against night-time symptoms and are symptom **controllers**, used in conjunction with ICS (preventers) or long-acting muscarinic antagonists

Typical mechanisms of action of drugs on bronchial smooth muscle

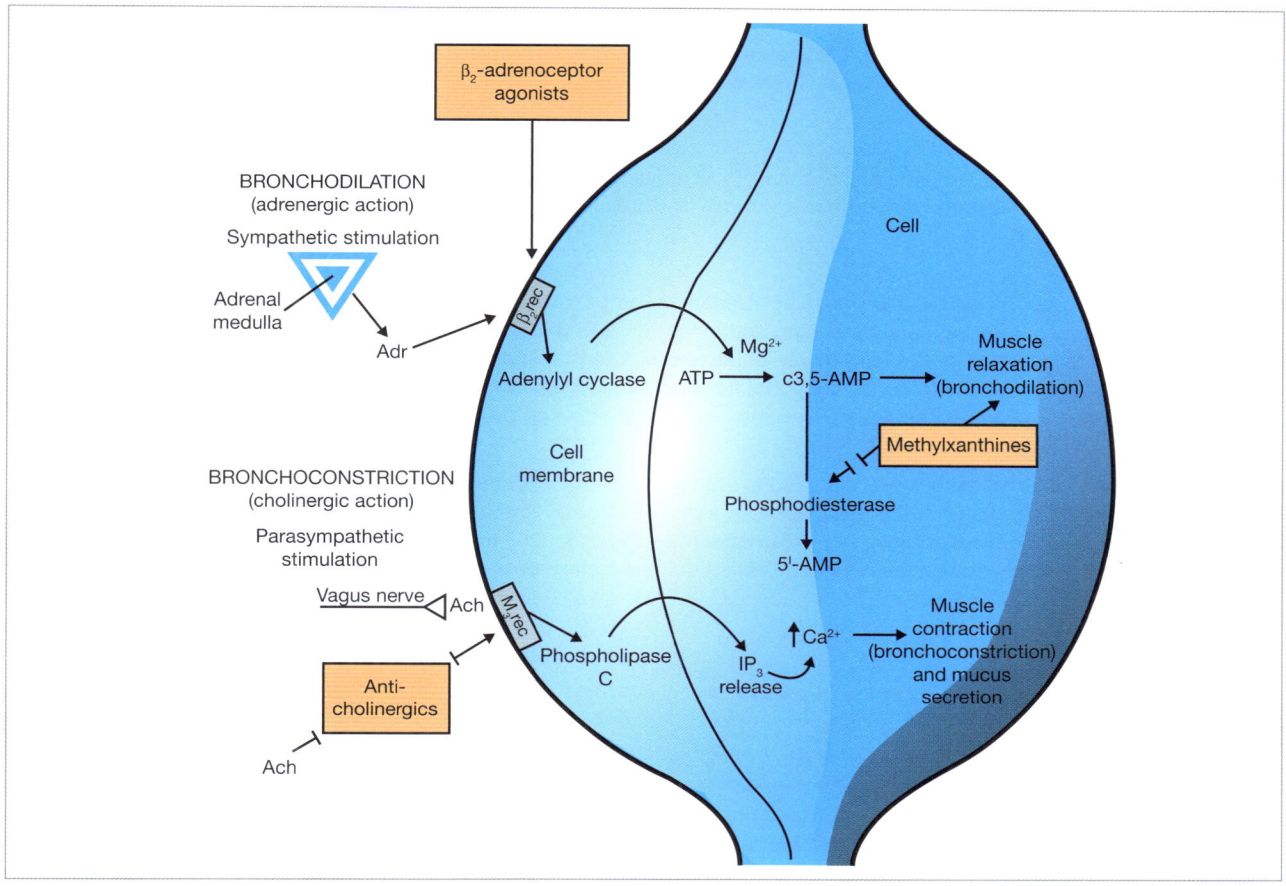

FIGURE 18.7 A Bronchodilation pathway. **B** Bronchoconstriction pathway. ACh = acetylcholine; Adr = adrenaline; $\beta_2$rec = β_2-adrenoreceptor; IP = inositol phosphate; M_3rec = M_3 muscarinic receptor; VIP = vasoactive intestinal peptide

---

DRUG MONOGRAPH 18.1
Salbutamol and terbutaline

Mechanism of action

These are SABA bronchodilators.

Indications

For the symptomatic relief of acute asthma and protection against exercise-induced asthma, and for uterine relaxation (tocolysis) during pregnancy.

Pharmacokinetics

- Onset of action by inhalation is rapid, within 5–15 minutes, with peak effect within 1–2 hours and duration of action of 3–6 hours.
- Salbutamol is metabolised in the liver and excreted in the kidneys.
- Terbutaline is excreted largely unchanged. Small amounts of either drug swallowed are rapidly metabolised.

Drug interactions

Concomitant therapy with other sympathomimetic amines will cause excessive sympathetic stimulation (tremor, tachycardia). β-blockers, including those for hypertension and in eyedrops for glaucoma antagonise the effects of β_2-agonists and may

Continued

DRUG MONOGRAPH 18.1
Salbutamol and terbutaline—cont'd

precipitate asthma, so they are contraindicated. Hypokalaemia resulting from β_2-agonist therapy may be potentiated by xanthine derivatives, steroids, or diuretics. Potassium levels should be monitored. Antidepressant drugs may potentiate cardiovascular effects.

Adverse effects

These include tremor, palpitations, anxiety, restlessness, headaches, muscle cramps, hyperglycaemia, tachycardia, and an unusual taste in the mouth. Symptoms of overdose are those of excessive α- or β_1-adrenoceptor stimulation – for example, hypertension or palpitations.

Precautions

Precautions are needed in people with cardiovascular disease, diabetes, or hyperthyroidism. Excessive use of bronchodilator aerosols, or lack of response, may indicate worsening asthma control. Both drugs are safe in pregnancy and when breastfeeding although care should be taken with use of intravenous terbutaline in the first 3 months of pregnancy. Treatment of asthma should be in accordance with current national treatment guidelines (in Australia, the National Asthma Council guidelines and in New Zealand, the Asthma and Respiratory Foundation – see Online resources).

Dosage and administration

The adult bronchodilator dose for both is 1–2 inhalations (100 micrograms salbutamol, 500 micrograms terbutaline), with the second inhalation at least 1 minute after the first, repeated every 4–6 hours. Both drugs can be administered by nebuliser, orally, or parenterally in acute severe attacks. For external cephalic version, 250 micrograms of terbutaline administered subcutaneously or intravenously can be used, with attention paid to maternal heart rate following administration.

(see below) in maintenance treatment of asthma. Formoterol (eformoterol) has a rapid onset of action (Table 18.1) and can also be used for quick relief.

There is some controversy about the safety of LABAs. Their use may increase tolerance to SABAs and increase exacerbations of asthma, especially if LABAs are used alone (i.e. without ICS). There may be a genetic component to this increased susceptibility. There is limited experience with the use of LABAs in pregnancy and lactation, but their use is considered safe in the second and third trimesters.

Methylxanthines

The xanthine group of drugs includes the methylxanthines: caffeine, theophylline, and theobromine. Beverages from the extracts of plants containing these alkaloids have been used by humans since ancient times, and strong coffee was historically used as a remedy for asthma. (CNS stimulation by xanthines and social use as drinks is discussed in Chapter 21.)

Xanthine derivatives relax smooth muscle (particularly bronchial muscle); stimulate cardiac muscle, diaphragm contractility, and the CNS (hence their social use); and produce diuresis, through increased renal perfusion and increased sodium and chloride excretion. The main medical use of these natural products and their synthetic analogues is as bronchodilators.

The most active xanthine bronchodilator is theophylline (DM 18.2), sometimes used as its derivative aminophylline (a more soluble but highly alkaline ethylene-diamine-theophylline derivative, given IV). It has a narrow therapeutic index and many drug interactions (DI 18.1). Monitoring of theophylline or aminophylline concentrations is advised in pregnancy, and there is limited data on the use of either drug in lactation. Although a weak bronchodilator, theophylline has useful anti-inflammatory effects and may increase responsiveness to corticosteroids in people resistant to steroids.

Mechanisms of action

Despite their long history and wide social and medical usage, the mechanism of action of xanthines is not well understood. One explanation for their bronchodilator effect is inhibition of phosphodiesterase (the enzyme that metabolises cAMP), leading to increased intracellular levels of cAMP, smooth muscle relaxation and bronchodilation (Fig 18.7). However, the concentrations of theophylline required to inhibit the enzyme in vitro are much greater than therapeutic levels. Other mechanisms proposed include inhibition of cyclic GMP-specific phosphodiesterase; competitive antagonism of adenosine at adenosine receptors (which activates adenylate cyclase, and has cardiac-depressant, bronchoconstrictor, pro-inflammatory and platelet-aggregation-suppressant effects); increased histone deacetylase 2 activity, which may help reverse corticosteroid resistance; and selective inhibition of phosphoinositide 3-kinase, a regulator of inflammation. In treatment of asthma, theophylline derivatives act as bronchodilators, provide inhibition of the late (inflammatory) phase of asthma, and directly stimulate the medullary respiratory centre.

DRUG MONOGRAPH 18.2
Theophylline

Theophylline is the prototype xanthine bronchodilator. It is typically prescribed as controlled-release tablets for maintenance treatment of poorly controlled moderate-to-severe asthma.

Mechanism of action

Theophylline is a phosphodiesterase inhibitor; the resultant cyclic AMP and cyclic GMP activation leads to bronchiolar smooth muscle relaxation. It is also an adenosine receptor antagonist thus reversing adenosine induced bronchoconstriction.

Pharmacokinetics

- Absorption is little altered by food. Sustained-release (SR) tablets are formulated to optimise absorption. Although enteric-coated tablets and sustained-release dosage forms have delayed and unreliable absorption patterns, most provide a bioavailability of 100%.
- Peak level of theophylline is reached in 1–2 hours with the oral solution, and in 4–13 hours for sustained-release products.
- Protein binding is moderate (50–70%), and theophylline distributes across the placenta (Pregnancy Category A) and into breast milk.
- Liver metabolism produces various uric acid and xanthine derivatives (some with low activity), which are excreted via the kidneys.
- The half-life of theophylline varies with age and with concurrent illness: in premature newborns the half-life is around 30 hours; it is 3.5 hours for children 1–9 years of age, and 3–12 hours for adult non-smokers with uncomplicated asthma. In an adult smoker it is only 3–4 hours. Theophylline has a narrow therapeutic window: trough plasma levels are between 10 and 20 mg/L; however, therapeutic responses are variable and close supervision is necessary.
- Excretion is by the kidney and about 10% of the dose is excreted unchanged in the urine.

Drug interactions

There are many drug interactions with theophylline (DI 18.1); reference databases should be consulted for specific drugs and therapy monitored closely.

Adverse effects

These are dose-dependent and are related to the other main actions of xanthines (CNS and cardiac stimulation and diuresis), and include nausea, headache, insomnia, increased anxiety, vomiting, gastro-oesophageal reflux, and increased urination. Tachycardia and convulsions may appear at high plasma levels (> 30 mg/L). Toxicity may occur even at therapeutic levels. People with reduced renal function have an increased risk of toxicity due to reduced clearance.

Precautions

Use with caution in people with fever, gastrointestinal or cardiovascular disorders, and thyroid or liver dysfunction. Monitoring plasma levels is strongly recommended. Consider the risk–benefit profile prior to use in pregnancy and lactation.

Dosage and administration

The dosage of theophylline preparations should be adjusted to maintain a serum concentration of 10–20 microgram/mL (= mg/L; see previous comments on serum levels). Doses are increased gradually over several days while monitoring for adverse effects, and plasma concentration should be measured.

DRUG INTERACTIONS 18.1
Theophylline

DRUG	POSSIBLE EFFECTS AND MANAGEMENT
Aciclovir, alcohol, allopurinol, cimetidine, cipro- and norfloxacin, disulfiram, fluvoxamine, interferon alpha, macrolide antibiotics, oral contraceptives, propranolol	Theophylline concentration may be increased, dose may need to be reduced
Phenobarbital (Phenobarbitone), phenytoin, rifampicin, ritonavir, sucralfate	Theophylline concentration may be decreased, dose may need to be increased
β_2-agonists or diuretics	Theophylline can potentiate hypokalaemia caused by these drugs
Lithium, macrolides, pancuronium, phenytoin	Theophylline may decrease concentration of or response to these drugs; dose of the other drug may need to be increased

Anticholinergics

Plants from the *Atropa* or *Datura* genera have been smoked or inhaled for relief of respiratory symptoms for hundreds of years. These plants contain the alkaloids atropine or stramonium, competitive antagonists acting on muscarinic receptors. **Anticholinergics** produce bronchodilation by blocking vagal tone and parasympathetic reflexes mediating bronchoconstriction (Fig 18.7). They may also decrease secretions and make them hard to expectorate. Typical 'atropinic side effects' are dry mouth and throat, urinary retention, and constipation. Anticholinergics include the short- and long-acting muscarinic antagonists (Matera et al 2020a).

Short-acting muscarinic antagonist: Ipratropium

The **short-acting muscarinic antagonist** (SAMA) ipratropium has useful bronchodilator actions after inhalation; and can be used as maintenance treatment in severe asthma (Table 18.1). Ipratropium is a quaternary (charged) ammonium compound, unlikely to cross the blood–brain, breast, or placental barriers after administration, so has fewer adverse effects than atropine. Ipratropium is available as an MDI or nebuliser and may be used 3–4 times daily.

Long-acting muscarinic antagonists

Long-acting muscarinic antagonists (LAMAs) include tiotropium, glycopyrronium bromide (glycopyrrolate), aclidinium, and umeclidinium. Only tiotropium is licensed for treatment of asthma. LAMAs cause bronchodilation, have a duration of action of over 24 hours and are used once daily. Tiotropium is more selective for M_3 receptors: it is inhaled via a DPI once daily and is longer acting than ipratropium. A newer product for tiotropium, Spiriva Respimat, is a solution for inhalation. There is less experience with the use of LAMAs in pregnancy and lactation.

Short- and long-acting muscarinic antagonists should not be used prophylactically or for relief of symptoms, except in severe asthma (e.g. ipratropium bromide [Atrovent]). Instead, they are used as adjunctive controller therapy with corticosteroids (ICS). They can be used in combination with LABAs. Interactions with other drugs with anticholinergic effects are common, and combinations should be avoided. They have a wide therapeutic margin when administered by inhalation, as there is little systemic absorption. However, if the aerosol mist or powder reaches the eyes, it can cause mydriasis, blurred vision, and risk of glaucoma.

> **KEY POINTS**
>
> **Bronchodilator drugs**
>
> - Asthma relievers/bronchodilators include β_2-receptor agonists, methylxanthines, and anticholinergics.
> - β_2-receptor agonists relax smooth muscle in airways by activation of β_2-adrenoceptors.
> - β_2-receptor agonists include the non-selective agonist adrenaline, SABAs including salbutamol and terbutaline and the LABAs or symptom controllers, formoterol (eformoterol) and salmeterol. LABAs may be combined with corticosteroids or anticholinergics.
> - The methylxanthines, caffeine and theophylline induce bronchial smooth muscle relaxation.
> - Anticholinergics block the M_3 muscarinic receptors on bronchial smooth muscle leading to smooth muscle relaxation. Ipratropium is short-acting and tiotropium is long acting.

18.5 Prophylactic antiasthma drugs (preventers)

These drugs are collectively known as **preventers**. They include corticosteroids and newer drugs that prevent inflammatory responses.

Corticosteroids

Corticosteroids are used in chronic asthma to decrease airway obstruction. The anti-inflammatory and immunosuppressant actions of glucocorticoids such as cortisone and prednisolone are useful in asthma. Prophylactic use of ICS, preventing the late-phase inflammatory response and decreasing bronchial hyper-reactivity, has revolutionised the management of asthma. The products available now as DPI, pMDI, or nebuliser forms (ICS) are beclometasone (DM 18.3), budesonide, ciclesonide, and fluticasone (furoate and propionate forms) – see Table 18.1, and Figure 18.5 (earlier) for stepwise adjustment of dosage in asthma management according to level of symptom control. A spacer should be used with a pMDI to enhance drug delivery to the airways. Inhaled or oral corticosteroids appear to pose no risk to mother or child. Budesonide may be preferred as there is more experience with its use in pregnancy.

Mechanism of action

Corticosteroids enter the cytoplasm of cells, bind to specific glucocorticoid receptors, then translocate into the nucleus where they bind to response elements in target genes and bring about induction or repression of gene transcription. They also inhibit the enzyme phospholipase A2, thereby inhibiting the production of COX enzymes and subsequently the production of PGE_2 and PGI_2. Overall, glucocorticoids reduce both the early and late (proliferative) stages of the inflammatory response. They are indicated prophylactically in maintenance treatment of severe asthma (e.g. LABA + long-acting anticholinergic + ICS), and in acute asthma

DRUG MONOGRAPH 18.3
Beclometasone inhaled

Mechanism of action

As a glucocorticoid, beclometasone inhibits both inflammatory cells and release of inflammatory mediators associated with the pathophysiology of asthma.

Indications

ICS are indicated for maintenance treatment and prophylaxis in persistent asthma.

Pharmacokinetics

A considerable proportion (up to 80%) of an inhaled dose of beclometasone is likely to be swallowed, then absorbed from the intestinal tract. QVAR breath-activated formulations automatically release the metered dose through the mouthpiece and overcome the need for people to coordinate actuation with inspiration. There is increased lung deposition and reduced oropharyngeal deposition compared with chlorofluorocarbon-propelled devices.

Peak plasma concentrations are reached 3–5 hours after administration. The drug is subject to metabolism in the liver and excretion in faeces and urine.

Adverse effects

Local adverse effects include dysphonia (changed voice), oropharyngeal candidiasis (oral thrush) and allergic reactions. Systemic effects are rare.

Drug interactions

None are clinically significant. Other antiasthma medications may be continued.

Warnings and precautions

- Oral deposition of drug (and hence oral infections and systemic absorption) can be reduced by use of a spacer and by rinsing the mouth and throat after each dose.
- The drug is not useful for acute asthma attacks because it is not a bronchodilator.
- If prescribed with an inhaled bronchodilator, the β_2-agonist or anticholinergic should be inhaled (to open the airways) before the corticosteroid.
- Dosage should not be reduced or stopped unless advised.
- QVAR is Category B3 in pregnancy and there is inadequate clinical evidence on safety. The therapeutic benefits of QVAR should be weighed against the potential hazards to the mother and baby.

Contraindications

Hypersensitivity to any ingredient.

Dosage and administration

Dosage starts at levels likely to be effective, then reduced to the minimum dose that controls symptoms, and is 'stepped down' by 25% every 3 months if possible. Dosage may be doubled if asthma worsens, or respiratory tract infection occurs.

---

and croup. The maximum improvement in pulmonary function may take 1–4 weeks.

Systemic administration and adverse effects

Systemic (oral) administration of corticosteroids can cause significant adverse 'cushingoid' effects, including adrenal suppression and growth suppression; altered deposition of muscle, fat, skin, hair, and bone; ocular changes, infections, mineralocorticoid effects, and psychological disturbances. Systemic corticosteroids are still used (e.g. short courses of prednisolone orally) when inhaled medications (corticosteroids, β_2-agonists, anticholinergics) and oral theophylline cannot adequately control asthma. In emergencies, corticosteroids may be administered parenterally (e.g. IV hydrocortisone, dexamethasone).

Chemical modifications of the steroid molecule produced compounds such as beclometasone with enhanced absorption after inhalation and reduced risk of systemic adverse effects.

Local effects of inhaled steroids include hoarse voice and oral or oesophageal candida infections. To prevent fungal infections, users are advised to rinse their mouth out with water after use of a corticosteroid inhaler.

Frequent, long-term use of ICS may lead to a dose-related decrease in bone mineral density and increased risk of osteoporosis.

Glucocorticoid resistance

Resistance to steroid therapy can develop and increase asthma severity without impairing the other metabolic effects of steroids.

18.6 Other drug groups

Leukotriene-receptor antagonists (LTRAs)

The only **leukotriene-receptor antagonist** (Fig 18.3) currently used clinically is montelukast. The mechanism of action of this drug group is blockade of receptors for the cysteinyl leukotrienes (LTC_4, LTD_4 and LTE_4), which are components of the 'slow-reacting substance of anaphylaxis (SRS-A)' as it is historically known. SRS-A is thought to be a mediator of inflammation in both early and late phases of asthma. LTRAs also inhibit other pro-inflammatory cytokines, so they reduce the inflammation, mucus secretion, and bronchoconstriction associated with asthma.

Montelukast is not indicated for reversal of bronchospasm in acute asthma attacks but has additive effects to β_2-agonists and is useful adjunctive therapy for people whose asthma is inadequately controlled with ICS, as it may allow a reduction in corticosteroid dosage. Improvement in asthma symptoms should be noted within a few days.

Administered orally, montelukast is rapidly absorbed and has a rapid onset of action. Adverse effects include headache, nausea, and abdominal upset or pain. Adverse neuropsychiatric events, including suicidal ideation, depression, aggressive behaviour, and hallucinations may occur. People should be warned in advance to seek medical advice if this occurs. There appears to be limited evidence for congenital defects due to use in pregnancy and it is safe in breastfeeding women.

New drugs for asthma

New drugs are constantly being developed and tested for use in asthma, particularly as the pathogenesis is better understood. It has been reported that 5–10% of people have various subtypes of inadequately controlled and difficult to treat asthma. Newer, 'add on' therapies include biological therapies including monoclonal antibodies and drugs that target innate cytokines. In future, for severe asthma, therapies will target different phenotypes and endotypes (Palaia et al 2021).

Drugs to be used with caution for pregnant and postpartum women with asthma

Ergometrine: Typically used alone or in combination with oxytocin to prevent and manage postpartum haemorrhage because of the drug's ability to cause contraction of uterine smooth muscle. There are rare case reports of severe bronchospasm occurring after administration of ergometrine, so it should be used with caution in women with asthma.

Prostaglandin F 2 alpha: Used in the treatment of postpartum haemorrhage. It is a potent bronchoconstrictor and should be avoided in women with asthma.

Morphine and other opioids: During an acute exacerbation of asthma, opioid analgesia should be used with caution. Opioids can reduce respiratory drive and may lead to worsening hypoxia in a woman with an acute episode of asthma.

Aspirin and NSAIDs: About 10% of people with asthma are at risk for an acute exacerbation in symptoms after exposure to aspirin or non-steroidal anti-inflammatory drugs (Hamad et al 2004). Before prescribing aspirin during pregnancy for prevention of preeclampsia or growth restriction, or non-steroidal anti-inflammatory drugs, the woman's previous experiences in relation to her symptom control with such medications should be reviewed. For women with asthma who do not have a history of uncomplicated use of aspirin and non-steroidal anti-inflammatory drugs, the risk–benefit balance of using the medication should be carefully considered. If the decision is made to prescribe the medication, then close monitoring of the impact on respiratory symptoms should be in place.

18.7 Therapies and management of asthma in pregnancy

Combination therapy

Combined inhalers containing both a long-acting symptom controller and a corticosteroid preventer are now considered the 'gold standard' for asthma management. These combined formulations reduce the risk of severe asthma exacerbations. A combination is indicated for regular treatment of asthma when use of both drugs is appropriate. In Single-inhaler Maintenance and Reliever Therapy (SMART), a budesonide (ICS)–formoterol (eformoterol; LABA) inhaler can be used as a reliever therapy as required, with the same inhaler used twice daily as maintenance therapy (Global Initiative for Asthma 2016; National Asthma Council Australia 2020).

The pharmacokinetic parameters of each drug appear to be unaffected by co-administration, and adverse reactions, precautions, and interactions are as for each component drug. The advantages are the convenience of using only one inhaler, cost reduction, better control of asthma, regular use of a low-dose steroid, and likely better compliance with therapy.

Some people will wish to also explore complementary and alternative medicine approaches to manage their asthma symptoms (CFB 18.2). These typically work through the same pathways as conventional medical approaches.

Suboptimal therapy

Despite the availability of several groups of drugs for the treatment of asthma, asthma therapy is frequently not optimal, and there is still an unacceptably high level of mortality and morbidity. Possible reasons for unsuccessful therapy include:

- overreliance on short-acting bronchodilator relievers
- under-use of controller medications or inhaled corticosteroid preventers
- poor control over MDIs
- poor inhaler technique (Harris et al 2016)
- lack of understanding that asthma is a chronic condition
- anxiety about the safety of asthma medications in pregnancy
- lack of objective measurements of severity of asthma
- inadequate monitoring of therapy and compliance
- pharmacogenetic differences.

Stepwise management

Guidelines have been published to encourage appropriate evidence-based treatment. The emphasis in guidelines is on stepwise management, with treatment stepped up to stronger drugs to achieve good control of symptoms, and cautious stepping down after improvement and review of therapy. Asthma is classified and treated according to symptoms and severity. Pregnant women with asthma are managed in the same manner as other people with asthma. It is also important to assess future risk of adverse outcomes. Severity is determined retrospectively, after 2–3 months of treatment of specific symptoms. An example of the stepwise approach for management of asthma is shown in Figure 18.5 (earlier) (Global Initiative for Asthma 2016; National Asthma Council Australia 2020).

Chronic asthma

As treatment of chronic asthma begins, severity needs to be assessed with spirometry/peak-flow meters testing and trigger factors identified and managed. Treatment is tailored to suit the individual and the severity of their asthma. ICS are started at a dose sufficient to be effective, as monitored by peak-flow meter readings, then reduced to the minimum required to maintain control.

Acute asthma

Acute asthma is a life-threatening situation and may require systemic corticosteroids, adrenaline, aminophylline, oxygen, nebulised bronchodilators, and close monitoring of lung function, blood gases, and CNS function. Drugs also administered include ipratropium bromide and salbutamol.

Asthma action plans

Each person should have an individualised written action plan, including education and self-management aspects, so they can recognise their own symptoms, start and step-up treatment, and promptly reach medical attention. Action plans need to consider factors such as closeness to hospital help, as people living in rural locations face added risk factors (isolation, lack of support networks, and seasonal high levels of environmental allergens).

The various action plans proposed by Australian and New Zealand groups through the National Asthma Council advise people to:

- ensure they know when and where to get medical care including in emergencies, who wrote the plan and its date
- achieve best lung function (regularly monitor FEV_1)
- assess the severity of the condition and symptom control
- identify and avoid trigger factors
- optimise their medication programs (minimise the number of drugs, doses, and adverse effects)
- ensure they know their usual asthma and allergy medications and have clear instructions on how to

change medications (example: when asthma is getting worse or substantially worse or when peak flow falls below an agreed rate)

- follow action plans
- undertake self-education about how to assess and understand lung function, and good inhaler technique.

CLINICAL FOCUS BOX 18.2

CAMS for respiratory disorders

There are good pharmacological rationales for many traditional, complementary, and alternative medicine treatments for asthma:

- Garlic and horseradish contain several antiallergy compounds.
- Coffee and tea contain xanthine bronchodilators.
- Saltpetre (potassium nitrate) is a smooth muscle relaxant.
- The herb *Ephedra sinica* (ma huang), from traditional Chinese medicine, contains the bronchodilator ephedrine.
- New Zealand green-lipped mussels have anti-inflammatory actions.
- Echinacea extracts may stimulate phagocyte activity in the non-specific immune system.
- Fijian plants traditionally used for asthma are weleti (*Carica papaya*, pawpaw).
- Various other Chinese, Japanese, Indian and Native American herbs are used, some of which may have steroidal components with anti-inflammatory activities.

Also tried are dietary methods (avoidance of allergenic foods, and supplementation with fish oils, vitamin C, magnesium, selenium, or zinc) and mind–body techniques, including meditation and biofeedback.

Indigenous Australians use native plants to treat cough and respiratory tract congestion, either by inhalation or drinking a decoction (tea) containing plant oils and cineoles with mucolytic and decongestant properties. These are present in eucalypt species, the liniment tree (*Melaleuca symphocarpa*), lemon grasses (Cymbopogon) and river mint (*Mentha australis*).

Sources: Adapted from Braun & Cohen 2015; Cambie & Ash 1994.

KEY POINTS

Overview of asthma management in pregnancy

- Combined inhalers containing both a long-acting symptom controller and a corticosteroid preventer are now considered the 'gold standard' for asthma management.
- Good asthma control when pregnant is critical for the best possible health of woman and baby.
- Despite the availability of several groups of drugs for the treatment of asthma, asthma therapy is frequently not optimal, and there is still an unacceptably high level of mortality and morbidity.
- Management plans for asthma involve education, regular monitoring of lung function and compliance, avoiding trigger factors, and evidence-based stepwise management with antiasthma drugs guided by individualised written asthma action plans.

REVIEW EXERCISES

1. Katerina, a 26-year-old woman, has just been admitted to the maternity unit for planned induction at 37 weeks gestation for moderately severe preeclampsia. Katerina has mild asthma that has been well controlled through her pregnancy. She uses budesonide 100 micrograms with formoterol 6 microgram in a combined MDI (Symbicort 100/6), using one or two inhalations when required. Her blood pressure on admission was 170/110 and her obstetrician is planning to use an antihypertensive to better control this. What would be the possible impact on her asthma of using the antihypertensive labetolol? What other antihypertensive agents commonly used in the management of preeclampsia would be a preferable choice with respect to her asthma?

2. Julia, a 30-year-old woman, is transported to the emergency department in acute respiratory distress with tachycardia, tachypnoea, moderately severe increased work of breathing with oxygen saturations 87% in room air and widespread wheeze. She is speaking in two- to three-word phrases. Julia is 6 weeks pregnant and has a past history of severe asthma. After medical assessment, 10 mg of nebulised salbutamol and supplemental oxygen 8 L/minute are delivered via face mask, then nebulised ipratropium bromide 500 micrograms. The salbutamol/ipratropium nebules are repeated at 20-minute intervals for a further two doses, with only temporary improvement in her breathing difficulties. IV access is obtained, and full cardiac monitoring is commenced. Hydrocortisone 100 mg is administered IV stat. She is then loaded with IV aminophylline 5 mg/kg over 1 hour, and ambulance transfer is arranged to the nearest tertiary hospital for further care. Over the following 12 hours, Julia's air entry, respiratory effort, and oxygen requirements begin to improve. What are the mechanisms of action of ipratropium bromide, hydrocortisone, and aminophylline? Should Julia's daily inhaled corticosteroid preventer be continued while she is in hospital receiving intravenous corticosteroids?

REFERENCES

Australian Bureau of Statistics 2022. National Health Survey 2020-21: Asthma. https://www.abs.gov.au/statistics/health/health-conditions-and-risks/asthma/latest-release

Australian Medicines Handbook 2020. Australian medicines handbook 2020. Adelaide: AMH.

Braun L, Cohen M. Herbs and natural supplements: an evidence-based guide, 4th ed. Sydney: Elsevier, 2015.

Cambie RC, Ash J. Fijian medicinal plants. Australia: CSIRO, 1994.

Centre of Excellence in Treatable Traits. 2023. Asthma in Pregnancy Toolkit. https://asthmapregnancytoolkit.org.au

Clifton V, Das J, Flenady V, Rae K. 2022. Neonatal death is a major concern for Indigenous women with asthma during pregnancy and could be prevented with better models of care. Australian and New Zealand Journal of Obstetrics & Gynaecology, 62, 160–63.

Conte T, Bergeron C, FitzGerald J. 2018. Asthma and pregnancy: a review of management strategies with an emphasis on medication safety and outcomes. Canadian Journal of Respiratory, Critical Care, & Sleep Medicine, 2, 3, 155–165. https://doi.org/10.1080/24745332.2017.1409090

Global Initiative for Asthma. Global Strategy for Asthma Management and Prevention, 2016. Available at: http://www.ginasthma.org.

Hamad A, Sutcliffe A, Knox A. Aspirin-induced asthma: clinical aspects, pathogenesis and management. Drugs. 2004;64(21):2417–2432. doi: 10.2165/00003495-200464210-00004.

Harris K, Mosler G, Williams S, et al. Suboptimal asthma control and asthma medication adherence in UK secondary school children. American Journal of Respiratory and Critical Care Medicine. 2016;193:A2162.

Kuruvilla ME, Lee FE, Lee GB. Understanding asthma phenotypes, endotypes, and mechanisms of disease. Clin Rev Allergy Immunol. 2019;56(2): 219-233. doi: 10.1007/s12016-018-8712-1

Matera MG, Belardo C, Rinaldi M, et al., 2020a. Emerging muscarinic receptor antagonists for the treatment of asthma. Expert Opinion in Emergency Drugs. 2020;25:2:123-130. doi: 10.1080/14728214.2020.1758059

Matera MG, Page CP, Calzetta L, et al, 2020b. Pharmacology and therapeutics of bronchodilators revisited. Pharmacological Reviews 72(1):218-252. doi: 10.1124/pr.119.018150. PMID: 31848208.

Ministry of Health. 2018. Annual Data Explorer 2018/19: New Zealand Health Survey. Wellington: Ministry of Health. https://minhealthnz.shinyapps.io/nz-health-survey-2018-19-annual-data-explorer.

Murphy V. Asthma in pregnancy–management, maternal co-morbidities, and long-term health. Best Practice & Research Clinical Obstetrics and Gynaecology, in press. 2022. https://doi.org/ 10.1016/j.bpobgyn.2022.06.005

NAC (National Asthma Council Australia) 2018. National Asthma Strategy 2018. Melbourne: National Asthma Council Australia. AIHW.

National Asthma Council Australia. Australian Asthma Handbook. Version 2.1. Melbourne: National Asthma Council Australia; 2020. http://www.asthmahandbook.org.au (accessed 15 October 2021)

Page C, O'Shaughnessy B, Barnes P. Pathogenesis of COPD and asthma. Handbook of Experimental Pharmacology 2017; 237:1–21.

Popa M, Peltecu G, Gica N, Ciobanu A, Botezatu R, Gica C, Steriade A, Panaitescu A. 2021. Asthma in pregnancy. Review of current literature and recommendations. Maedica – a Journal of Clinical Medicine, 16(1):80-87. https://doi.org/10.26574/maedica.2021.16.1.80

Respiratory Expert Group. Therapeutic guidelines: respiratory, 6th ed. Melbourne: Therapeutic Guidelines Limited, 2020.

Trivedi R, Richard N, Mehta R, et al. Umeclidinium in patients with COPD: a randomised, placebo-controlled study. European Respiratory Journal. 2014;43:72–81.

Waugh A, Grant A. Ross & Wilson anatomy & physiology in health and illness, 12th ed. London: Churchill Livingstone, 2014.

ONLINE RESOURCES

Asthma and Respiratory Foundation (New Zealand): http://www.asthmafoundation.org.nz/ (accessed 20 January 2022)

Asthma Australia: https://www.asthmaaustralia.org.au (accessed 20 January 2022)

Asthma in Pregnancy Toolkit 2023: https://asthmapregnancytoolkit.org.au

Australian Bureau of Statistics 2022: https://www.abs.gov.au/statistics/health/health-conditions-and-risks/asthma/latest-release (accessed 28 February 2023)

Australian Government Department of Health (search keyword 'asthma'): http://www.health.gov.au/ (accessed 20 January 2022)

Global Initiative for Asthma: http://www.ginasthma.org/ (accessed 20 January 2022)

Medsafe (for specific New Zealand drugs): http://www.medsafe.govt.nz/ (accessed 20 January 2022)

National Asthma Council – Australian asthma handbook: https://www.nationalasthma.org.au/health-professionals/australian-asthma-handbook (accessed 20 January 2022)

National Asthma Council Australia – Action plans: https://www.nationalasthma.org.au/health-professionals/asthma-action-plans/asthma-action-plan-library (accessed 20 January 2022)

National Asthma Council Australia – Asthma cycle of care: https://www.nationalasthma.org.au/living-with-asthma/resources/health-professionals/reports-and-statistics/asthma-cycle-of-care (accessed 20 January 2022)

National Asthma Council Australia – Asthma mortality statistics: https://www.nationalasthma.org.au/living-with-asthma/resources/health-professionals/reports-and-statistics/asthma-mortality-statistics (accessed 20 January 2022)

National Asthma Council Australia – Inhaler technique: https://www.nationalasthma.org.au/living-with-asthma/resources/health-professionals/information-paper/hp-inhaler-technique-for-people-with-asthma-or-copd (accessed 20 January 2022)

World Health Organization: http://www.who.int/tb/en/ (accessed 20 January 2022)

CHAPTER 19

MENTAL HEALTH

Kirsten Small, Maryam Bazargan, Roslyn Donnellan-Fernandez

Key Abbreviations

CAM	complementary and alternative medicine
CNS	central nervous system
ECT	electroconvulsive therapy
GABA	gamma-aminobutyric acid
5-HT	5-hydroxytryptamine (serotonin)
MAO	monoamine oxidase
MAOI	monoamine oxidase inhibitor
PTSD	posttraumatic stress disorder
SNRIs	serotonin noradrenaline reuptake inhibitors
SSRIs	selective serotonin reuptake inhibitors
TCA	tricyclic antidepressant

Key Terms

Chapter Focus

Mental health disorders occur across the life span. They can arise for the first time during pregnancy and the postnatal period, or preexisting mental health issues may change. Anxiety and depression are the most common mental health issues seen during the childbearing year. Both can be appropriate short-term responses to cues in the woman's environment. However, excessive anxiety or low mood that interferes with daily functioning and sleep is counterproductive and usually benefits from assessment and treatment. Bipolar disorder, with shifts between depression and mania, is less common. Deciding on the use of lithium in pregnancy and breastfeeding, commonly used to prevent episodes of mania, is challenging due to safety concerns. Postnatal psychosis is uncommon and is a distressing event. Short-term pharmacological management is often beneficial. This chapter reviews the psychotropic drugs likely to be used in pregnancy and the postnatal period to treat anxiety, depression, mania, and psychotic disorders.

Key Drug Groups

Anti-anxiety agents:

- Benzodiazepines: diazepam (DM 19.1), lorazepam, midazolam
- Benzodiazepine antagonists: flumazenil

Antidepressants:

- Monoamine oxidase inhibitors: phenelzine, tranylcypromine, moclobemide
- Selective serotonin reuptake inhibitors: escitalopram, fluoxetine (DM 19.2), sertraline, paroxetine
- Serotonin noradrenaline (norepinephrine) reuptake inhibitors: duloxetine, venlafaxine, desvenlafaxine
- Tricyclics: imipramine, nortriptyline

Antimania drugs:

- lithium (DM 19.3)

Antipsychotic agents:

- Atypical: olanzapine (DM19.4), quetiapine
- Conventional: chlorpromazine

Learning Outcomes

- Describe the typical features of common mental illnesses that can complicate the childbearing year.
- Describe the major classes of drugs used to manage mental illness and their mechanisms of action.
- Consider the therapeutic approaches for mental health disorders experienced during the childbearing continuum, including factors that influence decision making for specific pharmacotherapeutic agents.
- Outline the drug safety profiles in pregnancy and lactation for medications used to manage mental disorders and describe additional measures to enhance safety.
- Discuss the potential effects on the neonate from exposure to medications used in the management of mental illness during the third trimester.

CRITICAL THINKING SCENARIO

Sara is a 36-year-old mother of two. Her partner Phillip was diagnosed with cancer about a year ago. Sara developed anxiety and reactive depression related to the stress of having to return to the workforce to support the family's finances, while still managing the household and caring for her partner. Her GP referred her for counselling and recommended a trial of fluoxetine, which she found very helpful. Around the time Sara recognised she was pregnant again, her partner's cancer recurred with the expectation he would be unlikely to survive to the end of her pregnancy.

Sara discussed her antidepressant medication with her GP, who advised that she continue with fluoxetine, but not breastfeed. Sara's midwife suggested Sara ask her psychiatrist whether it might be better to change to a different antidepressant, one considered more appropriate for use in breastfeeding. Sara's neighbour suggested she try St John's wort to help get her through this tough time.

1   Outline the reasons why Sara's GP may have advised against breastfeeding.

2   Describe the potential risks and benefits to mother and baby of changing an effective antidepressant during pregnancy.

3   Identify the antidepressants with a more favourable safety profile for use in lactating women than fluoxetine.

4   List the symptoms commonly seen in neonates adjusting to the withdrawal of selective serotonin reuptake inhibitors and describe approaches that can minimise these.

5   What is serotonin syndrome and how might the use of St John's wort in addition to fluoxetine precipitate symptoms of this condition for Sara?

Introduction: Mental health and illness

Mental health is defined by the World Health Organization (2018) as 'a state of well-being in which the person realises his or her own abilities, can cope with the normal stresses of life, can work productively and fruitfully, and is able to make a contribution to his or her community'. This definition involves subjective, sociological, and philosophical aspects of mental health, encompassing a broader perspective than 'psychiatric' illness.

Mental illness in the childbearing year

Mental illness is common, with women more likely to experience a mental illness than men (Biaggi Pariente 2020). Psychosocial factors play a role in this sex-difference. For example, in some societies girls and women have inferior status and roles; less opportunity for education, paid employment or healthcare; and are at risk for violence and abuse. These psychosocial factors interact with differences in hormones – along with physical stressors due to pregnancies, breastfeeding, and the burden of childcare – to increase the risk of mental illness.

The following mental illnesses can complicate the perinatal period (O'Hara et al 2014; Nillni et al 2018; Sharmaet al et al 2020):

- Depression is the most common mental illness, with approximately 15% of women experiencing depression during or after pregnancy. Suicide continues to be a leading cause of death in pregnancy and the 12 months following birth (Chin et al 2022).
- Anxiety disorders impact around 13% of women in the childbearing year and can occur in combination with depression.
- Bipolar disorder affects around 3% of women in the childbearing year.
- Major postpartum psychosis is a rare disorder. It can occur within 1–4 weeks of childbirth with an incidence of 1–2 per 1000 births, often due to underlying bipolar disorder.

In addition to the symptoms women experience relating to their mental illness, these disorders lead to higher risks of pregnancy complications and impact on parenting.

Women with serious mental illness are more likely to develop gestational hypertension, gestational diabetes, or have their infant admitted to the nursery in the

TABLE 19.1 Drugs used in managing mental health conditions and their safety in pregnancy and lactation

DRUG	CLINICAL USE	PREGNANCY SAFETY*	LACTATION SAFETY**
Benzodiazepines: e.g. diazepam	Anxiety, sedation, seizures	• Neonatal adjustment syndrome may occur after use in third trimester • Categories B3 or C	• Most are L2 or L3
Monoamine oxidase inhibitors (MAOIs): e.g. phenelzine	Depression	• Rarely used • Category B3	• Rarely used • L4
Tricyclic antidepressants (TCAs): e.g. imipramine	Depression	• Rarely used • Category C	• Most are L2 or L3
Selective serotonin reuptake inhibitors (SSRIs): e.g. fluoxetine, sertraline, paroxetine	Depression	• Neonatal adjustment syndrome may occur after use in third trimester • Paroxetine associated with congenital cardiac defects – category D • Fluoxetine associated with persistent pulmonary hypertension – category C	• Most are L2
Serotonin noradrenaline reuptake inhibitors (SNRIs): e.g. duloxetine, venlafaxine	Depression	• Category B2 or B3	• L3
Reversible inhibitors of MOAI-A (RIMAs): e.g. moclobemide	Depression	• Category B3	• L4
Lithium	Mania in bipolar disorder	• Small increased risk of cardiac and other anomalies • Category D	• Avoid dehydration of the neonate • L4
First-generation antipsychotics: e.g. chlorpromazine	**Psychosis**	• Rarely used • Category D	• L3
Second-generation antipsychotics: e.g. olanzepine	Psychosis	• Monitor for hyperglycaemia • Category C	• L2

* Therapeutic Goods Administration – Prescribing medicines in pregnancy database
** Dr Hale's Lactation Risk Categories

perinatal period (Galbally et al 2019). Preterm birth, low birth weight, and unplanned caesarean section are also more common among women with serious mental illness (Edvardsson et al 2022). The degree to which the mental illness or the medications used to manage it contributes to these outcomes is unclear. Drugs reviewed in this chapter for their use in the management of mental health conditions and their potential effects during pregnancy and lactation are summarised in Table 19.1.

Mental illness in Indigenous populations

Indigenous communities worldwide have suffered disruptions after colonisation, with subsequent discrimination, dispossession, poverty, poor health, suppression of traditional cultures and family supports, and lack of educational and employment opportunities. These are established risk factors for psychological distress and mental illness, particularly for depression, anxiety, and substance abuse.

KEY POINTS

Mental illness in the childbearing year

- Mental illnesses, such as depression, anxiety, bipolar disorder, and psychosis can complicate the childbearing year.
- Women with significant mental illness are at increased risk of pregnancy complications.

19.1 Pathophysiology of mental health disorders

It should be noted the causes and pathophysiology of mental illness are still relatively poorly understood, and research continues. Drugs used in the management of mental illness target one or more neurotransmitters. To understand the actions of the medications in this chapter, it is important to review current knowledge of neurotransmitters.

Monoamine neurotransmitters

The monoamine neurotransmitters (acetylcholine, catecholamines, dopamine, histamine, and serotonin or 5-HT), are particularly involved in the aetiology, pathogenesis, and pharmacological treatment of psychosis and depression. GABA receptor sites are the target for antianxiety agents. While there may be evidence that a transmitter is depleted in a condition (e.g. 5-HT in depression), or is present in increased levels (e.g. dopamine in schizophrenia), or that enhancement of a transmitter improves people's symptoms (e.g. selective serotonin reuptake inhibitors [SSRIs] in depression), many links in the cause–effect–treatment chain remain to be completed.

Dopamine

Dopamine is both a neurotransmitter and a precursor for noradrenaline. It is particularly important in psychosis. D_1 and D_2 receptors are the main types involved with movement disorders in the basal ganglia and are influenced by antipsychotic agents with **extrapyramidal effects** due to dopamine receptor antagonism. Newer antipsychotic agents with low affinity for D_2 receptors are less apt to cause extrapyramidal effects. Further research may produce more specific agents with fewer adverse effects.

Noradrenaline

Noradrenergic pathways are thought to have global activating functions in response to sensory stimuli. Noradrenaline has important roles in arousal, autonomic control, and mood and reward systems. Noradrenergic neurons innervate virtually the entire CNS, from the cerebral cortex to all spinal levels. Many antidepressants enhance noradrenergic transmission by inhibiting reuptake of noradrenaline into nerve terminals.

5-hydroxytryptamine (5-HT; serotonin)

5-HT usually decreases the discharge rate in neurons and hence is inhibitory. Many drugs that mimic or block actions of 5-HT produce changes in mood and behaviour. The efficacy of the SSRIs in treating major depression provides evidence that 5-HT function is impaired in depressive illness.

Histamine

Histamine, although not a catecholamine, is included among the monoamine transmitters. Systemically administered antihistamines cause CNS effects (sedation, hunger), evidence for roles of histamine in the brain. Many antidepressants have antagonistic activity on histamine receptors. They therefore frequently cause sedation, weight gain, and antiemetic effects.

GABA

Gamma amino butyric acid (GABA) is the main inhibitory transmitter in the brain, at about 30% of all CNS synapses, in many pathways and brain areas. The limbic system, associated with the regulation of emotional behaviour, contains a highly dense area of GABA binding sites in the amygdala, suggesting the antianxiety effects occur there. Stimulation of GABA receptors produces decreased excitability of the neuron leading to sedative, anxiolytic, muscle relaxant, or cognitive effects.

KEY POINTS

Mental illness and CNS neurotransmitters

- There are several individual disorders, such as anxiety, depression, psychosis, and bipolar affective disorder, that can be managed with pharmacological intervention.

- Psychoactive drugs may affect balances in CNS neurotransmitter levels, especially the monoamines noradrenaline, dopamine, and **5-HT (serotonin)**. These neurotransmitters are involved in the pathogenesis and clinical manifestations of mental illnesses.

- For many mental illnesses there may be evidence that a transmitter is depleted in a condition or that enhancement of a transmitter improves the condition. A neurotransmitter may be present in increased levels and blockade of receptors alleviates symptoms.

- Many antidepressants have antagonistic activity on histamine receptors and therefore frequently cause sedation, weight gain, and antiemetic effects.

19.2 Approaches to therapy

It is important that all maternity services provide further assessment, support, referral, and management for women with perinatal mental health disorders. Women with well-managed and mild symptoms from preexisting mental illness can typically be managed by their primary care provider (midwife, general practitioner, or obstetrician). Women with more serious or less stable mental illnesses benefit from a multi-disciplinary approach with the involvement (where available) of a dedicated specialist perinatal mental health service (Schofield et al 2019).

Non-drug therapy

In mild mental disorders, non-drug therapies are used first. In this context, drugs may be no more effective than placebos. Psychotherapies include treatments based on a relationship between a person needing help for psychological distress or disturbed behaviour, and a trained health professional (e.g. psychologist, psychiatrist, social worker) who uses interventions to deal with a crisis, improve specific symptoms, facilitate self-awareness, or provide long-term supportive help. Types of therapies include psychoanalysis, group psychotherapy, self-help groups, counselling, behaviour modification therapy, and cognitive behaviour therapy.

DRUGS AT A GLANCE
Drugs used in the management of mental health conditions

PHARMACOLOGICAL GROUP AND EFFECT	KEY EXAMPLES	CLINICAL USE
Antianxiety Agents		
Benzodiazepines • Facilitate GABA binding	Diazepam	Sedation, anxiety
Antidepressants		
Tricyclic antidepressants (TCAs) • Block reuptake of noradrenaline and 5-HT into nerve terminals	Imipramine Amitryptiline Nortryptiline	Depression, bipolar disorder, generalised anxiety disorder
Monoamine oxidase inhibitors (MAOIs); non-selective • Inhibit both MAO-A and MAO-B enzymes for 2–3 weeks • Desensitise the α_2- or β-adrenoceptors and 5-HT receptors (downregulation) • Increase levels of monoamine neurotransmitters	Tranylcypromine	Moderate-to-severe depression, bipolar disorder
Selective serotonin reuptake inhibitors (SSRIs) • Block reuptake of serotonin (5-HT) into nerve terminal via the transporter (SERT)	Fluoxetine (es) citalopram	Depression, bipolar disorder, generalised anxiety disorder
Serotonin noradrenaline reuptake inhibitors (SNRIs) • Block reuptake of noradrenaline and 5-HT into nerve terminals via blockade of the serotonin transporter (SERT) and NET	Venlafaxine, desvenlafaxine	Moderate-to-severe depression, bipolar disorder, generalised anxiety disorder
Antimanic Agents		
Lithium • Mechanism generally unknown. It inhibits G-protein coupling with receptors, adenylate cyclase activity, phosphoinositol cycling and various phosphokinase activities inhibits transmitter release (especially dopamine) at synapses, increases the turnover of noradrenaline and 5-HT, and decreases postsynaptic receptor sensitivity		**Mania** in bipolar disorder
Mood stabilisers • Various mechanisms as per antiepileptics including blockade of sodium channels to reduce neuronal firing	Antiepileptic drugs, sodium valproate	Acute mania
Antipsychotic Agents		
Phenothiazines – conventional (typical) • Antagonism of D_1 and D_2 dopamine receptors	Chlorpromazine	Schizophrenia Behavioural emergencies
Atypical antipsychotics • Partial agonist at D_2 and 5-HT_{1A} receptors, and antagonist at 5-HT_{2A} receptors • Antagonises D_1, D_2 and D_4 dopamine receptors, with less affinity for D_2 receptors, so is less apt to induce extrapyramidal effects • α_1-adrenoceptors and histamine H_1 receptors • Antagonist at both 5-HT_{2A} and dopamine D_2 receptors	Olanzapine	Psychosis
Antimanic Agents		
Lithium Mechanism generally unknown. It inhibits G-protein coupling with receptors, adenylate cyclase activity, phosphoinositol cycling and various phosphokinase activities inhibits transmitter release (especially dopamine) at synapses, increases the turnover of noradrenaline and 5-HT in the brain, and decreases postsynaptic receptor sensitivity		Mania
Mood stabilisers Various mechanisms as per antiepileptics, including blockade of sodium channels to reduce neuronal firing	Antiepileptic drugs, sodium valproate	Acute mania

Pharmacotherapy

While people with mild mental illnesses may be treated successfully with non-drug psychotherapies, those with moderate-to-severe disorders are more likely to benefit from additional drug therapy. Drug therapy reduces mood and behaviour symptoms and allows the person to participate more fully in other non-pharmacological forms of treatment.

Risks for the woman and her fetus from untreated mental illness during pregnancy need to be weighed against the risk of exposing the fetus to pharmacological agents. A single drug generally considered safest in pregnancy and/or lactation, in the lowest effective dose should be used, with appropriate follow-up and support. Polytherapy may be necessary when co-morbid conditions exist (such as anxiety and depression), or if a single agent has not achieved the desired result. Most drugs used in the management of mental illness cross the placenta and can cause clinical effects, or after birth lead to adjustment symptoms in the neonate. Decision making in the postnatal period is more complex as the options include either breastfeeding or not, while using medications or not. (See Chapter 10.)

The following are general guidelines for prescribing drugs for the management of mental illness in the childbearing year:

- Thorough diagnostic assessment is necessary.
- Drugs should be used only if essential, in addition to, not in place of, other therapies.
- Drug therapy needs to be tailored to the specific woman.
- Information about the expected time-course of response and likely adverse effects should be shared as part of an informed decision-making conversation.
- The simplest and lowest effective dose regimen and regular follow-up are important.

CLINICAL FOCUS BOX 19.1

Complementary and alternative medicines and mental illness

Many natural products and techniques from complementary and alternative medicine (CAM) have been used to attain relief from symptoms of mental illness. Enquiry about the prior use of these approaches is important during assessment of a woman with new or changed symptoms of mental illness.

In the treatment of anxiety, music therapy, massage, acupuncture, selenium, yoga, and many herbs have been shown to be effective. Some herbs act via the same pathways as conventional medications – such as St John's wort with its action similar to a tricyclic antidepressant (see CFB 19.2). The neuropharmacological effects of ginseng, peony extract, albizia, perilla, fuzi, rhodilia rosea, saffron, gingko biloba, valerian, lemon balm, angelica, and lavender oil; and the Chinese herbs chai hu, and suan zo ren have all been studied. Each has some potential for effectiveness in mental health disorders (Liu et al 2015).

Informed decision making in mental illness

Decision making requires balancing the risks and benefits of proposed interventions against those of untreated mental illness (Anderson et al 2020). The SAFEDLCT mnemonic is one way to consider structuring conversations about medication use (Sprague et al 2020):

- *Supply:* Does the drug impact milk supply?
- *Alternatives:* Are there other effective medications/therapies?

- *Formula:* Consider the potential risks of not breastfeeding
- Effectiveness of the drug for the woman's condition
- Duration of treatment anticipated
- *Levels:* Consider pharmacokinetics impacting drug levels in fetus and infant
- *Child characteristics:* Consider gestation, infant age, prior exposure to drug therapy, or health issues that might impact on pharmacokinetics
- Talk with the woman and her family to assess and address concerns.

In the context of mental illness, the concept of informed decision making can be difficult. People may need support and assistance to make decisions about their treatment. Negotiations should be documented, which may involve signing appropriate consent forms. Some of these medications have unpleasant and disabling adverse effects, and initially treatment might seem worse than the disease. Adhering to drug therapy is sometimes an issue for this reason. A combination of good prescribing choices (such as drugs with simple daily dosing and lower rates of adverse events), along with professional and social support (regular reminders and monitoring of the effectiveness of therapy) can assist.

Discontinuation of therapy and rebound effects

Withdrawal effects after discontinuing therapy are related more to rebound phenomena than to dependence on the drug. For example, after cessation of antidepressant therapy, there may be agitation and insomnia. These effects may be avoided by slow tapering off the drug. Because of the long-term nature of many mental health conditions, relapse may occur, and the recommencement of drug treatment be appropriate at a future point (Henssler et al 2019).

KEY POINTS

Clinical aspects of drug therapy in psychiatry

- People with mild mental disorders may be treated successfully with non-drug psychotherapies.
- Drug therapy reduces mood and behaviour symptoms and allows people to participate in other forms of treatment.
- General guidelines for prescribing psychotropic drugs include:
  - carrying out a thorough diagnostic assessment
  - using drugs only if essential, in addition to other therapies
  - tailoring drug therapy to the specific woman
  - sharing information about the expected time-course of response and likely adverse effects.

- Adherence to long-term antipsychotic drug therapy is sometimes an issue due to the wide-ranging side effects of these drugs. Many of these medications have unpleasant and disabling adverse effects.

- Adherence can be enhanced by using the simplest and lowest effective dose regimen and using regular follow-up.

- After discontinuing therapy, withdrawal effects are often related to rebound phenomena rather than dependence on the drug. Effects may be avoided by slow tapering.

19.3 Anxiety

Anxiety is a state of apprehension, agitation, uncertainty, and fear resulting from the experience or anticipation of some stress or danger. It may impact sleep and interfere with day-to-day activities. Anxiety is usually a natural psychological and physiological response to a personally threatening situation such as a threat to one's health, loved ones, job, or lifestyle. Generally, this anxiety stimulates constructive actions to counteract the perceived threat. In its extreme form, anxiety can be characterised by autonomic nervous system responses including rapid heart rate, dry mouth, sweaty palms, insomnia, loss of appetite, muscle tremor, diarrhoea, and dyspnoea.

Anxiety in the childbearing year

Anxiety disorders are common, impacting about 13% of women during pregnancy and the postnatal period (Nillni et al 2018). Women may have specific anxieties about aspects of pregnancy or birth, or more generalised concerns that are difficult to control and persist over a long period of time (Harp 2021). Worries are often accompanied by other symptoms such as restlessness, fatigue, poor concentration, tense muscles, and poor sleep. A subset of women with anxiety experience panic attacks. These involve sudden onset of fear or discomfort accompanied by physical symptoms such as shortness of breath, tachycardia, chest pain, dizziness, trembling, and numbness. Some women use compulsions (behaviours or mental acts) to manage anxiety symptoms, such as repeatedly checking on the baby, or arranging and rearranging items in the baby's room.

When excessive anxiety interferes with daily functioning, it may be beneficial to offer treatment. Non-pharmacological treatments such as counselling and behaviour modification therapies are available, while **anxiolytic** drugs (**antianxiety agents**) are sometimes prescribed for the short-term treatment of anxiety. These drugs reduce feelings of excessive anxiety, such as apprehension, fear, and panic, and reduce the physiological responses, such as dyspnoea and insomnia, thus improving sleep patterns. While benzodiazepines and tricyclic antidepressants may sometimes be used in pregnancy, selective serotonin reuptake inhibitors and serotonin and norepinephrine reuptake inhibitors are preferred antianxiety medications during pregnancy.

Benzodiazepines

Benzodiazepines are among the most widely prescribed drugs, primarily because of their advantages over older agents such as barbiturates, chloral hydrate, and alcohol; and their action as anxiolytics. These advantages include:

- specific dose-related anxiolytic action
- lower fatality rates following acute toxicity and overdose
- lower potential for abuse
- more favourable adverse effect profiles
- fewer potentially serious drug interactions when administered with other medications
- the availability of a specific antidote (flumazenil).

Diazepam (Valium; see DM 19.1) is the prototype benzodiazepine. Newer and safer shorter acting benzodiazepines have replaced its use for many indications. As the various benzodiazepines have similar pharmacodynamic effects, they will be discussed as a group.

Flumazenil is an antagonist at the benzodiazepine binding site on the $GABA_A$ receptor, where it decreases the binding of GABA. Flumazenil is anxiogenic and is used to treat benzodiazepine overdoses.

Management of benzodiazepine overdose

Benzodiazepine overdose is manifest as CNS depression, ranging from confusion and drowsiness through to coma, hypotonia, hypotension, and respiratory depression. Overdose is not usually life-threatening unless multiple other CNS-depressant drugs have been taken. Supportive treatment is necessary and may include maintaining an adequate airway with oxygen for depressed respiration, monitoring vital signs, and promoting diuresis by administering IV fluids. Hypotension must be monitored and might require vasopressors such as noradrenaline (norepinephrine) or dopamine. Flumazenil can reverse the effects of benzodiazepines at the GABA receptor.

Tolerance and dependence associated with benzodiazepine use

With chronic administration, tolerance develops to the sedative effects but less often to the anxiolytic effects. Dependence is common and leads to craving, overuse, and abuse of these drugs, and drug-seeking behaviours. Dependence can develop after only a few days' use of benzodiazepines, and withdrawal from chronic use of the drugs can be difficult. Gradual withdrawal from hypnotic drugs is recommended, for example dose reductions of 10–20% per week, with a few days to stabilise at each dose level.

DRUG MONOGRAPH 19.1
Diazepam

Diazepam is the prototype benzodiazepine and, as such, has anxiolytic, sedative–hypnotic, muscle relaxant, and antiseizure actions.

Mechanism of action

Diazepam acts on $GABA_A$ receptors leading to more neuronal inhibition. This results in the clinical effects of diazepam.

Indications

Diazepam is indicated for short-term (a few days) management of anxiety, acute withdrawal from alcohol or benzodiazepines, acute behavioural disturbance, muscle spasm and spasticity, premedication and conscious sedation, and as adjunctive treatment for seizures such as in status epilepticus and eclampsia.

Pharmacokinetics

Diazepam is one of the longest-acting benzodiazepines because it is very lipid-soluble and has active metabolites. Other benzodiazepines may be better options when short-acting sedation is the aim, for example temazepam or midazolam.

Adverse reactions

All benzodiazepines can cause excessive CNS depression, dependence, and neurological dysfunction. Diazepam is likely to cause fatigue, drowsiness, and muscle weakness. Less common adverse effects include disturbances of memory, gastrointestinal tract function, genitourinary functions, and vision and skin reactions. Paradoxical CNS stimulation can occur. Tolerance and dependence develop readily.

Drug interactions

Diazepam has additive CNS-depressant effects when used with any other CNS depressants, including alcohol, other sedative–hypnotics, antihistamines, anaesthetics, antidepressants, and antiepileptic agents. Many drugs can inhibit the metabolism of diazepam and hence prolong its effects, for example cimetidine and fluconazole (see also DI 19.1).

Warnings and contraindications

Diazepam is contraindicated in people with chronic obstructive airways disease, severe respiratory or liver disease, sleep apnoea, myasthenia gravis, dependence on other substances, or hypersensitivity to benzodiazepines. It should be prescribed only for short periods. Dependence develops readily and a long withdrawal period may be necessary to avoid withdrawal seizures. Diazepam should be used with caution in people with glaucoma, impaired kidney or liver function, depression or psychosis, and during pregnancy or lactation. In pregnancy shorter acting benzodiazepines are preferred.

Dosage and administration

Dosage should be individualised, depending on the indication for which the drug is prescribed and the clinical condition of the person it is prescribed for:

- Agitation and anxiety: diazepam is normally given orally, the adult dose being 2–5 mg up to a maximum of 10 mg daily. It can also be administered IV or by rectal solution.
- Acute severe anxiety, agitation, behaviour disturbance, seizures: IV, 5–10 mg, repeated if necessary every 5–10 minutes to a maximum of 30 mg.

DRUG INTERACTIONS 19.1
Benzodiazepines

DRUG OR DRUG GROUP	LIKELY EFFECTS AND MANAGEMENT
CNS depressants such as alcohol, antihistamines, antianxiety agents, opioids, other sedatives/hypnotics, psychotropic agents (especially clozapine), and antidepressants	Enhanced CNS-depressant effects, sedation, and respiratory depression. Monitoring is necessary because the dosage of one or both drugs may need adjustment
Many drugs can inhibit the metabolism of benzodiazepines (especially drugs that inhibit CYP3A4). Examples are azole antifungals (itraconazole), cimetidine, verapamil, omeprazole, macrolide antibiotics (erythromycin, clarithromycin), fluoxetine, and some HIV antivirals	CNS depression and respiratory depression effects of benzodiazepines are prolonged. Reduce dose or substitute a non-interacting drug
Drugs can increase benzodiazepine metabolism (carbamazepine, phenytoin, rifampicin, St John's wort)	Higher dose of benzodiazepine may be required
Stimulant drugs such as theophylline may reduce the sedative effects of benzodiazepines	Increase benzodiazepine dose if necessary
Drugs that lower the seizure threshold, including many antipsychotics, antivirals, and antimicrobials	Benzodiazepines used cautiously, if at all

Withdrawal is characterised by CNS stimulation: anxiety, sleep disorders, aching limbs, palpitations, and nervousness. These symptoms reflect those seen in neonates born to mothers who regularly used benzodiazepines in the third trimester. Seizures can occur in people who previously used high doses.

Warnings and contraindications

Benzodiazepines are contraindicated in people with respiratory depression or sleep apnoea, severe hepatic impairment, or myasthenia gravis. They should be used with caution during pregnancy or lactation and in people with renal impairment.

KEY POINTS

Anxiety and the benzodiazepines

- Anxiety is a state of apprehension, agitation, uncertainty, and fear resulting from the experience or anticipation of some stress or danger. It can impact on sleep cycles and interfere with day-to-day activities.

- Anxiety disorders affect approximately 13% of women and may present either as generalised anxiety or specific worries related to pregnancy and birth.

- Anxiolytic drugs (antianxiety agents) are commonly prescribed for the short-term treatment of anxiety. Drugs used for anxiety include benzodiazepines, antidepressants, and antipsychotics.

- Benzodiazepines, such as diazepam, are used to treat anxiety and insomnia, as preoperative medication, and for seizure disorders. They act by facilitation of GABA-mediated CNS inhibitory pathways.

- Drug interactions frequently occur with other CNS depressants and with drugs that affect the metabolism of benzodiazepines. Common adverse reactions include excessive CNS depression, tolerance, and dependence.

- Benzodiazepine overdose is manifest as CNS depression. Overdose is not usually life-threatening. Supportive treatment is necessary.

- With chronic administration, tolerance develops to the sedative effects of the benzodiazepines but less often to the anxiolytic effects. Dependence is common. Withdrawal can be difficult.

19.4 Depression

Criteria for a major depressive disorder include the presence of:

- *mood changes* (sadness, guilt feelings, self-pity, pessimism, and loss of interest in life and social activities). These are often worse in the morning.
- *psychological symptoms* (low self-esteem, poor concentration, hopeless or helpless feelings, indecisiveness, and suicidal tendencies or increased focus on death)

- *physiological manifestations* (sleep disturbances, decreased interest in sex, loss of energy, menstrual dysfunction, headaches, palpitations, constipation, loss of appetite, and weight loss or gain)
- *thought alterations* (a decreased ability to concentrate, poor memory, confusion; or delusions relating to health, persecution, or religion).

Depression in the childbearing year

Depression is as common in the antenatal period as it is postpartum (Molenaar et al 2018). While not the only effective therapeutic approach, antidepressants are commonly used, with around 70% of women with depression managed with medication (Molenaar et al 2018). Other treatments include reducing environmental stressors, psychotherapy, treatment with **electroconvulsive therapy** (ECT), and transcranial magnetic stimulation. Herbal remedies like St John's wort are popular. Referral to a specialist perinatal mental health service is advisable in severe depression when psychotherapy and first-line pharmaceutical measures have been ineffective.

Decisions about whether to use antidepressants during and after pregnancy are complex. Untreated depression increases the rate of preterm birth, low birth weight, gestational hypertension; and behavioural, emotional, cognitive, and motor problems in the infant, along with issues with mother–child bonding (Molenaar et al 2018). These balance against documented associations between antidepressant use in pregnancy with cardiovascular malformations, persistent pulmonary hypertension, neonatal adaptation syndrome, preterm birth, low birth weight, and psychiatric disorders in later life (Molenaar et al 2018).

Antidepressant drugs

The first **antidepressant** drugs were discovered by chance. Iproniazide, a tuberculosis treatment, and imipramine, a drug being tested for schizophrenia, were found to elevate the mood. This led to studies of the actions and mechanisms of similar drugs, called 'first-generation' antidepressants: the **monoamine oxidase inhibitors** (MAOIs, iproniazide-like) and the **tricyclic antidepressants** (TCAs, such as imipramine), respectively. Second-generation antidepressants include SSRIs, **serotonin noradrenaline reuptake inhibitors** (SNRIs) and **reversible inhibitors of MAO-A** (RIMAs). Third-generation antidepressants are those not confined to serotonin reuptake inhibition. These include venlafaxine, reboxetine, and mirtazapine.

Mechanisms of action of antidepressants

The following mechanisms of action are generally accepted:

- MAOIs (e.g. moclobemide) inhibit MAO enzymes found in neuronal mitochondria responsible for metabolising noradrenaline, dopamine and 5-HT, thus allowing a buildup of the neurotransmitter available for release.

- Many antidepressants (including the tricyclics) inhibit the reuptake of noradrenaline or 5-HT, increasing the amount of the neurotransmitter available. These drugs have many sympathetic nervous system side effects. They also have significant anticholinergic actions, and can cause sleepiness, weakness, and impaired cognition.
- SSRIs (e.g. fluoxetine) are more potent inhibitors of 5-HT reuptake than of noradrenaline. They have fewer side effects and are less lethal in overdose than the TCAs. SSRIs now dominate antidepressant prescribing in Australia and New Zealand.
- SNRIs (e.g. venlafaxine) act by inhibiting reuptake of both 5-HT and noradrenaline.

Antidepressant drug therapy: Clinical aspects

Indications for antidepressant drugs

Antidepressants are administered in moderate-to-severe depressive disorder to relieve psychological and physical symptoms, improve general functioning, and reduce self-harm or suicide. They are also useful in a range of other conditions including posttraumatic stress disorder, some anxiety disorders, premenstrual syndrome, and as adjunctive therapy in neuropathic pain and migraine. People with mild depressive disorders are unlikely to benefit from antidepressant drugs, with non-drug therapies a better option.

Selecting an antidepressant

Antidepressants appear to have similar efficacies, although there is a wide variability in individual responses. The *Australian Medicines Handbook* (2023) and *Therapeutic Guidelines: Psychotropic* (2021) recommend the SSRIs (other than paroxetine and fluoxetine) as first-line therapy for the treatment of perinatal depression. Women who are already stabilised on an antidepressant are advised to continue with the same agent when planning pregnancy (Molenaar et al 2018), though some may wish to switch from paroxetine, or fluoxetine if breastfeeding is planned, to an SSRI considered safer.

Selecting an antidepressant is empirical, taking into consideration any concurrent conditions and medications, the adverse effect or drug interaction potential of the drug, and the person's previous responses. Potential toxicity in overdose is also important, especially if suicide is a risk – SSRIs are safer than TCAs in this regard.

In the context of safety in pregnancy and breastfeeding, the risks of depression to mother and baby must be considered, as well as risks from antidepressants.

All antidepressants readily cross the placental barrier (Ray et al 2014). Paroxetine is considered contraindicated in pregnancy, as it has been associated with a higher rate of congenital cardiac defects following first trimester exposure (Hanley et al 2014). Some women choose to continue paroxetine and have detailed cardiac morphology assessment on ultrasound during pregnancy, and pulse oximetry assessment of the baby after birth to detect any defects.

Increasing blood volume and glomerular filtration with advancing gestational age results in higher clearance rates and lower serum concentrations of antidepressants (Ray et al 2014). Dose increases may need to occur to maintain efficacy.

After birth, levels of antidepressant medication in the newborn fall. This reduction can lead to a constellation of short-term symptoms, known as neonatal adjustment syndrome. Symptoms include respiratory distress, feeding difficulty, jitteriness and seizures, temperature instability, sleep problems, irritability, jaundice, and hypoglycaemia (Hanley et al 2014). Approximately 30% of infants with third trimester exposure to an SSRI show signs of neonatal adjustment syndrome, but the symptoms are mostly mild and pass within 2 weeks of birth. Third trimester exposure to SSRIs, in particular fluoxetine, appears to increase the incidence of persistent pulmonary hypertension in the neonate (Hanley et al 2014). The risk is small, and findings about the risk are inconsistent across different studies.

The SSRIs appear to be safe with respect to transfer into breast milk, except for fluoxetine. Fluoxetine has a longer half-life than other SSRIs and achieves higher breast milk concentrations (Molenaar et al 2018), therefore increasing risks for adverse impacts in the breastfed infant.

Delayed onset of action

Antidepressants have a long-delayed onset of action. Some improvement in clinical symptoms may be apparent in 2–3 weeks and full effects may not appear for 6–8 weeks. The initial drug should be commenced at low dose, increasing over 2–4 weeks, then in recommended doses for an adequate period and compliance checked before changing to another class. During this period, people are at risk of deepening depression and increased suicidal thoughts and may need additional psychotherapeutic and practical support. After symptoms improve, therapy for a major depressive episode should be continued for at least 6 months or into the postnatal period for women first diagnosed during pregnancy.

Stopping therapy

Rebound effects may occur on withdrawal. Withdrawal from TCAs with strong anticholinergic actions leads to typical parasympathetic effects (salivation, urination, diarrhoea), while withdrawal from SSRIs, SNRIs or mirtazapine may lead to anxiety, agitation, and confusion. Withdrawal effects may occur after missing just one or two doses of drugs with a short half-life.

Tricyclic antidepressants

Tricyclic antidepressants were the first major group of drugs successful in treating depression and tend to have names ending in -mipramine or -tryptyline (e.g. imipramine and amitriptyline, respectively). Their chemical structures have three rings, hence their group name. All TCAs act by the same mechanism, inhibition of reuptake of noradrenaline and 5-HT into nerve terminals, and appear to have similar efficacies, leading to improved mood.

Other actions include antagonism of receptors for other transmitters, acetylcholine (muscarinic), histamine H_1, noradrenaline α_1 and 5-HT, leading to adverse drug reactions in many body systems, including anticholinergic effects, sexual dysfunction, weight gain, and sedation, and these actions make the drugs particularly unsafe in overdose. TCAs have been largely overtaken by safer drugs such as the SSRIs for this reason. They are rarely used in pregnancy and lactation.

The herbal remedy St John's wort has been shown to have a similar mechanism of action to the TCAs, acting by inhibition of monoamine reuptake and metabolism. Hence, it has some similar actions, adverse reactions, and interactions (CFB 19.2).

CLINICAL FOCUS BOX 19.2

St John's wort

Extracts of the plant St John's wort (*Hypericum perforatum*) have been used for more than 2000 years for their medicinal properties ('wort' is an old English word for herb). It is believed to be the most widely prescribed herbal medicine worldwide, with about 450 products containing St John's wort listed for sale in Australia. St John's wort has been shown to block reuptake of monoamine neurotransmitters, bind to GABA receptors, upregulate 5-HT receptors, and inhibit MAO and COMT enzymes.

Double-blind, randomised controlled trials subjected to meta-analysis have shown St John's wort to be more effective than placebo in depression but less effective than tricyclic antidepressants. Rates of adverse effects are low, but serotonin syndrome and drug interactions can occur, so it should not be taken with other antidepressants. Hypericum extracts are potent inducers of hepatic drug-metabolising enzymes and can reduce the levels and efficacy of important drugs such as oral contraceptives. Women should be asked about their use of all remedies – prescription, non-prescription, and complementary.

Sources: Braun et al 2014; Sarris 2014.

Monoamine oxidase inhibitor antidepressants

MAO, an enzyme found in mitochondrial membranes in nerve terminals, the liver, and the brain, inactivates and degrades various monoamines. Tyramine, catecholamines (noradrenaline, adrenaline, and dopamine), 5-HT and several amine drugs are all substrates for the enzyme. MAOIs inhibit the enzyme and thus impair inactivation of amine neurotransmitters and may potentiate their actions, particularly the vasopressor effects, causing high blood pressure. Members of this drug class include phenelzine, tranylcypromine, and moclobemide.

The early MAOIs are irreversible and non-selective in their inhibitory effects. They raise levels of monoamines, but there is a long delay in mood improvement. There are many serious adverse reactions, including autonomic and sexual dysfunction, orthostatic hypotension or severe hypertension, serotonin syndrome, and insomnia. Because of serious adverse drug reactions and interactions, MAOIs are now indicated only as second- or third-line antidepressants for depression that does not respond to other, safer drugs. They are rarely used in pregnancy and lactation.

Selective serotonin reuptake inhibitors

SSRIs are as effective as other antidepressants and considerably safer than TCAs. They have become first-line treatment, including during pregnancy and lactation. SSRIs are indicated to treat depression and anxiety disorders, eating disorders, and premenstrual syndrome. They have similar delayed onset of action to the TCAs. Unlike the TCAs, which often cause weight gain, the SSRIs (except paroxetine) can cause anorexia and weight loss. They are the least toxic antidepressants in overdose.

SSRIs block reuptake of serotonin (5-HT). The first, fluoxetine (DM 19.2), was so successful that it rapidly took over the market for antidepressants. Fluoxetine was soon followed by sertraline, fluvoxamine, paroxetine, and citalopram, then the active S-isomer of the latter, escitalopram. There are potential drug interactions, especially with other antidepressants and with drugs implicated in serotonin syndrome. SSRIs can also inhibit the metabolism of many drugs (DI 19.2).

Serotonin noradrenaline reuptake inhibitors

The relatively new SNRIs act like the old TCAs via inhibition of reuptake of noradrenaline and 5-HT but are more specific. This group includes duloxetine, venlafaxine, and its metabolite desvenlafaxine. They are indicated in major depression, and some also in generalised anxiety and panic disorder. Their use is uncommon in pregnancy and lactation.

Adverse effects include autonomic, CNS, and sexual dysfunctions. They may provoke manic episodes or seizures, and reduced platelet aggregation can cause GIT bleeding. Venlafaxine has been associated with stress cardiomyopathy as an adverse effect. In theory, there

DRUG MONOGRAPH 19.2
Fluoxetine

Mechanism of action

Fluoxetine (well known by its original trade name, Prozac) is an SSRI antidepressant, inhibiting reuptake of 5-HT more than of noradrenaline. It is less effective at antagonism of acetylcholine, histamine, and α-adrenergic receptors than tricyclic antidepressants.

Indications

Fluoxetine is indicated in major depression, obsessive–compulsive disorder, and premenstrual syndrome. It can also be used for bulimia nervosa, panic disorder, and posttraumatic stress disorder. It helps elevate mood, relieve other symptoms, and reduce social impairment.

Pharmacokinetics

Fluoxetine is readily absorbed after oral administration and reaches peak plasma levels after about 6–8 hours. It is highly protein-bound and has a very high volume of distribution. It is extensively metabolised in the liver but has non-linear kinetics as it inhibits its own metabolism. With chronic administration the half-lives of fluoxetine and its metabolite norfluoxetine are, respectively, 4–6 and 9–16 days. Hence, it takes some weeks to achieve steady-state concentration or to eliminate the active metabolite after discontinuation of the drug, and there is an extended period for drug interactions. Metabolites are excreted via the kidneys.

Drug interactions

Fluoxetine inhibits metabolism by the CYP2D6 and CYP3A4 isoenzymes. It raises plasma levels of drugs metabolised by these enzymes, including many antiepileptic drugs, antipsychotics, benzodiazepines, tricyclic antidepressants, and St John's wort. It interacts with other serotonergic agents implicated in serotonin syndrome (DI 19.2).

Adverse reactions

Common reactions include rashes, anxiety, dizziness, weight loss, nausea, and headaches. Seizures are rare. There is debate as to whether antidepressants increase the risk of suicide in depression, or whether this relates to worsening symptoms while waiting for the drug effects to begin.

Warnings and contraindications

People need to be warned of possible adverse effects, of the delay before therapeutic effects, and of caution required if driving or operating machinery. The dose needs to be reduced in severe liver disease. Fluoxetine readily crosses the placenta and can cause neonatal adjustment syndrome. It is not recommended during lactation due to its lipid solubility and long half-life.

Dosage and administration

The usual starting dose is 20 mg/day taken in the morning, which may be increased after several weeks' trial gradually to a maximum of 80 mg/day in divided doses. It is available in capsule and dispersible tablet formulations.

---

might be fewer drug interactions with desvenlafaxine than with the parent drug; however, the precautions are similar for both drugs.

Adverse drug reactions of antidepressants

Antidepressants have many adverse effects, as they enhance monoamine neurotransmission in many areas of the peripheral, enteric, and central nervous systems. Common adverse effects are gastrointestinal and sexual dysfunctions. Simple strategies may help manage adverse effects: for example, for dry mouth – adequate fluid intake, lip balm and sugarless gum; for constipation – adequate fluid and fibre intake and physical activity; for orthostatic hypotension – care when standing or sitting up suddenly; for insomnia – taking medication in the morning; and for weight gain – taking medications at bedtime, and encouraging healthy eating and physical activity.

Antidepressants can be dangerous when taken in high dose. Least toxic in overdose are the SSRIs. The most toxic, and to be avoided when suicide risk is high, are the TCAs and MAOIs.

Serotonin syndrome

Excessive stimulation of 5-HT_{2A} receptors by serotonergic drugs can cause **serotonin syndrome**, or serotonin toxicity, characterised by mental state changes (confusion, delirium, and hypomania), GIT effects (diarrhoea), neuromuscular hyperactivity (hyperreflexia, incoordination, tremor, and ocular clonus), autonomic instability, sweating, fever, and shivering. It occurs particularly when MAOIs are combined with SSRIs or SNRIs. Other drugs enhance 5-HT transmission, including antimigraine drugs, opioid analgesics, CNS stimulants, St John's wort and many illicit drugs, and these can also cause the syndrome. Implicated drugs must be stopped immediately as serotonin syndrome is serious and deaths have occurred. Moderate-to-severe cases require hospitalisation for stabilisation, sedation, and hydration. Serotonin antagonists such as cyproheptadine or chlorpromazine may be administered.

Drug interactions

With antidepressants, there are potentially many drug interactions due to their interactions with multiple neurotransmitter systems (DI 19.2). Reference texts should be consulted for specific interactions, especially for effects on CYP drug-metabolising enzymes.

....

DRUG INTERACTIONS 19.2
Antidepressants

DRUG	POSSIBLE EFFECTS AND MANAGEMENT
Other serotonergic drugs	With TCAs, SSRIs, SNRIs or MAOIs: risk of serotonin syndrome; implicated drugs must be discontinued
Other CNS depressants	Enhanced CNS depression and orthostatic hypotension
Drugs that lower seizure threshold	With TCAs, SNRIs or SSRIs: may cause seizures; avoid combination
Other drugs with sympathomimetic effects	With TCAs or MAOIs: additive effects, including hypertension
Drugs with anticholinergic effects	With TCAs: concurrent drug use may result in an increase in anticholinergic adverse effects, including delirium
Other drugs that prolong the QT interval	With TCAs: increased risk of cardiac dysrhythmias; avoid combination
Other drugs affecting blood glucose	With SSRIs: can increase blood glucose concentration; monitor blood glucose level. MAOIs may decrease blood glucose concentrations affecting control of diabetes
Drugs affecting platelet aggregation	With SSRIs or SNRIs: added risk of bleeding
Other drugs that lower blood pressure	With MAOIs: can cause hypotension; monitor closely when co-administered
Tyramine-containing foods and drinks	Potentially dangerous drug–food interactions with MAOIs; avoid those foods and drinks
Fluoxamine	Interacts with many drugs at specific liver enzymes, increasing concentration and toxicity; consult reference lists for specific interactions

KEY POINTS

Depression

- Depression occurs commonly in women during pregnancy and the postnatal period, and the use of antidepressant medications is common.

- Antidepressants are classified by their mechanism of action as TCAs, MAOIs, SSRIs and SNRIs with SSRIs being the most prescribed class in pregnancy and lactation. TCAs are the least safe option with respect to overdose.

- Antidepressants cross placental and breast barriers readily and generate pharmacological effects for the fetus and newborn. Paroxetine has been associated with a higher incidence of congenital heart defects and is not recommended for use in pregnancy. Fluoxetine has a long half-life and is the least favourable SSRI during lactation. All antidepressants have the potential for neonatal adjustment syndrome.

- Common side effects include dry mouth, constipation, insomnia, weight gain, and orthostatic hypotension. Drug interactions are common and can lead to serotonin syndrome.

19.5 Posttraumatic stress disorder

Posttraumatic stress disorder (PTSD) describes a constellation of symptoms arising after a traumatic event. That event could be related to pregnancy, birth, or the postnatal period (e.g. major postpartum haemorrhage) or unrelated life experiences (e.g. childhood sexual abuse). Symptoms include intrusive negative thoughts, typically leading to attempts to avoid places, people, or activities that trigger these thoughts. Depressed moods may occur, and it can be difficult to distinguish perinatal depression from PTSD. Arousal symptoms are also common, such as irritability, nightmares, and heightened responses to external stimuli leading to feelings of panic.

PTSD affects 3.3% of pregnant women and 4% of the postnatal population (Yildiz et al 2017). The COVID pandemic has seen an increased incidence of the disorder in women during pregnancy and the postnatal period (Liu et al 2021), particularly for women with other preexisting mental health issues. Non-pharmacological management with psychotherapy is the preferred option for treatment. There has been little research to guide pharmacological management of PTSD during pregnancy and the postnatal period (Thomson et al 2021). Antidepressants are typically used as first-line treatment when medication is considered appropriate with the addition of second-generation antipsychotics if there has been inadequate response to the antidepressant.

Bipolar affective disorder

Bipolar (affective) disorder, previously called manic–depressive psychosis, involves shifts between depression and manic episodes. **Mania**, the opposite pole of depression, is characterised by excessive energy, high pressure of speech, extravagant gestures and gifts, and a seeming lack of need for sleep. Approximately 3% of women in the childbearing year have a diagnosis of bipolar disorder (Sharma et al 2020). Other mental illnesses, such as anxiety disorders, often co-exist, and substance use is common (Thomson et al 2018). Unlike other mental illnesses, pregnancy appears to have a protective or neutral impact on the occurrence of relapse in women with bipolar disorder, but postpartum relapse is common (Thomson et al 2018). Mania in the postpartum period can appear as postpartum psychosis and can be the first presentation of bipolar disorder.

Managing bipolar disorder in pregnancy and the postnatal period

Counselling, psychotherapy, and drug therapy are useful for treating bipolar disorders. Lithium is specific for acute mania and prevention of recurrences of manic episodes (DM 19.3), but there have been historical concerns about its safety in pregnancy and lactation. The effectiveness and safety of medications in the treatment of bipolar disorder in women during pregnancy, the postpartum period, and lactation is an area that has been significantly under-researched. Other medications commonly used in the management of bipolar disorder include the antiepileptic drug lamotrigine (see Chapter 20), and the antipsychotic drugs quetiapine and olanzapine (discussed later in this chapter). Antidepressants and antianxiety agents are also sometimes used to manage symptoms.

Pregnancy should, ideally, be planned. The preconception period is the optimal time to counsel women about the likely impact of pregnancy and birth on symptom relapse. If feasible, the preconception period can be used to achieve symptom control with only one agent without known potential for teratogenesis (Thomson et al 2018). If an antiepileptic agent is being used for mood stabilisation, folate supplementation should be advised (see Chapter 20).

The use of medication for bipolar disorder during pregnancy is best managed with comprehensive planning across all stages of the childbearing continuum, considering the impact on both mother and fetus/baby. Women's priorities in relation to the balance between the risk to the fetus and for relapse should be considered. Mood instability is associated with the use of alcohol, tobacco, and other drugs, poor self-care, lack of engagement with health services, poor parenting, and the possibility of suicide (Hermann et al 2019), so undertreatment is not without consequence. Postpartum relapse is more common when medications have been ceased during pregnancy (Thomson et al 2018). Drug doses may need to be increased as pregnancy progresses to achieve stable serum concentrations. Options for modifying drug therapy during pregnancy are (Thomson et al 2018):

1 Discontinue all medications if symptoms have previously been mild, the woman is currently stable and has good social support.

2 Selective discontinuation of medications to achieve monotherapy.

3 Stop all or most medications in the first trimester and recommence in the third trimester. This reduces fetal exposure during organogenesis and the risk of postpartum relapse, but leaves the woman at risk for relapse during pregnancy.

4 Continue medications but swap to one or more drugs with a better pregnancy safety profile.

Lithium: The antimanic drug

Chemically, lithium is a simple metal, first isolated in 1817. It is the third-lightest element, related in its properties to the other alkali metals, sodium and potassium. Lithium salts were once used for gout, as **sedatives**, and as a salt substitute. It was known that excess lithium caused cardiac depression, nausea, and mental depression. In 1948, Dr John Cade, a Melbourne psychiatrist researching the chemical basis of mania, considered it as a potential treatment. By the 1960s, lithium had been evaluated and its efficacy in reducing the prevalence, severity, and duration of recurrent manic episodes was proven. There is an 80–85% response rate when lithium is used prophylactically in bipolar disorder (Cade 1979).

Lithium use in pregnancy

Lithium is known to be effective for preventing relapse during pregnancy and the postpartum period, but there are concerns about safety for the fetus and neonate (Thomson et al 2018). Historical evidence showed a very high risk of congenital heart defects – Ebstein's anomaly in particular – in infants exposed to lithium during the first trimester. More recent research indicates these previous concerns were overestimated, with the increased incidence of cardiac malformation being reported at 1 in 100 (Hermann et al 2019). There is also a small increased risk of non-cardiac anomalies and miscarriage.

Lithium use appears to not alter the risk of pregnancy and birth complications, other than higher rates of low Apgar scores and admission to the nursery (Hermann et al 2019). Neurodevelopment in offspring exposed to lithium in utero has been studied up to 15 years of age, and growth, behaviour, and development have been shown to be within normal range (Hermann et al 2019).

Some women previously well controlled on lithium may elect to continue it during pregnancy. High-quality cardiac ultrasound during pregnancy is advised, aiming to identify any cardiac anomalies so early treatment can be

---

DRUG MONOGRAPH 19.3
Lithium

Mechanism of action

The mechanism of action of lithium has not been established. Sodium in cells has been reported to increase as much as 200% in people with mania. Lithium and sodium are both actively transported across cell membranes, but lithium cannot be pumped out of the cell as effectively as sodium can. Lithium can impair sodium actions in many physiological processes. Overall, it inhibits transmitter release (especially dopamine) at synapses, increases the turnover of noradrenaline and 5-HT in the brain, and decreases postsynaptic receptor sensitivity, with the result that the presumed overactive catecholamine systems in mania are corrected. It has little effect in people without mania.

Indications

Lithium is indicated for preventing manic or depressive episodes in bipolar affective disorder and to treat acute mania, and as adjunctive therapy in schizophrenia and treatment-resistant depression. It is a difficult drug, clinically, due to its low therapeutic index. It must be monitored closely.

Pharmacokinetics

Apart from the slow-release dosage form, lithium is rapidly absorbed and reaches peak plasma concentrations in 1–3 hours. It has a long half-life of 24 hours in adults, so steady-state plasma concentrations are not reached for 5–7 days. Lithium is excreted unchanged by the kidneys and plasma concentrations are sensitive to changes in renal function. Because of the increased glomerular filtration rate seen in pregnancy, half-life and plasma concentrations fall, while the volume of distribution remains unchanged (Clark et al 2022).

Therapeutic drug monitoring

Lithium has a very narrow therapeutic range, so plasma levels must be monitored regularly. Samples are taken 12–24 hours post-dose to measure trough levels. During pregnancy lithium levels should be tested every 2–4 weeks until 34 weeks of gestation, then weekly to birth (Hermann et al 2019). They should be checked 24 hours following birth, then twice a week for 2 weeks, then 4 weeks post-birth, reflecting the rapid changes in renal function occurring in the postnatal period.

Drug interactions

Lithium has specific interactions with other drugs affecting the kidneys, such as diuretics, sodium salts, and non-steroidal anti-inflammatory agents (DI 19.3). Levels are elevated by renal dysfunction, diarrhoea, vomiting, fluid or salt loss, diuretics, dehydration, low-salt diets, excess sweating, high fever, or strenuous exercise. Conversely, high intake of sodium chloride, sodium bicarbonate or potassium citrate, and theophylline can result in lowering of lithium levels. During pregnancy, increased glomerular filtration results in increased clearance of lithium, a shorter half-life, and lower serum levels (Clark et al 2022). In addition, lithium interacts with drugs affecting thyroid function or 5-HT levels.

Adverse effects

These include tremor, thirst, nausea, increased urination, diarrhoea, and irregular pulse rate. Long-term effects include acne, psoriasis, hypothyroidism, weight gain, hyperparathyroidism, and renal damage. A specific adverse reaction is nephrogenic diabetes insipidus, in which lithium inhibits the actions of antidiuretic hormone on the distal tubule cells, leading to polyuria. Early signs of lithium toxicity include confusion, vomiting, tremors, slurred speech, and drowsiness.

Warnings and contraindications

Lithium should be used with caution in people with diabetes mellitus, hypothyroidism, goitre, psoriasis, and people on a sodium-restricted diet. Avoid use in people with a history of lithium hypersensitivity or with severe dehydration or renal impairment, and during lactation. Calcium levels should be monitored for hyperparathyroidism.

Dosage and administration

Lithium, as the carbonate salt, is available as tablets and controlled-release tablets. For acute mania, the dose is initially 70–1000 mg daily in divided doses, increasing the dose by 250–500 mg daily as necessary. Adjust dosage according to serum concentration. For prophylaxis, the maintenance dose is 200–1000 mg per day in one or two doses. The dose is adjusted according to the response.

---

planned (Thomson et al 2018). It is important to maintain good hydration, so care should be taken for women with hyperemesis and during long labour. At birth, reduce the dose to the pre-pregnancy dose or 600 mg.

Lithium use in breastfeeding

The risk of relapse during the postpartum period is high. Of women with type I bipolar disorder with a previous episode of postpartum mania, 43% will have another, while the rate is 9% for women with no previous history of postpartum mania (Di Florio et al 2018), and 90% of relapses occur in the first 6 weeks after birth.

Sleep deprivation increases the possibility for relapse. As breastfeeding requires frequent night feeds during the early postpartum weeks when relapse risk is high, the decision about choice of infant feeding method is not only about risks related to neonatal drug exposure.

DRUG INTERACTIONS 19.3
Lithium

DRUG	POSSIBLE EFFECTS AND MANAGEMENT
Antithyroid drugs or iodides	Can enhance the hypothyroid goitrogenic effects of lithium on these medications; monitor closely for lethargy or intolerance to cold
Non-steroidal anti-inflammatory agents; ACE inhibitors; sartans; topiramate	Can decrease excretion of lithium, leading to raised lithium levels and toxicity; monitor closely for blurred vision, confusion, and dizziness
Phenothiazines, fluoxetine, haloperidol	Lithium levels may be altered, with risk of neurotoxicity; monitor physical symptoms and drug serum levels
Diuretics (loop; thiazide)	Decreased lithium excretion results in a raised lithium level and toxicity; a reduction in lithium dosage may be indicated; monitor closely
Drugs increasing 5-HT levels	Enhanced risk of serotonin toxicity
Ziprasidone	Interacts with lithium to augment the prolongation of the cardiac QT interval

Lithium levels in the serum of breastfed infants are 25–50% of the levels in their mothers (Hermann et al 2019). Lithium can reach toxic levels in the neonate if they become dehydrated but appears otherwise safe. If the mother chooses to continue lithium therapy while breastfeeding, adequate social support to prevent sleep deprivation and monitoring of serum levels in the infant are advised (Hermann et al 2019). Lamotrigine and second-generation antipsychotics are generally considered safer options for the management of bipolar disorder during lactation.

KEY POINTS
Treatment of bipolar disorder

- Lithium is the drug of choice for prophylaxis and treatment of mania and bipolar affective disorder but may increase the risk of congenital heart defects.
- Dose increases of lithium for the treatment of bipolar disorder are commonly required during pregnancy.
- Breastfeeding increases the risk of symptom relapse and concomitant use of lithium is associated with a risk of lithium toxicity in the neonate.

19.6 Postpartum psychosis

Postpartum psychosis typically presents suddenly in the first 2 weeks after birth, and in about 50% of cases the acute episode represents their first experience of psychosis (Gressier et al 2020). It is uncommon, impacting one or two women per 1000 who give birth (Albers et al 2023). Symptoms include the presence of delusions (typically centred on the birth and/or the baby, such as a conviction that the baby is dead or was never born) or hallucinations, typically accompanied by labile mood, confusion, and irritability. Both suicide and infanticide have been reported (Sharma et al 2022).

Postpartum psychosis is more common for women with a personal or family history of mental illness, particularly bipolar disorder. Cessation of pharmacotherapy previously used to stabilise mental health increases the risk of relapse. Other risk factors include primiparity, traumatic birth experiences, and sleep deprivation (Osborne 2018).

Postpartum psychosis is an emergency and requires rapid assessment and management to prevent harm to the woman and/or her infant. Hospitalisation or admission to a dedicated mother/baby unit is advised. Treatment should be tailored to address the specific presentation. Multiple drugs may be required, including a sedative/anxiolytic (e.g. lorazepam), an antipsychotic, and a mood stabiliser such as lithium or lamotrigine to prevent recurrence of symptoms. Breastfeeding is generally contraindicated, both for the potential risk to the infant from the woman, and the risk of harm from the medications used.

Antipsychotic agents

Antipsychotic, or **neuroleptic**, agents are the mainstay of treatment of psychosis and in the manic phase of bipolar disorder. The first effective **tranquilliser** (to calm an agitated or anxious person) without serious sedating actions was chlorpromazine (Largactil). It revolutionised treatment when released in the early 1950s and is still the prototype antipsychotic. Based on chronology, antipsychotics are classified as **typical antipsychotics** or first-generation antipsychotics (the phenothiazines, thioxanthines, and haloperidol-type drugs); and the **atypical antipsychotics**, also referred to as second-generation agents (clozapine, olanzapine, and risperidone). Atypical antipsychotics are less likely to induce extrapyramidal side effects but more likely to cause metabolic effects, such as weight gain and diabetes. Antipsychotic agents decrease hallucinations, delusions, initiative, emotion, aggression, responses to external stimuli, and thought disorder, and can prevent relapses. Drowsiness is common, but people remain readily rousable without confusion.

Formulations and routes

Most antipsychotics are administered orally, as tablets or capsules, oral liquid, or sublingual wafers. Controlled-release tablets are useful for drugs with short half-lives. Some are available only in parenteral formulations, either as a short-acting injection or a long-acting depot preparation.

Mechanisms of action

There is good evidence that antipsychotics act by antagonism of dopamine receptors at the D_2 receptor type. This antidopaminergic action leads to useful therapeutic effects (slower thinking, movement, and antiemetic actions), and common adverse reactions, including extrapyramidal effects. Dopamine antagonism also causes hyperprolactinaemia. In men and non-pregnant women this infrequently results in breast enlargement and milk secretion. Some dopamine antagonists are specifically used to enhance lactogenesis (e.g. domperidone).

In addition to acting at D_2 receptors, antagonism to 5-HT_{2A} and partial agonism of 5-HT_{1A} receptors contribute to the clinical effects seen. Adverse effects are mainly due to antagonism at α-adrenoceptors (hypotension) and muscarinic ACh receptors (**anticholinergic effects**).

Conventional (typical) antipsychotics

Chlorpromazine was the first – and is still the prototype – phenothiazine antipsychotic drug, a member of the typical class of antipsychotics. It is rarely prescribed in pregnancy and lactation so it will not be further explored here.

Atypical antipsychotic agents

Atypical antipsychotics have less potential to cause extrapyramidal effects, **tardive dyskinesia**, neuroleptic malignant syndrome, or sedation, so are more commonly prescribed. However, they are more likely to prolong the cardiac QT interval, cause metabolic adverse effects, or weight gain. They are not a homogeneous class, having widely differing adverse effect profiles. Clozapine and olanzapine are most likely to cause hyperglycaemia and weight gain.

Use in pregnancy and lactation

Due to the relative rarity of postpartum psychosis and other indications (such as bipolar disorder) for the use of antipsychotics in pregnant or lactating women, there is little evidence to guide practice. Monitoring for metabolic changes, such as hyperglycaemia secondary to the use of atypical antipsychotics, is important (Betcher et al 2019). Quetiapine and olanzapine (see DM 19.4), both atypical antipsychotics, are typically recommended when use of an antipsychotic is planned (Thomson et al 2018). Although data are limited, olanzapine appears to have

---

DRUG MONOGRAPH 19.4
Olanzapine

Mechanism of action
Olanzapine is a dopamine inhibitor, and the antagonism of central dopaminergic function may be related to the therapeutic effect in psychotic conditions.

Indications
Olanzapine is indicated in bipolar disorder, schizophrenia, postpartum psychosis, and nausea and vomiting in terminal illness.

Pharmacokinetics
Olanzapine is well absorbed orally but subject to first-pass metabolism, with about 40% of the dose inactivated on first pass. Approximately 93% of the drug is protein-bound. Peak plasma levels are reached 4–8 hours after oral administration. Onset of antipsychotic effect is achieved gradually over several weeks, and peak effects occur around 2–3 months. Olanzapine's longer half-life (around 30 hours) makes it suitable for once-a-day dosing. Olanzapine is metabolised in the liver and 60% of a given dose is excreted by the kidneys and 30% in faeces.

Adverse effects
Common adverse effects include hyperglycaemia, dyslipidaemia, and oedema. Orthostatic hypotension, sedation, anticholinergic and extrapyramidal effects, and tardive dyskinesia can occur. The incidence of extrapyramidal effects is lower with olanzapine than most other antipsychotics. Neuroleptic malignant syndrome may be seen after months or years of treatment.

Drug interactions
Olanzapine is a substrate of CYP1A2, so interactions with inducers, inhibitors or other substrates of this enzyme are likely. Tobacco smoking induces CYP1A2 and reduces serum concentrations per dose of olanzapine due to increased metabolism.

Warnings and contraindications
Use with caution in people with cardiovascular disease, moderate-to-severe liver impairment, hyperthyroidism, Parkinson's disease, chronic respiratory disease, epilepsy, and conditions involving problems of parasympathetic control. Avoid use in people with olanzapine hypersensitivity. See Use in Pregnancy and Lactation for more details.

Dosage and administration
Dosage of antipsychotic agents varies according to the individual, indication for treatment, and the person's response to the medication. It is best to titrate from a low dose, increasing when necessary for therapeutic response. When stopping therapy, dosage should be reduced gradually over 2–3 weeks, otherwise rebound nausea, vomiting, dizziness, tremors, and dyskinesias may occur. Olanzapine is available in tablet, oral wafer, and short- or long-acting injection formulations. The starting oral dose is 5–10 mg once daily, and then adjusted according to response by 2.5–5 mg each week. The maximum daily dose is typically 20 mg.

no detrimental fetal effects (Brunner et al 2013). The transfer of quetiapine into cord blood is lower than for olanzepine, and breast milk concentrations (while still low) are lower with olanzapine than quetiapine (Schoretsanitis et al 2020; Zheng et al 2022). Maternal serum levels fall during pregnancy due to increased metabolism and volume of distribution, so upward dose adjustments may be needed to maintain efficacy (Badhan et al 2020).

Adverse effects of antipsychotics

Many antipsychotic drugs affect several transmitters and their receptors – particularly in the autonomic and enteric nervous systems – so it is inevitable they will have adverse effects. Adverse effects on blood pressure (orthostatic hypotension), GIT functions (dry mouth, constipation, and weight gain), sexual function (decreased libido), and eye functions (blurred vision) are common.

Because typical antipsychotic drugs also block receptors for a wide range of receptors (ACh [muscarinic], noradrenaline [α-], histamine [H_1], 5-HT and dopamine), there are wide-ranging adverse CNS and peripheral effects. Adverse effects include movement disorders, dizziness, constipation, dry mouth, confusion, and drowsiness.

All groups of antipsychotics can cause metabolic disturbances such as weight gain, diabetes, and dyslipidaemia. Olanzapine and quetiapine particularly are associated with weight gain and diabetes.

Extrapyramidal effects

Common adverse effects from antipsychotics are the extrapyramidal effects, due to blockade of D_2 receptors and subsequent overactivity of cholinergic (motor) pathways or extrapyramidal pathways. Extrapyramidal effects include dystonia (painful muscular spasms), akathisia (motor restlessness), pseudoparkinsonism (rigidity and tremor), and tardive dyskinesis (involuntary muscle movements).

Neuroleptic malignant syndrome

This rare but potentially fatal syndrome occurs in 0.5–1% of people using typical antipsychotics. It may occur months or years after starting treatment with the drug, then progress rapidly over 1–3 days. It involves high temperature, muscle rigidity, altered consciousness, and impaired autonomic homeostasis. Treatment requires withdrawal of the drug, hydration and sometimes bromocriptine (a dopamine agonist) and dantrolene to control muscle spasms.

Drug interactions

With all antipsychotics, there are a multitude of potential drug interactions and long lists of potential interactions. Common interactions are listed in DI 19.4. Consult tables in the *Therapeutic Guidelines: **Psychotropics*** and *Australian Medicines Handbook* for specific interactions. Antipsychotic

drugs are likely to interact with all other drugs affecting the central or autonomic nervous systems; for example, those that depress the CNS (opioids, anxiolytics, anaesthetics, sedatives, antiepileptics, antiemetics), alter the cardiac QT interval, cause hypotension, lower the seizure threshold, are dopamine agonists or antagonists, have anticholinergic effects, affect blood glucose concentration, or either inhibit or enhance the metabolism of the antipsychotic agent (e.g. social drugs such as alcohol and tobacco).

DRUG INTERACTIONS 19.4
Antipsychotic drugs

DRUG	POSSIBLE EFFECTS AND MANAGEMENT
Other CNS depressants such as benzodiazepines, anaesthetics, lithium, antihistamines, opioids, and alcohol	Additive CNS depression (may be useful if sedation desired), respiratory depression, and hypotensive effects. Drug dosage should be reduced
Drugs that lower seizure threshold	May cause seizures – avoid combination
Antihypertensive agents	Concurrent drug use with the antipsychotics may result in an exacerbation of hypotensive effects
Drugs with anticholinergic effects	Concurrent drug use may result in an increase in anticholinergic adverse effects, including delirium
Drugs that prolong the QT interval, such as antidysrhythmic agents, many antimicrobials (e.g. clarithromycin), tyrosine kinase inhibitors (antineoplastics)	Additive prolongation with antipsychotics droperidol, haloperidol, amisulpride, sertindole, ziprasidone – potentially fatal ventricular dysrhythmia
Drugs affecting blood glucose concentrations	Many antipsychotic drugs cause hyperglycaemia, so alter the actions of other drugs

---

KEY POINTS

Antipsychotic agents

- Antipsychotic agents include (typical) phenothiazine derivatives, and the atypical antipsychotics, acting mainly by dopamine blockade in specific areas of the CNS.

- Major adverse effects of antipsychotics occur in the central, autonomic, and motor nervous systems, including sedation, hypotension, metabolic changes, extrapyramidal effects, and neuroleptic malignant syndrome.

- There are many potential drug interactions with antipsychotics.

REVIEW EXERCISES

1 Nina is a 38-year-old mother of four, including her newborn son Tyson. Nina was diagnosed with bipolar disorder in the postnatal period after the birth of her third child when she had an episode of acute mania. Her symptoms responded well to lithium, but lithium was ceased when her pregnancy was diagnosed due to concerns about the risk of congenital cardiac anomalies. What is Nina's risk of another episode of mania in the next few weeks? Explain the discussion you would have with Nina about the issues relating to infant feeding, and the use of lithium in the postnatal period.

2 Patrick is 2 days old and was admitted to the special care nursery. He was born at 38 weeks of gestation after an uncomplicated labour and birth. His mother, Zoe, has major depression and her symptoms had been well managed during pregnancy. She uses sertraline 50 mg daily. Last night, Patrick was unsettled and difficult to get to sleep, and Zoe struggled to get him to feed at the breast. When he was assessed, he was noted to be hypoglycaemic and hypothermic. Both resolved quickly with oral glucose gel and a radiant heater over his cot. He remains irritable this morning. Zoe wants to know if Patrick's symptoms could be due to her use of sertraline? Would stopping sertraline, or ceasing breastfeeding, help? How long might Patrick's symptoms last?

3 You are attending a postnatal home visit for Alyssa. She gave birth seven days ago. As you arrive at the house you can hear the baby crying and there is no answer at the door. You look over the fence and can see Alyssa at the clothesline, removing clothes and throwing them on the ground. You open the side gate and go to speak to her. She does not seem to recognise you, even though you have been her midwife through the entire pregnancy. She tells you a demon has possessed her baby. Outline the next steps you would take to ensure Alyssa's safety and that of her baby. Which medication classes might be useful in the acute management of Alyssa's symptoms?

REFERENCES

Albers S, Wen T, Monk C, et al. Postpartum psychosis during delivery hospitalisations and postpartum readmission, 2016–2019. Am J Obstet Gynecol MFM. 2023;5:100905. doi. org/10.1016/j.ajogmf.2023.100905

Anderson KN, Ailes EC, Lind JN, et al. Atypical antipsychotic use during pregnancy and birth defect risk: National Birth Defects Prevention Study, 1997-2011. Schizophrenia Research. 2020;215:81-88. doi: 10.1016/j.schres.2019.11.019

Australian Medicines Handbook 2023. Australian Medicines Handbook. Adelaide: AMH.

Badhan R, Macfarlane H. Quetiapine dose optimisation during gestation: a pharmacokinetic modelling study. J Pharm Pharmacol. 2020;72: 670-681. doi: 10.1111/jphp.13236

Betcher HK, Montiel C, Clark CT. Use of antipsychotic drugs during pregnancy. Curr Treat Options Psychiatry. 2019 Mar;6(1):17-31. doi: 10.1007/s40501-019-0165-5. Epub 2019 Jan 30. PMID: 32775146; PMCID: PMC7410162

Biaggi A, Pariante C. Risk factors for depression and anxiety during the perinatal period. In, Quatraro R, Grussu P (eds.), Handbook of perinatal clinical psychology: from theory to practice, Ch 13, pp 316–346. Taylor Francis Group, 2020.

Braun L, Cohen M. Herbs and natural supplements: an evidence-based guide, 4th edn. Sydney: Elsevier Mosby, 2014.

Brunner E, Falk D, Jones M, et al. Olanzapine in pregnancy and breastfeeding: a review of data from global safety surveillance. BMC Pharmacol Toxicol. 2013;14:38. doi. org/10.1186/2050-6511-14-38

Cade JF. Mending the mind: a short history of twentieth century psychiatry. Melbourne: Sun Books, 1979.

Chin K, Wendt A, Bennett I, Bhat A. Suicide and maternal mortality. Curr Psychiatry Rep. 2022;24:239-275. doi.org/10.1007/s11920-022-01334-3

Clark C, Newmark R, Wisner K, et al. Lithium pharmacokinetics in the perinatal patient with bipolar disorder. J Clin Pharmacol. 2022;62(11):1385-1392. doi:10.1002/jcph.2089

Di Florio A, Gordon-Smith K, Forty L, et al. Stratification of the risk of bipolar disorder recurrences in pregnancy and postpartum. Br J Psychiatry. 2018;213:542-547. doi: 10.1192/bjp.2018.92

Edvardsson K, Hughes E, Copnell B, et al. Severe mental illness and pregnancy outcomes in Australia. A population-based study of 595 792 singleton births 2009–2016. PLoS One. 2022;17(2):e0264512. doi.org/10.1371/journal.pone.0264512

Galbally M, Frayne J, Watson S, et al. Psychopharmacological prescribing practices in pregnancy for some with severe mental illness: a multi centre study. Eur Neuropsychopharmacol. 2019;29:57-65. doi.org/10.1016/j.euroneuro.2018.11.1103

Gressier F, de Cordova I, Glatigny E, et al. Postpartum psychosis, bipolar disorders, and mother-baby unit. In, Quatraro RM, Grussu P. (eds.), Handbook of perinatal clinical psychology: from theory to practice, Ch 15, pp.374–386. Taylor Francis Group, 2020.

Hanley G, Oberlander T. The effect of perinatal exposures on the infant: antidepressants and depression. Best Pract Res Clin Obstet Gynaecol. 2014;28:37-48. doi.org/10.1016/j.bpobgyn.2013.09.001

Harp, AG. Perinatal patients with symptoms of anxiety. In, Cox E. (ed.), Women's mood disorders. Springer Cham, 2021. doi-org.libraryproxy.griffith.edu.au/10.1007/978-3-030-71497-0_10

Henssler J, Heinz A, Brandt L, et al. Antidepressant withdrawal and rebound phenomena. Deutsches Ärzteblatt International. 2019 May 17;116(20):355-361. doi: 10.3238/arztebl.2019.0355. PMID: 31288917; PMCID: PMC6637660.

Hermann A, Gorun A, Benudis A. Lithium use and non-use for pregnant and postpartum women in bipolar disorder. Curr Psychiatry Rep. 2019;21:114. doi.org/10.1007/s11920-019-1103-3

Liu CH, Erdei C, Mittal L. Risk factors for depression, anxiety, and PTSD symptoms in perinatal women during the COVID-19 pandemic. Psychiatry Research, 2021, 113552. doi.org/10.1016/j.psychres.2020.113552

Liu L, Liu C, Wang Y, et al. Herbal medicine for anxiety, depression and insomnia. Curr Neuropharmacology. 2015;13:481–193. doi: 10.2174/1570159X1304150831122734

Molenaar N, Kamperman A, Boyce P, et al. Guidelines on treatment of perinatal depression with antidepressants: an international review. Aust NZ J Psychiatry. 2018;52(4):320-327. doi: 10.1177/0004867418762057

Nillni Y, MehralizadeA, Mayer L, et al. Treatment of depression, anxiety, and trauma-related disorders during the perinatal period: a systematic review. Clin Psychology Rev. 2018;66:136-148. doi.org/10.1016/j.cpr.2018.06.004

O'Hara M, Wisner K. Perinatal mental illness, definition, description and aetiology. Best Pract Res Clin Obstetrics Gynaecol. 2014;28:3-12. doi.org/10.1016/j.bpobgyn.2013.09.002

Osborne L. Recognising and managing postpartum psychosis: a clinical guide for obstetric providers. Obstetric Gynecol Clinical N Am. 2018;45:455-468. doi.org/10.1016/j.ogc.2018.04.005

Psychotropic Expert Group. Therapeutic guidelines: psychotropic, version 7, Melbourne, 2021 Therapeutic Guidelines Limited. eTG complete [digital]. Melbourne: Therapeutic Guidelines Limited, 2019. https://www.tg.org.au

Ray S, Stowe Z. The use of antidepressant medication in pregnancy. Best Pract Res Clin Obstetrics Gynaecol. 2014;28:71-83. doi.org/10.1016/j.bpobgyn.2013.09.005

Rowland T, Marwaha S. Epidemiology and risk factors for bipolar disorder. Ther Adv Psychopharmacol. 2018;8(9): 251-269. doi: 10.1177/2045125318769235

Sarris J. Nutrients and herbal supplements for mental health. Aust Prescr. 2014;37(3):90-93.

Schofield Z, Kapoor D. Pre-existing mental health disorders and pregnancy. Obstet Gynaecol Reproductive Med. 2019;29(3):74-79. doi.org/10.1016/j.ogrm.2019.01.005

Schoretsanitis G, Westin A, Deligiannidis K, et al. Excretion of antipsychotics into the amniotic fluid, umbilical cord blood, and breast milk: a systematic critical review and combined analysis. Ther Drug Monitoring. 2020;42(2):245-254.

Sharma V, Mazmanian D, Palagi L, Bramante A. Postpartum psychosis: revisiting the phenomenology, nosology, and treatment. J Affect Disord. 2022;10:100378. doi.org/10.1016/j.jadr.2022.100378

Sharma V, Sharma P, Sharma S. Managing bipolar disorder during pregnancy and the postpartum period: a critical review of current practice. Exp Rev Neurother. 2020 Apr;20(4):373-383. doi.org/10.1080/14737175.2020.1743684

Sprague J, Wisner K, Bogen D. Pharmacotherapy for depression and bipolar disorder during lactation: a framework to aid decision making. Semin Perinatol. 2020;44: 151224. doi.org/10.1016/j.semperi.2020.151224

Thomson M, Sharma V. Weighing the risks: the management of bipolar disorder in pregnancy. Curr Psychiatry Rep. 2018;20:20. doi.org/10.1007/s11920-018-0882-2

Thomson M, Sharma V. Pharmacotherapeutic considerations for the treatment of post traumatic stress disorder during and after pregnancy. Expert Opin Pharmacother. 2021;22(6):705-714. doi.org/10.1080/14656566.2020.1854727

World Health Organization 2018. Mental health: strengthening our response. Online. https://www.who.int/news-room/fact-sheets/detail/mental-health-strengthening-our-response

Yildiz PD, Ayers S, Phillips L. The prevalence of posttraumatic stress disorder in pregnancy and after birth: a systematic review and meta-analysis. J Affect Disord. 2017;208:634-645.

Zheng L, Yang H, Dallmann A. Antidepressants and antipsychotics in human pregnancy: transfer across the placenta and opportunities for modeling studies. J Clin Pharmacol. 2022;62(S1):S115-S128. doi: 10.1002/jcph.2108

ONLINE RESOURCES

Beyond Blue, the national depression initiative: https://www.beyondblue.org.au/home

Marcé Society for Perinatal Mental Health (International): https://marcesociety.com/

Mental Illness Fellowship of Australia: https://www.mifa.org.au/en/ (accessed January 2022)

HalesMeds.com Dr Hale's Lactation Risk Categories. Springer Publishing: https://www.halesmeds.com/mnemonics/47704 (accessed 4 October 2023)

New Zealand Medicines and Medical Devices Safety Authority: https://www.medsafe.govt.nz/ (accessed January 2022)

Perinatal Anxiety and Depression Aotearoa: https://pada.nz

Post and Antenatal Depression Association Inc (Australia): https://panda.org.au/

Therapeutic Goods Administration. Prescribing medicines in pregnancy database: https://www.tga.gov.au/products/medicines/find-information-about-medicine/prescribing-medicines-pregnancy-database (accessed 4 October 2023)

Wellways Australia Limited – a leading not-for-profit mental health and disability support organisation with services in Queensland, New South Wales, the Australian Capital Territory, Victoria and Tasmania: https://www.wellways.org/ (accessed January 2022)

CHAPTER 20

EPILEPSY

Kirsten Small, Maryam Bazargan, Roslyn Donnellan-Fernandez

Key Abbreviations

AED   antiepileptic drug
CA   carbonic anhydrase
GABA   gamma-aminobutyric acid

Key Terms

antiepileptic
    (anticonvulsant)
    drugs 382
antiepileptic
    hypersensitivity
    syndrome 389
drug interaction 389
eclampsia 387
epilepsy 380

non-linear
    pharmacokinetics
    390
primary, or idiopathic,
    epilepsy 380
secondary
    epilepsy 380
seizures 380
status epilepticus
    382

Chapter Focus

Epilepsy is one of the most common chronic neurological illnesses, involving recurrent epileptic seizures that may affect parts or the whole of the cerebral cortex, and that cause muscle twitching and impaired consciousness. Approximately 50 million people worldwide have epilepsy, affecting one in every 200 adults in Western societies, although mild seizures in children are much more common. Prior to conception, during pregnancy, and in the postpartum period, women with epilepsy have special considerations regarding medication choice and overall management of their seizure disorder.

This chapter discusses classifications of the types of epilepsy and a selection of the antiepileptic drugs available to treat this disorder. Clinical aspects of therapy of epilepsies are considered, including choice of drug, compliance, therapeutic drug monitoring, lifestyle aspects and drug use in pregnancy and lactation.

Key Drug Groups

Antiepileptic drugs

Acting by blockade of sodium channels:
- phenytoin (DM 20.1), carbamazepine, lamotrigine (DM 20.2), sodium valproate

Acting by enhancement of GABA inhibition:
- barbiturates: phenobarbital (phenobarbitone)

- benzodiazepines: clonazepam, diazepam, midazolam
- other drugs: topiramate

Acting by other mechanisms:
- gabapentin, levetiracetam (DM 20.3), magnesium sulfate
- folic acid

Learning Outcomes

- Define epilepsy and describe different seizure types that may occur.
- Outline the major drug classes used to manage epilepsy in pregnancy and their mechanisms of action, their contraception and pregnancy considerations, and the safety profile of these drugs on embryo, fetus, and neonate.
- Describe core principles of pharmacological and non-pharmacological management of epilepsy.
- Discuss priorities for management of epilepsy in women of reproductive age.
- Name the drugs commonly used in the management of epilepsy in pregnancy and describe the following for each: mechanism of action; potential for teratogenesis and behavioural impact on the neonate; dose; adverse effects; therapeutic monitoring during pregnancy and after birth; and suitability for use in lactation.

CRITICAL THINKING SCENARIO

Petrina is a 23-year-old nulliparous woman with a history of generalised (tonic–clonic) epilepsy. Her seizures have been well controlled on carbamazepine. She is on the combined oral contraceptive pill (levonorgestrel 150 microgram, ethinylestradiol 30 microgram) and is not planning pregnancy. However, she missed two periods and has a positive pregnancy test. An ultrasound scan confirms a viable 7-week pregnancy. She decides to continue the pregnancy with the support of her partner and immediate family. After consultation with her neurologist, Petrina decides to continue taking carbamazepine to minimise the dangers from uncontrolled epilepsy and because the risk to the fetus does not necessarily reduce if the antiepileptic drug is stopped at this stage of the pregnancy.

Her GP starts her on high-dose folic acid (5 mg daily). At her routine 20-week morphology ultrasound a mild spina bifida is noted. Petrina has multi-disciplinary care from a team including her midwife, her local obstetrician and GP, and the maternal fetal medicine and neurology teams at the nearest tertiary facility. The rest of Petrina's pregnancy is uncomplicated, and she remains seizure-free. She has a spontaneous labour and vaginal birth at 39 weeks. The baby undergoes corrective spinal surgery at 1 month of age, with no long-lasting neurological deficits.

1 Is the low-dose contraceptive pill appropriate for a woman also taking carbamazepine? If not, what are the recommended contraceptive methods?

2 Why did Petrina's doctor suggest she take high-dose folic acid?

3 To benefit most from folic acid, when should it be started?

4 If Petrina's pregnancy had been planned, might changing to another antiepileptic drug prior to conception have reduced the risk of a congenital malformation?

Introduction

Epilepsy is a group of chronic neurological disorders consisting of many syndromes or diseases. It is characterised by sporadic, recurrent episodes of convulsive seizures resulting from occasional, excessive disorderly discharges in neuronal pathways across the cerebral cortex. It has been known for more than 3000 years, including in ancient Babylonian and Chinese civilisations, and was described as 'the falling sickness'.

About 5% of people will experience seizures at some stage in their lives, while about 1% of people are diagnosed with recurrent epilepsy. Seizure disorders affect 0.3–0.8% of pregnant women (Li & Meador 2022). Around 50 million people worldwide have epilepsy. Between 4 and 10 per 1000 people in the general population are estimated to have active epilepsy (i.e. continuing seizures or with the need for treatment), and rates are even higher (up to 139 per 1000 people) in low- and middle-income countries (World Health Organization [Who] 2024). According to the International League Against Epilepsy (ILAE) (see Online resources) epilepsy is a disease of the brain defined by any of the following conditions:

- at least two unprovoked (or reflex) seizures occurring more than 24 hours apart

- one unprovoked (or reflex) seizure and a probability of further seizures similar to the general recurrence risk (at least 60%) after two unprovoked seizures, occurring over the next 10 years
- diagnosis of an epilepsy syndrome (Fisher et al 2017b).

Seizures can lead to loss of consciousness, muscle jerking, sensory disturbances, and abnormal behaviour. Although nearly 70% of seizures do not have an identifiable cause (**primary, or idiopathic, epilepsy**), around 30% have an underlying cause (**secondary epilepsy**) that may be treatable – for example, eclampsia, traumatic head injury, cerebrovascular infarct or haemorrhage, infection, brain tumour, drug toxicity, or metabolic imbalance. There is evidence of genetic links, particularly in familial focal epilepsy (Fisher et al 2017a).

The aim of therapy is to avoid factors that can trigger attacks and choose a drug or drugs that effectively control seizures and restore physiological homeostasis with a minimum of undesirable side effects or drug interactions.

Classification of seizures

The choice of appropriate AEDs has depended on accurate diagnosis and classification of the seizure type, although there has been a recent shift to treatment with first-line agents and then classification. The types of seizures are outlined below. Identifying specific seizure types is critical in developing a treatment plan.

The classification of epileptic seizures is complex and still evolving. The ILAE provides definitions for key concepts and classification schemes. Figure 20.1 shows earlier terminologies, as well as a revised operational (practical) classification recently introduced by the ILAE (Fig 20.2; Scheffer & Mullen 2013). The purpose of the

Classification of seizures, based on the system proposed by the International League Against Epilepsy and showing some earlier terminology. See also the classification diagram at www.epilepsy.org.au/about-epilepsy/

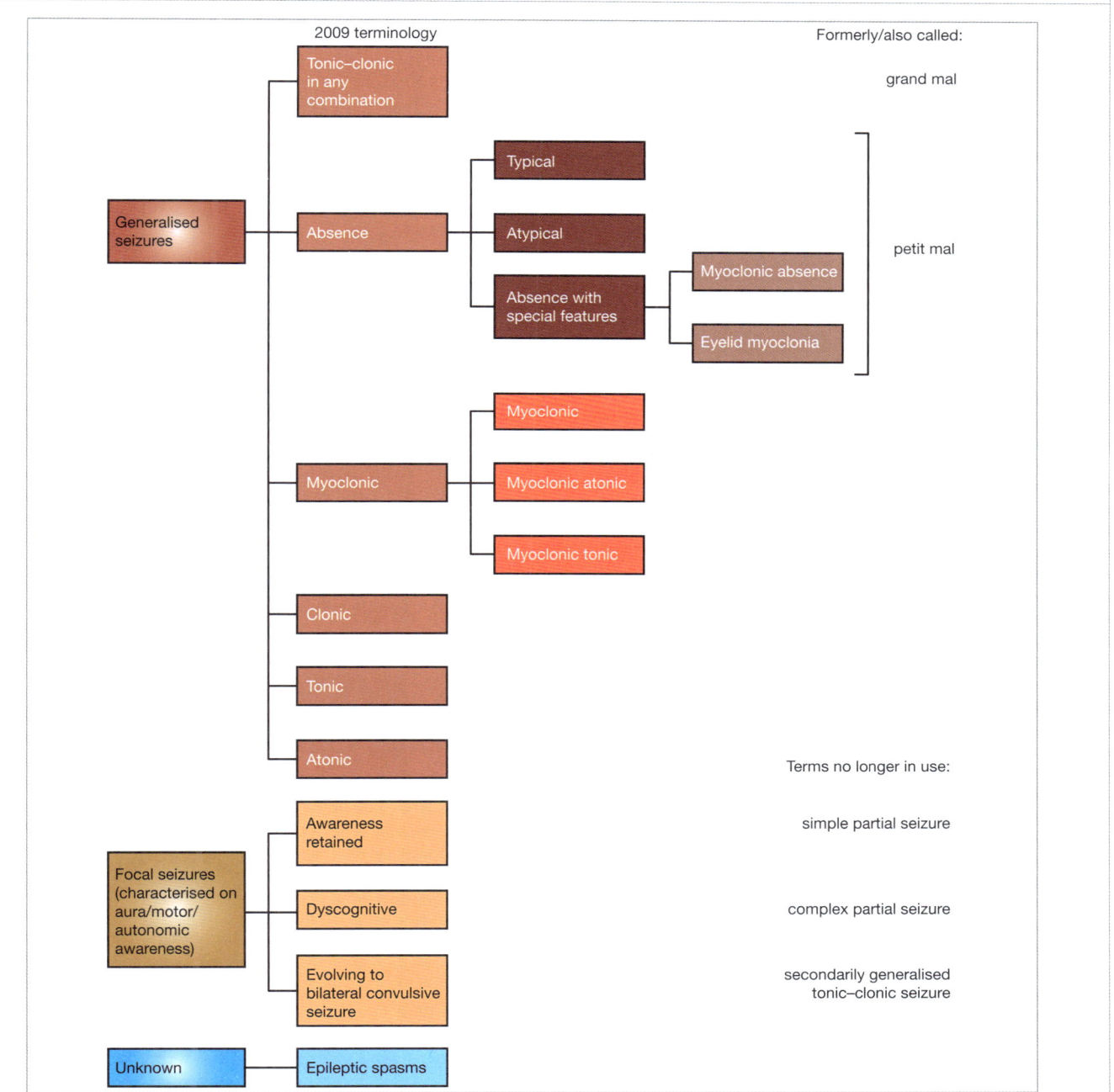

FIGURE 20.1

Source: Fisher et al 2017a; with permission of John Wiley & Sons.

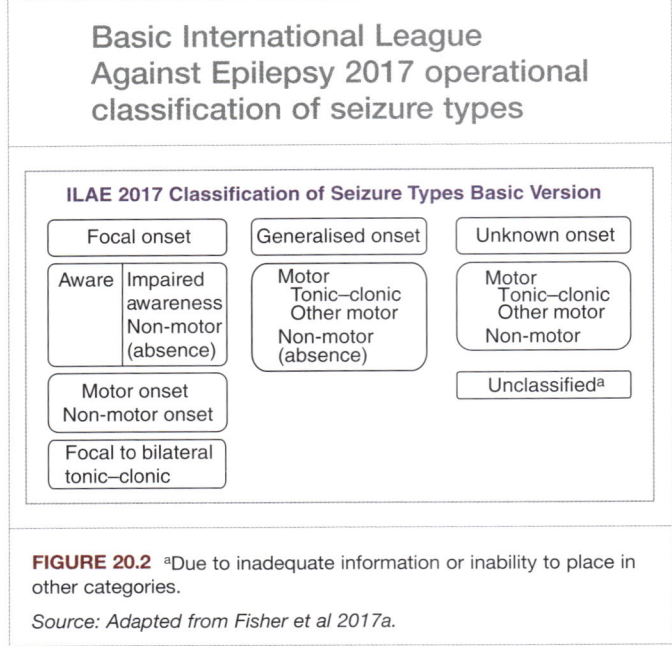

Basic International League Against Epilepsy 2017 operational classification of seizure types

ILAE 2017 Classification of Seizure Types Basic Version

Focal onset	Generalised onset	Unknown onset
Aware / Impaired awareness Non-motor (absence)	Motor Tonic–clonic Other motor Non-motor (absence)	Motor Tonic–clonic Other motor Non-motor
Motor onset Non-motor onset		Unclassified[a]
Focal to bilateral tonic–clonic		

FIGURE 20.2 [a]Due to inadequate information or inability to place in other categories.

Source: Adapted from Fisher et al 2017a.

update is to enable transparency and clarification of nomenclature, classification of some seizure types as either focal or generalised, and indication when onset is unknown.

Focal onset seizures

Focal onset seizures (formerly known as partial) are associated with irritation of a specific part of the brain. A single body part may be affected. Consciousness may not be lost unless the seizure develops into a generalised convulsion.

Dyscognitive seizures are a type of focal seizures and are characterised by brief alterations in consciousness. They may include unusual, stereotyped movements (e.g. chewing or swallowing movements) repeated over and over, changes in temperament, confusion, and feelings of unreality. Focal seizures may spread and evolve to generalised tonic–clonic seizures.

Generalised onset seizures

Generalised onset seizures arise within the central nervous system (CNS) and rapidly involve bilaterally distributed networks in the brain. They start in both hemispheres simultaneously. Generalised non-motor or '**absence seizures**', simple or complex (formerly known as petit mal), are most often seen in childhood and consist of temporary lapses in consciousness that last a few seconds. They may have many episodes in a single day. Sometimes a generalised absence seizure is followed by a generalised **tonic–clonic seizure**.

Myoclonic seizures, a type of generalised onset motor seizure, are characterised by sudden shock-like muscle jerks, often with loss of consciousness. They may be atonic (with loss of muscle tone), tonic (with sudden muscle stiffening), or tonic–clonic (alternating muscle stiffening and jerking).

The most common type of epilepsy is tonic–clonic generalised epilepsy (formerly known as grand mal). Seizures of this type may be characterised by a warning aura (numbness, visual disturbance, or dizziness), followed by sudden loss of consciousness and motor control. The person falls forcefully due to continuous tonic spasm (stiffening, increased muscle tone), which may be followed by a series of clonic (rapid, synchronous jerking) muscular contractions. The eyes roll upwards, the arms flex, and the legs extend. Respiration is suspended temporarily, the skin becomes sweaty and cyanotic, incontinence may occur, saliva flows, and the person may bite the tongue. No pain is felt, as the person is deeply unconscious. When the seizure subsides, the person regains partial consciousness, may complain of aching, and then tends to fall into a deep sleep. High frequency of tonic–clonic seizures is associated with a high risk of sudden unexplained death in epilepsy due to seizure-induced hypoxia, cardiac dysrhythmias, and autonomic dysfunction.

Status epilepticus is a clinical emergency. It is the state of continuous seizure activity or repeated seizures without an intervening period of consciousness. A 10% mortality rate results from hypoxia in this state (Choi et al 2022). The major cause of status epilepticus is untreated or under-treated epilepsy. Other causes include cerebral infarction, CNS tumour or infection, trauma, or low blood concentration of calcium or glucose (Trinka et al 2015).

CLINICAL FOCUS BOX 20.1

Drugs that may cause seizures

Drugs that reduce the seizure threshold via their action in the CNS are potentially dangerous in people predisposed to or who have epilepsy. Groups of drugs known to have this effect include some anticholinesterases, antipsychotics, antihistamines, interferons, monoamine oxidase inhibitors, quinolone antibiotics and some other antimicrobials, selective serotonin reuptake inhibitors and other serotonergic drugs, tricyclic antidepressants, general anaesthetics, vaccines, narcotic analgesics, bronchodilators, social drugs (alcohol, caffeine, cocaine, cannabis), and even some **antiepileptic (anticonvulsant) drugs** (AEDs) themselves (clonazepam, sodium valproate), plus many individual drugs. The metabolites of pethidine (norpethidine) also cause seizures. Such drugs should be used cautiously, if at all, in conjunction with AEDs.

Triggers to seizures

Idiopathic epilepsy has no known organic cause, but many factors are likely to act as triggers to an attack. These include hyperventilation, trauma, lack of sleep, poor nutrition, excess alcohol, fever, stress, bright lights – especially flashing lights of a TV set or strobe lights such as in a nightclub – or changes in blood levels of hormones, fluids, or electrolytes. Catamenial epilepsy describes the pattern of more frequent seizures during specific times in the menstrual cycle (Bui 2022). A high estrogen to progesterone ratio favours seizure activity. See Clinical Focus Box 20.1 for drugs that may cause seizures.

20.1 Antiepileptic drug therapy

Clinical aspects

The main goal of antiepileptic drugs is to control or prevent the recurrence of the seizure disorder while ensuring unwanted drug effects do not limit the person more than further seizures would. When deciding whether to treat epilepsy with drugs, the severity of the seizures and the person's circumstances are taken into consideration. Factors to consider when choosing an antiepileptic drug include:

- efficacy in treating the syndrome
- certainty of syndrome diagnosis
- current or future pregnancy
- adverse effects including body weight changes, impaired cognition and sedation, cosmetic changes such as hirsutism, gingival hyperplasia
- age
- cost
- ease of use
- need for measuring serum drug concentration
- pharmacokinetics
- drug interactions
- preparations available.

While secondary epilepsy usually responds to correction of the underlying condition and perhaps short-term use of drugs, primary generalised epilepsy requires long-term AED therapy (Neurology Expert Group 2017).

DRUGS AT A GLANCE
Antiepileptic drugs

PHARMACOLOGICAL GROUP AND MECHANISM OF ACTION	KEY EXAMPLES	CLINICAL USE
Antiepileptic drugs (= anticonvulsants)		
GABA inhibition enhancers *Benzodiazepines* *Barbiturates* • Occupy specific allosteric binding sites in the GABA receptor complex to facilitate GABA-mediated inhibition of neural activity via activation of chloride ion channels	Diazepam, midazolam Phenobarbitone	Treatment of acute seizure activity and status epilepticus
Others		
• Blocks sodium channels • Enhances GABA inhibition • Antagonises the action of kainate at excitatory glutamate receptors • Weak carbonic anhydrase (CA) inhibitor • Selective inhibitor of both neuronal and glial GABA (gamma-aminobutyric acid) uptake, resulting in an increase in GABA-mediated inhibition in the brain • Irreversible inhibitor of GABA transaminase, thereby allows a buildup of the neurotransmitter in synapses	Topiramate	Management of seizure activity (preventative)
Sodium channel function inhibitors • Blocks neuronal sodium channels decreasing excitability	Sodium valproate, phenytoin, carbamazepine, lamotrigine	Management of seizure activity (including acute and preventative)
Miscellaneous/others • Raises brain GABA levels and inhibits glutamate synthesis	Gabapentin	Management of seizure activity (preventative), neurogenic pain
• Binds to synaptic vesicle glycoprotein SV2A and inhibits presynaptic calcium channels, thus reducing neurotransmitter release	Levetiracetam	Management of seizure activity (preventative)

Monotherapy and subsequent therapy

The aim of treatment is to control epilepsy with one AED (monotherapy), introduced slowly. Approximately 70% of people become seizure-free with the first AED tried. If maximum tolerated doses of one drug are not effective, another drug is added and the first drug is gradually withdrawn. If seizure control cannot be achieved with the two drugs, a different drug may be tried. Up to 70% of children and adults with epilepsy can be successfully treated (i.e. their seizures completely controlled) with AEDs (WHO 2024). About 14% become seizure-free with the second or third drug. Furthermore, after 2–5 years of successful treatment and being seizure-free, drugs can be withdrawn in about 60% of adults without subsequent relapse (Bastos et al 2020).

Choice of antiepileptic drug

Different types of seizure may respond best to specific antiepileptic agents, although levetiracetam and sodium valproate are considered first-line treatment for most seizure types in people who are not likely to become pregnant. Specific subsets of epilepsy require individualised treatment (e.g. in absence seizures in childhood, ethosuximide is better tolerated and therefore is the drug of first choice). Drug treatment should be individualised according to the seizure type, co-morbidities, current drug treatment, and the preferences of the individual. Second-line agents may be tried if the first-line drugs are not successful in controlling seizures. (See tables in Therapeutic Guidelines: Neurology 2021, for details and dose regimens.)

Drug-resistant epilepsy

Drug-resistant (refractory or uncontrolled) epilepsy is defined as a failure of adequate trials of two (or more) tolerated, appropriately chosen and used AED regimens (whether administered as monotherapy or in combination) to achieve freedom from seizures. About 75% of people can be well controlled with drugs. The other 25% – especially those who had many seizures before treatment, had inadequate response to the first drug tried, or in whom there was a known cause of epilepsy – may remain refractory to treatment for a period and should be referred to a specialist epilepsy centre for careful re-examination and treatment. Common reasons for the failure of first AED treatment are lack of efficacy or intolerable side effects, particularly severe skin reactions.

Status epilepticus

Generalised convulsive status epilepticus is fortunately rare and results from failure of normal mechanisms to terminate an isolated seizure. First-line drugs are fast-acting benzodiazepines, such as diazepam given IV (2 mg/minute to maximum of 10 mg) or rectally, clonazepam (IV 1–2 mg over 2–5 minutes), or midazolam (IV, IM, intranasal, buccal), followed by a long-acting AED such as IV phenytoin, sodium valproate, phenobarbital, or levetiracetam. If these are ineffective, general anaesthetics are required (thiopental, midazolam, or propofol), with assisted ventilation to ensure adequate ventilation and oxygenation is achieved (AMH 2024).

Medication adherence and therapeutic drug monitoring

As seizures may occur at irregular intervals, epilepsy can be difficult to control clinically. Clinical response to treatment is the mainstay of monitoring, in line with ILAE guidelines. People should be encouraged to keep a simple diary, recording all drugs taken and seizures experienced. As with other conditions in which relapses and remissions occur, therapeutic monitoring can be useful in optimising drug therapy while minimising adverse drug reactions.

It is important to individualise epilepsy treatment to achieve seizure control with the least adverse effects. Therapeutic drug monitoring involves measuring serum concentrations of drugs to examine the relationship between dosage prescribed, concentration in body fluids, and pharmacological effect. Published therapeutic plasma 'reference ranges' of various AEDs are used as a guide to therapy. Measurement of plasma antiepileptic drug concentrations is particularly recommended for carbamazepine, phenobarbital, and phenytoin. It is a valuable tool for assessing individual variability in responses to doses and for studying variations in pharmacokinetics.

Discontinuing antiepileptic therapy

A diagnosis of epilepsy no longer implies a lifetime of drug therapy: as noted before, AEDs may be safely withdrawn from up to 60% of people who are seizure-free for at least 2 years. In long-term studies (Lamberink et al 2017), seizures recurred in about 50% of people, particularly in those who had:

- an onset of seizures after 18 years of age
- a family history of seizure activity
- a longer duration before seizure control was achieved
- a large total number of seizures
- an abnormal EEG even with therapy
- the presence of an organic neurological disorder or intellectual disability.

Withdrawal from phenytoin or sodium valproate is associated with a higher rate of recurrence than for other drugs. Abrupt discontinuation of an AED may provoke seizures or status epilepticus. Medications should be tapered down slowly (in a non-emergency situation) to avoid risks. If the person is taking more than one AED, each drug is withdrawn separately and slowly over several months.

Principles of epilepsy management for women in their reproductive years

While many of the underlying management principles for women in their reproductive years who might possibly become pregnant are the same as for the general population, there are additional specific considerations (Speigel et al 2020). Overall, seizure control is of the highest priority because hypoxia and trauma from seizures during pregnancy generally pose a greater risk to mother and fetus than do AED adverse effects (Vajda et al 2020). Unplanned pregnancy is common and should be avoided. Pregnancy is best planned when the woman has remained free from seizures for 9–12 months, on an AED with a lower risk for teratogenic and neurobehavioural issues affecting the baby.

The principles of managing epilepsy for women in their reproductive years are:

1 Choose the best AED for the seizure type.

2 Choose an AED with the lowest rate of teratogenesis and neurobehavioural issues for the infant.

3 Use one drug when this is sufficient and in the lowest effective dose to maintain seizure control.

4 Do not wait until after pregnancy diagnosis to shift to a pregnancy appropriate AED. Doing so results in teratogenic risk during the critical early period of organogenesis and places the woman and her fetus at risk for seizure complications while determining whether the new AED will adequately prevent seizures.

5 All women with epilepsy who might become pregnant, not only those actively attempting conception, should supplement with folic acid. Neural tube defects are more common in infants born to women using AEDs. While there is no direct evidence folic acid interrupts this higher risk, it is effective at preventing neural tube defects in the general population (Benson & Pack 2020). Dose recommendations vary between 2–5 mg, with higher doses advised for women using AEDs associated with higher rates of neural tube defects or where there is another risk factor. This is higher than the dose in most pregnancy multivitamins.

6 Lamotrigine and levetiracetam are the most used AEDs for women in their reproductive years, as they balance high levels of effectiveness as a monotherapy against lower fetal risks. Plasma concentrations of some AEDs, especially carbamazepine, lamotrigine, and phenytoin, may fall during pregnancy, putting mother and fetus at risk. Baseline measurements should be taken before or early in pregnancy and then regularly to maintain drug levels close to optimum (Jacob et al 2016).

Clinical trials and treatment in pregnancy and lactation

Clinical trials of drugs do not usually include pregnant or lactating women as subjects. Consequently, there is relative absence of data about the effectiveness of new drugs for pregnant and lactating women, and the risks of teratogenesis. Large registries collate data from women exposed to AEDs during pregnancy, such as the European Registry of Antiepileptic Drugs and Pregnancy (EURAP), the UK epilepsy and pregnancy register, the Irish epilepsy and pregnancy register, and the USA epilepsy and pregnancy register. In Australia, women with epilepsy who are pregnant or have given birth in the previous 12 months (regardless of whether they are currently using AEDs or not) are invited to contribute to the Australian pregnancy register for women on AEDs – www.apr.org.au.

AEDs and teratogenesis

Many AEDs are potentially teratogenic or can affect cognitive development of the child. Fetal abnormalities are two to three times more likely in babies whose mothers took AEDs during pregnancy (Güveli et al 2017; Tomson et al 2019). Treatment of epileptic women of childbearing age must include consideration of these risks. In women planning pregnancy, only continue treatment if needed to prevent seizures (Veroniki et al 2017; Weston et al 2016). Common AED associated malformations include cardiovascular defects (like atrial or ventricular septal defects, tetralogy of Fallot, patent ductus arteriosus) and musculoskeletal defects. Valproate use in the first trimester increases the likelihood of spina bifida 12 times, while for carbamazepine the increased risk is 2.6 times above the population risk (Li & Meador 2022).

All the 'old' AEDs are implicated, especially high-dose sodium valproate (Table 20.1). Recommendations for sodium valproate now include a maximum daily dose of 600 mg for women of childbearing potential, lower than was previously advised. At this dose the teratogenic risk is like other AEDs. Some of the second-generation AEDs, such as tiagabine, gabapentin, pregabalin, and levetiracetam, appear to have higher fetal safety.

AEDs and neurobehavioural effects for the infant

Infants born to women using AEDs have lower intelligence quotient (IQ) scores and are more likely to be diagnosed with autism or attention deficit hyperactivity disorder (Li & Meador 2022). Levetiracetam and topiramate appear to be best options to reduce the possibility of these problems. Unlike teratogenesis, the risk period for development of neurobehavioural disorders is the third trimester. Therapeutic drug monitoring plays a role in ensuring the minimum effective dose is used during this trimester.

TABLE 20.1 Central nervous system adverse effects of some antiepileptic drugs

DRUG	BEHAVIOURAL ALTERATIONS	COGNITIVE EFFECTS
Phenobarbital (phenobarbitone)	Physical dependence, altered mood. May cause a paradoxical effect (e.g. increased activity or excitement, irritability, altered sleep patterns, increased tiredness)	Confusion, impaired judgement, short-term memory impairment, decreased attention span
Carbamazepine	Drowsiness, anorexia, increased irritability, insomnia, behavioural changes, depression	Less than phenytoin, phenobarbital (phenobarbitone) or primidone
Diazepam	Drowsiness, dizziness, ataxia, impaired speech and vision, hysteria, tolerance, dependence and withdrawal symptoms after cessation, paradoxical reactions (excitement, insomnia, agitation)	Anterograde amnesia, memory impairment, confusion, impaired concentration
Lamotrigine	Dizziness, ataxia, somnolence, hyperkinesia	
Phenytoin	Insomnia/sedation, fatigue, increased clumsiness, mood alterations, agitation, vertigo	Decreased attention span, decreased ability to solve problems, impaired learning, confusion
Sodium valproate	Sedation, ataxia, depression, increased appetite and weight, tremor	Stupor (associated with excess dosage or polytherapy)

Contraception

Epilepsy itself appears to carry no risk for infertility; however, higher rates of infertility have been reported for women using valproate or phenobarbitone, or who require a polypharmacy approach to maintain seizure control. Planning pregnancy is important, so consider the use of highly effective contraception for any women not actively attempting pregnancy. All women with epilepsy who have the potential for pregnancy (in that they have not had permanent sterilisation or hysterectomy and are sexually active with a male partner) should be counselled and supported to access effective contraception to reduce the incidence of unplanned pregnancy.

AEDs may reduce the effectiveness of the oral contraceptive pill due to the enzyme-inducing capabilities of most AEDs, leading to breakthrough bleeding, ovulation, and pregnancy. (See DI 20.1 and Critical Thinking Scenario.) Drugs that are known to induce enzymes are: phenytoin, phenobarbital, primidone, carbamazepine, eslicarbazepine acetate, oxcarbazepine, rufinamide, topiramate (in doses of $\geq$ 200 mg/d), perampanel (in doses of $\geq$ 12 mg/d), cenobamate, and felbamate (Benson & Pack 2020).

Women treated with an AED who wish to use the oral contraceptive pill are advised to use a high-dose option along with condoms to improve contraceptive efficacy (Li & Meador 2022). Progestin releasing and copper intrauterine devices maintain their efficacy as enzyme induced metabolism does not impact on the mechanism of action for either (Benson & Pack 2020). Higher failure rates occur with hormone implants and injections, and these should be replaced or repeated at a shorter interval than is usually advised.

The converse can also occur. Estrogen induces the metabolism of lamotrigine, decreasing plasma concentration of the drug and can lead to seizure breakthrough (Benson & Pack 2020). The four- to seven-day hormone free interval typical of most oral contraceptive pills is problematic for women using AEDs with shorter half-lives due to the fluctuating levels of their medication that occur. Avoiding the hormone-free interval and taking 'active' pills daily avoids this.

Pregnancy and epilepsy

It is difficult to differentiate between the risk of epilepsy on pregnancy outcomes and the risk relating to AED use. The risk of pregnancy complications appears to be higher among women with epilepsy and preventing seizures is believed to reduce this risk, though it is challenging to prove this in research. Higher rates of perinatal mortality, miscarriage, antepartum haemorrhage, hypertensive disorders of pregnancy, breech presentation, and preterm birth have been reported (Li & Meador 2022). Hypoxia during seizures clearly presents a risk for concurrent fetal hypoxia.

Most women experience no change in their seizure frequency during labour, unless their medication regime is changed. One or two percent of women experience seizures during labour, and an agreed and written management plan for what to do in this event is preferable. Epilepsy in the absence of a specific pregnancy complication is not considered an indication for caesarean section.

The puerperium and epilepsy

Although breastfeeding is not usually contraindicated in mothers taking AEDs, CNS-depressant drugs may pass into breast milk, so breastfed infants should be monitored for drowsiness and feeding difficulties. Sleep deprivation can trigger seizure activity. Women and their immediate family should have a plan to avoid sleep deprivation and to manage any seizures in the early postnatal period. Adjustments to parenting, such as changing nappies on the floor rather than a change table, or never bathing the baby when alone, may be required to avoid the risk of harm to the infant should the mother experience a seizure during this activity.

Falling estrogen levels reverse the enzyme induction seen during pregnancy, reducing the metabolism of many AEDs. Stepped dose reductions in the first week after birth are advised, returning to the pre-pregnancy dose to avoid adverse effects from higher serum levels (Benson & Pack 2020). Monitoring drug levels during this period of adjustment may be helpful. Rates of anxiety and depression have been reported to be higher in the postnatal period for women with epilepsy (Li & Meador 2022). Screening and appropriate early management of perinatal mental health concerns are important (CFB 20.2).

CLINICAL FOCUS BOX 20.2

Counselling

The risks of antiepileptic drug therapy to the fetus, and the risks of suboptimally treated epilepsy to the mother and fetus, should be considered and discussed with the woman (Stephen et al 2019). Sudden cessation of an AED during early pregnancy risks loss of seizure control. Women with epilepsy do not always discuss this decision with their care provider in advance, so it is important to proactively discuss this and advise against medication cessation.

Important aspects of living with epilepsy, including issues related to emergency management of seizures, sleep patterns, employment, driving and other hazardous activities, use of social drugs, and participation in sport and other recreational activities, also need to be discussed. While these may have been addressed prior to pregnancy, it may be beneficial for the woman and those close to her to renew this discussion with their neurologist during the pregnancy.

Eclampsia

Eclampsia is a serious complication of the pregnancy specific disorder of pre-eclampsia. The occurrence of seizures marks the distinction between the two conditions, with eclampsia representing a severe form of the condition. Pre-eclampsia is characterised by elevated blood pressure, proteinuria, and evidence of dysfunction in other organ systems such as elevated liver enzymes and low platelet counts (see Chapter 15 – Hypertension). Treatment of pre-eclampsia aims to control elevated blood pressure, prevent seizures, maintain organ function, and generally provide optimal conditions for the woman and her fetus while planning for birth and postpartum recovery to occur.

Women with moderate-to-severe pre-eclampsia who are at risk for eclamptic seizures should be offered prophylaxis with magnesium sulphate (see Chapter 15). Eclamptic seizures are usually self-limiting tonic–clonic seizures, and last 60 to 90 seconds. If the seizure is prolonged, intravenous diazepam clonazepam may be given while the magnesium sulphate is being prepared if the seizure is prolonged. The mother should continue to be monitored closely after birth, as seizures may still occur in the postpartum period.

KEY POINTS

Antiepileptic drug therapy

- Antiepileptic drug therapy to control seizures may be lifelong. The choice of drug is determined by the type of seizure, likely adverse drug reactions, other drugs that may interact, and individual aspects such as pregnancy and adherence.

- Therapeutic monitoring is regularly carried out for some AEDs by measuring drug concentration in plasma samples. This helps in checking whether levels are in the therapeutic range, in monitoring adverse drug reactions, and adherence. It is important to individualise epilepsy treatment to achieve seizure control with the least adverse effects.

- AEDs may reduce the risk of pregnancy complications, but this must be balanced against the risk of teratogenesis or neurobehavioural disorders.

- Contraception and pregnancy planning are important and may reduce risks associated with epilepsy and AED use in pregnancy.

20.2 Antiepileptic drugs

The ideal antiepileptic drug

Although there is no ideal antiepileptic drug, the following characteristics are desirable:

- highly effective, with a low incidence of toxicity
- effective against more than one type of seizure and for mixed seizures
- long-acting and non-sedating so the person is not inconvenienced by the need for multiple daily drug dosing or by excessive drowsiness
- not highly protein-bound and not involved in significant drug interactions
- inexpensive, as people may have to take it for years or for the rest of their lives
- not resulting in the development of tolerance to the therapeutic effects.

The major first-line drugs used in the treatment of focal seizures and generalised tonic–clonic seizures in people who are not likely to become pregnant are sodium valproate and levetiracetam. Newer AEDs include gabapentin, lamotrigine, vigabatrin, tiagabine, topiramate, and levetiracetam. As no one antiepileptic agent is ideal, there is considerable current research into new mechanisms of action of AEDs. It is very expensive to carry out large-scale, high-powered clinical trials, particularly in a chronic condition such as epilepsy in which the manifestations (seizures) occur occasionally and randomly, so there is little level-one evidence on the comparative efficacy and safety of the newer AEDs from randomised controlled clinical trials. There is even less research on the safety of these drugs in pregnancy and lactation.

General considerations

Adverse drug reactions are common with AEDs. In particular, CNS depression is likely (Table 20.2) and there are behavioural and cognitive effects. While each drug has its own adverse-effect profile, common reactions include excessive sedation, ataxia and confusion, and depression of the cardiovascular and respiratory centres. Paradoxical reactions (excitation rather than depression) sometimes occur with benzodiazepines and barbiturates. A possible association between some AEDs and suicidal thoughts or behaviours has been flagged and should be monitored.

Some AEDs enhance the metabolism of vitamin D and reduce bone mineral density (Khoo et al 2023). Along with the increased risk of falls with seizures and with the CNS-depressant effects of AEDs, this compounds the risk of fractures, so levels of calcium and vitamin D may need monitoring. This is particularly the case for women with dark skin, those with reduced sun exposure, or who live well south of the equator. Vitamin D supplementation may be advisable during pregnancy for women at higher risk of deficiency.

TABLE 20.2 Properties of long-established antiepileptic drugs

DRUG	SITE OF ACTION				MAIN USES	MAIN UNWANTED EFFECT(S)	PHARMACOKINETICS
	SODIUM CHANNEL	GABA$_A$ RECEPTOR	CALCIUM CHANNEL	OTHER			
Carbamazepine	+				All types except absence seizures Most widely used antiepileptic drug	Sedation, ataxia, blurred vision, water retention, hypersensitivity reactions, leukopenia, liver failure (rare)	Half-life 12–18 h (longer initially) Strong induction of liver enzymes, so risk of drug interactions
Phenytoin	+				All types except absence seizures	Ataxia, vertigo, gum hypertrophy, hirsutism, megaloblastic anaemia, fetal malformation, hypersensitivity reactions	Half-life ~24 h Saturation kinetics therefore unpredictable plasma levels Plasma monitoring often required
Valproate	+	?+	+	GABA transaminase inhibition	Most types, including absence seizures	Generally less than with other drugs Nausea, hair loss, weight gain, fetal malformations	Half-life 12–15 h
Phenobarbital (phenobarbitone)	?+	+			All types except absence seizures	Sedation, depression	Long plasma half-life (> 60 h) Strong induction of liver enzymes, so risk of drug interactions (e.g. with phenytoin)
Benzodiazepines (e.g. diazepam)		+			Used intravenously to control status epilepticus	Sedation Withdrawal syndrome	See Chapter 19

Source: Dale MM, Rang HP: *Rang & Dale's pharmacology*. Edinburgh; Churchill Livingstone 2007.

Antiepileptic hypersensitivity syndrome

Antiepileptic hypersensitivity syndrome is a rare but potentially serious reaction related to the CYP450 metabolites of barbiturates, carbamazepine, and phenytoin. It can occur 1–4 weeks after treatment initiation and involves fever, rash that can develop into Stevens-Johnson syndrome, toxic epidermal necrolysis, and impairment of systemic organs. Administration of the drug must be stopped.

Drug interactions

Many AEDs are metabolised by CYP450 enzymes, and/or either induce or inhibit these enzymes, so drug interactions with AEDs are common, variable, and unpredictable. Interactions need to be anticipated. A good general rule is 'see an antiepileptic drug, think **drug interactions**'. Therapeutic monitoring is important whenever adding or withdrawing an antiepileptic drug, as drug concentrations and efficacies may be increased or reduced (Johannessen et al 2020). Typical examples are shown in Drug Interactions 20.1. As it is difficult to generalise drug interaction effects with AEDs, a reference text should be consulted for details of adverse drug interactions with individual antiepileptic agents, for example AMH 2024 (Fisher et al 2017b).

KEY POINTS

General considerations for antiepileptic drugs

- While all CNS-depressant drugs may reduce seizure incidence, most are too sedating to be useful. The major drugs used to treat seizures act by enhancing GABA-mediated inhibition of neural transmission, or inhibit neurotransmission by blocking sodium channel functions.

- The most common adverse effects are those of CNS depression. Antiepileptic hypersensitivity syndrome is a rarer but serious reaction affecting particularly the skin.

- Drug interactions are common because of the effects of antiepileptic agents in increasing or decreasing the metabolism of other drugs. The possibility of drug interactions must always be borne in mind by health professionals providing care for people with epilepsy.

20.3 Mechanisms of action of currently used antiepileptics

The aim of using a drug to prevent seizures is to decrease the likelihood of excessive neuronal transmission in CNS pathways, without causing excessive sedation. The exact modes and sites of action for effective AEDs are complex and incompletely understood. A common mechanism of action relates to stabilisation of the nerve cell membrane by altering cation transport, especially that of sodium, potassium, or calcium (e.g. sodium valproate, phenytoin, or carbamazepine) and enhancing the effect of **gamma-aminobutyric acid** (GABA) (e.g. benzodiazepines).

The main mechanisms of action of currently used antiepileptics are:

- enhancement of GABA inhibition
- inhibition of sodium channel function
- other mechanisms, including inhibition of calcium channel function, inhibiting glutamate release, antagonism of AMPA-induced neuronal excitability, and inhibition of carbonic anhydrase (CA) in the CNS causing intracellular acidification.

Note that some drugs may have more than one proposed mechanism of action (Tables 20.1 and 20.3).

Antiepileptics that enhance GABA inhibition

Neuronal activity is reduced by drugs that enhance GABA-mediated inhibition. Possible pathways to achieving this are by facilitating GABA-mediated opening of chloride channels, inhibiting GABA transaminase (the enzyme that inactivates GABA), or by inhibiting the GABA reuptake processes. The benzodiazepines (midazolam, clobazam, and clonazepam), and barbiturates (phenobarbital) act by facilitating GABA-mediated opening of chloride channels (see Chapter 19). Some newer drugs (vigabatrin, tiagabine, and topiramate) act by mechanisms relating to GABA inhibition.

Benzodiazepines

The benzodiazepines used as AEDs are those with long half-lives, such as diazepam, and midazolam (Table 20.1). These drugs are sedative–hypnotic and antianxiety agents. Their mechanism of action is to occupy specific benzodiazepine-binding sites on the GABA receptor and facilitate GABA-mediated inhibition via activation of chloride ion channels (see DM 19.1, Chapter 19 for details on diazepam). This suppresses the propagation of seizure activity. Long-term benzodiazepine use is not recommended due to sedative effects, dependence, tolerance, and withdrawal reactions after cessation.

Diazepam and other benzodiazepines can be given orally or IV, or rectally when IV injection is not possible – for example, in prolonged eclamptic convulsions that do not respond to magnesium sulphate. It has rapid onset but short duration of antiepileptic action because it redistributes rapidly out of the CNS, then has a long elimination half-life. Drug interactions with other CNS depressants (including alcohol) are common. Dosage is usually individualised and titrated for effectiveness.

TABLE 20.3 Properties of newer antiepileptic drugs

DRUG	SITE OF ACTION				MAIN USES	MAIN UNWANTED EFFECT(S)	PHARMACOKINETICS
	SODIUM CHANNEL	GABA$_A$ RECEPTOR	CALCIUM CHANNEL	OTHER			
Lamotrigine	+		?+	Inhibits glutamate release	All types	Dizziness, sedation, rashes	Plasma half-life 24–36 h
Gabapentin			+		Focal seizures	Few side effects, mainly sedation	Plasma half-life 6–9 h
Topiramate	+	?+	?+	AMPA receptor block	Focal and generalised tonic–clonic seizures Lennox–Gastaut syndrome	Sedation Fewer pharmacokinetic interactions than phenytoin Fetal malformation	Plasma half-life −20 h Excreted unchanged
Levetiracetam				Binds to SV2A protein	Focal and generalised tonic–clonic seizures	Sedation (slight)	Plasma half-life −7 h Excreted unchanged

SV2A = synaptic vesicle protein 2A
Source: Rang et al 2016, Table 45.2.

Barbiturates

The mechanism of action for barbiturates is non-selective depression of the CNS via facilitation of chloride entry into cells at GABA$_A$ receptors (acting at a different site from those where GABA or benzodiazepines bind), enhancing inhibitory systems that use GABA as a neurotransmitter (see Chapter 19). Barbiturates selectively act on the motor cortex even in small doses, which explains their use as AEDs. Barbiturates, especially phenobarbital (phenobarbitone), have been used for many decades. However, their use is limited by initial sedative effects, a reduced safety margin, and a high incidence of tolerance to anticonvulsant activity developing over time (Table 20.1). Drug interactions are frequent, especially with other CNS depressants, including alcohol.

Topiramate

This relatively new AED is indicated as adjunctive therapy in seizures not well controlled by other drugs. Topiramate has four useful mechanisms of action (Table 20.3) and is used for focal and generalised seizures in adults. The main adverse reactions are CNS-depressant effects.

KEY POINTS

Antiepileptics that enhance GABA inhibition

Drugs that act by enhancement of GABA inhibition include:

- barbiturates (phenobarbital [phenobarbitone]),
- benzodiazepines (diazepam, midazolam) that act to facilitate the action of GABA at the GABA receptor complex
- topiramate, which has four mechanisms of action.

Antiepileptics that inhibit sodium channel function

Drugs that inhibit sodium channel function appear to preferentially block the excitation of cells that are firing repetitively. Refer to Tables 20.1 and 20.3 for the properties of long-established and newer antiepileptic drugs. Phenytoin blocks sodium channels and possibly also calcium influx, thus stabilising cell membrane excitability and reducing the spread of seizure discharge. Carbamazepine also inactivates sodium channels, which alters neuronal excitability and decreases synaptic transmission. Other examples of drugs acting by this mechanism are sodium valproate and lamotrigine.

Phenytoin

Phenytoin (diphenylhydantoin) (DM 20.1; Table 20.1) was developed by searching for an AED that would cause less sedation than the barbiturates. Phenytoin is recommended for treating all types of epilepsy except absence seizures. It is particularly interesting from the pharmacokinetic point of view, as it has **non-linear pharmacokinetic** parameters, which often make clinical use of phenytoin difficult. There is a genetic variability in metabolism.

DRUG MONOGRAPH 20.1
Phenytoin

Mechanism of action and indications

Phenytoin acts by blocking sodium channels. It is more effective for generalised and focal seizures than for generalised absence seizures. It is also frequently prescribed in combination with phenobarbital (phenobarbitone) and may be prescribed to prevent seizures after surgery on the brain, after head trauma, and for status epilepticus.

Pharmacokinetics

Because of saturable metabolism, the non-linear pharmacokinetics of phenytoin means that the dose–plasma concentration relationship is complex, and a small rise in dose may cause an unexpectedly large rise in plasma drug levels. Oral absorption of phenytoin is slow and variable. The drug is highly bound to plasma albumin. The time to peak serum level is 1.5–3 hours and the half-life varies with dose and serum level, ranging from 7–42 hours, with an average of about 24 hours. Steady-state levels are achieved after 7–10 days. It is inactivated in the liver and metabolites are excreted in the bile and in urine.

Drug interactions

There are many important drug interactions with phenytoin (DI 20.1; AMH 2024). Drugs including chloramphenicol, cimetidine, disulfiram, isoniazid, oral anticoagulants, allopurinol, omeprazole, imipramine, azole antifungals, and sulfonamides may inhibit the metabolism of phenytoin and hence prolong the half-life, leading to neurotoxic effects.

Adverse reactions

There are many dose-related neurotoxic effects (drowsiness, dizziness, confusion) at plasma concentrations higher than 80 micromol/L (20 mg/L), as well as idiosyncratic reactions such as hirsutism, gingival hyperplasia with bleeding, sensitive gum tissue or overgrowth of gum tissue, acne, and facial coarsening. Signs of overdose or toxicity include blurred or double vision, slurred speech, clumsiness, dizziness, confusion, and hallucinations.

Warnings and contraindications

Use with caution in pregnancy (Category D) and in people with drug allergies, diabetes mellitus, cardiac arrhythmias, or liver or renal impairment. Women relying on estrogen-containing contraceptives may require higher doses or should use non-hormonal contraception. Regular dental care is important to detect gum problems. Avoid use in people with hydantoin hypersensitivity, and exercise caution when used in combination with similar compounds such as phenobarbital (phenobarbitone) and carbamazepine. In long-term use, bone mineral density should be monitored, and vitamin D and calcium supplements may be required.

Dosage and administration

The usual adult dosage is 200–500 mg daily. Careful monitoring and titration of dose is required to keep the plasma concentration within the therapeutic range of 40–80 micromol/L (10–20 mg/L). Free phenytoin levels may need to be measured at steady state during pregnancy as lower concentrations of albumin impairs protein binding.

In status epilepticus in adults, phenytoin is given IV 15–20 mg/kg and an additional 5 mg/kg is given after 12 hours if necessary. Phenytoin has very low water solubility and is provided in specially formulated IV solutions, which should not be administered IM or mixed with other drugs or glucose solutions.

Carbamazepine

Carbamazepine also blocks sodium channels, preventing repetitive neuronal discharges and decreasing the propagation of seizures (Table 20.1). Oral absorption is slow, and onset of action may range from hours to days, depending on the individual. Due to auto-induction of metabolism (i.e. it induces higher levels of the enzymes that metabolise it) it may take a month to reach a stable therapeutic serum level. Carbamazepine is metabolised in the liver (it has one active metabolite) and excreted primarily by the kidneys.

Adverse reactions include CNS depression, possible severe hypersensitivity reactions including skin reactions (particularly in people of Asian ancestry), depressed white cell counts, GIT disorders, and antidiuretic hormone-like effects. There are many clinically significant drug interactions with carbamazepine. Its half-life is prolonged by drugs that inhibit CYP3A4 enzymes and by grapefruit juice. It enhances the metabolism and thus decreases the effectiveness of many drugs, including anticoagulants (warfarin), other AEDs and carbamazepine itself, corticosteroids, and oral contraceptives (see a typical example in the Critical Thinking Scenario at the beginning of the chapter). Plasma concentration should be monitored whenever any of these medications is added or discontinued, as dosage adjustment may be necessary.

Sodium valproate

The mechanism by which sodium valproate exerts its antiepileptic effects has not been fully established (Table 20.1). It may enhance brain levels of GABA and

DRUG INTERACTIONS 20.1

Antiepileptics

DRUG	POSSIBLE INTERACTION AND MANAGEMENT
Barbiturates, benzodiazepines, phenytoin	Can cause raised plasma concentrations of other AEDs and of many other drugs, and increase toxicity. Dosages of these drugs may need to be lowered.
Barbiturates, carbamazepine, phenytoin, topiramate	Can induce drug-metabolising enzymes and cause lowered plasma concentrations of other AEDs and even of themselves (and of other drugs, including hormones, cardiovascular drugs, and antimicrobial agents), and reduce seizure control. Drug dosages may need to be raised. Increased metabolism of vitamin D increases risk of fractures. Induce hepatic enzymes and increase metabolism of many hormonal contraceptives, excluding the levonorgestrel intrauterine device and medroxyprogesterone depot, which are preferred hormonal contraceptives.
Drugs that lower the convulsive threshold (including antidepressants, antipsychotics, and anticholinesterases) – usually contraindicated in epilepsy	Potential danger. AED requirements are altered.
Drugs that inhibit CYP3A4, including cimetidine, -conazole antifungals, protease inhibitors, grapefruit juice and fluoroquinolone antibiotics	May inhibit metabolism of benzodiazepines and carbamazepine and prolong their effects. Reduce dose of AED.
Drugs that induce CYP3A4, including corticosteroids, rifampicin, some antivirals, and St John's wort	May increase metabolism of benzodiazepines and carbamazepine and reduce their effects. Increase dose of AED or use another drug.
Sodium valproate	May reduce platelet aggregation and prolong bleeding time. Monitor effects if giving with other drugs that affect bleeding times. Regular use increases concentration and toxicity of lamotrigine, phenobarbitone, and phenytoin.

also block sodium, potassium and/or calcium channels. By competitive inhibition, it may prevent the reuptake of GABA by glial cells and axonal terminals.

Sodium valproate is indicated for treating absence seizures, including generalised absence seizures, and for people with multiple seizure types. It is also useful in bipolar disorder and migraine. Its suitability for women of reproductive age is limited by its association with increased risk of congenital malformations, including spina bifida. Valproate is in Pregnancy Safety Category D for this reason. Adult doses start at 300 mg twice daily and can be increased gradually up to a maximum of 2.5 g/day.

Sodium valproate is converted in the stomach to valproic acid, which is rapidly absorbed from the GIT. Food delays absorption. Sodium valproate has variable onset time and half-life (6–16 hours), depending on the formulation administered.

Adverse effects include drowsiness, tremors, mild gastric distress, hair thinning, weight gain, irregular menstruation, skin reactions and hepatotoxicity (especially in infants), or pancreatitis. Drug interactions occur, particularly with: CNS depressants (alcohol, general anaesthetics, barbiturates); anticoagulants and aspirin (increased risk of bleeding); carbapenem antibiotics (reduce sodium valproate levels and increase risk of seizures); drugs that lower the seizure threshold; and combinations of AEDs because of drug metabolism interactions. Levels should be monitored to check toxicity or compliance.

Lamotrigine

Lamotrigine is believed to stabilise seizures by blocking sodium channels and thus inhibiting the release of excitatory neurotransmitters (glutamate and aspartate) (DM 20.2; Table 20.3). It is indicated as adjunctive therapy for treating focal seizures and generalised epilepsy. It is one of the two most commonly used AEDs for women of reproductive age. It has a long half-life (30 hours) that may be reduced by enzyme-inducing drugs and female sex hormones but increased by sodium valproate. Dosage regimens are complicated, depending on whether or not other drugs affecting the metabolism of lamotrigine are also being taken.

Early clinical experience with lamotrigine has shown that there is a high risk of severe, potentially life-threatening skin reactions, including toxic epidermal necrolysis – in particular, with high dosage or when drug interactions prolong the half-life. Administration must be ceased if any rashes or skin reactions occur.

DRUG MONOGRAPH 20.2
Lamotrigine

Mechanism of action

Lamotrigine stabilises neuronal membranes by blocking voltage-dependent and use-dependent sodium channels and inhibits glutamate release, thus reducing the frequency of action potentials.

Indications

Used for monotherapy and as add-on therapy in the treatment of focal (partial) onset seizures, and generalised tonic–clonic seizures. It is also used for treatment of bipolar disorder.

Pharmacokinetics

Lamotrigine is administered orally, and readily bioavailable with limited first-pass metabolism. Peak plasma concentration is reached by 1–3 hours. It is extensively metabolised in the liver with a mean plasma elimination half-life of 25–35 hours. Steady state is not reached for several days.

Drug interactions

As with all AEDs, there are potential additive effects with other CNS depressants. Metabolism may be increased by drugs that induce drug-metabolising enzymes, including other AEDs such as carbamazepine, necessitating dose increase. Phenytoin may increase the concentration of lamotrigine by enzyme inhibition.

Adverse reactions

The most common adverse effects are due to CNS depression and include cognitive impairment, ataxia, and speech disorders. Women should be warned against driving or operating machinery. Other possible adverse effects include headache, fatigue, nausea and vomiting, photosensitivity, blurred vision, and thrombocytopaenia. Serious skin reactions (Stevens-Johnson syndrome and toxic epidermal necrolysis) have been reported in people receiving lamotrigine, usually when concurrently taking other AEDs associated with these disorders.

Warnings and contraindications

Precautions are required before prescribing to women predisposed to the adverse effects, especially those with hepatic impairment, or a history of serious skin reactions to other AEDs.

The drug is classified D with respect to pregnancy safety, due to increased risk of cleft lip and/or palate. While the incidence of malformations is higher for women using lamotrigine than those using no AED, it is lower than for sodium valproate (Vajda et al 2010). There is no evidence for lower intelligence quotient scores in infants exposed to lamotrigine in utero (Bromley et al 2014).

Dosage and administration

Lamotrigine is available as tablets. Dispersible and chewable options are available for people who have difficulty swallowing tablets. The usual starting monotherapy dose in adults is 25 mg/day, taken at night, gradually increasing to a maximum of 200 mg.

KEY POINTS

Antiepileptics that inhibit sodium channel function

- Drugs that inhibit sodium channel function appear to block preferentially the excitation of cells that are firing repetitively.

- Phenytoin blocks sodium channels and possibly also calcium influx, thus stabilising cell membrane excitability and reducing the spread of seizure discharge.

- Carbamazepine also inactivates sodium channels, which alters neuronal excitability and decreases synaptic transmission.

- Other examples of drugs acting by this mechanism are sodium valproate and lamotrigine.

Antiepileptics that act by other mechanisms

There are other antiepileptics operating via a variety of mechanisms of action. These antiepileptics include levetiracetam and gabapentin, and some drugs that are more commonly used in other clinical conditions but have useful membrane-stabilising actions such as magnesium sulphate.

Levetiracetam

Levetiracetam is a relatively new AED (DM 20.3; Table 20.3). Its mechanism of action is as yet unknown; however, it binds to synaptic vesicle glycoprotein SV2A and inhibits presynaptic calcium channels, thus reducing neurotransmitter release. It is well tolerated. Common adverse effects include somnolence, headache, and altered behaviours, but long-term safety has not yet been established. There are few significant drug interactions.

> ## DRUG MONOGRAPH 20.3
> ## Levetiracetam
>
> ### Mechanism of action
> The exact mechanism is unknown but binding to synaptic vesicle protein 2A has been proposed as how neuromodulation is achieved.
>
> ### Indications
> Used for monotherapy and as an adjunct in the treatment of focal (partial) onset seizures and for generalised tonic–clonic seizures.
>
> ### Pharmacokinetics
> Levetiracetam is rapidly absorbed after oral administration. Peak plasma concentration occurs at 1.3 hours. Levetiracetam does not bind to plasma proteins. One third of the dose is metabolised and the remainder excreted in urine without alteration. It has a mean plasma elimination half-life of 6–8 hours. Metabolism occurs in the bloodstream rather than the liver.
>
> ### Drug interactions
> Levetiracetam is less prone to drug interactions given the lack of hepatic metabolism.
>
> ### Adverse reactions
> Adverse effects are like other AEDs, and include lethargy, poor concentration, insomnia, double vision, and ataxia. People should be warned against driving or operating machinery. Serious skin reactions have been reported but are rare. Levetiracetam can impact mental health with depression, anxiety, and aggression reported.
>
> ### Warnings and contraindications
> Precautions are required before prescribing to people with renal impairment. The drug is classified B3 with respect to pregnancy safety.
>
> ### Dosage and administration
> Levetiracetam is available as tablets. Oral liquid is available for people who have difficulty swallowing tablets. The usual starting monotherapy dose in adults is 250 mg twice daily, gradually increasing to a maximum of 1500 mg twice a day.

Gabapentin

Gabapentin is an AED that was designed as a GABA analogue but unexpectedly appears not to mimic the actions of GABA. The mechanism for its antiepileptic action is not yet established (Table 20.3). Absorption is reduced with high doses and by antacids.

Magnesium sulphate

Magnesium sulphate has a depressant effect on the CNS and reduces striated muscle contractions. The mechanism of action is unclear but possibly involves the blockade of glutamate receptors. It is used to treat and prevent seizures associated with hypertensive disorders of pregnancy and for neuroprotection of the preterm fetal brain when early birth is anticipated. (See discussion of use under 'Eclampsia' earlier and Chapter 15.)

Adverse effects include flushing, nausea, and vomiting. These are most pronounced during the loading dose. Hypermagnesaemia leads to progressive neuromuscular blockade with loss of deep tendon reflexes and respiratory depression with eventual arrest at high doses. Close monitoring of renal output, tendon reflexes, and respiratory rate, along with serum magnesium levels is advised. Calcium gluconate is used to reverse the effects in cases of overdose.

Magnesium is administered intravenously. It is excreted via the kidney without prior metabolism and is sensitive to changes in renal function. The half-life is 2–4 hours. It is considered safe to use in pregnancy and lactation.

> **KEY POINTS**
>
> **Antiepileptics that act by other mechanisms**
> - Newer drugs act by other mechanisms, including calcium channel blockade and membrane stabilisation. Some of the mechanisms are yet to be elucidated.

CONCLUSION

Epilepsy is characterised by sporadic recurrent episodes of convulsive seizures and is classified by extent (generalised / focal) and signs exhibited (loss of consciousness; muscle tone and twitching). Pharmacotherapy with an AED is the mainstay of treatment for epilepsy. For pregnant women, risks of teratogenesis and neurobehavioural disorders in the infant must be weighed against the risk of hypoxia during seizures. Lamotrigine (sodium channel blocker) and levetiracetam (mechanism unknown) are the most commonly used agents for women of reproductive age. During pregnancy and the postpartum period, women with epilepsy should have multi-disciplinary care.

REVIEW EXERCISES

1 Laura is 29 years old and has idiopathic epilepsy. Over the past 3 years her seizures have been well controlled with a combination of phenytoin and levetiracetam. She and her partner would like to attempt pregnancy. Outline the discussion you would have with her about pharmacological and non-pharmacological management of epilepsy in pregnancy.

2 Pippa used lamotrigine during her pregnancy. Prior to conception, her seizures were controlled by a dose of 100 mg daily. During pregnancy, she increased the dose to 75 mg twice a day to maintain her serum levels close to those that were typical for her prior to pregnancy. Pippa gave birth yesterday.

   a. What issues specific to the postnatal period could increase Pippa's chance of incurring seizures?

   b. What safe practices can Pippa's midwife promote for her as a new mother with a diagnosis of epilepsy?

   c. Describe the approach you would take to managing the dosage of her lamotrigine during the early postnatal period.

REFERENCES

Australian Medicines Handbook 2024. Australian medicines handbook. Adelaide: AMH.

Bastos F, Cross H. Epilepsy. Handb Clin Neurol. 2020;174: 137-158. doi.org/10.1016/B978-0-444-64148-9.00011-9

Benson R, Pack A. Epilepsy. Handb Clin Neurol. 2020;172: 155-167. https://doi.org/10.1016/B978-0-444-64240-0.00009-X

Bromley R, Weston J, Adab N, et al. Treatment for epilepsy in pregnancy: neurodevelopmental outcomes in the child. Cochrane Database Syst Rev. 2014 Oct30; 2014(10):CD010236. doi: 10.1002/14651858.CD010236.pub2.

Bui W. Women's issues in epilepsy. Continuum (Minneap Minn). 2022;28(2);399-427. doi: 10.1212/CON.0000000000001126

Choi S, Lee H, Kim K, et al. Mortality, disability, and prognostic factors of status epilepticus. Neurology. 2022;99(13);e1393-1401. doi.org/10.1212/WNL.0000000000200912

Dale MM, Rang HP. Rang & Dale's pharmacology. Edinburgh: Churchill Livingstone, 2007.

Fisher RS, Cross JH, D'Souza C, et al. Instruction manual for the International League Against Epilepsy: operational classification of seizure types. Epilepsia. 2017 April;58(4):531-542. doi:10.1111/epi.13671

Fisher RS, Cross JH, French JA, et al. Operational classification of seizure types by the International League Against Epilepsy: Position paper of the ILAE Commission for Classification and Terminology. Epilepsia. 2017 Apr;58(4):522–530. doi:10.1111/epi.13670

Güveli BT, Rosti RÖ, Güzeltaş A, et al. Teratogenicity of antiepileptic drugs. Clin Psychopharmacol Neurosci. 2017 Feb 28;15(1):19-27. doi.org/10.9758/cpn.2017.15.1.19

Jacob S, Nair AB. An updated overview on therapeutic drug monitoring of recent antiepileptic drugs. Drugs in R&D. 2016;16:303.

Johannessen Landmark C, Johannessen SI, et al. Therapeutic drug monitoring of antiepileptic drugs: current status and future prospects. Expert Opin Drug Metab Toxicol. 2020; Mar;16(3):227-238. doi: 10.1080/17425255.2020.1724956. Epub 2020 Feb 13. PMID: 32054370.

Khoo C, Shukor M, Tan J, et al. Prevalence and predictors of vitamin D deficiency among adults with epilepsy: a cross-sectional study. Epilepsy Behav. 2023 Oct;147:109432. doi.org/10.1016/j.yebeh.2023.109432

Lamberink H, Otte W, Geerts A, et al. Individualised prediction model of seizure recurrence and long-term outcomes after withdrawal of antiepileptic drugs in seizure-free patients: a systematic review and individual participant data meta-analysis. Lancet Neurol. 2017;16:523-531. doi: 10.1016/S1474-4422(17)30114-X

Li Y, Meador K. Epilepsy and pregnancy. Continuum (Minneap Minn). 2022;28(1):34-54. doi: 10.1212/CON.0000000000001056

Rang HP, Dale MM, Ritter JM, et al: Rang & Dale's pharmacology, 8th edn. Edinburgh: Churchill Livingstone, 2016.

Scheffer IE, Mullen SA. Epilepsy in 2012: advances in epilepsy shed light on key questions. Nat Rev Neurol. 2013 Feb;9(2):66-68. doi: 10.1038/nrneurol.2012.272

Spiegel R, Merius H. Principles of epilepsy management for women in their reproductive years. Front Neurol. 2020;11(322):1-5. doi:10.3389/fneur.2020.00322

Stephen LJ, Harden C, Tomson T, et al. Management of epilepsy in women. Lancet Neurol. 2019 May;18(5):481-491. doi: 10.1016/S1474-4422(18)30495-2. Epub 2019 Mar 8. PMID: 30857949.

Therapeutic guidelines 2017. Neurology, version 5, Melbourne: Therapeutic Guidelines Limited. eTG complete [digital]. https://www.tg.org.au.

Therapeutic Guidelines Limited 2021. Neurology [published 2021 Mar]. In: Therapeutic Guidelines [digital]. Melbourne: Therapeutic Guidelines Limited. https://www.tg.org.au.

Tomson T, Battino D, Perucca E. Teratogenicity of antiepileptic drugs. Curr Opin Neurol. 2019 Apr;32(2):246-252. doi: 10.1097/WCO.0000000000000659. PMID: 30664067.

Trinka E, Cock H, Hesdorffer D, et al. A definition and classification of status epilepticus—Report of the ILAE Task Force on Classification of Status Epilepticus. Epilepsia. 2015 Oct;56(10):1515-1523. doi: 10.1111/epi.13121. Epub 2015 Sep 4. PMID: 26336950.Au

Vajda F, Graham J, Hitchcock A, et al. Is lamotrigine a significant human teratogen? Observations from the Australian Pregnancy Register. Seizure. 2010;19(9):558-561. https://doi.org/10.1016/j.seizure.2010.07.019.

Vajda FJE, O'Brien TJ, Graham JE, et al. The outcome of altering antiepileptic drug therapy before pregnancy. Epilepsy Behav. 2020 Oct;111:107263. doi: 10.1016/j.yebeh.2020.107263.

Veroniki AA, Cogo E, Rios P, et al. Comparative safety of anti-epileptic drugs during pregnancy: a systematic review and network meta-analysis of congenital malformations and prenatal outcomes. BMC Med. 2017;15(1):95. doi:10.1186/s12916-017-0845-1

Weston J, Bromley R, Jackson CF, et al. Monotherapy treatment of epilepsy in pregnancy: congenital malformation outcomes in the child. Cochrane Database Syst Rev. 2016 Nov; 11(11): CD010224. doi:10.1002/14651858.CD010224.pub2

World Health Organization. Fact sheet: Epilepsy. 2024. https://www.who.int/news-room/fact-sheets/detail/epilepsy

ONLINE RESOURCES

Epilepsy Action Australia: https://www.epilepsy.org.au/ (accessed January 2022)

Epilepsy Foundation: https://epilepsyfoundation.org.au/ (accessed January 2022)

Epilepsy support groups (Australia): https://www.epilepsy.org.au/how-we-can-help/our-services/ (accessed January 2022)

Health Navigator New Zealand: Anti-seizure medication: https://www.healthnavigator.org.nz/medicines/a/anti-seizure-medication/ (accessed March 2023)

International League Against Epilepsy – an organisation of more than 100 national chapters: https://www.ilae.org/ (accessed January 2022)

Ministry of Health NZ – Manatu Hauora: Epilepsy – Information for people taking medicines for epilepsy who could get pregnant: https://www.health.govt.nz/your-health/conditions-and-treatments/diseases-and-illnesses/epilepsy (accessed March 2023)

New Zealand Medicines and Medical Devices Safety Authority: https://www.medsafe.govt.nz/ (accessed January 2022)

CHAPTER 21

DRUGS OF DEPENDENCE

Kirsten Small, Roslyn Donnellan-Fernandez, Maryam Bazargan

Key Abbreviations

5-HT   5-hydroxytryptamine (serotonin)

MDMA 3,4-methylenedioxymethamphetamine

THC   tetrahydrocannabinol

Key Terms

addiction 398

alcohol 407

alcoholism 405

dependence 398

designer drugs 403

drug abuse 398

drug misuse 398

ethanol 407

illicit drugs 399

legal highs 403

methadone 405

tolerance 398

withdrawal
        syndrome 399

Chapter Focus

Drugs likely to produce dependence have two characteristics: they act fast, and either make you feel good or stop you feeling bad. Drug use and abuse is widespread in societies despite legislation, enforcement, medical treatments, and educational efforts. Other drugs are culturally accepted when used for purely social reasons and in moderation, such as caffeine and alcohol. The use of social drugs, drug dependence, and drug abuse disorders can pre-date or arise during pregnancy and the postnatal period.

The most commonly used drugs of dependence are central nervous system stimulants (e.g. cocaine, amphetamines, ecstasy, nicotine, and caffeine), opioids (e.g. heroin, morphine, and codeine), central nervous system depressants (e.g. alcohol and benzodiazepines), and psychotomimetics (cannabis and hallucinogens). This chapter describes the use and misuse of caffeine, nicotine, amphetamines, alcohol, and marijuana, and the pharmacological management of opioid dependence.

Key Drug Groups

Central nervous system stimulants:

- amphetamines, caffeine, cocaine
- designer drugs, ecstasy, 'legal highs'
- nicotine (DM 21.1) and smoking

Opioids:

- morphine, codeine, heroin
- drugs for opioid dependence: buprenorphine, methadone (DM 21.2), naltrexone

Central nervous system depressants:

- alcohol (DM 21.3)

Cannabinoids:

- cannabis, marijuana, Δ^9-tetrahydrocannabinol

CRITICAL THINKING SCENARIO

Lucy is 26 years old and planning her first pregnancy. She has chronic migraines and fibromyalgia. Chronic pain impacts her daily life. After several other unsatisfactory trials of managing her pain pharmacologically, her pain specialist has prescribed tetrahydrocannabinol (THC) 40 mg (2 mL of 20 mg/mL) as an oral oil each evening. Lucy's THC is dispensed by a reputable pharmacy with high standards of quality control. This dose of THC has been effective for Lucy, with minimal side effects. She consults with you during a pre-conception visit.

1   Describe the potential fetal risks from THC use during pregnancy.

2   Would you advise any dose adjustment to Lucy's THC if she continues it during pregnancy? What, if any, modifications to routine antenatal care would you advise?

3   If Lucy continues with THC during her pregnancy, what impact might it have on her baby's health and behaviour during the first month of life?

4   Lucy plans to breastfeed. Does THC enter breast milk? What advice would you give Lucy about the risks and benefits of breastfeeding while continuing to use THC?

Introduction

The use of drugs with the potential for dependence operates on a scale, from medically indicated, prescribed, and supervised use; to drug dependence disorders where drug use is one aspect of a constellation of social and psychological challenges. Research on the impact of drug use is highly contextual – a woman using a standardised prescribed dose of dexamphetamine for management of attention-deficit hyperactivity disorder will have different health outcomes to a woman with a drug dependence disorder involving the same drug as an unregulated street drug (where dose and constitution are not guaranteed). It is important to consider this when interpreting research findings and counselling women.

21.1 Drug abuse and misuse

Drug abuse refers to the self-administration of a drug in chronically excessive quantities, in a manner that deviates from approved medical or social patterns in each culture, resulting in physical or psychological harm. Abuse is therefore defined by what is accepted in a society based on its laws, history, religion, and ethos. It depends on accepted medical practice; for example, opiates are approved on medical prescription for pain but not for relief of anxiety. The term **drug misuse** refers to inappropriate or indiscriminate use of drugs.

Drug dependence

In drug **dependence**, the administration of a drug is compulsively sought in the absence of a therapeutic indication and despite adverse psychological, social, or physical effects. Dependence may lead to disturbed behaviour to ensure further supplies. Drug abuse does not always entail dependence on the drug: people may abuse simple analgesics or megadoses of vitamins without developing dependence. Dependence does not always cause problems. A person may be dependent on caffeine, which is safe and cheap, without breaking laws or suffering serious adverse or withdrawal reactions.

Governments regulate most drugs of dependence (see Chapter 2). However, some drugs (alcohol, nicotine, caffeine) are considered differently and are readily available in most countries. In Australia, drugs of dependence are generally listed in Schedule 8: Controlled Drugs of The Poisons Standard (SUSMP), and are subject to the strictest controls of availability, storage, labelling, and prescribing. Thus, most drugs of dependence are **illicit** (illegal) outside of approved medical use on prescription.

Addiction (a term sometimes used synonymously with 'dependence') is a behavioural pattern of drug use with overwhelming involvement in procurement and use of the drug, and a high tendency to relapse back into dependence.

Tolerance is a physical state in which repeated doses of the drug cause decreasing effects, and doses must be increased to maintain the same effects. Not all drugs of dependence induce tolerance. Tolerance develops rapidly to most effects of morphine (but not to constipation or pupil constriction), whereas there is little tolerance to marijuana. In receptor-site (pharmacodynamic) tolerance, receptor synthesis may be downregulated, receptors may be lost or desensitised, or there may be exhaustion of chemical mediators or transmitters. In metabolic (pharmacokinetic) tolerance, prolonged exposure increases drug clearance.

Withdrawal syndromes

The **withdrawal syndrome** after drug cessation is due to uncompensated adaptive changes induced by chronic drug administration. Withdrawal frequently manifests as a rebound in the systems affected. Thus, withdrawal from benzodiazepines (CNS depressants) may lead to anxiety and agitation, whereas withdrawal from amphetamines (CNS stimulants) leads to depressed mood and drowsiness.

Patterns of drug abuse in Australia

To estimate the extent of drug abuse, attitudes, and behaviours in Australia, large-scale population surveys have been carried out every 3–4 years since 1985. Data collected underpin policies for Australia's response to drug-related issues. Some emerging facts and trends are (Australian Institute of Health and Welfare 2022a; 2022b):

- Australians are reducing their alcohol intake, with 5.4% of the population consuming alcohol daily (down from 6.2% in 2016). Only 2% of women reported consuming alcohol in the first half of pregnancy in 2020.
- Fewer Australians are smoking tobacco daily (down from 24% in 1991, to 12.2% to 2016 to 11% in 2019). However, more Australians are using e-cigarettes, with 11.3% of the population having ever used an e-cigarette in 2019 (up from 8.3% in 2016). One in 10 women reported smoking at any time in pregnancy in 2020, a rate that has been falling slowly over the past decade.
- In 2019, 17.4% of Australians had used an illicit drug at some time in that year, with marijuana the most common, then ecstasy, methamphetamines, and cocaine (up from 15.6% in 2016).
- The people most likely to experience drug-related risks are residents of remote and very remote areas, Aboriginal and Torres Strait Islander people, and people who are unemployed, homosexual, or bisexual.

Patterns of drug abuse in New Zealand

The 2019–20 New Zealand Health Survey reported that most New Zealanders report being in good health – however, Māori, Pacific Islander peoples, and those living in the most deprived areas generally report poorer health. Results relating to use of specific drugs are summarised below:

- Alcohol is the most consumed drug in New Zealand: 81.5% of adults consumed alcohol in the past year. One in five adults drank alcohol in a way that could harm themselves or others.
- The 2019–20 Health Survey showed that 13.4% of adults were current smokers; approximately 31.4% of Māori adults, and 22.4% of Pacific Islander people. Smoking rates during the postnatal period

have fallen in the past decade, with 9% of women in 2020 reporting some tobacco use (Health New Zealand/Te Whatu Ora 2022).

- Marijuana is the most popular illegal drug in New Zealand, with 14.9% of people having used cannabis in the past year.
- In 2019–20, 1.1% of adults self-reported using amphetamines in the preceding year.

Drug abuse during pregnancy and breastfeeding

Most drugs of dependence, being lipid-soluble, can cross the placental barrier and adversely affect the fetus, potentially causing altered gene expression, drug dependence, or long-term behavioural and psychiatric disorders in the infant. **Illicit drugs** such as heroin, cannabis, and ecstasy do not have pregnancy safety classifications, nor do non-scheduled substances such as caffeine, alcohol, and tobacco. Drug abusers often use many different drugs, and lifestyle factors may contribute to poor antenatal care.

The benefits of breastfeeding generally outweigh any potential risks to the baby from drugs the mother takes, so ongoing exposure to moderate amounts of caffeine, alcohol, and tobacco may be preferable to withdrawal syndromes or to weaning the infant.

Care of the woman with drug dependence complicating the childbearing year

Contact with healthcare professionals during pregnancy and the postnatal period can provide women and their partners with an opportunity to re-evaluate their use of nicotine, alcohol, and other substances. Screening questions about current and past use of nicotine, alcohol, and other drugs should be asked early in pregnancy and repeated at later visits to assist in identifying women who would benefit from additional support (World Health Organization 2014). Where available, women with alcohol or other substance use disorders should be offered referral to specialised drug and alcohol services. Smoking cessation services are available online and via telephone from Quitline (see www.quit.org.au or www.quit.org.nz).

Women who use nicotine, alcohol, and/or other substances should be treated with respect and dignity. Establishing a therapeutic relationship through continuity of carer is likely to be particularly beneficial. Multi-disciplinary care with effective case management is important. In some instances, child protection issues may need to be addressed. Depending on the specific circumstances, additional fetal surveillance during pregnancy may be warranted. The neonate should be assessed and monitored for withdrawal symptoms and other effects of maternal drug use. Counselling regarding breastfeeding should be informed by evidence and by weighing the known harms of formula use against the risk of neonatal exposure to drugs through breast milk, and any risk of direct harm from breastfeeding while intoxicated (such as dropping or smothering the infant).

21.2 Central nervous system stimulants

CNS stimulants include amphetamines (and related 'designer drugs' such as ecstasy), nicotine, cocaine, and caffeine. Stimulants achieve their effects through interactions with dopamine, and the neurotransmitters NA, 5-HT, GABA, and glutamate. Some stimulants are socially approved and available for sale without prescription, some are prescribed for therapeutic use, and some are illegal and have a high potential for abuse.

Caffeine and the xanthine alkaloids

The xanthine alkaloids caffeine, theophylline, and theobromine are found naturally in plants used for making the stimulating beverages coffee, tea, and cocoa. Xanthines have medical uses as CNS stimulants and bronchodilators, with mild diuretic and cardiac-stimulant effects, and are used to treat respiratory failure in premature infants. Caffeine, the most powerful CNS stimulant of the xanthine alkaloids, is present in many non-prescription medications, in some prescribed medicines, and in coffee, tea, cocoa, cola, and 'energy drinks'.

Pharmacological mechanisms and effects

Chemically, xanthines are closely related to the purine bases adenine and guanine (building blocks for DNA and RNA). Xanthines are thought to act through antagonist effects on adenosine receptors, disinhibiting the effects of endogenous adenosine on ascending dopamine and arousal systems. At higher concentrations, xanthines also inhibit phosphodiesterase, raising intracellular levels of cyclic adenosine monophosphate (cAMP).

Caffeine is a mild stimulant, reducing fatigue and improving concentration, intellectual, and motor tasks. Large doses (300–600 mg) can cause insomnia, anxiety, palpitations, tremor, headache, increased gastric secretion, and seizures.

Social use of caffeine

Caffeine is the most widely used psychoactive substance worldwide. About 20% of the world's population drink a caffeinated beverage every day. Typical daily caffeine intake of adults is 180–250 mg. Tea accounts for about 43% of caffeine consumption worldwide. Sales of energy drinks are specifically targeted at young adults.

Caffeine is metabolised by CYP1A2. Habitual consumers and smokers are faster metabolisers. Two to three cups of strong coffee are sufficient to raise caffeine levels in the plasma or brain to approximately 100 µM, a concentration at which adenosine-receptor blockade and some phosphodiesterase inhibition occurs. Caffeine is also present in many foodstuffs and may not be noted on the labelling if it is in cocoa, coffee, tea, chocolate, or guarana products. The maximum recommended daily intake for caffeine is 300–400 mg.

Caffeine and pregnancy

Caffeine use is common during pregnancy, with rates of use of up to 70% reported in some countries (Qian et al 2020). Caffeine metabolism is reduced during pregnancy, extending the half-life from 2.5 to 4.5 hours (Qian et al 2020). Caffeine's lipophilic nature means it crosses the placental barrier readily. Caffeine and its metabolites paraxanthine, theophylline, and theobromine are all secreted in breast milk in levels proportional to the level of caffeine consumed (Purkiewicz et al 2022).

Caffeine consumption in pregnancy is associated with increased rates of miscarriage, stillbirth, low birth weight and small for gestational age babies, acute leukaemia in childhood, and childhood obesity (James 2021). There is no demonstrable association with preterm birth. A dose–response relationship has been demonstrated for miscarriage, stillbirth, low birth weight and being small for gestational age (Greenwood et al 2014), with higher risks for women who consume more caffeine. The effects of caffeine consumption during breastfeeding have received little attention in research. Hale's Medications and Mothers' Milk database lists it as L2.

Food Standards Australia New Zealand (2019) advises that no more than 200 mg of caffeine be consumed daily by women who are pregnant and/or breastfeeding. The Royal Australian and New Zealand College of Obstetricians and Gynaecologists (2022) recommends pregnant women avoid excess consumption, defined as more than 300 mg daily. The TGA lists the pregnancy safety category for caffeine as A. The advice of these organisations is at odds with the evidence, which suggests there may be no risk-free level of caffeine consumption in pregnancy (James 2021).

Caffeinated energy drinks

Gaining prominence in the soft-drink market are pre-mixed 'formulated caffeinated beverages', marketed to 'sustain energy levels' and 'improve mental acuity'. These drinks may also contain guarana, another natural source of caffeine, and can cause agitation, palpitations, tremor, and GIT upset, as well as the serious effects of hallucinations, dysrhythmias, and seizures. The dose of caffeine varies but can be up to 500 mg in a single drink (Kelly et al 2016).

Nicotine and tobacco smoking

Daily tobacco smoking among the general population has more than halved since 1991 (down from 24.3% to 11% in 2019) (AIHW 2023). This is mainly the result of younger people not taking up smoking. The ever-increasing cost of cigarettes is associated as a motivational reason to quit. In 2011, Australia became the first country in the world to introduce and legislate plain packaging of cigarettes. The intervention, aimed to reduce the attractiveness of smoking, saw all tobacco products packaged in a certain colour (drab green) and free from branding logos and text, has worked at reducing smoking rates (White et al 2019). Interestingly, the use of electronic or e-cigarettes is increasing. In large part, this is because they are perceived to have less harmful health impacts.

Smoking rates are also falling for pregnant women – from 14% in 2010 to 9% in 2020 (AIHW 2022b). Many women cease smoking during pregnancy, so the rate of smoking after 20 weeks of pregnancy was lower at 7% in 2020. Indigenous women, women under the age of 25 years, those with four or more previous births, living in remote communities, and of lower socioeconomic status are more likely to smoke during pregnancy.

Nicotine is the chief alkaloid in the tobacco plant *Nicotiana tabacum*. It is an oily liquid that turns brown on exposure to air and is freely soluble in both organic solvents and water. Nicotine has no therapeutic use (other than in nicotine replacement therapy for smokers trying to quit) but is of great pharmacological and public health importance. Nicotine is commonly self-administered by smoking cigarettes (containing about 1 g of nicotine each), cigars or pipes, and liquid nicotine vaping (electronic cigarettes). Smoking has major toxic effects, while the absorbed nicotine induces dependence.

Pharmacological effects of nicotine

- *Peripheral effects – autonomic:*
  - Low doses stimulate all sympathetic and parasympathetic ganglia, while higher doses depress responses at all autonomic pathways.
  - Effects on the cardiovascular system are complex: heart rate may be slowed then accelerated, small blood vessels constrict but later dilate, the blood pressure rises then falls.
  - Nicotine has an antidiuretic action and decreases gastrointestinal motility.
- *Peripheral effects – neuromuscular:*
  - At neuromuscular junctions, nicotine exerts a curare-like action (flaccidity) on skeletal muscle.
  - Large doses may cause tremor.
- *CNS effects:*
  - Nicotine stimulates acetylcholine receptors in medullary centres (respiratory, emetic, and vasomotor). Convulsions may occur at high dose.
  - Stimulation is followed by depression. First-time smokers may become anxious and nauseated.
  - Euphoria and antidepressant effects are commonly reported. Increased alertness and concentration, and reduced boredom and anxiety. Learning and performance may improve.

Tobacco smoking

Tobacco smoke is an aerosol containing about 4×10^9 particles per mL, about 10–80 mg per cigarette; nicotine accounts for about 0.14–1.21 mg. Burning tobacco generates around 4,000 chemicals, including 60 known carcinogens such as tars, formaldehyde, hydrogen cyanide, benzene, and nitrosamines, implicated in causing cancers of the lung, bladder, buccal cavity, oesophagus, and pancreas. Other smoking-related problems include pulmonary emphysema, chronic bronchitis, coronary heart disease, strokes, myocardial infarction, chronic dyspepsia, peripheral vascular disease, and vasospasm in retinal blood vessels.

Tobacco smoking and pregnancy

Tobacco smoking presents significant risks to women during their reproductive life, increases the incidence of pregnancy complications, and has consequences for the infant that extend well beyond the perinatal period. The TGA gives it a pregnancy safety rating of D and Hale's Medications and Mothers' Milk database lists nicotine as L3. Risks include (Gould et al 2020):

- Reduced fertility, particularly when advanced reproductive technology is used
- Miscarriage and ectopic pregnancy
- 10–30% higher rates of congenital abnormalities – particularly spina bifida, cryptorchidism, and cleft lip and/or palate
- Stillbirth and neonatal death
- Sudden unexplained death in infancy
- Abruption
- Placenta praevia
- Folate and vitamin B12 deficiency
- Preterm birth and low birth weight

- Earlier discontinuation of breastfeeding
- Neonatal illnesses including non-Hodgkin's lymphoma, acute lymphoblastic leukaemia, neuroblastoma, wheezing illnesses including asthma, respiratory tract infections.

Similar risks have been noted for smokeless forms of tobacco (chewing or snuff) but there is currently little data about the risk profile of electronic cigarettes (also known as vaping) (Glover et al 2020).

Drug interactions

Pharmacodynamic interactions can occur between nicotine and any drug affecting acetylcholine functions in the autonomic, motor, or central nervous systems (DI 21.1). Tobacco smoking induces the drug-metabolising enzymes CYP1A2 and CYP2B6, causing numerous pharmacokinetic drug interactions with other inducers, inhibitors, or substrates of the enzymes. Smokers have greater rates of clearance of many drugs, and people who stop smoking abruptly may have altered metabolism of other drugs

....

DRUG INTERACTIONS 21.1
Nicotine (or tobacco)

DRUG	POSSIBLE EFFECTS AND MANAGEMENT
CYP substrates: paracetamol, duloxetine, fluvoxamine, imipramine, caffeine, oxazepam, melatonin, propranolol, clozapine, mirtazapine, zolmitriptan olanzapine, methadone, and theophylline (and others)	Cigarette smoking induces the activity of CYP1A2, and increases the metabolism of substrates, lowering substrate blood concentrations and efficacy. Higher or more frequent drug dosing of CYP1A2 substrates may be required
Adrenergic agonists or blocking agents, catecholamines, corticosteroids	Smoking and nicotine raise catecholamine and cortisone levels; therapy with adrenoceptor agonists or antagonists or corticosteroids may require dosage adjustment
Insulin	Smoking cessation may result in an increased insulin effect; dosage reduction may be necessary; monitor closely for symptoms of hypoglycaemia
Autonomic drugs, including antihypertensives, bronchodilators and vasodilators	Effects of nicotine on autonomic ganglia are complicated and dose-dependent; doses of other autonomic drugs may need adjusting
Vasoconstrictors	Nicotine decreases myocardial oxygen supply and increases demand, effects compounded by other vasoconstrictors
Acidic beverages (coffee, soft drinks)	May decrease buccal absorption of nicotine
Nicotine (in other forms, e.g. cigarettes, patches)	Additive effects, leading to chest pains and palpitations

Sources: Australian Medicines Handbook 2023; Lucas et al 2013.

(see databases for individual potential interactions) (AMH 2023; Lucas et al 2013).

Supporting smoking cessation in pregnancy

Smoking is notoriously hard to quit. The withdrawal syndrome – consisting of craving, irritability, hunger, anxiety, and headaches – continues for several days. The craving can persist for years. Medical advice and behavioural therapy, with follow-up by QuitLine (see Online resources) can significantly enhance quit rates. Smoking cessation programs are most effective when they are flexible and tailored to specific communities (e.g. for Indigenous populations). Anti-smoking campaigns effectively reduce the prevalence of smoking, and by preventing thousands of cases of cancers, cardiovascular and pulmonary diseases can bring significant healthcare savings.

Treatment of nicotine dependence during pregnancy aims to relieve the symptoms of nicotine withdrawal, help women to stop smoking, and reduce morbidity and mortality for both the woman and her baby. Research specifically focusing on smoking cessation in pregnancy demonstrates that financial incentives work, and a combination of counselling with biological feedback (such as monitoring carbon monoxide levels) is highly effective (Gould et al 2020). Evidence for the effectiveness of nicotine replacement therapy, such as nicotine gum (see DM 21.1), is weak, with higher rates of smoking cessation but little impact on clinical outcomes.

Nicotine by other routes

Nicotine patches, gum, lozenges, sublingual tablets, oral spray, or inhaler are formulated in a range of doses. Many are available in supermarkets (unscheduled) and some are subsidised on the Pharmaceutical Benefits Scheme.

Electronic cigarettes are designed to mimic the act of smoking while delivering a small dose of nicotine but not burning tobacco, and may help with quitting. Electronic cigarettes are Schedule 4 Prescription Only in Australia. That is, they can only be legally supplied by a pharmacist on presentation of a prescription and evidence of Therapeutic Goods Administration (TGA) approval (under the Special Access Scheme B or authorised prescriber scheme). Electronic cigarettes containing nicotine, or nicotine liquid, are also being accessed illegally via the internet from overseas.

Amphetamines

Amphetamines have rapid euphoriant effects and are strongly addictive. They are prescribed for the management of conditions such as attention-deficit hyperactivity disorder or are used illicitly as social drugs. Natural amphetamine-type compounds include ephedrine from *Ephedra sinica* and cathinone (khat) from *Catha edulis*.

DRUG MONOGRAPH 21.1
Nicotine gum

When used medically in nicotine replacement therapy by smokers trying to quit, nicotine facilitates smoking cessation and decreases severity of the withdrawal syndrome. Dependence on nicotine replacement therapy is considered easier to break than the smoking habit.

Actions and mechanism of action

Nicotine released from the gum mimics the actions of nicotine absorbed from smoking. (For the mechanism of action and effects, see text.)

Pharmacokinetics

Nicotine is very lipid-soluble so is rapidly absorbed across lipid membranes of the mouth, airways, and GIT. When chewed as a gum, it is steadily released and absorbed through buccal mucosa more slowly than if inhaled while smoking. When saliva containing nicotine is swallowed, the drug is absorbed from the GIT. Peak plasma concentration is reached at 45–60 minutes. Nicotine is metabolised primarily in the liver. Most metabolites are inactive, but cotinine, the main oxidation product, may have antidepressant and psychomotor stimulant properties. The half-life is 1–3 hours. Elimination is primarily renal, with 10% excreted unchanged. The drug is excreted in breast milk.

Drug interactions

Cimetidine slows the elimination of nicotine. Nicotine potentiates the effect of adenosine. While cigarette smoke induces hepatic enzymes CYP1A1, CYP1A2, and 2E1, nicotine has no effect on the enzymes. Tobacco smoking has many more drug interactions than nicotine alone.

Adverse reactions

Adverse effects of nicotine have been described in the text. Reactions to nicotine gum include local injury to mouth, teeth or dental work, and jaw muscle ache. Some symptoms may be due to stopping smoking rather than to nicotine gum. Signs of overdose include nausea and vomiting, increased salivation and abdominal pain, diarrhoea, cold sweat, severe headache and dizziness, disturbed hearing and vision, confusion, and severe weakness.

Warnings and contraindications

Use with caution in people with cardiovascular disease, insulin-dependent diabetes mellitus, hyperthyroidism, peptic ulcer disease, or phaeochromocytoma. Avoid use in people with nicotine hypersensitivity, and moderate hepatic or renal impairment. Use is not recommended in pregnancy or breastfeeding. The gum contains significant amounts of sodium.

Dosage and administration

Nicotine gum comes in two strengths, 2 mg or 4 mg nicotine per piece, and various flavours. The person should be instructed to stop smoking before using nicotine replacements. The gum is chewed intermittently when the person has the craving to smoke, controlling the dose by biting the gum to release nicotine. Dosage is 2 or 4 mg as chewing gum, repeated as needed to a maximum of 40 mg/day, tapering off over several weeks.

Actions and pharmacokinetics

Chemically, amphetamines are like the natural catecholamines adrenaline, noradrenaline (Fig 1.3A), and dopamine, but have fewer hydroxyl groups so are more lipid-soluble and CNS-active. They cause release of catecholamines into synapses and inhibit their reuptake. Central effects include increases in alertness and mental and physical capacities, and decreased appetite and sleep. Euphoria and stereotyped behaviours also occur. There is a rapid fall-off in drug effects, followed by periods of sleep. On waking the person feels hungry, lethargic, and profoundly depressed (anhedonia, 'crashing'), which enhances intense craving and rapidly leads to addiction and risk of suicide.

Amphetamines are generally taken orally but can also be inhaled after vaporisation, inhaled as fine powders ('snorted'), or injected. They cause rapid marked euphoria – a 'rush'.

Designer drugs, new psychoactive substances and 'legal highs'

The classic **designer drug** is MDMA (better known as 'ecstasy') and was originally synthesised in 1914 as an appetite suppressant. Related compounds have varying chemical substituents (methoxy-, methyl-, halogen or sulfur) on the phenyl ring of the amphetamine. **'Legal highs'** refers to hundreds of new psychoactive substances, semi/synthetic drugs designed to mimic the actions of cannabis or amphetamines. People designing the drugs aim to keep a step ahead of drug policymakers and law-enforcement officers. New psychoactive substances are based on the phenylethylamine molecule (as are catecholamines and amphetamines) or on cocaine, tryptamine, phencyclidine, or cannabinoids. Their number more than doubled between the mid-2000s and the mid-2010s (Miliano et al 2016). They all increase dopamine signalling in the nucleus accumbens, causing reward and dependence. Complex mixtures of synthetic drugs with unknown additives and side effects pose new threats: they are highly addictive, causing long-lasting, severe toxicities.

Amphetamines and pregnancy

While less common than tobacco, alcohol, and cannabis use, amphetamine use continues to be an issue in pregnancy. Even when used as prescribed for attention-deficit hyperactivity disorder, rates of congenital malformations are higher (Huybrechts et al 2018). Dexamfetamine is listed as B3 in terms of safety in pregnancy by the TGA, and Hale's Medications and Mothers' Milk database lists it as L3. Other risks include abruption, preeclampsia, preterm birth, and reduced growth in childhood. Rates of maternal and neonatal morbidity and mortality are higher in amphetamine users (Admon et al 2019; Garey et al 2020; Huybrechts et al 2018).

KEY POINTS

Dependence on CNS stimulants

- Caffeine is very commonly consumed in beverages such as coffee, tea, and sports/energy drinks. Despite its widespread acceptance, it can have adverse effects in pregnancy, particularly at high dose.

- The most problematic drug of dependence is nicotine, taken by smoking. Tobacco has significant adverse effects during pregnancy and breastfeeding, in addition to well-established longer-term harms.

- CNS stimulants commonly abused for their euphoriant effects include amphetamines, ecstasy, and similar designer drugs.

21.3 Dependence on opioids

Opioid abuse and dependence

Morphine and codeine are opium alkaloids from natural sources (Fig 1.2A). The term 'opioid' refers to products with morphine-like agonist effects on enkephalin (opioid) receptors, including semi/synthetic drugs such as pethidine and oxycodone.

Opioids rapidly relieve pain and anxiety, change or elevate mood, and produce feelings of peace and euphoria, so they are particularly likely to lead to dependence, abuse, and chronic adverse effects. Prior to 2018, codeine was available in Australia without prescription and was often taken with other opioids and CNS depressants, leading to deaths from codeine overdose.

Opioids generally have low oral bioavailability. Sniffing (snorting), subcutaneous injection (skin popping), or direct IV injection (mainlining, 'shooting up'), are favoured when the drug is abused as these routes produce almost immediate effects.

Opioid dependence and pregnancy

Opioid dependence in pregnancy is more common than for amphetamines and cocaine, and the use of more than one of these drugs of dependence is common. Opioids are listed as Category C in relation to safety in pregnancy by the TGA, and L3 by Hale's Medications and Mothers' Milk database. There are three common scenarios for opioid dependence in the perinatal period (McCarthy et al 2017):

1 Untreated opioid dependence disorder
2 Prescribed opioid use for chronic pain management
3 Medication-assisted management of opioid dependence disorder.

Women with opioid dependence disorders have higher rates of severe maternal morbidity and mortality during the childbearing year (Admon et al 2019). Acute withdrawal is particularly problematic in pregnancy. Whether due to cessation of opioid consumption or abrupt reversal with an opioid antagonist, acute withdrawal presents with excitation and diarrhoea, 'cold turkey' skin, and pupil dilation. Catecholamine levels rise, and consequently, uterine contractions can be stimulated (Holzman et al 2009), along with reduced uterine blood flow and oxygenation. Fetal withdrawal causes hyperactivity, increased oxygen demand and increased noradrenaline. The combination of maternal and fetal withdrawal can precipitate labour, fetal hypoxia, and stillbirth (McCarthy et al 2017). Withdrawal also increases corticosteroid production. This may have epigenetic consequences and increase the vulnerability of the child to stress-related disease in later life, with possible intergenerational effects.

The maintenance of stable opioid levels during pregnancy is therefore important. Long-acting opioids, such as methadone, help avoid rapid shifts in serum levels and are therefore preferred over morphine and other opioids. Opioid metabolism increases during pregnancy, so dose increases may be required over time to maintain stable serum levels.

Babies born to women who are dependent on an opioid (whether prescribed or not) may experience neonatal abstinence syndrome after birth (CFB 21.1). Typical symptoms include irritability, tremors, hyperactive reflexes, sweating, increased muscle tone, poor feeding, and difficulty settling (Grossman et al 2019). Non-pharmacological approaches include avoiding overstimulation in a dark, quiet room, extended periods of skin-to-skin contact, and frequent, small volume feeds to minimise symptoms. If this is insufficient, pharmacological management with an opioid, followed by an extended period of slow weaning is used.

Managing women with pharmacological dependence on opioids

Women who use opioids during pregnancy are a diverse population. Those using opioids orally under medical supervision for chronic pain conditions present far lower risk for poor outcomes than women who self-administer intravenous opioids obtained illegally and lack good social support networks. Care must be tailored to the specific needs of the woman.

The main aim of treatment during pregnancy is to avoid acute withdrawal, while addressing the social, psychological, and medical needs of the woman. For women using illicit and/or short-acting opioids, substitution with a long-acting opioid like methadone (see DM 21.2) or buprenorphine is recommended.

Methadone or buprenorphine maintenance

Methadone or buprenorphine maintenance programs are cost-effective harm-minimisation options. In Australia, programs must comply with requirements of the state health department. The person attends the pharmacy for supervised oral dosing of methadone (daily) or buprenorphine (daily or alternate days). Maintenance doses that avoid withdrawal syndrome and deter cravings are in the order of 60–80 mg/day oral methadone, or 12–24 mg/day sublingual buprenorphine. Occasional take-away doses are allowed.

Buprenorphine is a partial agonist at μ- and antagonist at κ-opioid receptors so is safer in overdose and can block the effects of any heroin taken simultaneously. It

---

DRUG MONOGRAPH 21.2
Methadone oral syrup

Indications

Methadone is a synthetic, orally active, opioid agonist formulated as a syrup for short-term management of withdrawal symptoms during opioid detoxification programs or long-term use in methadone maintenance programs. It is also used as tablets or parenteral solution for pain relief. Oral administration reduces the risk from IV drug administration and can be readily supervised.

Pharmacokinetics

Methadone is well absorbed orally and has good bioavailability but variable pharmacokinetics. Peak plasma levels are reached in 1–5 hours; it is widely distributed via the bloodstream, with protein binding in the range 60–90%. Metabolism occurs in the liver to at least two inactive metabolites. Auto-induction of metabolising enzymes leads to a shorter half-life and tolerance. Methadone and metabolites are excreted in urine and faeces. The half-life is long (15–60 hours), so steady-state levels take several days.

Adverse drug reactions

The adverse-reaction profile of methadone is typical of opioids: euphoria, CNS and respiratory depression, gastrointestinal tract (GIT) and cardiovascular disturbances, and spasm of biliary and renal tract smooth muscle. Tolerance develops in a few weeks to most adverse effects, so people on methadone maintenance can live their normal lifestyle.

Drug interactions

Women using methadone maintenance should alert health professionals so other drugs can be prescribed appropriately. Other CNS depressants have additive effects. Enzyme inducers, including many antiepileptic drugs and antivirals, can precipitate a withdrawal syndrome, requiring higher methadone doses. There is increased risk of dysrhythmias with drugs that prolong the cardiac QT interval.

Warnings and contraindications

Methadone is contraindicated in respiratory depression, acute **alcoholism**, head injury, and severe hepatic or gastrointestinal diseases. Prolonged use leads to dependence, but it is usually easier to wean off methadone than off heroin or morphine. There are cautions against driving or operating machinery. Methadone is in Category C with respect to pregnancy safety classification; however, it remains safer than unregulated and unsupervised opioid use. Higher doses are generally required in pregnancy because of faster metabolism, and a prompt dose reduction at birth to avoid overdose effects. Methadone enters breast milk where it can minimise neonatal withdrawal symptoms. Provided there are no other contraindications, breastfeeding can be an effective therapy for neonatal abstinence syndrome.

Dosage and administration

Methadone syrup is classified as Schedule 8 and there are strict regulations about prescribing, dispensing, and administration. The strength of the formulation is 5 mg/mL. Initial oral dose is 20–30 mg/day, with dosage increased gradually to the minimum required maintenance dose, usually 30–60 mg/day to a maximum 80 mg/day. Due to the shorter half-life in pregnancy, twice daily dosing may sometimes be required. Some women eventually come off methadone by gradually reducing their daily dosage after pregnancy, but most remain on methadone programs indefinitely.

also helps suppress craving and withdrawal symptoms. Due to its longer half-life, it is a useful alternative to methadone, but it can precipitate withdrawal symptoms at commencement. Sublingual 'film' formulations also contain a low dose of naloxone to deter IV usage. If injected, naloxone can precipitate an unpleasant withdrawal reaction. There is some evidence that neonatal abstinence syndrome occurs less often when buprenorphine rather than methadone is used in the antenatal period (McCarthy et al 2017).

Similar maintenance programs operate in New Zealand to minimise the harms associated with misuse of opioid drugs. The *New Zealand Practice Guidelines for Opioid Substitution Treatment 2014* emphasises moving from maintenance treatment to recovery while deterring substance misuse and diversion (see Online resources).

Acute overdosage

The signs and symptoms of acute opioid overdose are altered consciousness (lethargy, unresponsive, or unconscious), pupil constriction, vomiting, slow shallow breathing or respiratory arrest, hypotension, and bradycardia. The lethal dose depends on the tolerance. The treatment of choice for acute overdosage is administration of an antagonist (e.g. naloxone), respiratory and cardiovascular support, and rehydration. Naloxone is commonly administered by paramedics to treat opioid overdose. It is now available OTC as a Pharmacist-Only drug and can safely be administered IM by laypeople in emergencies (Jauncey et al 2017). Onset of effect after IM or IV injection is 1–3 minutes. As the duration of action of naloxone (30–45 minutes) may be shorter than that of the opioid, multiple doses of naloxone may be required. Adverse effects are those of acute opioid withdrawal.

CLINICAL FOCUS BOX 21.1

An overdose in an opioid-dependent newborn

An infant was born at a large regional hospital at 34 weeks gestation to a mother who was taking prescribed methadone and illicit heroin. Routine medical and nursing care of the baby included supportive treatment of anticipated opioid withdrawal: swaddling, frequent small feeds, and 4-hourly narcotic abstinence syndrome scoring to monitor withdrawal symptoms. Scores increased rapidly over the first 48 hours, indicating the onset of abstinence symptoms. The baby was started on 4-hourly doses of oral morphine (0.5 mg/kg/day in six divided doses) to manage these symptoms. Unfortunately, the baby received two six-fold overdoses of morphine. Due to a prescribing error the morphine dose was documented as 0.5 mg/kg *per dose* rather than *per day*. The withdrawal symptoms stopped immediately but the baby developed sedation and respiratory depression and

overdose was diagnosed. Oxygen was administered and the senior paediatrician was called.

Normally, an opioid antagonist such as naloxone would be contraindicated in this situation, but the baby needed an antagonist to overcome adverse effects of the morphine overdose. Naloxone was administered IV and IM, carefully titrating effects on opioid receptors of the antagonist (naloxone) against the agonists (morphine, plus any remaining methadone or heroin). The baby survived the iatrogenic morphine overdose, the abstinence syndrome was controlled over the coming days using oral morphine, and the slow process of weaning the baby off oral morphine began, determined by the baby's abstinence scores.

Source: Dr Philippa Shilson, paediatrician.

Analgesia for women with opioid abuse disorders

Providing adequate analgesics to manage labour or other acute pain in women with an opioid dependence disorder is difficult. Women may be tolerant to opioids, or in withdrawal. It is important to provide effective relief of acute pain and to prevent opioid withdrawal. Continuation of usual medications is required, with short-term use of additional opioid if indicated, plus maximisation of non-opioid analgesics and adjuvant therapies.

KEY POINTS

Opioid dependence and its treatment

- Most opioids are subject to abuse and dependence, particularly heroin, codeine, and pethidine.

- While ongoing opioid use presents risks to the woman and her fetus, acute withdrawal can precipitate preterm labour, fetal compromise, or stillbirth, and is best avoided.

- Infants born to women who use opioids regularly during pregnancy should be screened for neonatal abstinence syndrome.

- In the treatment of opioid dependence, methadone or buprenorphine are used for long-term maintenance.

21.4 Alcohol

While more Australians are abstaining or reducing alcohol intake, 25% still drink to risky levels on a single occasion at least monthly (AIHW 2022b). Alcohol consumption during pregnancy is not recommended, and strong public health campaigns and product labelling have been effective in reducing use. Only 2% of pregnant women reported consuming alcohol in the first 20 weeks of their pregnancy in 2020, with the rate falling to under 1% after 20 weeks (AIHW 2022b). Reflecting the pattern for tobacco smoking, alcohol use was more commonly reported by women who were Indigenous, younger, and living in remote areas, but unlike tobacco use, alcohol consumption rose as socioeconomic status improved.

Chemically, alcohol is a hydrocarbon derivative in which one or more of the hydrogen atoms (–H) has been replaced by a hydroxyl group (–OH) (Fig 1.2E). In a medical or social context, the term usually refers to ethanol (ethyl alcohol). Alcohol is naturally produced by the fermentation of cereals and fruits: wine from grapes, beer from grains, and spirits distilled after fermentation of sugar cane, grains, fruits, or vegetables.

Ethanol (ethyl alcohol, 'alcohol')

Ethanol (**alcohol**) is the only alcohol used extensively in medicine and in alcoholic beverages. Therapeutically, ethanol has been used as an appetite stimulant, a mild hypnotic, an antidote for acute methanol or ethylene glycol poisoning, and in many oral pharmaceuticals as a solvent, preservative, or flavour. In pregnancy, alcohol was historically used for hyperemesis and preterm labour (Killian Thomas 2020). Ethanol denatures proteins by precipitation and dehydration, hence its effects as a skin antiseptic and disinfectant.

Alcohol use in pregnancy

Alcohol is highly lipid-soluble and readily crosses the placenta. The fetus has limited capacity to metabolise alcohol, and alcohol-induced vasoconstriction of fetal placental vessels reduces the back diffusion of alcohol (Price 2021). There are multiple complex mechanisms through which paternal and/or maternal alcohol consumption has an impact on the fetus and infant (Aiton 2021). These help to explain why there is a broad range of variable effects seen in response to alcohol consumption, broadly gathered under the term fetal alcohol spectrum disorder (FASD). These mechanisms include:

- Paternal – Chronic alcohol exposure impacts spermatogenesis, reducing sperm quality, and has epigenetic impacts.
- Grand-maternal – exposure to alcohol in utero while fetal oogenesis is in progress potentially has epigenetic impacts on the second generation of children.
- Maternal – heavy alcohol consumption alters metabolism, diet, behaviour, and relationships.
- Pregnancy – chronic alcohol consumption modifies the hormonal environment of pregnancy and impacts on placental development and function. This mechanism may be responsible for the higher rates of low birth weight and prematurity in infants born to women with heavy chronic consumption of alcohol.

- Fetal – alcohol has direct teratogenic effects on fetal development. The impact of alcohol consumption is modified by the timing of exposure in relation to fetal developmental stages.
- Neonate – exposure to heavy chronic alcohol use in pregnancy leads to withdrawal after birth, with modifications in behaviour that can impact on mother–infant interactions.

Fetal alcohol syndrome (FAS) is diagnosed when an infant has evidence of pre- and postnatal growth deficiency, reduced head size or structural brain abnormality, characteristic facial abnormalities, and a history of maternal alcohol consumption (Spohr 2018). Typical facial features include small eyes, a thin upper lip, and a smooth philtrum. Many affected individuals have cognitive and neurobehavioural challenges. Other morphological abnormalities can co-occur with FAS or without the other diagnostic criteria and are then included in the broader diagnostic category of FASD. These include congenital heart defects, scoliosis, renal and genital abnormalities, hearing loss, and others.

In addition to FASD, alcohol use in pregnancy is associated with miscarriage, preterm labour, placental dysfunction, hypertensive disorders, and low birth weight (Aiton 2021). National guidelines in both Australia and New Zealand advise against alcohol consumption of any level during pregnancy (Australian Government Department of Health and Aged Care 2022; New Zealand Government Ministry of Health 2018). While there is clear evidence of a dose-response relationship, no clear safe minimum dose has been established. In breastfeeding women, ethanol partitions into breast milk and can cause CNS depression in the infant proportional to the level of maternal consumption. Hale's Medications and Mothers' Milk database lists alcohol as L4.

Pharmacological mechanisms and actions of ethanol

Mechanisms of action

Alcohol impairs transmission of nerve impulses at synaptic connections. A proposed mechanism for the euphoria, feelings of reward, and relief of stress and pain, is the release of endorphins in the nucleus accumbens and activation of mesolimbic dopaminergic pathways.

CNS depression

Alcohol causes progressive depression of the cerebrum, cerebellum, medulla, and spinal cord. What may appear as behavioural stimulation results from depression of higher faculties and loss of inhibitions. Pharmacological effects vary with the blood alcohol level, pharmacological tolerance, the presence or absence of extraneous stimuli, the rate of ingestion, and the presence of other gastric contents.

DRUG MONOGRAPH 21.3
Alcohol (ethanol)

Taken orally, alcohol is a sedative and euphoriant. Alcohol is the most used and abused drug in Australia, usually taken in the form of alcoholic drinks.

Pharmacokinetics

Being a very small lipophilic molecule (molecular weight 46), alcohol diffuses readily into cells. Most is absorbed from the small intestine, with peak blood alcohol levels after 30–60 minutes. Alcohol is distributed into every tissue.

About 90% of absorbed alcohol is metabolised in the liver to acetaldehyde, which is oxidised to acetic acid, and thence to carbon dioxide and water. Remaining alcohol is excreted via lungs, sweat, and kidneys.

As plasma ethanol levels rise, the hepatic alcohol dehydrogenase pathway becomes saturated. Clearance and half-life are therefore dose-dependent. Hence, blood alcohol levels remain high if the person keeps drinking steadily. Plasma levels tend to be higher in women than in men after equivalent doses due to lower levels of dehydrogenase enzymes and a relatively smaller volume of distribution for water-soluble drugs. Chronic administration (i.e. in people who have a dependence on alcohol) initially increases the rate of metabolism, but as liver damage and cirrhosis develop, metabolism becomes impaired.

Adverse drug reactions

See the chapter text below for pharmacological effects.

Drug interactions

Ethanol interacts with many prescription and OTC drugs – in particular, with other CNS depressants, so there are frequent adverse drug interactions (DI 21.2).

Warnings and contraindications

Alcohol is not recommended during pregnancy or lactation, for people with liver disease or psychiatric problems, or who are taking any of the many drugs with which it interacts.

DRUG INTERACTIONS 21.2

Alcohol

SUBSTANCES INTERACTING WITH ALCOHOL	MECHANISM	POSSIBLE EFFECTS
All CNS depressants, including antihistamines, antidepressants, opioid analgesics, hypnotics, antianxiety agents, antipsychotics, chloral hydrate	Additive	Enhanced CNS-depressant effects
Disulfiram, some cefalosporins, oral antidiabetic agents, griseofulvin, metronidazole, procarbazine, tinidazole, chloral hydrate	Inhibition of alcohol metabolism by aldehyde dehydrogenase, leading to acetaldehyde accumulation (a 'disulfiram-type reaction')	Most severe effects seen with disulfiram and alcohol: flushing, stomach pain, head throbbing, raised heart rate, hypotension, sweating, nausea, and vomiting; with antidiabetic agents, mild-to-severe hypoglycaemia
Phenytoin, warfarin	Increase or decrease in liver metabolism	Chronically: possible decrease in effect due to enzyme induction; acutely: possible decrease in metabolism, causing raised serum level and toxicity
Salicylates	Additive	Increased gastrointestinal irritability and bleeding
Nitrates, glyceryl trinitrate	Additive	Vasodilation leading to hypotension, syncope
Anticholinergics, antispasmodics	Slowed gastrointestinal functions	Slowed absorption of alcohol
Paracetamol	Additive	Enhanced hepatic toxicity of paracetamol
Acitretin (an oral retinoid)	Alcohol may increase metabolism of acitretin to etretinate, which is teratogenic	Women of childbearing age should avoid alcohol while taking acitretin and for 2 months afterwards

Source: Australian Medicines Handbook 2023.

Effects on other systems

Some effects of alcohol on other body systems are:

- *Cardiovascular system – depression:* vasodilation; chronically: hypertension, dysrhythmias, and cardiomyopathy
- *Gastrointestinal system:* secretion of saliva and gastric juice rich in acid; nutritional deficiencies, gastritis, thiamine deficiency, pancreatitis; fatty liver, hepatitis, irreversible fibrosis, and cirrhosis
- *Endocrine system:* raised levels of adrenocorticotrophic hormone; lowered levels of antidiuretic hormone (ADH; hence diuresis and dehydration) and oxytocin (delayed labour during childbirth)
- *The fetus:* risk of fetal alcohol syndrome.

Hangover and alcohol withdrawal syndrome

A 'hangover' is a mild withdrawal syndrome after acute intoxication. The symptoms are craving for alcohol, headache, nausea, tremor, anxiety, vertigo, pallor, tachycardia, and nystagmus (rapid jerky eye movements). A more severe withdrawal reaction includes hallucinations, flushes, GIT disturbances and in severe cases delirium tremens ('DTs') requiring hospitalisation. Symptoms are caused by hypoglycaemia, dehydration, electrolyte imbalances, and persistence of lactic acid and acetaldehyde in the bloodstream.

KEY POINTS

Dependence on CNS depressants

- Alcohol use is common in Australian society and ranges from occasional problem drinking through to chronic alcoholism.
- Alcohol is a known teratogen, leading to fetal alcohol syndrome (FAS) and other neurobehavioural and morphological problems in offspring of women who consume moderate-to-high levels of alcohol.

21.5 Cannabis drugs (marijuana, hashish)

Cannabis is the most widely used illicit drug, with about 11.6% of Australians admitting to having used it in the previous 12 months (AIHW 2022a). In some states, laws against cannabis have been relaxed, and medical marijuana may now be prescribed.

Cannabis drugs are derived from hemp plants (*Cannabis sativa*), probably originally native to Central Asia. The plants have historically been grown for their strong fibres and fast growth (up to 5 m in length), used for weaving into fabric (canvas), for twisting into ropes (hemp), and for making paper. Hempseed is used as birdseed and a source of oil. There are also dermatological preparations (oils, soaps, lotions), foods, and fabrics based on cannabis. The active drugs used for mental relaxation and euphoria are from the resin of the plant, exuded from the leaves and flowering tops.

Preparations and active constituents

Marijuana (cannabis prepared for smoking) and hashish (the compressed form of the plant resin) are the most common forms. Cannabis plants contain chemicals termed phytocannabinoids, with complex three-ring structures. The main psychoactive ingredient is Δ^9-tetrahydrocannabinol (THC); typical leaves contain 3–10% THC, hashish 7–12%, and marijuana cigarettes about 0.5–2 g. Other components are cannabidiol (CBD) and cannabinol. Cannabis smoked for recreational use is high in Δ^9-THC.

Administration and pharmacokinetics

Cannabinoids are highly lipid-soluble so are readily absorbed. They are most potent when inhaled. Cannabis may be smoked in pipes or cigarettes, with smoke retained in the lungs for maximal absorption. About 15–50% of THC is absorbed from the respiratory tract, with peak plasma level occurring within minutes. Topical and oral administration routes are also used. Onset of action after ingestion is around 30–60 minutes with a duration of action of 6–8 hours (Thompson et al 2019).

THC is highly protein-bound, so only a small proportion enters the CNS. It persists in adipose tissue (for over 4 weeks) and in lungs and liver, with a long half-life. It is metabolised in the liver by CYP2C9 and 3A4 enzymes to hydroxylation products, some pharmacologically active. Metabolites are excreted in urine, bile, and faeces. The long half-lives of cannabinoids make it difficult to correlate blood cannabinoid concentration with impaired driving performance.

Mechanism and pharmacological effects

Cannabinoid receptors

Two cannabinoid (CB) receptors have been isolated. CB1 occurs mainly in presynaptic membranes of neurons regulating transmitter release including glutamate and GABA, and CB2 in immune and haemopoietic cells.

The actions of cannabinoids have been extensively studied: Δ^9-THC is a partial agonist at CB1 and CB2 receptors, mainly causing euphoria and distorted perceptions. Cannabidiol is an agonist at CB2 and antagonist at CB1 receptors, causing relaxation, and is used for pain management. It does not impair cognition and may have antipsychotic effects. Cannabinol is an agonist preferentially at CB2 receptors with no psychoactive effects. Synthetic cannabinoids include dexanabinol, dronabinol, nabilone, and nabiximol.

Effects

Cannabinoids act as CNS depressants and as mild hallucinogens. Responses are subjective, with a high placebo reaction. THC has effects on lipid membranes: at low doses, relief of anxiety, disinhibition, and excitement, then anaesthesia. At high doses, respiratory and vasomotor depression occur.

Cannabinoids affect most body systems:

- *CNS* – euphoria, reduced anxiety, distorted perceptions, loss of concentration, impaired decision making, tremors, incoordination, sedation; antiemetic, anticonvulsant, and analgesic effects; hypothermia; and with high doses, hallucinations, anxiety, acute psychoses, and increased risk of schizophrenia
- *cardiovascular system* – palpitations, tachycardia then bradycardia, postural hypotension, atherosclerosis
- *GI tract* – dry mouth and throat, decreased gastrointestinal motility, enhanced appetite and flavour appreciation, gum overgrowth
- *respiratory tract* – bronchodilation, sore throat, bronchitis, emphysema, and increased risk of lung cancer from heavy long-term smoking
- *ocular effects* – reddening of eyes, ptosis (drooping of eyelids), decreased intraocular pressure (useful antiglaucoma effect)
- *endocrine system* – diuretic effect, estrogenic effects
- *other actions* – reported antibacterial, immunosuppressant, and antineoplastic effects
- *toxic effects* – low acute toxicity, with few if any human deaths attributed solely to its use.

Medical uses of cannabinoids

Synthetic cannabinoids have been tested in the treatment of nausea and vomiting, migraine, insomnia, anorexia, epilepsy, opioid withdrawal, glaucoma, and asthma. They have also been tested in the symptomatic relief of neuropathic and cancer pain; as an adjunct in treating people with wasting conditions and in chronic pain syndromes; and for neurological diseases with spasticity, such as stroke and multiple sclerosis.

All Australian states have legalised the use of medical marijuana for defined groups of people, including people with a terminal illness and children with intractable epilepsy. The use of social marijuana remains illegal in all Australian jurisdictions, except for the ACT.

Long-term cannabis use

With regular low doses, no tolerance develops. Approximately 9% of users develop dependence.

Withdrawal causes mild rebound anxiety, sleep disturbances, muscle weakness and tremor. Craving can recur intermittently for months.

Overall health risks from regular use of cannabinoids are less than from some legal drugs of dependence, notably alcohol and tobacco. Heavy daily use over many years may cause cannabis dependence, cognitive and occupational impairment, diseases associated with smoking including cancers, and increased risk of moving on to other drugs (tobacco, amphetamines, ecstasy, cocaine).

There is strong evidence associating cannabis use with psychosis, as CB1 agonists increase activity of dopaminergic neurons. Acute cannabis intoxication can cause brief psychotic symptoms and, in people with established psychosis, the use of cannabis causes more frequent relapses. Endocannabinoids function as crucial molecular signallers in the development of the fetal nervous system.

Cannabis use in pregnancy and lactation

Most research on the use of cannabinoids in relation to pregnancy and childbearing examines the impact of their use when smoked, with some research from jurisdictions where use remains illegal while other research relates to medically prescribed marijuana. Some of the research is confounded by concomitant use of tobacco in marijuana cigarettes. The importance of the social context in which research has been performed should not be underestimated.

The lipid solubility of all cannabinoids means they all rapidly pass the placental and breast barriers. Renal clearance increases during pregnancy. THC levels remain detectable in breast milk up to 6 days after the last reported inhalation of cannabis but are much lower for other routes of administration (Bertrand et al 2018).

Cannabis is perceived to be effective for the management of nausea and vomiting in pregnancy, postpartum depression, and pain (Thompson et al 2019). The Royal Australian and New Zealand College of Obstetricians and Gynaecologists guidance advises women to discontinue cannabis use when planning or during pregnancy (RANZCOG 2018). Despite this, women who use medically prescribed cannabinoids to successfully manage chronic conditions such as migraines, fibromyalgia, posttraumatic stress disorder, or seizures may choose to continue treatment (Metz et al 2018).

Most research has not identified any teratogenic risk associated with cannabis use in pregnancy (Thompson et al 2019). There are conflicting findings about whether there is an association between marijuana use and pregnancy loss, fetal growth restriction, or preterm birth. CB1 receptors are expressed by trophoblastic cells so it is biologically plausible that cannabis use may lead to compromised placental function (Metz et al 2018). The TGA lists cannabidiol as B2 but has no listing for THC.

There is also limited evidence about the postnatal effects of antenatal cannabis use for the infant (Navarrete et al 2020). There is some evidence for increased tremors and startle responses in the neonatal period, and poorer attention and cognitive function during early education (Metz et al 2018; Thompson et al 2019). Breastfeeding initiation and continuation rates are lower in cannabis users, but the extent to which this is due to advice to not breastfeed rather than a pharmacological effect is unknown (Thompson et al 2019). Hale's Medications and Mothers' Milk database lists cannabidiol as L3, and chronic use of THC as L4.

KEY POINTS

Cannabis

- Cannabis and its synthetic derivatives are the most frequently used illicit drugs. It is used socially to produce euphoria, distorted perceptions, and freedom from anxiety. Chronic use can precipitate psychotic episodes.

- Medical marijuana is used to treat severe vomiting, chronic pain disorders such as migraine and fibromyalgia, glaucoma, and epilepsy.

- There is limited evidence available regarding the safety of cannabis products during the childbearing year.

REVIEW EXERCISES

1 Paul, a 3-day-old neonate, has been admitted to the nursery exhibiting signs of neonatal abstinence syndrome. Which drug family is his mother likely to have used during pregnancy? Does the timing of onset of his symptoms provide information about the pharmacology of the drug she was using? Describe non-pharmacological management options you can use as a midwife to reduce the severity of his symptoms.

2 Margarite has recently purchased e-cigarettes from an online store. She is 12 weeks pregnant and was advised by a friend that vaping is safer than smoking cigarettes during pregnancy. Is vaping legal in the jurisdiction you live in? Are there any pregnancy-specific harms associated with smoking e-cigarettes? Compare these harms with tobacco smoking. What advice would you give Margarite about using e-cigarettes during pregnancy?

3 Louisa works night shifts at an aged-care facility. She drinks a caffeinated energy drink containing 160 mg of caffeine per can, and typically has four per day when she is working to stay alert. Now that Louisa is pregnant, what advice would you give her about the risks of caffeine consumption in pregnancy?

REFERENCES

Admon L, Bart G, Kozhimannil K, et al. Amphetamine- and opioid-affected births: incidence, outcomes, and costs, United States, 2004–2015. Am J Public Health. 2019;109(1):148-154. doi: 10.2105/AJPH.2018.304771

Aiton N. How does alcohol affect the developing fetus? In Mukherjee R, Aiton N (eds.), Prevention, recognition and management of fetal alcohol spectrum disorders, Ch 3. Springer Nature, 2021. doi.org/10.1007/978-3-030-73966-9_4

Australian Government Department of Health and Aged Care 2022. Pregnancy Care Guidelines. https://www.health.gov.au/resources/pregnancy-care-guidelines

Australian Institute of Health and Welfare, 2022a. Illicit drug use. Online. https://www.aihw.gov.au/reports/australias-health/illicit-drug-use.

Australian Institute of Health and Welfare 2022b. Australia's mothers and babies. Online. https://www.aihw.gov.au/reports/mothers-babies/australias-mothers-babies.

Australian Institute of Health and Welfare 2023. Alcohol, tobacco other drugs in Australia. Online. https://www.aihw.gov.au/reports/alcohol/alcohol-tobacco-other-drugs-australia/contents/drug-types/tobacco.

Australian Medicines Handbook 2023. Australian Medicines Handbook. Adelaide: AMH.

Bertrand K, Hanan N, Honerkamp-Smith G, et al. Marijuana use by breastfeeding mothers and cannabinoid concentrations in breast milk. Pediatrics. 2018;142(3):e20181076. doi.org/10.1542/peds.2018-1076

Food Standards Australia New Zealand 2019. Caffeine. https://www.foodstandards.gov.au/consumer/generalissues/Pages/Caffeine.aspx

Garey J, Lusskin S, Scialli A. Teratogen update: amphetamines. Birth Defects Res. 2020;112:1161-1182. 10.1002/bdr2.1774

Glover M, Phillips C. Potential effects of using non-combustible tobacco and nicotine products during pregnancy: a systematic review. Harm Reduct J. 2020;17:16. doi.org/10.1186/s12954-020-00359-2

Gould G, Havard A, Lim L, et al. Exposure to tobacco, environmental tobacco smoke and nicotine in pregnancy: a pragmatic overview of reviews of maternal and child outcomes, effectiveness of interventions and barriers and facilitators to quitting. Int J Environ Res Public Health. 2020;17:2034. doi: 10.3390/ijerph17062034

Greenwood D, Thatcher N, Ye J, et al. Caffeine intake during pregnancy and adverse birth outcomes: a systematic review and dose-response meta-analysis. Eur J Epidemiol. 2014;29:725-734. doi:10.1007/s10654-014-9944-x

Grossman M, Berkwitt A. Neonatal abstinence syndrome. Semin Perinatol. 2019;43:173-186. doi.org/10.1053/j.semperi.2019.01.007

Health New Zealand/Te Whatu Ora. Maternity clinical indicator trends in New Zealand. 2022. https://tewhatuora.shinyapps.io/maternity-clinical-indicator-trends/

Holzman C, Senagore P, Tian Y, et al. Maternal catecholamine levels in midpregnancy and risk of preterm delivery. Am J Epidemiol. 2009;170(8):1014–1024. doi.org/10.1093/aje/kwp218

Huybrechts K, Bröm G, Christensen L, et al. Association between methylphenidate and amphetamine use in pregnancy and risk of congenital malformations: a cohort study from the International Pregnancy Safety Study Consortium. JAMA Psychiatry. 2018;75(2):167-175. doi: 10.1001/jamapsychiatry.2017.3644

James J. Maternal caffeine consumption and pregnancy outcomes: a narrative review with implications for advice to mothers and mothers to be. BMJ Evidence-Based Medicine. 2021;26:114-115. doi: 10.1136/bmjebm-2020-111432

Jauncey ME, Nielsen S. Community use of naloxone for opioid overdose. Aust Prescr. 2017;40(4):137.

Kelly CK, Prichard JR. Demographics, health, and risk behaviors of young adults who drink energy drinks and coffee beverages. J Caffeine Res. 2016;6(2):73-81. doi. org/10.1089/jcr.2015.0027

Killian C, Thomas E. Fetal alcohol syndrome warnings: policing women's behavior distorts science. J App Soc Science. 2020;14(1):5-22. doi: 10.1177/1936724419898885

Lucas C, Martin J. Smoking and drug interactions. Aust Prescr. 2013;36(3):102-104.

McCarthy J, Leamon M, Finnegan L, et al. Opioid dependence and pregnancy: minimizing stress on the fetal brain. Am J Obstet Gynecol. 2017;216(3):226-231. http://dx.doi. org/10.1016/j.ajog.2016.10.003

Metz T, Borgelt L. Marijuana use in pregnancy and while breastfeeding. Obstet Gynecol. 2018;132(5):1198-1210. doi: 10.1097/AOG.0000000000002878

Miliano C, Serpelloni G, Rimondo C, et al. Neuropharmacology of new psychoactive substances (NPS): focus on the rewarding and reinforcing properties of cannabimimetics and amphetamine-like stimulants. Front Neurosci. 2016;10:153. doi: 10.3389/fnins. 2016.00153

Navarrete F, García-Gutiérrez MS, Gasparyan A, et al. Cannabis use in pregnant and breastfeeding women: behavioral and neurobiological consequences. Front Psychiatry. 2020;11:586447. doi: 10.3389/fpsyt.2020.586447

New Zealand Government Ministry of Health. 2018. Alcohol: pregnancy and babies. https://www.health.govt.nz/your-health/healthy-living/addictions/alcohol-and-drug-abuse/alcohol/alcohol-pregnancy-and-babies

Price A. Overview of FASD: how our understanding of FSAD has progressed. In, Mukherjee R, Aiton N (eds.). Prevention, recognition and management of fetal alcohol spectrum disorders, Ch2, pp 9–22. Springer Nature, 2021. doi. org/10.1007/978-3-030-73966-9_2

Purkiewicz A, Pietrzak-Fiećko R, Sörgel F, et al. Caffeine, paraxanthine, theophylline, and theobromine content in human milk. Nutrients. 2022;14:2196. doi.org/ 10.3390/nu14112196

Qian J, Chen Q, Ward S, et al. Impacts of caffeine during pregnancy. Trends Endocrinol Metab. 2020;31(3):218-227. doi. org/10.1016/j.tem.2019.11.004

Royal Australian and New Zealand College of Obstetricians and Gynaecologists. 2018. Substance use in pregnancy. https://ranzcog.edu.au/wp-content/uploads/2022/05/Substance-use-in-pregnancy.pdf

Royal Australian and New Zealand College of Obstetricians and Gynaecologists. 2022. Pre-pregnancy counselling. https://ranzcog.edu.au/wp-content/uploads/2022/05/Pre-pregnancy-Counselling-C-Obs-3a-Board-approved_March-2022.pdf

Spohr H-L. Fetal alcohol syndrome. De Gruyter, 2018.

Thompson R, DeJong K, Lo, J. Marijuana use in pregnancy: a review. Obstet Gynecol Surv. 2019;74(7):415-428. doi: 10.1097/OGX.0000000000000685

White VM, Guerin N, Williams T, et al. Long-term impact of plain packaging of cigarettes with larger graphic health warnings: findings from cross-sectional surveys of Australian adolescents between 2011 and 2017. Tob Control. 2019 Aug;28(e1):e77-e84. doi: 10.1136/tobaccocontrol-2019-054988.

World Health Organization. 2014. Guidelines for the identification and management of substance use and substance use disorders in pregnancy. https://www.who.int/publications/i/item/9789241548731

ONLINE RESOURCES

Alcohol and Drug Foundation: https://www.adf.org.au/ (accessed 10 August 2021)

Australian Government National Drugs Campaign: https://campaigns.health.gov.au/drughelp/about-this-campaign/ (accessed 10 August 2021)

Australian Institute of Health and Welfare (AIHW): National Drug Strategy Household Survey Detailed Report: 2013. Drug statistics series no. 28. Cat. no. PHE 183. Canberra: AIHW: https://www.aihw.gov.au/reports/australias-health/illicit-drug-use/ (accessed 10 August 2021)

Australian Institute of Health and Welfare (AIHW): https://www.aihw.gov.au/publications/ (accessed 10 August 2021) [For many relevant reports and publications, follow links to Drugs and substance abuse, then to Program/Initiatives, Publications, Tobacco control, National Drug Strategy, etc.]

Commonwealth of Australia Department of Health Drugs: https://www.health.gov.au/health- topics/drugs?utm_source=health.gov.auutm_medium=redirectutm_campaign=digital_transformationutm_content=drugs (accessed 10 August 2021)

Family Drug Support Australia: https://www.fds.org.au/ (accessed 10 August 2021)

Prescription Shopping Programme: https://www.humanservices.gov.au/organisations/health-professionals/services/medicare/prescription-shopping-programme (accessed 10 August 2021)

Quit: https://www.quit.org.au/ (accessed 10 August 2021)

CHAPTER 22

ROLE OF THE MIDWIFE

Roslyn Donnellan-Fernandez, Clare Davison, Michelle Gray,
Maryam Bazargan, Kirsten Small

Key Abbreviations

ACM	Australian College of Midwives
ACSQHC	Australian Council for Safety and Quality in Healthcare
AHPRA	Australian Health Practitioner Regulation Agency
AMH	Australian Medicines Handbook
ANMAC	Australian Nursing and Midwifery Accreditation Council
CPD	continuing professional development
HPCAA	Health Practitioners Competence Assurance Act
HPPP	Health Professions Prescribing Pathway
Medsafe	New Zealand Medicines and Medical Devices Safety Authority
NMBA	Nursing and Midwifery Board of Australia
NZCOM	New Zealand College of Midwives
MBS	Medicare Benefits Schedule
NMP	National Medicines Policy
NPS	National Prescribing Service
PBAC	Pharmaceutical Benefits Advisory Committee
PBS	Pharmaceutical Benefits Scheme
Pharmac	(Te Pātaka Whaioranga)
PII	professional indemnity insurance
QUM	quality use of medicines
Te Tatau o te Whare Kahu	Midwifery Council (New Zealand)
TG	Therapeutic Guidelines
TGA	Therapeutic Goods Administration

Chapter Focus

This chapter focuses on the role and responsibilities of the midwife regarding pharmacological management, including authorised prescribing, when caring for women and their babies across the childbirth continuum. It provides an understanding of current midwifery contexts of practice specific to the Australian and New Zealand health systems, including the maternity models of care available to women within these countries. The regulatory environment and relevant legislation, and the professional standards, guidelines, competencies and decision making frameworks that support autonomous midwifery practice, prescribing and multi-disciplinary collaboration across a range of settings are covered. An overview of the safety and quality systems that support access to and quality use of medicines in Australia and New Zealand is provided. Requirements for continuing professional development are considered as well as future challenges and opportunities that impact midwives' role and responsibilities in pharmacology and prescribing practice when providing care for women and their babies.

Learning Outcomes

- Understand the role and responsibilities of the midwife related to pharmacologic management when caring for women and their babies across the childbirth continuum.

- Understand clinical assessment, medication review, and decision making in relation to midwife prescribing and medication management.

- Review principles of medication selection and prescription writing.

- Describe the governance in place (legislative and regulatory) for midwifery prescribing in Australia and New Zealand.

- Identify and describe the professional standards, guidelines, competencies, and decision making frameworks that support medication management (administration, supply, prescription) by midwives during their practice.

- Outline the systems that exist to support safe, quality use of medicines and universal access in Australia and New Zealand.

- Identify and discuss current and future challenges and opportunities that impact midwives' role and responsibilities in pharmacology and prescribing practice: educational and regulatory contexts; mutual recognition; cross-border practice; telehealth; electronic prescribing, and midwifery/maternity models of care.

Key Terms

administering 420
authorised
    prescriber 415
dispensing 414
endorsed midwife 421
medication review 415
midwife standards for
    practice 420
possessing 420

prescribing 420
prescribing
    competencies 418
prescription 419
regulation 419
scheduled
    medicine 416
supplying 420

CRITICAL THINKING SCENARIO

Bridie is an experienced midwife who has recently gained her Endorsement for Scheduled Medicines for Midwives with the Nursing and Midwifery Board of Australia. She is excited to be commencing employment within the midwifery group practice of a newly established, freestanding birthing unit in a major capital city where midwives provide continuity of care. Bridie is seeking professional support to develop her confidence in midwifery prescribing across the care continuum, as her previous context of practice was mainly focused on the provision of intrapartum care in a public tertiary hospital. She approaches her service manager for advice and assistance for access to support, resources, and professional development with prescribing practice.

1   What advice should Bridie's manager provide regarding assistance and ongoing professional support and/or professional development for a midwife prescriber?

2   What are the basis and parameters for establishing a mentoring relationship with another health professional for support for an autonomous prescriber? How should this be established and facilitated?

Introduction

Historically, midwives have possessed specialised knowledge of the effects and side effects of a vast range of pharmaceuticals and conventional medicines. Many have also remained skilled in herbal lore and folk remedies, including the effects, indications, and contraindications for use of these preparations by women and their babies during pregnancy, childbearing, and lactation. However, during the social shift to increased medical management of pregnancy and childbearing in the nineteenth and twentieth centuries there was a diminished focus on the importance of formalised pharmacologic knowledge for the broader profession of midwifery. Following this shift, midwives practised within institutional settings and enacted administration of prescribed drugs and treatments for women and their babies as 'ordered' by their medical colleagues. In some institutions and hospitals this extended to **dispensing** and 'supply' of medication on discharge. In contemporary times, the requirement for enhanced roles, extended scope of practice, and expansion of midwifery models of maternity care in diverse settings – including the

provision of quality care for greater numbers of women experiencing complexities – provides renewed impetus for augmenting access to midwifery prescribing practice.

Midwives play a vital role in delivering comprehensive care to women and their families throughout pre-pregnancy, antenatal care, education and counselling, birth support and postnatal care. Midwives' practise in many settings including the home, community, public and private hospitals, birth centres, clinics or health units – including Māori, and Aboriginal Community Controlled Health Organisations – and are spread across metropolitan, regional, and rural areas. As autonomous practitioners, midwives work in partnership with women, and collaboratively with other health professionals, to develop comprehensive treatment plans for women and babies in their care. However, midwifery practice is broader than providing direct clinical care and may extend to any role where midwifery skills and knowledge apply. This includes working within clinical settings or community services, and non-clinically through research, professional development, regulatory and advisory roles. Having midwives with authority to prescribe the medicines associated with maternity care, including women's health, sexual and reproductive health, and child and family healthcare, enables women to access a greater range of midwifery services. A broader range of midwifery services and models improves access to an expanded range of birthing options for women close to home, enables greater continuity of care in evidence-based, best practice models, and fully utilises the skills, knowledge, and scope of the midwifery workforce at start of life and across the first 2000 days (Sandall et al 2024; Chung et al 2022).

Scope of practice

Scope of practice refers to the range of roles, responsibilities, activities, and interventions that midwives are educated, trained, and authorised to perform within the context of their profession. Midwives' scope of practice is dependent on the area in which they practise. As well as maternity care, midwifery practice encompasses women's health, sexual and reproductive health, and child and family healthcare. Midwives use their knowledge to provide advice, assessment, health education, diagnostic review, emotional and wellbeing support, and manage referrals to other health professionals as required.

As per the Essential Competencies for Midwifery Practice (see Online resources; ICM 2019) all midwives, regardless of their context of practice, are required to demonstrate robust knowledge of the basic principles of pharmacology, pharmacokinetics and pharmacodynamics, including the impact on maternal, fetal and neonatal physiology for those who are healthy, as well as those who experience co-morbidities and chronic health challenges. Foundational knowledge and complex key concepts on pharmacokinetics and pharmacodynamics have been covered in previous chapters as applied across the childbearing continuum for women who are healthy and for those who experience complexities. This understanding is essential for both undergraduate midwifery students and for experienced midwives who are **authorised prescribers**. This knowledge encompasses understanding the role and responsibilities of the midwife related to comprehensive history taking and assessment; **medication review** and diagnostic investigations associated with pharmacologic management provided for the care of women and their babies across the continuum of pregnancy, birth, and the postpartum period; and includes preconception care, unplanned pregnancy, sexual healthcare, lactation, and contraception.

International prescribing context

Prescribing by nurses and midwives is now well established internationally in either independent or collaborative prescribing models and is legislated in the United States, Sweden, United Kingdom, Canada, Ireland, New Zealand and Australia (ANZCCNMO 2017). International examples of nurse and midwife models of prescribing have provided valuable guidance to inform the development of prescribing by nurses and midwives in Australia. Many of the prescribing models were developed to support health reform objectives, including improving safe access to medicines for the community and improving access to care for consumers. Evidence from evaluation of these models is that nurses and midwives who are educated to prescribe do so safely and effectively within their scope of practice (Casey et al 2020; Fong et al 2015; Hart 2013; Pritchard & Kendrick 2001; Smith et al 2014).

22.1 Governance of midwifery prescribing

In the last few decades midwifery practice in New Zealand and Australia has undergone many changes, including authorisation for midwife prescribing. In New Zealand, midwives have been authorised to prescribe since 1990 (*Nurses Amendment Act 1990*). It was not until after the 2009 Commonwealth Report: Improving Maternity Services in Australia that federal health reforms were enabled in 2010 through legislative amendments permitting midwives to access the Medicare Benefit Schedule (MBS) and Pharmaceutical Benefits Scheme (PBS). Prior to 2010, in Australia, responsibility for prescribing medications was limited to medical practitioners and dentists. However, during the past 15 years there has been a shift where non-medical professionals have assumed this role within their field of practice, including endorsed midwives.

Midwifery prescriptive authority in New Zealand

NZ midwifery prescriptive authority realised through the *Nurses Amendment Act 1990* included amendments to the *Misuse of Drugs Act 1975* and the *Medicines Act 1981*. The Medicines Amendment Regulations (2011) superseded the 1990 amendment to the Medicines Regulations (1984). The education of midwives in NZ to prescribe medicines is embedded in the four-year undergraduate Bachelor of Midwifery program. This enables all midwives to provide lead maternity care for childbearing women and prescribe autonomously within their scope of practice in accordance with the relevant **legislation**, the *Health Practitioners Competence Assurance Act 2003* (the HPCAA). There is no defined list of medicines that a NZ midwife may prescribe except for controlled drugs. At professional entry a midwife must demonstrate the ability to prescribe, supply and administer medicine, vaccines, and immunoglobulins safely within the midwife's scope of practice. Since the Misuse of Drugs Amendment Regulations in July 2014, this prescribing authority now includes the controlled drugs morphine, fentanyl, and pethidine (see Online resources: NZCOM Consensus Statement: Midwife Prescribing 2014; Te Tatau o te Whare Kahu Midwifery Council 2023; Hunter & Davis 2023).

Midwifery prescriptive authority in Australia

In contrast, in Australia, prescriptive authority currently requires midwives to undertake an approved postgraduate program of study to become endorsed as an authorised prescriber (NMBA 2017; Hull et al 2023; Hull et al 2024). In November 2009, the *Health Legislation Amendment (Midwives and Nurse Practitioners) Act 2010* was introduced. Under Section 94 of the Health Practitioner Regulation National Law (the National Law) as in force in each state and territory, the Nursing and Midwifery Board of Australia (NMBA) has the power to endorse the registration of suitably qualified midwives to administer, obtain, possess, prescribe, supply, or use NMBA-approved Schedule 2, 3, 4 and 8 medicines for the management of women and their infants in the antenatal, intrapartum and postnatal periods (Medway et al 2021). In 2010, the Australian Health Workforce Ministerial Council approved the Registration Standard: Endorsement for Scheduled Medicines for Midwives, enabling endorsed midwives to prescribe medicines in accordance with the relevant state or territory poisons legislation.

In Australia, midwives who meet the criteria set out by the NMBA can apply to be endorsed for **scheduled medicines** (substances listed in the schedules of the Commonwealth Poisons Standard).

Midwives who hold the endorsement for scheduled medicines are considered by the NMBA to be qualified to:

- administer, obtain, possess, prescribe, or supply specified Schedule 2, 3, 4 and 8 medicines to the extent authorised under the relevant legislation that applies in the state or territory in which they practise
- use those medicines appropriately for the management of women and infants during the pregnancy, birth, and postnatal periods, and
- apply to Medicare Australia for a PBS prescriber number.

The endorsement means:

'... that the midwife has met the requirements of the NMBA Registration Standard: Endorsement for scheduled medicines for midwives and is qualified to prescribe scheduled medicines and provide associated services required for midwifery practice in accordance with relevant state and territory legislation.'

(NMBA 2017).

In Australia, as the prescribing authority is dependent on variation in state and territory drug and poisons legislation (see Chapter 2, Table 2.1), it is important for midwives to be aware that the scope of midwifery prescribing also varies by state and territory (Hope et al 2016). Many Australian jurisdictions have implemented regulatory or legislative adjustments to enable endorsed midwives to prescribe within their scope of practice, thereby enabling them to practise in alignment with their qualifications; New South Wales, South Australia, Northern Territory, Western Australia; Australian Capital

TABLE 22.1 NPS prescribing competencies

THE PERSON-CENTRED PRESCRIBING PROCESS (COMPETENCY AREAS 1–5)
Competency Area 1: Understand the person and their needs
1.1 Ensure competence to assess the person's needs 1.2 Discuss with the person their medical and treatment history 1.3 Assess the person according to the clinical context and the health professional's scope of practice 1.4 Consider the person's cultural history and identity when gathering information to understand their needs 1.5 Review and interpret information in the person's health records to contribute to an understanding of their needs and current treatment 1.6 Explore with the person their adherence to prescribed medicines and the treatment plan 1.7 Make or review and understand the diagnosis and key clinical issues including those that are, or may be, medicine-related 1.8 Discuss with the person the clinical issues and implications for treatment
Competency Area 2: Understand the management options
2.1 Recognise when it is clinically appropriate not to prescribe medicines 2.2 Review current medicines and consider the possibility of a contribution to current health issues 2.3 Where treatment is indicated, consider both non-pharmacological and pharmacological options 2.4 Identify suitable medicine options 2.5 Obtain, interpret, and apply current reliable evidence and information about medicines to inform decision making 2.6 Consult other health professionals about potential medicines and the treatment plan, where appropriate 2.7 Tailor medicines for the person, considering relevant potential benefits, harms, medicine and person-specific factors 2.8 Consider the financial cost and affordability of the medicines to the person 2.9 Consider the implications to the wider community of prescribing a particular medicine 2.10 Refer the person for further assessment or treatment when the suitable treatment options are outside the health professional's scope of practice

TABLE 22.1 NPS prescribing competencies—cont'd

Competency Area 3: Agree on a plan for medicines
3.1 Explore the person's opinions and preferences concerning medicines and the treatment plan
3.2 Negotiate therapeutic goals that enhance self-management
3.3 Discuss the possible medicines options with the person and allow them time to make an informed decision
3.4 Explore and respond appropriately to the person's concerns and expectations about their health and the use of medicines to maintain their health
3.5 Develop the medicines plan in partnership with the person
3.6 Identify the need for, and develop with the person, a plan to review treatment

Competency Area 4: Prescribe medicines and communicate the agreed treatment decision
4.1 Ensure adequate and current knowledge of medicines prior to prescribing
4.2 Prescribe medicines compliant with relevant legislation, regulatory frameworks, guidelines, codes of practice, scope of practice and organisational policies and procedures
4.3 Where prescribing relies on electronic (e.g. telehealth) or telephone services (e.g. verbal prescription or medication order), ensure compliance with relevant legislation, guidelines and policies
4.4 Provide accurate and complete information to other health professionals in a timely manner when implementing new medicines or modifying existing medicines or treatment plans
4.5 Discuss and document the treatment plan with the person and ensure they understand both the plan and how to use the medicine/s safely and effectively

Competency Area 5: Review the outcomes of treatment
5.1 Explore with the person their response to treatment including adherence to the medicines and treatment plan
5.2 Gather objective information, using appropriate indicators, to assess the response to medicines, where appropriate
5.3 Synthesise information provided by the person, other health professionals and from the assessment, to determine the response to medicines
5.4 Stop or modify existing medicines and other treatments, where appropriate
5.5 Discuss with the person the benefits of a comprehensive medicines review, where appropriate
5.6 Work with the person and other health professionals to modify the treatment plan to optimise the safety and effectiveness of treatment, where appropriate
5.7 Discuss the findings of the review and recommendations with other health professionals, where appropriate

PROFESSIONAL PRACTICE THAT SUPPORTS PRESCRIBING (COMPETENCY AREAS 6 & 7)
Competency Area 6: Prescribe safely and effectively
6.1 Understand and prescribe medicines according to relevant legislation, regulatory frameworks and organisational requirements
6.2 Practise within the limits of the health professional's education, training and scope of practice as applied to prescribing
6.3 Understand common causes of incidents and error associated with prescribing and medicines use and implement strategies to reduce the risk of these occurring
6.4 Detect and report errors, incidents and adverse events involving medicines
6.5 Apply quality use of medicines principles when prescribing medicines
6.6 Critically evaluate information about medicines and make evidence-based decisions in the context of the person's needs

Competency Area 7: Prescribe professionally
7.1 Understand and comply with applicable professional standards, codes of conduct and guidelines relevant to prescribing
7.2 Demonstrate appropriate professional judgement when interpreting and applying prescribing guidelines and protocols to the person's situation
7.3 Maintain accurate and complete records of the interaction
7.4 Accept responsibility and accountability for prescribing decisions
7.5 Engage in ongoing professional development and education to improve prescribing practice
7.6 Ensure the person's needs take precedence over all considerations in all prescribing decisions
7.7 Demonstrate respect for other health professionals and their contributions within a collaborative care model

Source: Reproduced with permission from Prescribing Competencies Framework, developed by the Australian Commission on Safety and Quality in Health Care (ACSQHC). ACSQHC: Sydney 2021.

Territory; Queensland. In two states, Tasmania and Victoria (currently under review), midwife prescribing remains limited to a formulary of specified medicines. (See also Online resources: Unleashing the potential of our health workforce; Scope of practice review – Issues Paper 2: 2024). By June 2016 there were 250 midwives nationally who held the scheduled medicines endorsement (Small et al 2016[RD7]). As of March 2024, 1257 midwives held the scheduled medicines endorsement (3% of the midwifery workforce), contrasted with 32,491 'practising' midwives listed on the public register (NMBA 2024).

22.2 Educational preparation for prescribing

To ensure a sound knowledge base from which to prescribe medication, comprehensive preparatory education programs are required to support the safety, quality, and success of autonomous midwife prescribing. Courses in midwifery prescribing are designed to reflect the national approach to prescribing through the National Medicines Policy, the Health Workforce

Professionals Prescribing Pathway (HPPP) project and the National Prescribing Service (NPS MedicineWise) **Prescribing Competencies** Framework (see Online resources). Courses cover a range of topics such as legal and ethical frameworks; complete medical, obstetric and medication history; clinical assessment; pharmacology (including mechanisms of drug action, uses, potential side effects, drug interactions, and adverse effects); communication and shared decision making skills with women and their families; documentation, monitoring, consultation, collaboration, and referral (including emergency management); and follow-up. Midwifery prescribing courses aim to ensure that midwives are competent and confident in their ability to prescribe medications safely and effectively within their context of practice and practice setting.

Currently in Australia, postgraduate education accreditation standards ensure the attainment of competence to prescribe medicines in line with the National Prescribing Service Competencies (NPS MEDICINEWISE 2021) required to prescribe medicines (Australian Nursing and Midwifery Accreditation Council [ANMAC] Programs Leading to Endorsement for Scheduled Medicines for Midwives Accreditation Standards 2015). The midwifery prescribing framework that underpins midwifery prescribing curricula in Australia clearly articulates the role of the prescriber in the quality use of medicines as one of the central objectives of Australia's National Medicines Policy (see Online resources: Australian Government NMP 2022 and Box 22.1).

Additionally, the NMBA Registration Standard: Endorsement for Scheduled Medicines for Midwives covers:

- guidance specific to midwife practice; the Safety and Quality Guidelines for Privately Practising Midwives (2023)

- course accreditation standards for midwifery prescribing course
- accreditation standards for professional practice review programs
- guidelines for scope of practice decisions, and
- professional boundaries and professional ethics guidance.

For autonomous prescribing in Australia at professional entry level, a review of current undergraduate Bachelor of Midwifery and midwifery accreditation standards is required to support midwives to practise safely in the role of prescriber.

Australian requirements for endorsement for scheduled medicines as a midwife

When applying for endorsement for scheduled medicines as a midwife, a midwife must be able to demonstrate all of the following:

- *Current general registration* as a midwife in Australia with no conditions or undertakings relating to unsatisfactory professional performance or unprofessional conduct.
- Registration as a midwife that is *the equivalent of 3 years full-time clinical practice (5000 hours) in the past 6 years* that is either:
  - across the continuum of care, or
  - in a specified context of practice from the date when the complete application seeking endorsement for scheduled medicines is received by the NMBA.
- *Successful completion of an NMBA-approved program of study* leading to endorsement for scheduled medicines, or a program that is substantially equivalent to an NMBA-approved program of study leading to endorsement for scheduled medicines as determined by the NMBA.

For details of accredited courses visit the NMBA website.

BOX 22.1 Framework for autonomous midwife prescribing in Australia

MIDWIFE WITH SCHEDULED MEDICINES ENDORSEMENT – AUTONOMOUS PRESCRIBER	
Scope of prescribing	Able to independently diagnose and treat maternity related conditions within their scope of practice. Collaborates with other health practitioners as required
Education and experience	Postgraduate qualification in prescribing, including pathophysiology, assessment and based on the NPS prescribing competencies and QUM. Minimum 3 years (5000 hours)
Prescribing authority	Authorised prescriber in accordance with state and territory poisons legislation
Regulation	Endorsement by the NMBA. State and territory legislation and local policies

22.3 Legislation and regulations impacting prescribing and medication management

Legislation is a legal framework enacted by Acts of parliament to establish the legal obligations of members of society. The most relevant to midwifery practice are criminal law and civil law (common or tort). The midwife must be aware that lack of knowledge of legislation will not be considered a valid defence in the case of legal action. The midwife is responsible for ensuring that they have a working knowledge of the legislation relevant to the states in which they practise (see Chapter 2 for review and Box 22.2).

Criminal law

Under criminal law, an individual may be accused by government or other body of having broken a law (prosecution) and a trial takes place. If it is determined that the law has been breached fines or imprisonment may be ordered. Australian laws are made at both state and national levels.

Civil law

Civil law involves private individuals or businesses who may file a lawsuit against an individual or a business. Healthcare providers are more often involved in civil law cases than criminal. No fines or imprisonment generally result from these cases, but often 'damages' are paid to the injured party.

Three levels of legislation govern the midwife prescriber in Australia:

- international law
- Commonwealth law (Australian)
- state or territory law.

In New Zealand, both international law and NZ national law govern the midwife prescriber.

Commonwealth legislation

The Commonwealth legislation relevant to prescribing of medicines is the *National Health Act 1953* and the *Therapeutic Goods Act 1989*. The *National Health Act 1953* and the National Health (Pharmaceutical Benefits) Regulations specify who is authorised to prescribe different types of medicines under the PBS. The other main objects of these Acts is to promote and protect public health and safety by minimising:

1. accidental and deliberate poisonings by regulated substances; and
2. medicinal misadventures related to regulated substances; and

3. the diversion of regulated substances for abuse; and
4. the manufacture of regulated substances that are subject to abuse; and
5. harm from regulated therapeutic goods.

The objects of this Act also include ensuring that:

1. consumers of **prescription** medicines have adequate information and the understanding necessary to allow them to use the medicines safely and effectively; and
2. consumers of non-prescription medicines have adequate information and the understanding to allow them to select the most appropriate medicines for their condition and to use the medicines safely and effectively, considering the condition of their health.

State or territory legislation

As a federation, in Australia each state and territory has its own Drugs and Poisons Act, and the authority to prescribe by midwives is determined within the legislation of each state or territory. Legislation has been amended since the introduction of prescribing rights to include midwifery prescribing. It is important that as a midwife you are aware of the legislation for each state that you practise in, whether you are an authorised prescriber, or not. This is particularly relevant for midwives who engage in cross-border practice, whether in person or via virtual technologies or electronic means, for example telehealth services.

Regulation of midwifery prescribing

A **regulation** is a rule or directive made and maintained by an authority. In midwifery, regulations are set by such agencies as:

- The Australian Health Practitioners Agency (AHPRA)
- The Nursing and Midwifery Board of Australia (NMBA)
- The Australian Nursing and Midwifery Accreditation Council (ANMAC)
- Te Tatau o te Whare Kahu Midwifery Council (NZ).

Regulations may or may not be backed by legislation. In the case of regulations, failure to adhere may lead to loss of clinical privileges. The regulation of prescribing by midwives is shared between the NMBA, AHPRA and Commonwealth agencies (under Commonwealth legislation), and states/territories (prescribing authority under drugs and poisons legislation).

The NMBA Registration Standards define the requirements that applicants, registrants or students need to meet to be registered (see Online resources: NMBA).

Australian Midwifery Framework

The documents representing the current Australian Midwifery Framework that supports endorsed midwives are listed below. The midwife must ensure they are familiar with each of these:

- NMBA **Midwife Standards for Practice** 2018
- NMBA Code of Conduct for Midwives 2018
- ICM Code of Ethics for Midwives in Australia 2018
- NMBA Decision-making Framework for Nursing and Midwifery 2020
- ACM National Midwifery Guidelines for Consultation and Referral 2021
- NMBA Safety and Quality Guidelines for Privately Practising Midwives 2023.

More information on the Registration Standard: Endorsement for scheduled medicines, can be found on the NMBA website; and for midwifery prescribing in New Zealand – including the scope of midwifery practice, and prescribing of controlled drugs – on theTe Tatau o te Whare Kahu Midwifery Council website (see Online resources).

Box 22.2 below provides summary information on key professional standards and legislation relevant to midwife prescribers in Australia and New Zealand. Recent mapping of drugs and poisons legislation undertaken by the Australian Government is reported in 'Unleashing the potential of our health workforce – Scope of practice review', Issues paper 2 (2024), Appendix A: Summary of review of legislation and regulation. This paper identifies how primary health practitioners, including midwives, are enabled (or hindered) from participating in four different domains of competency in respect of drugs and poisons in each state and territory of Australia: **supplying**, **prescribing**, **possessing**, and **administering** (see Online resources).

BOX 22.2 Key professional midwifery standards, guidelines and legislation underpinning prescribing in New Zealand and Australia: A summary

INTERNATIONAL CONFEDERATION FOR MIDWIVES (ICM)

ICM International Definition and Scope of Practice of the Midwife https://internationalmidwives.org/resources/international-definition-of-the-midwife/
ICM Essential Competencies for Midwifery Practice 2019 https://internationalmidwives.org/resources/essential-competencies-for-midwifery-practice/
ICM Global Standards for Midwifery Education (Revised 2021) https://internationalmidwives.org/resources/global-standards-for-midwifery-education/

New Zealand Midwifery Standards/Competencies/Guidelines	Australia Midwifery Standards/Competencies/Guidelines
Te Tatau o te Whare Kahu Midwifery Council Competencies for Entry to the Register of Midwives 2007	Nursing and Midwifery Board of Australia Midwife Standards for Practice 2018 Code of Conduct for Midwives (2018) International Code of Ethics for Midwives (ICM 2014)
New Zealand College of Midwives, Midwife Standards of Practice (nd)	NMBA Registration Standard: Endorsement for Scheduled Medicines for Midwives 2017
New Zealand College of Midwives, Consensus Statement: Midwife Prescribing 2014	NMBA Safety and Quality Guidelines for Privately Practising Midwives 2023 NMBA Decision Making Framework for Nursing and Midwifery 2020
New Zealand College of Midwives (NZCOM) Consensus Statement. Prescribing and Administration of Opioid Analgesia in Labour 2014	Australian College of Midwives National Midwifery Guidelines for Consultation and Referral 2021

New Zealand Legislation	Australia Legislation
Health Practitioners Competence Assurance Act 2003 *Medicines Act 1981* Medicines Regulations 1984 Medicine Standing Orders Regulations 2002 Medicines (Standing Order) Amendment Regulations 2016 Medicines (Designated Prescriber: Nurse Practitioners) Regulations 2016 Medicines (Designated Pharmacist Prescribers) Regulations 2013	*Commonwealth* *Health Practitioner Regulation National Law Act 2009* Section 94 – Endorsement of health practitioner's registration in relation to scheduled medicines *Therapeutic Goods Act 1989 (Cth)* Therapeutic Goods Regulations 1990 (Cth) *National Health Act 1953 (Cth)* The National Health (Collaborative Arrangements for Midwives) Instrument 2022

BOX 22.2 Key professional midwifery standards, guidelines and legislation underpinning prescribing in New Zealand and Australia: A summary—cont'd

New Zealand Legislation	Australia Legislation
Misuse of Drugs Regulations 1977 Misuse of Drugs Amendment Regulations 2014	Health Legislation Amendment (Removal of Requirement for a Collaborative Arrangement) Bill 2024 Australian Capital Territory *Medicines, Poisons and Therapeutic Goods Act 2008* *Drugs of Dependence Act 1989* Drugs of Dependence Regulations 2009 New South Wales *Poisons and Therapeutic Goods Act 1966* Poisons and Therapeutic Goods Regulations 2008 *[This legislation is currently due to be automatically repealed under the* Subordinate Legislation Act 1989 *on 1 September 2024]* Northern Territory *Medicines, Poisons and Therapeutic Goods Act 2012 (NT)* Medicines, Poisons and Therapeutic Goods Regulations 2014 Queensland *Medicines and Poisons Act 2019* Medicines and Poisons (Medicines) Regulation 2021 Medicines and Poisons (Poisons and Prohibited Substances) Regulation 2021 South Australia *Controlled Substances Act 1984* Controlled Substances (Poisons) Regulations 2011 Tasmania *Poisons Act 1971* Poisons Regulation 2018 Poisons (Midwifery Substances) Order 2011 Victoria *Drugs, Poisons and Controlled Substances Act 1981* Drugs, Poisons and Controlled Substances Regulations 2017 Western Australia *Medicines and Poisons Act 2014* Medicines and Poisons Regulations 2016

Case study 1

Meredith undertook her initial midwifery education in New Zealand where she practised as a lead maternity care provider for 15 years. Meredith moved to Australia 2 years ago. She is a skilled midwife with prescribing authorisation (a current **endorsed midwife** with NMBA) and concurrently engaged in several professional midwifery roles. In addition to her substantive role (part-time 0.5 FTE employment within a tertiary public hospital in Victoria), Meredith also provides back-up as the second midwife attendant at planned homebirths for a small group of privately practising midwives in Victoria. Meredith also provides holiday relief for midwives employed with an emergency retrieval service, flying in and out of South Australia, the Northern Territory and Queensland. The latter service, headquartered in Queensland, provides a virtual postnatal midwifery review for women in rural and remote communities in those regions. Meredith provides occasional telehealth consultations involving cross-border practice for this service as part of her locum midwifery relief.

Questions

1 Discuss the factors that impact Meredith's ability to exercise her authorisation as a midwife prescriber in her various professional midwifery roles across these three contexts of practice.

2 Identify the challenges that Meredith may encounter and suggest strategies to assist in managing them.

3 What impact do legislation, professional guidelines, and consultation and referral with other health providers have in relation to Meredith's practice within each of the three professional roles in which she is engaged?

22.4 Quality and safety

Medicine use is an ever-increasing part of healthcare, and although medicines have the potential to improve health, their use is not without risk. Awareness of risks and benefits of medicines is important for all health professionals. The task of prescribing requires the application of specific knowledge, skills, and attitudes of a unique person at a given point in time. It is also complicated by the increasing availability of medicines designed to treat similar conditions.

Quality use of medicines

Competent prescribing contributes to the quality use of medicines, a central component of the National Medicines Policy. Prescribers are in a pivotal position to support the optimal use of medicines through effective partnerships with consumers and a collaborative, multi-disciplinary approach to medicines use.

The National Prescribing Service lists the four stages for best practice prescribing as follows:

1 information gathering
2 clinical decision making
3 communication
4 monitoring and reviewing.

These four stages are informed by a person's needs, their expectation of the prescribed medication/treatment, specific collaborative care, and drug therapy protocols.

Prescribing practice: Ensuring quality and safety

Prescribing has been defined as an iterative process involving the steps of information gathering, clinical decision making, communication and evaluation which results in the initiation, continuation, or cessation of medications (Nissen et al 2010). A prescriber is defined as a health practitioner authorised to undertake prescribing within the scope of their practice. See Chapter 2 for a review of the principles of prescribing, including requirements for valid written and electronic prescriptions; accepted abbreviations; and links to exemplars including PBS prescriptions, non-PBS/private prescriptions, Authority Streamlined prescriptions, the National Inpatient Medication Chart, and Special Authority Medicines in NZ. (See also Online resources; [Australia] Australian Commission on Safety and Quality in Healthcare 2024, PBS, PBAC, TGA; [NZ] (Pharmac, Medsafe).

Health Profession Prescribing Pathway

In 2013, Australian health ministers approved the Health Professions Prescribing Pathway (HPPP) (HWA 2013). The HPPP was developed to provide a nationally recognised, consistent approach to prescribing by health professionals. The HPPP provides guidance that describes the steps required for a health professional to prescribe, and considers the principles underpinning prescribing practice; the requirements for health professions to prescribe; the models of health professional prescribing; and the roles of stakeholders involved in health professional prescribing. Independent or autonomous prescribing occurs when the healthcare practitioner has the legal authority to issue prescription medicines.

The five key principles underpinning the HPPP are:

- The health, wellbeing and safety of the person taking a medicine must always be maintained.
- Health professionals who prescribe are accountable for their actions.
- Health professionals authorised to prescribe undertake prescribing within their individual and professional scope of practice and maintain the level of professional competence and ethical standards (including the separation of commercial interests) expected of their profession.
- Health professionals who prescribe commit to the safe and effective use of medicines as described by the *National Medicines Policy* (see Chapter 2 and Online resources: DOHA 2022).
- Health professionals involved in prescribing work in partnership with the person taking a medicine, their carers, and other members of the healthcare team.

NPS MedicineWise Prescribing Competencies Framework

Another key prescribing framework was developed by the National Prescribing Service in 2012 for all health professionals practising in Australia; the Prescribing Competencies Framework was revised in 2021 (see Online resources: NPS MEDICINEWISE 2021). The framework underpins current education programs for midwifery prescribing in Australia and is utilised by endorsed midwives to enhance their prescribing practices and ensure safe and effective medication management that is nationally consistent with other regulated health professions.

The aim of the National Prescribing Service (NPS) is to provide national leadership and services to the health sector. It is a useful education and starting point for prescribing for all Australian health professionals. NPS MedicineWise resources aim to improve the health of Australians through safe and wise use of medicines to:

- improve the use of medicines and other health technologies to optimise health outcomes for Australians
- improve the health literacy of Australians
- reduce misuse of medicines and other health technologies
- improve the sustainability of the Pharmaceutical Benefits Scheme and Medical Benefits Scheme.

Since 2023, NPS MedicineWise resources have been administered by the Australian Commission for Safety and

Quality in Health Care (2023). The intention of the NPS MedicineWise Prescribing Competencies Framework is to promote quality use of medicines by defining competencies for prescribers. The framework enables health professionals to prescribe judiciously, appropriately, safely, and effectively. The second edition released in 2021 offers a framework for all professional groups. This is in line with new professional groups now having the prescribing right, such as midwives. The second edition of the framework describes competencies prescribers can rely on to contribute to safe, person-centred, and quality medicine use.

The NPS Prescribing Competencies Framework has seven competency areas:

1–5 Person-centred Prescribing Process

1   Understand the person and their needs
2   Understand the management options
3   Agree on a plan for medicines
4   Prescribe medicines and communicate the agreed treatment decision
5   Review the outcome of treatment
6–7 Professional Practice that Supports Prescribing
6   Prescribe safely and effectively
7   Prescribe professionally.

(See Figure 22.1 for the NPS Prescribing Competencies Framework. See Table 22.1 NPS Prescribing Competencies and Table 22.2 Guidelines for Achieving NPS Prescribing Competencies.)

Person-centred use of medicines

Like woman-centred care, the person-centred ideal of the prescribing process emphasises the importance of a

NPS National Prescribing Competencies Framework

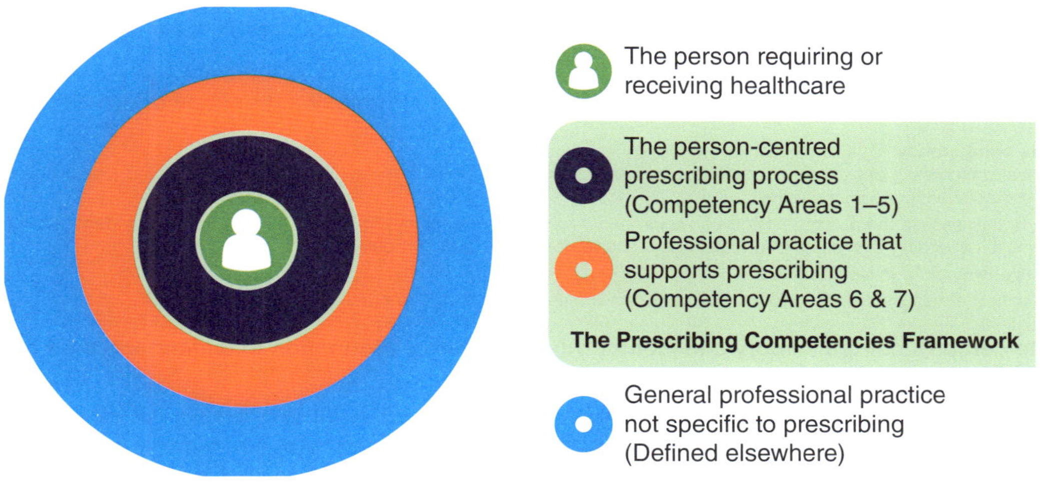

- The person requiring or receiving healthcare
- The person-centred prescribing process (Competency Areas 1–5)
- Professional practice that supports prescribing (Competency Areas 6 & 7)

The Prescribing Competencies Framework

- General professional practice not specific to prescribing (Defined elsewhere)

The person-centred prescribing process	Professional practice that supports prescribing
Competency Area 1 Understand the person and their needs	Competency Area 6 Prescribe safely and effectively
Competency Area 2 Understand the management options	Competency Area 7 Prescribe professionally
Competency Area 3 Agree on a plan for medicines	
Competency Area 4 Prescribe medicines and communicate the agreed treatment decision	
Competency Area 5 Review the outcomes of treatment	

FIGURE 22.1

Source: Reproduced with permission from Prescribing Competencies Framework, developed by the Australian Commission on Safety and Quality in Health Care (ACSQHC). ACSQHC: Sydney 2021.

TABLE 22.2 Guidelines for achieving NPS prescribing competencies

THE PERSON-CENTRED PRESCRIBING PROCESS (COMPETENCY AREAS 1–5)

Competency Area 1: Understand the person and their needs

1.1 Ensure competence to assess the person's needs

How to achieve this competency
- Consistent with the professional scope of practice, ensure your understanding of biomedical sciences (including anatomy, physiology, pathology, pathophysiology, microbiology, immunology, chemistry, biochemistry, clinical medicine) is adequate and current.
- Understand and be competent in the consultation process, including where relevant: establishing the person's medical and treatment history; undertaking a physical examination; interpreting information in the person's health records; accurately diagnosing or understanding a diagnosis of illness according to the professional scope of practice.

1.2 Discuss with the person their medical and treatment history

How to achieve this competency
- Integrate information obtained from the person and their health records with clinical knowledge and experience to refine and ask questions to determine the person's needs, with a focus on the priority issues for the person.
- Recognise the limitations of the information gathered, and verify the information given, where possible and with the person's consent, with other health professionals, family or carers.
- Recognise the risk of medicines errors at transitions of care (e.g. moving between wards or departments within a hospital or discharge from a hospital to the community) and conduct a medicines reconciliation. Reconcile the medicines history with the medical history, taking into consideration relevant social, cultural, and demographic details. Ensure the indications for current medicines are appropriate and understood by the person.
- Consider medicines as a possible cause of presenting symptoms.
- Verbally summarise the information for the person, where appropriate.
- Ask the person for more information or to clarify information provided, where required.
- Ascertain that sufficient information has been obtained about the person's co-existing conditions and current treatments to identify possible risks and contraindications for treatment.

1.3 Assess the person according to the clinical context and the health professional's scope of practice

How to achieve this competency
- According to the health professional's scope of practice, and with the person's consent, review the medical history and examination findings to inform appropriate further investigations, if required.
- Where required to further assess the person, perform an appropriate examination and arrange investigations, based on identified clinical issues and real and potential risks, according to the health professional's scope of practice and competence.
- Evaluate the clinical relevance of investigations.
- Refer the person for further assessment where outside the health professional's scope of practice.

1.4 Consider the person's cultural history and identity when gathering information to understand their needs

How to achieve this competency
- Discuss with the person their cultural identity and the aspects of their culture that may impact their treatment preferences.
- Acknowledge personal and system biases, including racism, assumptions, stereotypes and prejudices, and take steps to minimise the impact of these on prescribing practice.
- Recognise the importance of the individual, family and community in decisions about treatment and medicines use.
- Reflect on your prescribing practice and take steps to ensure you have the skills, knowledge and an appropriate attitude to incorporate cultural considerations in the prescribing process.

1.5 Review and interpret information in the person's health records to contribute to an understanding of their needs and current treatment

How to achieve this competency
- Identify, review and interpret relevant material in hard copy or e-Health records.
- Act cautiously in situations where there is concern that the information may be incomplete, inaccurate or biased.
- Source relevant missing information, with the person's consent, and record details.

1.6 Explore with the person their adherence to prescribed medicines and the treatment plan

How to achieve this competency
- Discuss with the person their views, beliefs, and perceptions of their current condition, health and wellbeing.
- Explore the person's psychological behaviours, health literacy and motivation for consulting a health professional.
- Use a non-judgemental approach to explore adherence to medicines and the treatment plan and understand barriers from the person's perspective, including possible cultural influences.
- Consider the risk factors for poor adherence, including social isolation, physical impairment, cognitive impairment or disturbance, low English proficiency, low health literacy, financial disadvantage.
- Recognise and respond to the potential misuse of medicines.
- Where relevant, and with the person's permission, discuss the person's adherence to medicines and treatment with a member of their family and/or their carer to better understand important issues.

TABLE 22.2 Guidelines for achieving NPS prescribing competencies—cont'd

1.7 Make or review and understand the diagnosis and key clinical issues including those that are, or may be, medicine-related

How to achieve this competency
- Evaluate the results of investigations in the context of the person's medical history and examination.
- Establish a list of possible conditions and explore their likelihood.
- Consider the possibility that the person's current medicines might be contributing to their presentation.
- Consider the possibility of non-disclosure of relevant information (e.g. high-risk behaviours or non-adherence to prescribed medicines).
- Understand the person's condition/s and the likely response to treatment, including medicines.
- Revisit the history with the person where results appear inconsistent with the original history.

1.8 Discuss with the person the clinical issues and implications for treatment

How to achieve this competency
- Understand and explain to the person the clinical relevance of the assessment findings, in the context of their co-existing conditions, medicines history, and current treatment plan, and the impact of these on prescribing decisions.
- Include the person's family and/or carer in these discussions where relevant and with the person's permission.
- Understand and explain to the person the likely natural progression of the condition with or without treatment.
- Consider the person's response to the clinical issues and work to maintain an effective therapeutic partnership that recognises the basis of rational prescribing.
- Refer clinical issues that are outside the health professional's scope of practice to other health professionals.

Competency Area 2: Understand the management options

2.1 Recognise when it is clinically appropriate not to prescribe medicines

How to achieve this competency
- Understand and explain to the person the clinical reasoning, including relevant potential benefits and harms, supporting the decision not to prescribe medicines.
- Where possible, confirm that the person understands the reason/s for not providing treatment.

2.2 Review current medicines and consider the possibility of a contribution to current health issues

How to achieve this competency
- Consider whether existing medicines have achieved the agreed goals and modifications are indicated (e.g. dose adjustment, discontinuation).
- Consider whether existing medicines may be causing adverse effects or may be ineffective and require modification (e.g. dose adjustment, discontinuation).
- Where polypharmacy is identified, specifically review the need for all medicines and consider discontinuation where appropriate and within the health professional's scope of practice to do so (refer to Competency 5.4 for further recommendations about ceasing medicines).
- Discuss potential modifications to medicines with the person.

2.3 Where treatment is indicated, consider both non-pharmacological and pharmacological options

How to achieve this competency
- Understand the clinical reasoning and/or evidence supporting treatment decisions.
- Identify non-pharmacological therapies and their relative outcome capacity in comparison with pharmacological interventions.
- Consider the potential benefits and harms of incorporating non-pharmacological and/or pharmacological therapies or a combination thereof.
- Discuss possible non-pharmacological options with the person in the context of other therapies and the person's preferences and goals.

2.4 Identify suitable medicine options

How to achieve this competency
- Integrate knowledge of pharmacology, other biomedical sciences, clinical medicine, and therapeutics, and identify medicines suitable for treating the condition.
- Understand the pharmacological basis supporting treatment decisions in the context of the person's current needs.
- Understand and consider factors specific to the medicine/s identified as suitable for treating the person's condition (e.g. availability, indications, contraindications, potential adverse effects and interactions).

2.5 Obtain, interpret and apply current, reliable evidence and information about medicines to inform decision making

How to achieve this competency
- Identify reliable information to inform decisions about medicines and other treatment options.
- Critically assess the findings of relevant studies. Review available evidence to identify the safety, efficacy, comparative effectiveness, and cost-effectiveness of medicines. Consider the hierarchy of evidence when assessing relevance.
- Apply study findings and medicines information in the context of relevant clinical considerations, the person's preferences, and their circumstances.
- Use clinical decision support tools and memory aids to support prescribing decision making. When prescribing unfamiliar medicines, use reliable and current sources of information and seek advice where unsure. Carefully apply information to the person's situation to enhance the safety and quality of prescribing decisions.

Continued

TABLE 22.2 Guidelines for achieving NPS prescribing competencies—cont'd

2.6 Consult other health professionals about potential medicines and the treatment plan, where appropriate

How to achieve this competency
- With the person's consent, engage with other health professionals to further understand medicines and/or other treatments previously prescribed.
- Consult other health professionals for advice about medicines choices in the interests of safety and optimal prescribing outcomes, where appropriate.
- Where appropriate, consult other health professionals to understand non-pharmacological therapies that are outside personal scope of practice. Consider implications for medicines management, if any.

2.7 Tailor medicines for the person considering relevant potential benefits, harms, medicine and person-specific factors

How to achieve this competency
- Apply knowledge of the differences between medicines in the same class to the person's situation to identify medicines for which the comparison of potential benefits and harms is favourable and to eliminate those medicines that are not suitable.
- Consider the possibility of drug–drug, drug–disease and/or drug–food interactions and the potential implication of these for the choice of medicine.
- Consider person-specific factors relevant to the choice of medicine, dose, frequency, route of administration, formulation and/or duration of therapy (e.g. lifestyle, preferences, beliefs, cultural influences, health literacy, pregnancy, breast feeding, co-existing conditions, current medicines, allergies, intolerances, genomic information, the ability to swallow, relevant fears or phobias, the potential for medicines abuse or misuse).
- Calculate the correct dose for the person according to relevant person-specific factors such as age, weight, renal function. Check and document all calculations.
- Avoid medicines that have caused previous adverse events or that are unsuitable because of the person's allergies or intolerances.
- Implement appropriate medicines strategies in situations where the diagnosis is ambiguous (e.g. pre-emptive treatment, defined trial periods).
- Act cautiously in situations where there is limited or no evidence for using the medicine with the person's particular co-morbidities or characteristics (e.g. age).
- Understand the clinical reasoning underpinning decisions about medicines.

2.8 Consider the financial cost and affordability of the medicines to the person

How to achieve this competency
- Consider the person's eligibility to access subsidised medicines (e.g. the Pharmaceutical Benefits Scheme [PBS], the Repatriation Pharmaceutical Benefits Scheme [RPBS], and the Quality Use of Medicines Maximised For Aboriginal and Torres Strait Islander Peoples [QUMAX] programs).
- Select a more affordable medicine in preference to one that is less affordable when the two medicines are therapeutically equivalent (e.g. a generic brand where clinically applicable).

2.9 Consider the implications to the wider community of prescribing a particular medicine

How to achieve this competency
- Understand and consider the principles of antimicrobial stewardship and antimicrobial resistance.
- Understand why generic medicines are an acceptable alternative to original brand medicines.
- Select a more cost-effective medicine in preference to a less cost-effective option.

2.10 Refer the person for further assessment or treatment when the suitable treatment options are outside the health professional's scope of practice

How to achieve this competency
- Arrange referrals to other health professionals as needed.

Competency Area 3: Agree on a plan for medicines

Where relevant, and with the person's permission, include the person's family and/or carer in decisions about medicines and the treatment plan.

3.1 Explore the person's opinions and preferences about medicines and the treatment plan

How to achieve this competency
- Respect the person's values, beliefs, expectations, opinions, and decisions about their treatment preferences.
- Consider the person's preferences for generic brands of medicines.
- Discuss with the person their capacity to pay for medicines.

3.2 Negotiate therapeutic goals that enhance self-management

How to achieve this competency
- Facilitate interactive negotiations about the goals of medicines as part of the treatment plan.
- Respect the person's beliefs and preferences during goal negotiations.

TABLE 22.2 Guidelines for achieving NPS prescribing competencies—cont'd

3.3 Discuss the possible medicines options with the person and allow them time to make an informed decision

How to achieve this competency
- Consider the person's priorities for treating their current and co-existing conditions, their readiness to address the current condition and their expectations of treatment.
- Discuss relevant lifestyle changes that will be required to support the effectiveness of the medicine/s.
- Provide sufficient necessary information about medicines options, including expected outcomes and possible side effects, in an appropriate format and language, to assist the person to make an informed choice about treatment. Ensure the person understands the information provided.
- Recognise and take steps to minimise the influence of personal bias when providing information about medicines to the person.
- Facilitate an interactive discussion and involve the person in the treatment decisions.
- Support the person to make an informed decision by providing additional time and/or resources according to their health literacy.
- Discuss the likely cost of the medicine options with the person and choose an option they agree to fund.
- Review the person's understanding of the treatment options.
- Discuss and work with the person to resolve discordant expectations or requests (e.g. the desire for a prescription where not warranted).
- Consider the potential for medicine misuse and discuss alternatives with the person. Identify, discuss and manage drug-seeking behaviour on the part of the person, where appropriate.
- Advise the person how they can access appropriate sources of medicines information in languages other than English, where appropriate.
- Provide the person with information about consumer support organisations, where appropriate.
- Use a consumer medicine information leaflet to help inform the person about medicines.
- Supplement verbal information with written information about the condition and treatment options, where appropriate.

3.4 Explore and respond appropriately to the person's concerns and expectations about their health and the use of medicines to maintain their health

How to achieve this competency
- Adopt a person-centred approach.
- Demonstrate appropriate empathy.
- Where applicable, explore and respond to the person's concerns and expectations about the consultation, their health, the role of health professionals and the person in managing their health, the health professional's scope of practice, and the role of medicines within the treatment plan.

3.5 Develop the medicines plan in partnership with the person

How to achieve this competency
- Respect the person's decision about the selection of medicines as part of the treatment plan.
- Respect the person's decisions about the use of medicines, including the decision to defer selection and initiation of medicines to a subsequent consultation, to obtain treatment from another health professional, or to not undergo treatment.
- Respect existing decisions made by the person about advance care planning.
- Establish a medicines management plan or add to a current one, making sure the person understands any changes made to previous plans.
- Recommend a dose administration aid if required.
- Consider the use of a medication management review where the person is taking multiple medicines regularly, has had significant changes to their medicines plan, has difficulty managing their medicines, or if it appears the person may not be adhering to their medicines plan.

3.6 Identify the need for and develop with the person a plan to review treatment

How to achieve this competency
- Discuss the need for a review with the person and identify and resolve potential barriers.
- Agree on the timing and details of the review with the person.
- Negotiate a prescribing contract with the person for medicines prone to abuse (e.g. opioids, benzodiazepines).
- Confirm the person's understanding of the review plan.

Competency Area 4: Prescribe medicines and communicate the agreed treatment decision

4.1 Ensure adequate and current knowledge of medicines prior to prescribing

How to achieve this competency
- Ensure the prescribing of medicines is justified within the context of professional scope of practice and the clinical needs of the person.
- Review the specifics of the medicine/s to be prescribed, including the likely effects, possible adverse effects, approved indications, dose, frequency, likely duration of therapy, contraindications, potential drug–drug, drug–food or drug–disease interactions and consider in the context of the person.
- Consider prescribing medicines for unlicensed indications (i.e. 'off label') only when a licensed medicine is unavailable or inappropriate, adequate information is available to support use and the potential benefits and harms have been considered.
- Consider current information about the availability and storage of medicines and the potential impact on prescribing decisions.

Continued

TABLE 22.2 Guidelines for achieving NPS prescribing competencies—cont'd

4.2 Prescribe medicines compliant with relevant legislation, regulatory frameworks, guidelines, codes of practice, scope of practice and organisational policies and procedures

How to achieve this competency
- Obtain approval to use medicines where appropriate. Comply with state, territory and federal legislative requirements, including restrictions required by the Pharmaceutical Benefits Scheme (PBS) and local approval processes.
- Adhere to legislative and regulatory requirements relevant to the profession and jurisdiction.
- Comply with local formularies, guidelines, restrictions, and protocols.
- Communicate appropriately, using unambiguous language, and/or symbolic representation.
- Use recommended terminology, abbreviations and symbols for prescribing medicines (e.g. use the active ingredient name of medicines, and the brand name if clinically necessary).
- Understand the concept of bioequivalence and its relevance to the prescription of generic or specific brand medicines. Be aware of situations where use of a consistent brand is preferred and consider in the context of the person.
- Prescribe using systems that support safe medicines use. Ensure competence to use prescribing systems and recognise the potential limitations of these systems (e.g. preferentially use electronic prescribing systems while maintaining competence to prescribe and/or order medicines using paper-based prescriptions/medication orders; use and understand the scope of computer decision support tools and automated medication alerts; complete the National Standard Medication Chart accurately and legibly, where appropriate).
- Where electronic medical records are used, ensure competence to use these systems.
- Ensure the prescription or medication order specifies the active ingredient name (and brand name where clinically appropriate), dose, route of administration and frequency of use. Where relevant, also include the duration of medicine use, the basis for dose calculations and the indication for the medicine.

4.3 Where prescribing relies on electronic (e.g. telehealth) or telephone services (e.g. verbal prescription or medication order), ensure compliance with relevant legislation, guidelines and policies

How to achieve this competency
- Understand the risks associated with prescribing medicines via electronic or telephone services and take steps to prevent or minimise.
- Communicate verbal medication orders appropriately using unambiguous language.
- Ascertain that the health professional receiving the verbal medication order has understood the instructions by asking them to repeat the instructions.
- Ensure that the verbal medication order is documented and signed for within legislative requirements and that this occurs as soon as practicable.
- Ensure that medicines prescribed under legislation applicable during emergencies are eligible and conform to all criteria, including requirements for documentation.

4.4 Provide accurate and complete information to other health professionals in a timely manner when implementing new medicines or modifying existing medicines or treatment plans

How to achieve this competency
- Provide an accurate and complete current list of the person's medicines for other health professionals, particularly the primary healthcare provider (usually their general practitioner), in support of maintaining continuity of care and when referring the person to another health professional. Include the details of, and reasons for, any changes made to the medicines.
- Provide information using secure means and an appropriate format that can be easily understood.
- Provide information about the person's history of allergies, intolerances and adverse drug reactions.

4.5 Discuss and document the treatment plan with the person and ensure they understand both the plan and how to use the medicine/s safely and effectively

How to achieve this competency
- Include the person's family and/or carer with their permission when discussing medicines and the treatment plan, where appropriate.
- Support the person's understanding of safe and effective prescribing, noting that sometimes no treatment is the better option.
- Summarise for, and discuss with, the person the rationale for the treatment plan and how to use and store medicine/s safely and the possible side effects of the medicine/s using language they can understand.
- Discuss the ongoing monitoring of the medicine and ensure there are no barriers to achieving this.
- Discuss and provide reliable, clear and relevant information in an appropriate format to support the person's understanding of the medicine/s and their self-management of the condition (e.g. the consumer medicine information leaflet, information from appropriate organisations).
- Provide pictorial or graphical information where helpful.
- Use the active ingredient name of the medicine and ensure the person understands the difference between the active ingredient and brand name.
- Discuss how to access information in languages other than English, where appropriate. Use resources in languages other than English where available and appropriate.
- Tailor information about medicines to ensure it is appropriate for the person's health literacy, language literacy and cultural needs.
- Discuss and provide practical guidance about what to do and who to contact if the person experiences signs and symptoms indicating an adverse event, if no improvement is noted over a defined period of time or if the person has other concerns about their medicines or condition.
- Discuss and provide information about support services (e.g. services for people with chronic conditions).
- Check the person's understanding by asking them to explain their treatment plan and to explain or demonstrate how they are to use the medicine.
- Update the person's current medicines list and encourage them to carry it with them and show it to other health professionals providing treatment.
- Recommend a medicines alert device where appropriate.
- Encourage the person to share information with other healthcare professionals involved in their care.

TABLE 22.2 Guidelines for achieving NPS prescribing competencies—cont'd

Competency Area 5: Review the outcomes of treatment

5.1 Explore with the person their response to treatment, including adherence to the medicines and treatment plan

How to achieve this competency
- Engage in interactive two-way communication with the person and, where relevant and permitted, their family and/or carer and other health professionals to review the outcomes of treatment.
- Ask the person to demonstrate how they take or use the medicine to ensure they are undertaking this correctly, where appropriate.
- Discuss with the person and/or family the person's experiences with the medicines, including perceived benefits, adverse effects, and adherence issues.
- Integrate information with clinical knowledge and experience to assess the progress towards attaining the planned therapeutic goals.

5.2 Gather objective information, using appropriate indicators, to assess the response to medicines, where appropriate

How to achieve this competency
- Gather observations at appropriate time intervals.
- Obtain additional information to assess whether the therapeutic goals have been achieved by observing and examining the person, requesting investigations and interpreting the findings, where appropriate and according to the health professional's scope of practice.
- Order and review therapeutic drug monitoring tests for medicines with a narrow therapeutic index.

5.3 Synthesise information provided by the person, other health professionals and from the assessment, to determine the response to medicines

How to achieve this competency
- Use information to determine whether: agreed therapeutic goals have been achieved; treatment should be discontinued, modified or continued (e.g. where adverse effects have been identified; the person should be referred to another health professional).
- Identify the key findings of the assessment (including history, examination and investigations) that indicate whether the therapeutic goals have, or have not been achieved.
- Act on the results of the findings to optimise the therapeutic outcome.
- Establish the clinical reasoning supporting the decision to discontinue, modify, or continue the treatment, and/or to refer the person to another health professional.
- Detect and manage adverse events experienced by the person and report them to the relevant authorities. Detect and manage adverse drug interactions.
- Report the abuse or misuse of medicines in accordance with relevant legislation and organisational policy and procedure.

5.4 Discontinue or modify existing medicines and other treatments, where appropriate

How to achieve this competency
- Consider discontinuing medicines where appropriate (e.g. where an adverse event has occurred, the treatment goals have been achieved and the medicine is no longer needed; new evidence suggests an alternative medicine should be used; the person is receiving palliative care).
- Adhere to protocols or guidelines for withdrawing medicines from a person's treatment plan.
- Negotiate with other health professionals to modify or discontinue treatments they have implemented, where appropriate.
- Discuss any changes to medicines and/or the treatment plan with the person and encourage them to return unwanted medicines to their community pharmacist for disposal.
- Reconcile and update the person's medicines record and/or health record with any changes made to their medicines.

5.5 Discuss with the person the benefits of a medication management review, where appropriate

How to achieve this competency
- Consider the use of a Home Medicines Review or Residential Medication Management Review where the person is taking multiple medicines regularly, has had significant changes to their medicines plan, has difficulty managing their medicines, or if it appears the person may not be adhering to their medicines plan.
- Complete a medicines management plan following a review.

5.6 Work with the person and other health professionals to modify the treatment plan to optimise the safety and effectiveness of treatment, where appropriate

How to achieve this competency
- Where appropriate, collaborate with and consider the input and expertise of other health professionals when deciding on changes to the treatment.
- Consider the possibility of adverse events or other concerns (e.g. cost) impacting adherence. Where it is likely these concerns will result in self-cessation or poor adherence, modify, substitute or discontinue the medicine in consultation with the person and, where relevant, other health professionals.
- Discuss with the person and ensure they understand the reasons for discontinuing, modifying, or continuing the treatment unchanged.
- Provide the person with an updated list of their medicines.
- Where an adverse event has occurred, discuss with the person the possible consequence of the adverse event (if any) and how to avoid medicines that have caused unwanted adverse events. Recommend a medicines alert device where appropriate.
- Communicate the details of any adverse events with relevant other health professionals in a timely manner.
- Where the expected outcomes of treatment have not been achieved as anticipated, consider referral to another health professional. Discuss with the person the reason/s for referral and provide all relevant information to the health professional in a timely manner to support their involvement.

Continued

TABLE 22.2 Guidelines for achieving NPS prescribing competencies—cont'd

5.7 Discuss the findings of the review and recommendations with other health professionals, where appropriate

How to achieve this competency
- Communicate, by secure means and in a timely manner, the details of the current treatment plan to other health professionals involved in the person's care.
- Inform other health professionals who provide clinical care for the person about changes to the treatment plan (e.g. dose alterations, medicines discontinued or initiated in response to the review) and whether the treatment plan appears to be achieving agreed goals.

PROFESSIONAL PRACTICE THAT SUPPORTS PRESCRIBING (COMPETENCY AREAS 6 & 7)

Competency Area 6: Prescribe safely and effectively

6.1 Understand and prescribe medicines according to relevant legislation, regulatory frameworks and organisational requirements

How to achieve this competency
- Achieve and maintain appropriate education, training and required endorsements (where applicable) prior to prescribing medicines.
- Implement procedures to address the medicolegal requirements that are relevant to the person, including those required for special or vulnerable populations.
- Comply with state, territory and federal legislative requirements, including restrictions with the Pharmaceutical Benefits Scheme (PBS) system, and local approval processes.
- Understand and comply with national, state and territory, and facility policies, procedures and standards relevant to prescribing (e.g. antimicrobial prescribing policy, shared care arrangements, national medicines management standards and guidelines).
- Prescribe according to required systems, including monitoring systems.

6.2 Practise within the limits of the health professional's education, training and scope of practice as applied to prescribing

How to achieve this competency
- Refer the person to other appropriate health professionals for further assessment or treatment when they require healthcare that is outside the health professional's education, training, and scope of practice.

6.3 Understand common causes of incidents and error associated with prescribing and medicines use and implement strategies to reduce the risk of these occurring

How to achieve this competency
- Conduct and document a comprehensive medicines assessment and understand the diagnosis prior to prescribing.
- Understand, maintain competence to use and recognise the limits of systems designed to improve prescribing.
- Confirm prescriptions and medication orders are accurate, particularly at points of transfer (e.g. between wards, between hospital and community).
- Ensure clear documentation is kept, including details of the person's allergies, intolerances and previous adverse drug reactions and any modifications made to the treatment plan.
- Report and learn from errors, incidents and near misses.
- Respectfully report, using appropriate methods, concerns about unsafe prescribing by colleagues.

6.4 Detect and report errors, incidents and adverse events involving medicines

How to achieve this competency
- Be aware of the systems that support the identification and reporting of incidents and errors associated with medicines, including those pertaining to the prescribing process.
- Report, using appropriate channels and according to legislative, professional and organisational requirements, the details of medicines misuse by persons receiving healthcare and/or colleagues and errors involving the prescribing process and/or medicines.
- Understand the importance of reporting potential as well as actual incidents and errors involving medicines, in order to improve prescribing practice.
- Detect and manage adverse events and report to the relevant authorities.
- Support other health professionals, particularly those who prescribe medicines for the person, and prevent prescribing errors by communicating complete and accurate information about prescribed medicines in a timely manner.

6.5 Apply quality use of medicines principles when prescribing medicines

How to achieve this competency
- Understand the principles of quality use of medicines as required. Further information is available here.
- Ensure medicines are prescribed judiciously, appropriately, safely and effectively and in accordance with the prescriber's authorisations and scope of practice.
- Contribute to quality health outcomes by committing to the fundamental tenets of quality medicines use, including:
  - recognising that medicines may not be the most appropriate management strategy
  - making wise medicines choices that align with the person's needs and preferences and medicine-specific factors
  - carefully monitoring the outcomes of medicines used
  - partnering with both the person and other healthcare professionals to optimise health outcomes.

TABLE 22.2 Guidelines for achieving NPS prescribing competencies—cont'd

6.6 Critically evaluate information about medicines and make evidence-based decisions in the context of the person's needs

How to achieve this competency
- Critically assess evidence and information about the safety, efficacy, comparative effectiveness, and cost-effectiveness of medicines.
- Apply study findings and medicines information in the context of relevant clinical considerations, the person's preferences, and their circumstances.
- Use feedback from the person prescribed new medicine to contribute to information about the safety and effectiveness of that medicine.

Competency Area 7: Prescribe professionally

7.1 Understand and comply with applicable professional standards, codes of conduct and guidelines relevant to prescribing

How to achieve this competency
- Adhere to relevant professional standards, codes of conduct and scope of practice statements or guidelines.
- Adhere to legislative and workplace requirements for obtaining and recording consent to access health records; obtain information from, and provide information to, other health professionals; conduct clinical examinations.

7.2 Demonstrate appropriate professional judgement when interpreting and applying prescribing guidelines and protocols to the person's situation

How to achieve this competency
- Identify prescribing guidelines and protocols that are relevant to the person and appropriate to the health professional's scope of practice.
- Interpret relevant guidelines and protocols according to the person's specific needs and the context in which they are accessing healthcare.

7.3 Maintain accurate and complete records of the interaction

How to achieve this competency
- Ensure records comply with legal, regulatory, and facility requirements and are completed in a timely manner.
- Include details of the consultation, clinical examinations and investigations, risk factors for medicines misadventure, the person's decision to decline treatment (where relevant), changes to the person's medicines treatment plan including the rationale behind the changes, the review plan, recommendations and date for next review and the outcomes of the treatment.
- Update the person's health record with details of changes to their medicines regimen or other relevant details, such as the occurrence of adverse events. Where available, and with the person's consent, include these details in the electronic health record.
- Discuss with the person the potential benefits and harms of treatment, the benefits of communicating with other health professionals about medicines and the treatment plan, and the financial costs associated with medicines use. Where appropriate, record the person's consent in relation to these matters.
- Where appropriate, record the person's request to withhold or withdraw consent for treatment.
- Consider the need to obtain consent in consultation with a third party about medicines and the treatment plan (e.g. for involuntary people, children, young people).

7.4 Accept responsibility and accountability for prescribing decisions

How to achieve this competency
- Audit adverse outcomes and respond appropriately.
- Understand and comply with the legal, ethical and professional responsibilities associated with prescribing.
- Understand the medicolegal risks associated with prescribing medicines and take appropriate professional precautions (e.g. professional indemnity insurance).

7.5 Engage in ongoing professional development and education to improve prescribing practice

How to achieve this competency
- Meet the registration requirements for continuing professional development.
- Use self-reflection to continually review prescribing practice and respond to feedback.
- Use audit data to benchmark personal prescribing practice, identify development areas, and plan appropriate learning activities.
- Continually update knowledge and skills required for medicines safety.
- Use available resources to improve prescribing practice in accordance with learning plans.

7.6 Ensure the person's needs take precedence over all considerations in all prescribing decisions

How to achieve this competency
- Maintain professional independence in prescribing decision making. Ensure prescribing decisions are made on the basis of providing safe and effective care.
- Prescribing decisions should be made consistent with the best available evidence, clinical expertise and professional judgement in the context of the person's needs. Ensure decisions align with safe and rational medicines use and are made independent of influences that are not focused on the person's needs.

Continued

TABLE 22.2 Guidelines for achieving NPS prescribing competencies—cont'd

• Where the person, their family and/or carer are unable to contribute to decisions about the person's treatment, or this is inappropriate, the prescriber must make decisions based exclusively on what is in the best interests of the person. • Recognise and implement strategies to minimise influences that may bias prescribing decisions, including: marketing influences; possible personal, professional, or financial gain; the health professional's own beliefs, values, culture, experiences and expectations; the views of colleagues, the media or consumers. • Adhere to professional and facility codes of conduct for interacting with the pharmaceutical industry and participating in industry-funded education sessions and research trials. • Avoid conflicts of interest. Should real or perceived conflicts of interest be identified, declare and address these in order to minimise the impact on prescribing decisions. • Audit the health professional's own prescribing to evaluate the impact of both external and internal influences on their prescribing practice and implement strategies to address identified issues.
7.7 Demonstrate respect for other health professionals and their contribution within a collaborative care model
How to achieve this competency • Contribute to effective communication and collaboration between health professionals, particularly the person's primary healthcare provider (usually their general practitioner) and others who prescribe medicines for the person, to support optimal medicines use and management outcomes. • Provide advice to colleagues who also care for the person including those who provide and administer medicines. • Understand the scope of practice of other health professionals.

Source: Reproduced with permission from Prescribing Competencies Framework, developed by the Australian Commission on Safety and Quality in Health Care (ACSQHC). ACSQHC: Sydney 2021.

knowledge of the individual's needs and the person–prescriber partnership in achieving quality health outcomes through optimal medicine use. The person-centred approach of the framework also describes the essential collaboration between the prescriber and other health professionals. Collaboration with the person's primary healthcare provider is essential to the prescribing process and to achieving optimal health outcomes from the use of medicines.

National safety and quality standards: Medication management

Medicines are the most common treatment used in healthcare. The National Medicines Policy (2022) aims to improve health outcomes for all Australians through access to, and the wise use of, medicines to achieve optimal health outcomes and economic objectives. The policy's four central objectives are to provide:

1 timely access to medicines that Australians need, at a cost that the person, facility, and community that funds the health system, can afford

2 medicines that meet quality, safety, and efficacy standards

3 quality use of medicines (judicious, appropriate, safe, and effective use of medicines)

4 the maintenance of a responsible and viable medicines industry.

(see Online resources Australian Government: NMP 2022)

Although appropriate use of medicines contributes to significant improvements in health, medicines can also be associated with harm. Medicines are associated with a higher incidence of errors and adverse events than other healthcare interventions (ACSQHC 2017). Various resources and supports are available to ensure safety and quality in medication management (see Online resources ACSQHC: various), including quality databases and prescribing sources, for example Therapeutic Goods Administration, Prescribing medicines in pregnancy database; MEDSAFE (NZ); Australian Medicines Handbook; and Therapeutic Guidelines (see Online resources).

The Australian Commission on Safety and Quality in Health Care (ACSQHC) has developed eight national safety and quality healthcare standards outlining the level of care consumers can expect when receiving health services (ACSQHC 2017). The primary aims of the standards are to protect the public from harm and to improve the quality of health service provision. They provide a quality assurance mechanism that tests whether relevant systems are in place to ensure that expected standards of safety and quality are met. The aim of the National Medication Safety Standard–Standard Four, is to ensure that health professionals, including midwives, should possess necessary credentials encompassing education and training to practise within their scope of practice. Standard Four also ensures that health professionals prescribe, dispense, and administer safe and appropriate medicines and monitor medicine usage. Midwives should consider issues such as health literacy to ensure consumers have knowledge about medicine, its use, and risks (ACSQHC 2014).

Midwives are required to comply with these standards to ensure the safe administration and management of medications in their practice. (See Box 22.3.)

BOX 22.3 NSQHS standards: Medication Safety Standard

Leaders of a health service organisation describe, implement, and monitor systems to reduce the occurrence of medication incidents, and improve the safety and quality of medicines use. The workforce uses these systems.

Intention of this standard

To ensure clinicians are competent to safely prescribe, dispense and administer appropriate medicines and to monitor medicine use. To ensure consumers are informed about medicines and understand their individual medicine needs and risks.

Criteria

Clinical governance and quality improvement to support medication management

Organisation-wide systems are used to support and promote safety for procuring, supplying, storing, compounding, manufacturing, prescribing, dispensing, administering and monitoring the effects of medicines.

Documentation of patient information

A patient's best possible medication history is recorded when commencing an episode of care. The best possible medication history, and information relating to medicine allergies and adverse drug reactions are available to clinicians.

Continuity of medication management

A patient's medicines are reviewed, and information is provided to them about their medicines needs and risks. A medicines list is provided to the patient and the receiving clinician when handing over care.

Medication management processes

Health service organisations procure medicines for safety. Clinicians are supported to supply, store, compound, manufacture, prescribe, dispense, administer, monitor, and safely dispose of medicines.

Source: Reproduced with permission from National Safety and Quality Health Service Standards (second edition), developed by the Australian Commission on Safety and Quality in Health Care (ACSQHC). ACSQHC: Sydney 2017.

22.5 Role of the midwife in prescribing

Holistic midwifery care is provided in partnership with a childbearing woman and her baby. Comprehensive assessment before prescribing includes a medical, psychosocial, and obstetric health history. Midwives should also consider factors such as preexisting chronic health conditions, current prescription or non-prescription medication use, gestational age, and breastfeeding status. Consideration of the possibility of differing responses, and potential side effects for woman and baby, and the potential for interaction with other treatments or therapies need to be assessed before prescribing any medications. In many situations, a medication may not be the best treatment approach or solution.

Consultation, referral and collaboration

The Australian College of Midwives (ACM) National Midwifery Guidelines for Consultation and Referral (ACM 2021) was developed to assist midwives in their decision making in situations where consultation and referral with another health provider may be indicated. Consultation and referral including escalation of care for medication management and/or review/further diagnostic investigations ensures the delivery of high-standard maternity care using evidence-based practices. Collaborative models of care involving general practitioners, obstetricians, and other healthcare professionals ensure women and babies receive the level of care required for their individual circumstances. Midwives can manage their needs, and refer women and babies experiencing complications to appropriate clinicians for support and management as soon as they are identified.

In all situations, informed consent requires that women and their families must receive comprehensive information and support about any proposed treatment, including prescribed medicines. They are better positioned to actively participate in their care and report any concerns, reducing the risk of adverse events.

CLINICAL FOCUS BOX 22.1

Midwifery health history assessment and medication review

Safe and effective use of medications begins with the initial assessment of the woman. A full medical and medication history must be taken by the midwife with careful consideration of the following:

- Is there an actual need for medication?
- Is this the most appropriate drug for the desired outcome?
- What is the normal dosage, route, possible interactions, contraindications, and side effects of the chosen drug?
- Do the benefits of the drug outweigh the potential side effects?
- Does the woman have any known allergies?
- Has sufficient information been given to the woman for her to make an informed choice?
- Has the woman given informed consent?
- Is the prescription clear, legible, and indelible, and signed by the appropriate practitioner?
- Is the correct name of the medication prescribed, the method of administration, dosage, frequency, drug commencement and completion date included on the prescription?

- Has the weight of the woman/baby been recorded, and does this influence the drug dosage?
- Does administration ensure that therapeutic blood levels are maintained?
- Is the drug to be added to a solution? Is the solution correct?

Other questions related to recent medication history must also be considered to enable a full assessment:

- Did she take any medications including vitamins or over-the-counter supplements or medicines during the early stage of pregnancy before she knew she was pregnant?
- Are there any medications that she took long term that she stopped as she intended to get pregnant?
- Are there any medications that she has used within the last month?

The midwife has an important role in communicating the need for prescribed medication to women. The woman needs to make an informed decision, and it is part of the role of the midwife to assist her to do this without coercion or manipulation. It is also critical that quality prescribing sources are consulted. Reputable quality sources within the Australian context include the Australian Medicines Handbook (2024) also online, and the Therapeutic Guidelines.

Pharmaceutical Benefits Scheme prescribing by midwives

The Pharmaceutical Benefits Scheme is a national government scheme that subsidises the cost of essential medicines for Australian citizens (see Chapter 2). Information for midwives to become authorised PBS prescribers is available from *Services Australia* (see Online resources: https://www.servicesaustralia.gov.au/). Endorsed midwives can utilise the Australian Government's Medicare Benefits Schedule (**MBS**) and the PBS for select items, to help women and their families receive benefits for services and obtain subsidies for prescribed Schedule 2, 3, 4 or 8 medicines. At present, 31 items (20 different medicines) qualify for a PBS subsidy when prescribed by an **endorsed midwife** (a midwife whose registration is endorsed under section 94 of the Health Practitioner Regulation National Law as being qualified to prescribe scheduled medicines required for midwifery practice).

The medicines listed for prescribing by authorised midwives are identified by 'MW' in the PBS Schedule (see Online resources: https://www.pbs.gov.au/browse/midwife summarised in Box 22.4). Midwives must not write PBS prescriptions for other medicines.

BOX 22.4 PBS prescription medicines able to be prescribed by authorised midwives (Australia)

PRESCRIBER CODE	ITEM CODE	NAME, MANNER OF ADMINISTRATION AND FORM & STRENGTH	MAX QTY PACKS	MAX QTY UNITS	NO. OF REPEATS
MP MW NP	1884E	AMOXICILLIN amoxicillin 250 mg capsule, 20	1	20	0
MP MW NP	1889K	AMOXICILLIN amoxicillin 500 mg capsule, 20	1	20	0
MP MW NP	1891M	AMOXICILLIN + CLAVULANIC ACID amoxicillin 500 mg + clavulanic acid 125 mg tablet, 10	1	10	0
MP MW NP	1775K	BENZYLPENICILLIN benzylpenicillin 600 mg injection, 1 vial	10	10	1
MP MW NP	11963P	CEFALEXIN cefalexin 250 mg capsule, 20	2	40	0
MP MW NP	3058Y	CEFALEXIN cefalexin 250 mg capsule, 20	1	20	0
MP MW NP	11934D	CEFALEXIN cefalexin 500 mg capsule, 20	2	40	0
MP MW NP	3119E	CEFALEXIN cefalexin 500 mg capsule, 20	1	20	0
MP MW NP	11112W	CHLORAMPHENICOL chloramphenicol 0.5% eye drops, 10 mL	1	1	2

BOX 22.4 PBS prescription medicines able to be prescribed by authorised midwives (Australia)—cont'd

PRESCRIBER CODE	ITEM CODE	NAME, MANNER OF ADMINISTRATION AND FORM & STRENGTH	MAX QTY PACKS	MAX QTY UNITS	NO. OF REPEATS
MP MW NP	3138E	CLINDAMYCIN clindamycin 150 mg capsule, 24	2	48	1
MP MW NP	1302M	DICLOFENAC diclofenac sodium 100 mg suppository, 20	2	40	3
MP MW NP	8121K	DICLOXACILLIN dicloxacillin 250 mg capsule, 24	1	24	0
MP MW NP	8122L	DICLOXACILLIN dicloxacillin 500 mg capsule, 24	1	24	0
MP MW NP	8487Q	ETONOGESTREL etonogestrel 68 mg implant, 1	1	1	0
MP MW NP	1526H	FLUCLOXACILLIN flucloxacillin 250 mg capsule, 24	1	24	0
MP MW NP	1527J	FLUCLOXACILLIN flucloxacillin 500 mg capsule, 24	1	24	0
MP MW NP	1440T	FRAMYCETIN SULFATE framycetin sulfate 0.5% eye/ear drops, 8 mL	1	1	2
MP MW NP	3192B	IBUPROFEN ibuprofen 400 mg tablet, 30	1	30	0
MP MW NP	2913H	LEVONORGESTREL levonorgestrel 30 microgram tablet, 112 tablets [4 x 28]	1	4	2
MP MW NP	2530E	LINCOMYCIN lincomycin 600 mg/2 mL injection, 5 x 2 mL vials	1	5	0
MP MW NP	11380Y	LINCOMYCIN lincomycin 600 mg/2 mL injection, 5 x 2 mL ampoules	1	5	0
MP MW NP	1206L	METOCLOPRAMIDE metoclopramide hydrochloride 10 mg/2 mL injection, 10 x 2 mL ampoules	1	10	0
MP MW NP	1207M	METOCLOPRAMIDE metoclopramide hydrochloride 10 mg tablet, 25	1	25	0
MP MW NP	10211K	MIFEPRISTONE (&) MISOPROSTOL mifepristone 200 mg tablet [1] (&) misoprostol 200 microgram tablet [4], 1 pack	1	1	0
MP MW NP	1644M	MORPHINE morphine sulfate pentahydrate 10 mg/mL injection, 5 x 1 mL ampoules	1	5	0
MP MW NP	1645N	MORPHINE morphine sulfate pentahydrate 15 mg/mL injection, 5 x 1 mL ampoules	1	5	0
MP MW NP	1086T	MORPHINE morphine hydrochloride trihydrate 10 mg/mL injection, 5 x 1 mL ampoules	1	5	0

Continued

BOX 22.4 PBS prescription medicines able to be prescribed by authorised midwives (Australia)—cont'd

PRESCRIBER CODE	ITEM CODE	NAME, MANNER OF ADMINISTRATION AND FORM & STRENGTH	MAX QTY PACKS	MAX QTY UNITS	NO. OF REPEATS
MP MW NP	1693D	NITROFURANTOIN nitrofurantoin 100 mg capsule, 30	1	30	1
MP MW NP	1692C	NITROFURANTOIN nitrofurantoin 50 mg capsule, 30	1	30	1
MP MW NP	12598C	PROGESTERONE progesterone 200 mg pessary, 42	1	42	3
MP MW NP	12465C	PROGESTERONE progesterone 200 mg pessary, 15	3	45	3
MP MW NP	1978D	RANITIDINE ranitidine 150 mg tablet, 60	1	60	5

Source: PBS Browse by midwife items.

PBS prescribing by midwives is limited by state and territory prescribing rights. It is also contingent on a prescriber being an *authorised midwife* and having collaborative arrangements in place, as required by amendments to the *National Health Act 1953*. However, as of May 2024 the Health Legislation Amendment (Removal of Requirement for a Collaborative Arrangement) Bill 2024 was passed by Parliament on 16 May 2024. The Governor-General provided Royal Assent on 31 May 2024. The date of effect of the legislation amendment is 1 November 2024. Compliance with existing legislation and maintenance of collaborative arrangements is required until 1 November 2024. How the legislative change will impact ongoing PBS prescribing across a range of settings may be variable depending on jurisdictional and organisational policy in both public and private sector workplaces.

The Pharmaceutical Benefits Advisory Committee (PBAC) is responsible for making recommendations to the Minister for Health regarding medicines for prescribing by authorised midwives. Within the New Zealand context, the relevant agency is Pharmac, the government agency that decides which medicines are funded in Aotearoa NZ. (See Online resources.) Some medicines are included in more than one section of the schedule, and for more than one prescriber type. For a prescription to be eligible for subsidy, prescribers must ensure that they prescribe under the PBS only those medicines, and in accordance with the restrictions listed for their prescriber type. Listing details for the same product may differ between sections, and different PBS item codes apply for each prescriber type.

Midwife PBS prescriptions are identifiable by colour and include the indicator 'MW' on personalised forms and a tick box on non-personalised (blank) forms. Prescriptions must include the midwife's PBS prescriber number. For unrestricted and restricted PBS medicines, midwives/nurse practitioners can use the personalised or non-personalised PBS prescriber forms. For authority required and authority required (streamlined) PBS medicines, midwives can use the authority personalised or non-personalised PBS prescriber forms. Midwife PBS prescriptions may include repeats.

Regulation 49 applies for midwife prescribing. A midwife can direct that original and repeat supplies of pharmaceutical benefits be supplied at the one time if certain conditions are satisfied.

- *Authority prescriptions:* For authority required items, or for increased quantities or repeats, prior approval is required from Services Australia for each prescription. (Refer to Prescribing Medicines—Information for PBS prescribers and Supplying Medicines—What Pharmacists Need to Know, for more information on authority prescriptions.)
- *State and territory requirements:* Midwives may prescribe medicines as private prescriptions according to their state/territory prescribing accreditation. The medicines which can be prescribed differ between states and territories. It is the midwife's responsibility to ensure adherence to state/territory law for all prescriptions (PBS and private) and additionally to all PBS requirements for PBS prescriptions (Box 22.4).

For women to be eligible to access the PBS they must be a resident in Australia, have a Medicare card, and the medicine must be for personal use. Medicare funds the

PBS. The Pharmaceutical Benefits Advisory Committee (PBAC) is responsible for deciding which medicines are included on the PBS list. In general, medicines that are used to treat significant medical conditions, with proven effectiveness and that are cost effective, are included on the list.

The PBS Schedule lists all the medicines available to be dispensed to persons at a government-subsidised price. The schedule is part of the wider PBS, managed by the Department of Health and administered by Department of Human Services. This schedule is now online and updated monthly.

This online searchable version contains:

- all the drugs listed on the PBS
- information on conditions of use for the prescribing of PBS medicines
- detailed consumer information for medicines that have been prescribed
- what you can expect to pay for medicines.

Health practitioners with PBS authority or a PBS prescriber number are sometimes referred to as PBS authorised prescribers. When health professionals with PBS authority write a prescription for medicines on the PBS list for that health professional group, the PBS rebate applies. Midwives can prescribe items not listed on the PBS (provided they do not contravene state or territory specific regulations) but these will be treated as a private script and the cost of medication will be applied to the client.

Activity 1

Access these websites and then consider the following questions:

https://www.pbs.gov.au/info/healthpro/explanatory-notes/section1/Section_1_2_Explanatory_Notes#PBS-prescribers

https://www.pbs.gov.au/browse/midwife

1 What restrictions exist around writing prescriptions?

2 What are the minimum legal requirements needed for a prescription to be dispensed?

3 How many medications can be written on one script?

Case study 2

You are an endorsed midwife employed in a large private midwifery group practice with clinical privileging and visiting access at the local regional hospital. You are providing relief caseload care for a group of women for one of your midwifery colleagues who commenced annual leave yesterday. You attend the local hospital for a postnatal consultation with Tabitha who gave birth to her first baby, Sammy, 48 hours ago by unplanned, emergency caesarean section.

The prescriptions on the NIMC have all been entered and signed by your midwifery colleague. As you review Tabitha's and Sammy's medical records and National Inpatient Medication Charts you note several prescribing errors, including:

- the maximum daily dose for an analgesic order of a controlled substance has been exceeded (Tabitha's chart)
- a prescription order entered for an antibiotic that is contraindicated postnatally (Tabitha's chart)
- the incorrect dose for intramuscular paediatric phytomenadione (vitamin K) is prescribed on the infant medication chart for Sammy.

Questions

1 What is your first and immediate response in this situation in relation to ongoing provision of midwifery clinical care for Tabitha and Sammy, including your professional responsibility as a prescriber?

2 What, if anything, do you discuss with Tabitha; when and how?

3 Are there any professional or reporting requirements and/or obligations in this situation? If so, what are they and to whom should reports be made?

4 From a systems safety and quality perspective, are there any other actions you would consider to be appropriate in these circumstances? Provide a rationale for your response.

22.6 Additional professional obligations for midwives

Continuing professional development

To renew professional registration in Australia, a midwife must fulfil a minimum of 20 hours CPD. However, for endorsed midwives with scheduled medicines endorsement, an additional 10 hours of CPD is necessary. These extra hours should be focused on the context of practice, including prescribing and administration of medicines, diagnostic investigations, as well as consultation and referral (see Online resources; NMBA).

Te Tatau o te Whare Kahu Midwifery Council of New Zealand requires all midwives to undertake a professional Midwifery Standards Review every 3 years (see Online resources).

Professional indemnity insurance

Professional indemnity insurance (PII) is a requirement of all midwives providing private care. PII is designed to assist in paying for legal costs and potential damages. In

New Zealand PII is offered through the New Zealand College of Midwives (see Online resources). In Australia, since 2010, a Commonwealth Government-legislated Professional Indemnity Contribution Scheme has been in place for the midwifery profession, including a Commonwealth Run-off cover Support Payment Scheme (see Online resources). Currently, the only insurance product for midwives is provided by Medical Insurance Group Australia (MIGA). As per NMBA Registration Standards, midwives who provide private midwifery services must hold PII (see Online resources).

Complaints

As with all areas of healthcare, there are several avenues through which a consumer, healthcare professional or hospital can institute a complaint against a health practitioner. In the case of the midwife a complaint can be made:

- to the midwife directly
- to the hospital in which the incident occurred
- to a state health complaints agency
- to the state coroner in event of maternal or infant death
- to AHPRA
- to a legal firm dealing in civil law.

Hospitals have their own processes and policies for investigation of complaints, which vary between institutions. Each state has a government agency dedicated to handling complaints from the healthcare users. State agencies aim to mediate complaints but have no authority to punish but will refer complaints onto AHPRA.

Each state also has a coroner's office that is responsible for investigating reportable deaths. A reportable death is where there are suspicious circumstances; where a doctor is unable to complete a death certificate as the cause is unknown; and for deaths related to healthcare (excluding stillbirths). The purpose of the coronial inquest is to determine the cause of death, and the coroner may then refer the case on to higher authorities if they feel the level of care provided was of concern.

Case study 3

You are concluding a routine antenatal visit with a pregnant woman, Sharna, whom you know well. This is Sharna's third pregnancy and you also provided care for her during the births of the family's previous two children. Sharna is aware you are an endorsed prescriber and requests two prescription items from you before you leave today's appointment. The first prescription request is for thyroxine. Sharna advises she has run out of medication due to missing her regular review visit with her obstetric physician and endocrinologist this month while the children were on school holidays, and it is impossible to get a replacement appointment. Sharna further confides that her 16-year-old daughter, Elsie, has recently confirmed she has an unplanned pregnancy and has requested access to the medical abortion pill. It is a very stressful time as Elsie's final high school examinations are coming up in 4 months. Sharna describes Elsie as stressed and isolated, and refusing to see the family GP as she is embarrassed and concerned about confidentiality.

Questions

What are your responses to Sharna in relation to these two prescription requests? Provide rationale and explanation for your responses, including your ongoing plan to address both issues.

REFLECTIVE THINKING EXERCISES

1 Discuss the benefits and challenges of written prescriptions versus electronic prescribing for midwives and the people they provide care and services for.

2 Explain prescriber responsibilities for antimicrobial stewardship considering increasing bacterial resistance. What specific actions are required of midwife prescribers re antimicrobial stewardship and where are they likely to have most impact?

3 Midwifery prescribing capability is currently underutilised in the public health system. Provide examples of how this may currently disadvantage timely medication access for women and their babies. Propose some future strategies that may address current barriers.

CRITICAL THINKING EXERCISES

1 Explain the physiological changes that may occur during a complex pregnancy – choosing from any of the chapters in Part 4, Pharmacology for special considerations – including how these could affect pharmacokinetics.

2 Locate the legislation for 'drugs and poisons regulation' for your state or territory/jurisdiction of midwifery practice and write a summary of the implications of this legislation on your prescribing practice.

3 Describe the quality prescribing resources you would use to ensure evidence-based, safe prescribing practice, including your plan to meet your continuing professional development requirements.

4 As a midwife seeking to gain endorsement to enable you to work in private practice you have a requirement to meet the expectations set out in the NMBA Safety and Quality Guidelines for Privately Practising Midwives https://www.nursingmidwiferyboard.gov.au/ Codes-Guidelines-Statements/FAQ/fact-sheet-safety-and-quality-guidelines-for-privately-practising-midwives.aspx. Read and make yourself familiar with these guidelines.

Activity 2

Access this website for information on the Pharmaceutical Benefits Scheme (PBS) : https://www.pbs.gov.au/info/about-the-pbs
Read the responses to the following questions you will find there:

• What is the PBS?

• Who is eligible for PBS?

When you have read all the information consider what you have learned about PBS. What aspects are relevant to your role of supporting women during the childbearing journey? If you are an endorsed midwife, you are eligible for Medicare benefits for specified midwifery services you provide privately. You can also request certain pathology and diagnostic imaging services and refer clients to an obstetrician and a paediatrician for a clinical need. See the Services Australia website for further information: https://www.servicesaustralia.gov.au/medicare-services-for-eligible-midwives
Make sure you read the relevant MBS item descriptions and explanatory notes on the MBS online website: https://www.mbsonline.gov.au/

CONCLUSION

This chapter focused on the role and responsibilities of the midwife related to pharmacological management, including authorised prescribing; and providing care for women and their babies across pregnancy, birth and the postpartum period in Australia and New Zealand. Midwives are accountable for their own practice, to the woman and her baby, to the hospital if the woman and baby were admitted to hospital under the care of the midwife, to the profession, and to society. As with all aspects of care, practitioners should only undertake medication management activities they are legally entitled , competent, and educationally prepared to perform, and for which they are willing to be accountable.

Models of maternity care and midwifery practice are subject to change; impacted by legislation, regulation, professional practice standards, guidelines, frameworks, educational requirements, research, and public expectations for safety and quality. The role of midwives, and the scope and context of professional practice includes care provided across the continuum of childbearing in partnership with women and their families; and in diverse contexts and settings supported by collaborative relationships with a range of other healthcare professionals. Safety and quality use of medicine as a preventative health strategy and in the pharmacological treatment of women and their babies during midwifery care is paramount, as is access to essential medicines for emergency treatment. Midwives are required to develop and maintain evidence-based specialised knowledge in the pharmacokinetics and pharmacodynamics of prescription medicines used during pregnancy, childbearing, and lactation. This knowledge extends to medication administration, supply, and possession, as well as awareness of community use of non-prescription/ OTC and complementary and alternative medicines, whether the midwife is an authorised prescriber or not.

Prescriptive authority as an *authorised prescriber* carries additional professional responsibilities for midwives. As stated in the introduction to this chapter, having midwives with authority to prescribe the medicines associated with maternity care – including women's health, sexual and reproductive health, and child and family healthcare – enables women to access a greater range of midwifery services. Developing your knowledge of pharmacology as a midwife and ensuring your knowledge is evidence-based and up to date is part of your professional responsibility in ensuring that you uphold high standards of safety in the provision of quality midwifery services to women and their families.

REVIEW QUESTIONS

1 Describe specific strategies used in your workplace and midwifery practice to reduce the risk of, identify, manage, and report adverse drug reactions.

2 Describe your approach to synthesising information provided by the woman, other healthcare professionals, and from clinical examinations and investigations to determine appropriate medication management. Provide an example of this from a clinical scenario in your recent midwifery practice. Did you use any quality prescribing sources and/or other evidence-based clinical guidelines or professional standards to inform your approach? How might this have impacted health outcomes for the woman and/or baby, and for you professionally?

3 Discuss the difference between active and passive monitoring of medication efficacy when used as treatment. How would you discuss this with a woman you are providing midwifery care for?

4 What guidance does the National Prescribing Competencies Framework for Health Professionals [NPS MEDICINE WISE 2021] https://www.nps.org.au/assets/NPS/pdf/NPS-MedicineWise_Prescribing_Competencies_Framework.pdf provide in this regard and which specific competencies may be useful here?

5 Select one competency area from Professional Practice that Supports Prescribing from the framework (Table 22.1). List the actions that will enable you to meet this competency in *your* midwifery prescribing practice and role.

6 How are *your* identified actions for Professional Practice that Supports Prescribing related to the national standards and guidelines for midwife practice in Australia and/or New Zealand?

7 Identify current differences between the Australian and New Zealand contexts of practice for midwives who are authorised to prescribe in each country. Describe how this may enhance or hinder midwifery role and models of maternity care provision in each setting, including timely access to assessment and treatment with prescription medicine for women and their babies. What needs to change? How should this be advanced?

REFERENCES

Australian College of Midwives. National midwifery guidelines for consultation and referral. 4th edn. Canberra: ACM, 2021. https://www.midwives.org.au/common/Uploaded%20files/_ADMIN-ACM/National-Midwifery-Guidelines-for-Consultation-and-Referral-4th-Edition-(2021).pdf

Australian Government Department of Health and Ageing. Improving maternity services in Australia: the report of the Maternity Services Review/Department of Health and Ageing. Commonwealth of Australia, 2009. https://parlinfo.aph.gov.au/parlInfo/search/display/display.w3p;query=Id:%22library/lcatalog/00151833%22

Australian Medicines Handbook 2024. Australian medicines handbook. Adelaide: AMH.

Australian and New Zealand Council of Chief Nursing and Midwifery Officers. Registered nurse and midwife prescribing – Discussion paper. ANZCCNMO, 2017.

Australian Nursing and Midwifery Accreditation Council. Programs leading to endorsement for scheduled medicines for midwives accreditation standards 2015. ANMAC, 2015. https://anmac.org.au/sites/default/files/documents/Accreditation_Standards_for_Programs_Leading_to_Endorsement_for_Scheduled_Medicines_for_Midwives_2015.pdf

Casey M, Rohde D, Higgins A, et al. Providing a complete episode of care: a survey of registered nurse and registered midwife prescribing behaviours and practices. J Clin Nurs. 2020;29(1-2):152-162. doi.org/10.1111/jocn.15073

Chung A, Hall A, Brown V, et al. The first 2000 days: synthesis of knowledge from the Australian Prevention Partnership Centre and CERI. Sydney, Australia: The Australian Prevention Partnership Centre, 2022. https://preventioncentre.org.au/wp-content/uploads/2022/08/First-2000-days-full-report-FINAL-1.pdf

Fong J, Buckley T, Cashin A. Nurse practitioner prescribing: an international perspective. J Nurs Res. 2015;5:99-108.

Hart M. Investigating the progress of community matron prescribing. Primary Health Care, 2013;23(2):26-31.

Health Practitioners Competence Assurance Act 2003 (New Zealand)

Hope DL, Dickfos ST, Ellerby RE, et al. Borderline health: jurisdictional variation in Australian medicines legislation poses potential risks to patients and healthcare practitioners. JPPR. 2016;46(3):201-208. doi.org/https://doi.org/10.1002/jppr.1179

Hull E., Donnellan-Fernandez R., Hastie C, et al. Endorsed midwives prescribing scheduled medicines in Australia: a scoping review. Women and Birth. 2024;37(2):288-295. doi.org/https://doi.org/10.1016/j.wombi.2023.10.009

Hull E, Hastie C, Bradfield Z, et al. Endorsed midwife prescribing in Australia: '[For] the women more than anything'. Women and Birth. 2024;37(5):101638. doi.org/10.1016/j.wombi.2024.101638

Hunter M, Davis D. Chapter 33 Pharmacology and prescribing. In: Pairman S, Tracy SK, Dahlen H, Dixon L (eds). Midwifery preparation for practice. 5th edn. Elsevier, 2022. ISBN:9780729597869

Health Workforce Australia. Health Professionals Prescribing Pathway (HPPP) Project – Final report. HWA; 2013.

Medicines Act 1981 (New Zealand)

Medicines Amendment Regulations 2011 (New Zealand)

Medicines Regulations 1984 (New Zealand)

Medway P, Sweet L, Muller A. Barriers and enablers for midwives to use the Nursing and Midwifery Board of Australia's Endorsement for scheduled medicines for midwives. Women and Birth. 2021;34(1):e57-e66. doi. org/10.1016/j.wombi.2020.06.001

Midwifery Council of NZ. Midwifery Council of NZ (MCNZ). Competencies for entry to the register of midwives. MCNZ, 2007. https://www.midwiferycouncil.health.nz/common/ Uploaded%20files/Midwifery%20Leaders/Competencies%20 for%20Entry%20to%20the%20register%20of%20Midwives%20 2007.pdf

Misuse of Drugs Act 1975 (New Zealand)

Misuse of Drugs Amendment Regulations 2014 (New Zealand)

Nissen L, Kyle G, Stowasser D, et al. Non-medical prescribing. an exploration of likely nature of, and contingencies for, developing a nationally consistent approach to prescribing by non-medical health professionals. Final Report 1 June 2010. National Health Workforce Planning and Research Collaboration, Australia. QUT, 2010.

NPS MedicineWise. Prescribing competencies framework: embedding quality use of medicines into practice. (2nd edn) Sydney: NPS MedicineWise, 2021. https://www.nps.org.au/ assets/NPS/pdf/NPS-MedicineWise_Prescribing_ Competencies_Framework.pdf

Nurses Amendment Act 1990 (New Zealand)

Nursing and Midwifery Board of Australia. Registrant data – Reporting period: 01 January 2024 to 31 March 2024. Australia: NMBA, 2024. https://www. nursingmidwiferyboard.gov.au/About/Statistics.aspx

Nursing and Midwifery Board of Australia. Midwife standards for practice. Australia: NMBA, 2018 https://www. nursingmidwiferyboard.gov.au/Codes-Guidelines-Statements/Professional-standards.aspx

Nursing and Midwifery Board of Australia. NMBA Registration standard: Endorsement for scheduled medicines for midwives. Australia: NMBA, 2017. https://www. nursingmidwiferyboard.gov.au/Codes-Guidelines-Statements/Codes-Guidelines/Guidelines-for-Midwives-applying-for-endorsement-for-scheduled-medicines.aspx

Nursing and Midwifery Board of Australia. Safety and quality guidelines for privately practising midwives. Australia: NMBA, 2023. https://www.nursingmidwiferyboard.gov.au/ Codes-Guidelines-Statements/Codes-Guidelines/Safety-and-quality-guidelines-for-privately-practising-midwives.aspx

Pritchard A, Kendrick D. Practice nurse and health visitor management of acute minor illness in a general practice. J Advanced Nurs. 2001;36(4):556-562.

Sandall J, Fernandez Turienzo C, Devane D, et al. Midwife continuity of care models versus other models of care for childbearing women. Cochrane Database Syst Rev. 2024;4:CD004667. doi: 10.1002/14651858.CD004667.pub6

Small K, Sidebotham M, Fenwick J, et al. Midwifery prescribing in Australia. Aust Prescr. 2016;39(6):215-218. doi. org/10.18773/austprescr.2016.070

Smith A, Latter S, Blenkinsopp A. Safety and quality of nurse independent prescribing: a national study of experiences of education, continuing professional development clinical governance. J Advanced Nurs. 2014;70(11):2506-2517.

ONLINE RESOURCES

Australian Commission on Safety and Quality in Health Care (ACSQHC) Medication Safety Standard: https://www. safetyandquality.gov.au/standards/nsqhs-standards/ medication-safety-standard

Australian Commission on Safety and Quality in Health Care. Health literacy: taking action to improve safety and quality. Sydney, 2014: https://www.safetyandquality.gov.au/sites/ default/files/migrated/Health-Literacy-Taking-action-to-improve-safety-and-quality.pdf

Australian Commission on Safety and Quality in Health Care. National Inpatient Medication Chart = NMIC user guide, 2024: https://www.safetyandquality.gov.au/publications-and-resources/resource-library/national-inpatient-medication-chart-nimc-user-guide

Australian Commission on Safety and Quality in Health Care. National Safety and Quality Health Service Standards. 2nd ed. Sydney, 2017: https://www.safetyandquality.gov.au/ sites/default/files/2019-04/National-Safety-and-Quality-Health-Service-Standards-second-edition.pdf

Australian Commission on Safety and Quality in Health Care. Quality use of medicines, 2024: https://www.safetyandquality. gov.au/our-work/medication-safety/quality-use-medicines

Australian Commission on Safety and Quality in Health Care. Safety and quality improvement guide, Standard 4: Medication safety (October 2012). Sydney, 2012: https:// www.safetyandquality.gov.au/sites/default/files/migrated/ Standard4_Oct_2012_WEB.pdf

Australian Government Department of Health and Aged Care. Browse by midwife items, Midwife PBS prescribing: https://www.pbs.gov.au/browse/midwife

Australian Government Department of Health and Aged Care. About prescriptions, 2024: https://www.health.gov.au/ topics/medicines/about-prescriptions

Australian Government Department of Health and Aged Care. Unleashing the potential of our health workforce – Scope of practice review – Issues Paper 2. 16 April 2024. Appendix A: Summary of review of legislation and regulation: https:// www.health.gov.au/resources/publications/unleashing-the-potential-of-our-health-workforce-scope-of-practice-review-issues-paper-2?language=en

Australian Government Department of Health and Ageing. Medication management for health practitioners. 2024: https://www.health.gov.au/topics/medicines/medication-management-for-health-practitioners

Australian Government Department of Health and Ageing. National Medicines Policy, 2022: https://www.health.gov.au/ resources/publications/national-medicines-policy?language=en

Australian Government Department of Health and Ageing. Therapeutic Goods Administration, Prescribing medicines in pregnancy database: https://www.tga.gov.au/prescribing-medicines-pregnancy-database/

Australian Government Department of Health and Ageing. Prescribing Medicines—information for PBS prescribers: http://www.pbs.gov.au/info/healthpro/explanatory-notes/ section1/Section_1_2_Explanatory_Notes.

Australian Prescriber 2024: https://australianprescriber.tg.org.au/

ICM Essential competencies for midwifery practice (2019 update): https://internationalmidwives.org/resources/essential-competencies-for-midwifery-practice/

ICM Global Standards for Midwifery Education (Revised 2021): https://internationalmidwives.org/resources/global-standards-for-midwifery-education/

ICM International Definition and Scope of Practice of the Midwife: https://internationalmidwives.org/resources/international-definition-of-the-midwife/

Medical Insurance Group Australia (MIGA): https://www.miga.com.au/insuring-with-us/midwives

Medsafe (New Zealand Ministry of Health) information on medicines: http://www.medsafe.govt.nz

Midwife Professional Indemnity (Commonwealth contribution) Scheme Act 2010: https://www.legislation.gov.au/Details/C2010A00030

Midwife Professional Indemnity (Run-off Cover Support Payment) Act 2010: https://www.legislation.gov.au/Details/C2011C00495

New Zealand College of Midwives (NZCOM). Consensus statement: Midwife prescribing. Christchurch, 2014a: https://www.midwife.org.nz/quality-practice/nzcom-consensus-statements

New Zealand College of Midwives (NZCOM). Consensus statement. Prescribing and administration of opioid analgesia in labour. Christchurch, 2014b: https://www.midwife.org.nz/quality-practice/nzcom-consensus-statements.

New Zealand College of Midwives (NZCOM). Midwife standards of practice: https://www.midwife.org.nz/midwives/professional-practice/standards-of-practice/

New Zealand Formulary: http://nzformulary.org/

New Zealand Ministry of Health – Prescribing statement – legal requirements and subsidisation, 13 February 2024: https://www.health.govt.nz/our-work/regulation-health-and-disability-system/medicines-act-1981/prescribing-statement-legal-requirements-and-subsidisation

New Zealand referral guidelines for maternity services: http://www.health.govt.nz/publication/guidelines-consultation-obstetric-and-related-medical-services-referral-guidelines

NPS MedicineWise: https://www.nps.org.au/

PBS Information Management Section. Department of Health. PBS expenditure and prescriptions report, 1 July 2022 to 30 June 2023: https://www.pbs.gov.au/info/statistics/expenditure-prescriptions/pbs-expenditure-and-prescriptions-report-1-july-2022-to-30-june-2023

Pharmac, Pharmaceutical Management Agency of New Zealand, online access to New Zealand Pharmaceutical Schedule detailing which pharmaceuticals attract subsidy: http://www.pharmac.govt.nz/

Services Australia: https://www.servicesaustralia.gov.au/

Te Tatau o te Whare Kahu Midwifery Council 2023, NZ. Midwifery Council statement on the Midwifery Scope of Practice and prescribing controlled drugs: https://www.midwiferycouncil.health.nz/common/Uploaded%20files/About%20Us/Midwifery%20Council%20on%20prescribing%20controlled%20drugs%20July%202023%20final%20(002).pdf

Therapeutic Guidelines Australia: www.tg.org.au

Index

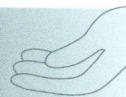